Structure and Function of SARS-CoV-2

Structure and Function of SARS-CoV-2

Editor: Zavier Kennedy

AMERICAN
MEDICAL PUBLISHERS
www.americanmedicalpublishers.com

AMERICAN
MEDICAL PUBLISHERS
www.americanmedicalpublishers.com

Cataloging-in-Publication Data

Structure and function of SARS-CoV-2 / edited by Zavier Kennedy.
p. cm.
Includes bibliographical references and index.
ISBN 979-8-88740-579-7
1. COVID-19 (Disease). 2. COVID-19 (Disease)--Epidemiology. 3. COVID-19 Pandemic, 2020- 4. Coronavirus infections. 5. Respiratory infections. I. Kennedy, Zavier.
RA644.C67 S77 2023
362.196 241 4--dc23

American Medical Publishers,
41 Flatbush Avenue,
1st Floor, New York,
NY 11217, USA

ISBN 979-8-88740-579-7 (Hardback)

Contents

Preface

I am honored to present to you this unique book which encompasses the most up-to-date data in the field. I was extremely pleased to get this opportunity of editing the work of experts from across the globe. I have also written papers in this field and researched the various aspects revolving around the progress of the discipline. I have tried to unify my knowledge along with that of stalwarts from every corner of the world, to produce a text which not only benefits the readers but also facilitates the growth of the field.

Severe acute respiratory syndrome coronavirus 2 (SARS-CoV-2) refers to a type of virus that belongs to the coronavirus family. Bats are the most plausible ecological reservoirs for SARS-CoV-2, although the virus is considered to have originated from an intermediate animal host and then crossed the species barrier to infect human beings. The SARS-CoV-2 genome encodes four main structural proteins, including the membrane (M) protein, the spike (S) protein, the envelope (E) protein and the nucleocapsid (N) protein, all of which are necessary to build the viral particle. In addition to four structural proteins, SARS-CoV-2 has sixteen non-structural proteins (nsp1–16). RNA replication and processing is mediated by Nsp1. It is crucial to comprehend the structure and function of SARS-CoV-2, as well as its variants, in order to develop viable treatments and vaccines to combat the COVID-19 disease. This book provides significant information to help develop a good understanding of the structure and function of SARS-CoV-2. Experts and students actively engaged in the research on this virus will find this book full of crucial and unexplored concepts.

Finally, I would like to thank all the contributing authors for their valuable time and contributions. This book would not have been possible without their efforts. I would also like to thank my friends and family for their constant support.

Editor

1

Perspectives and Challenges in the Fight Against COVID-19: The Role of Genetic Variability

Mariana Guilger-Casagrande[1,2]*, Cecilia T. de Barros*[2]*, Vitória A. N. Antunes*[2]*,*
Daniele R. de Araujo[3] *and Renata Lima*[2*]

[1] *Institute of Science and Technology, São Paulo State University–UNESP, Sorocaba, Brazil,* [2] *Laboratory for Evaluation of the Bioactivity and Toxicology of Nanomaterials, University of Sorocaba-UNISO, Sorocaba, Brazil,* [3] *Human and Natural Sciences Center, Federal University of ABC, Santo André, Brazil*

***Correspondence:**
Renata Lima
renata.lima@prof.uniso.br

In the last year, the advent of the COVID-19 pandemic brought a new consideration for the multidisciplinary sciences. The unknown mechanisms of infection used by SARS-CoV-2 and the absence of effective antiviral pharmacological therapy, diagnosis methods, and vaccines evoked scientific efforts on the COVID-19 outcome. In general, COVID-19 clinical features are a result of local and systemic inflammatory processes that are enhanced by some preexistent comorbidities, such as diabetes, obesity, cardiovascular, and pulmonary diseases, and biological factors, like gender and age. However, the discrepancies in COVID-19 clinical signs observed among those patients lead to investigations about the critical factors that deeply influence disease severity and death. Herein, we present the viral infection mechanisms and its consequences after blocking the angiotensin-converting enzyme 2 (ACE2) axis in different tissues and the progression of inflammatory and immunological reactions, especially the influence of genetic features on those differential clinical responses. Furthermore, we discuss the role of genotype as an essential indicator of COVID-19 susceptibility, considering the expression profiles, polymorphisms, gene identification, and epigenetic modifications of viral entry factors and their recognition, as well as the infection effects on cell signaling molecule expression, which amplifies disease severity.

Keywords: polymorphism, immune response, ACE2 receptor, cytokines, chemokines, X chromosome, SARS-CoV-2, coronaviruses

INTRODUCTION

COVID-19, the disease caused by the new coronavirus SARS-CoV-2, was first reported on December 29, 2019 in the city of Wuhan, China (WHO, 2020), and since then, more than a year later, we are living through a pandemic that has challenged doctors and scientists worldwide. SARS-CoV-2 has already infected 106,797,721 people and caused more than 2,341,145 deaths worldwide (WHO, 2021), with the main problem being the immune response that occurs in individuals. This is due to some peculiarities that SARS-Cov-2 presents, in particular the use of the angiotensin-converting enzyme 2 (ACE2) receptor to insert into human cells. Molecular study of the virus showed that it is a single-stranded RNA virus with a positive envelope (29.8 kb) that has six common open reading frames (ORFs) and several accessory genes (Mahmoudabadi and Phillips, 2018; Zheng, 2020) (**Figure 1**).

Sequence analysis showed that the viral genome found in different patients was highly conserved (Lu et al., 2020a; Zhou et al., 2020), indicating a recent evolution. The amino acid sequence of the experimental receptor binding domain of SARS-CoV-2 resembles that of SARS-CoV, the virus that triggered an outbreak in 2003, indicating that these viruses recognize the same receptor (Ren et al., 2020). Knowing the origin and structure of the new coronavirus, as well as its interaction with human cells, was a very important step for the confrontation that is currently being waged.

It is well known that while there are cases of individuals who are resistant to SARS-CoV-2 infection or asymptomatic, there is also a high rate of patients who progress to the severe form of the disease and die. This reality triggers several provocative questions.

WHAT LEADS SARS-COV-2 TO CAUSE PEOPLE MAJOR PROBLEMS?

ACE2 enzyme acts as a receptor responsible for viral binding to the cells (Wrapp et al., 2020; Xu et al., 2020). A peculiarity of SARS-CoV-2 is the surface protein (Spike, S) (**Figure 1**), which mediates virus recognition by human cells, that has a 10- to 20-fold higher affinity to ACE2 in comparison to the surface proteins of SARS-CoV, which contributes to its high infection and dissemination rates (Gheblawi et al., 2020). Such differences occur due to structural changes resulting from a four-residue motif (residues 482–485: Gly-Val-Glu-Gly) in the binding region, which makes the protein ridge more compact and allows better contact with the hACE2 N-terminal helix (Yan et al., 2020; Yi et al., 2020). Those structural features are essential to understand how ACE2-SARS-CoV-2 binding is processed.

In this scenario, the comprehension of ACE2 physiological functions and specific features could explain how comorbidities (hypertension, diabetes, obesity, and immunological diseases) and other biological factors (older age, male gender) can contribute to enhance the symptoms' severity, with progression to death, evoked by COVID-19.

The ACE2 receptor exerts a pivotal role by regulating the degradation of Ang II in Ang 1-7 *via* the G-protein accoupled Mas receptors axis, especially in the lungs. The protective functions associated with the ACE2 axis is a result of Ang 1-7 production, which leads to anti-inflammatory effects, the reduction of lymphocytes and neutrophils infiltration with decreased perivascular and bronchial inflammation. These effects are counter-regulated by AngII-mediated responses, such as myocardial and endothelial disfunction, hypertension associated with obesity, and coagulation alterations (Verdecchia et al., 2020).

Conversely, impaired ACE2 function in the lungs is responsible for increasing free-bradykinin levels, activating pro-inflammatory cytokines release, and pulmonary injury. Notably, Mas receptor activation stimulates prostacyclin and nitric oxide (NO) release in platelets, evoking anti-thrombotic effects. Additionally, Mas receptors are also expressed in the pancreas, improving perivascular blood flow, and in cardiac adipocytes, preserving cardiac function (Hoffmann et al., 2020;

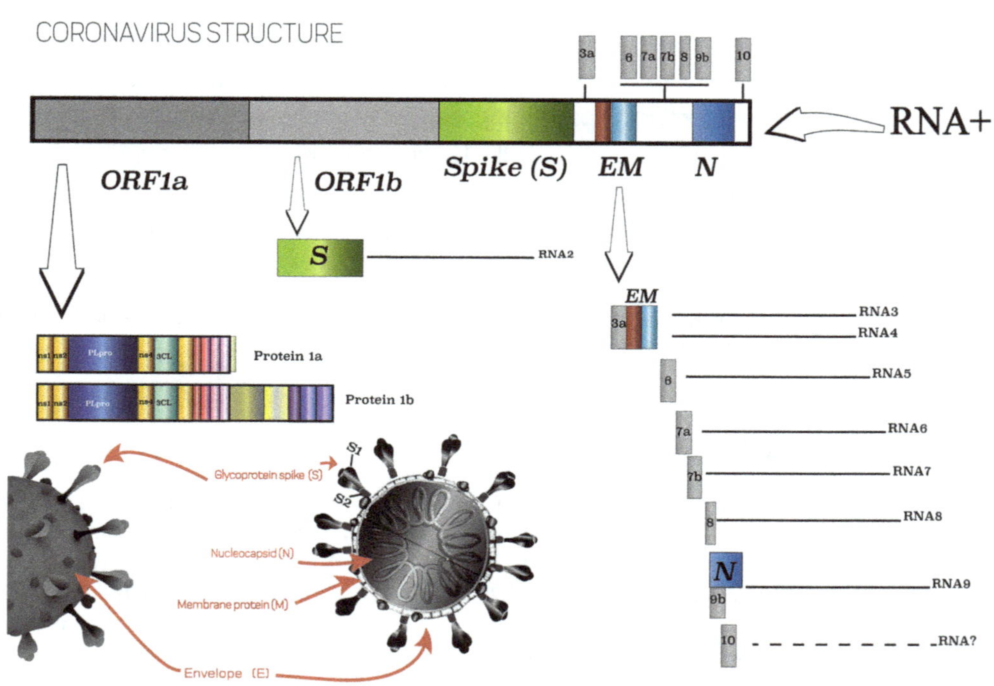

FIGURE 1 | Scheme of SARS-CoV-2 virus and its main characteristics. Based on ViralZone, 2020.

Liu et al., 2020). In this sense, it was possible to predict that the deficiency of or a reduction in the physiological function of ACE2 may favor pulmonary inflammation, thrombosis, obesity-induced hypertension, adipose tissue inflammation, and cardiac failure, which is especially detrimental to the baseline risk of COVID-19 patients (**Figure 2**).

Different morbidities, such as obesity, old age, and chronic obstructive pulmonary disease (COPD) are associated with severe COVID-19 symptoms, which, in general, are supra regulated by dipeptidyl peptidase-4 (DPP-4) (Roy et al., 2020). In addition, both DPP-4 and ACE2 are dysregulated proteins in diabetes, so it may be possible for diabetic patients to present more severe cases of COVID-19 due to the increased levels of these proteases (Valencia et al., 2020). Studies have also shown that ACE2 overexpression occurs in the nasal and oropharyngeal epithelium of individuals who are more vulnerable to severe COVID-19 symptoms (Chua et al., 2020; Li et al., 2020a; Ziegler et al., 2020).

Hamming et al. (2004) investigated the presence of ACE2 in different tissues and observed that this receptor is highly abundant in the lung and small intestine epithelium, as well as in the vascular endothelium. Those observations were reinforced by findings on the overexpression of ACE2 in alveolar epithelial cells and enterocytes, which compose potential target organs of SARS-CoV-2 (Zhou et al., 2020). Specifically, expression of the ACE2 gene is concentrated in type I (oxygen and carbon dioxide exchanges) and II pneumocytes (alveolar surfactant production), and the profile of gene expression varies from individual to individual (Zhao et al., 2020). In the presence of SARS-CoV-2 infection, pneumocyte types I and II are damaged, decreasing the production of alveolar surfactants, which implies reduced pulmonary elasticity and pneumocytes type I repair. These factors result in pulmonary fibrosis and inefficient gas exchange (Verdecchia et al., 2020).

The large contact surface of alveolar epithelial tissue associated with the high expression levels of SARS-CoV-2 entry factors in bronchial secretory cells and nasal epithelial cells emphasizes that some individuals are more vulnerable to respiratory failure than others. Additionally, microarray database analysis reported that infection-related factors are also highly expressed in the gastrointestinal system, explaining the diarrhea and virus isolation from stool samples (Gkogkou et al., 2020).

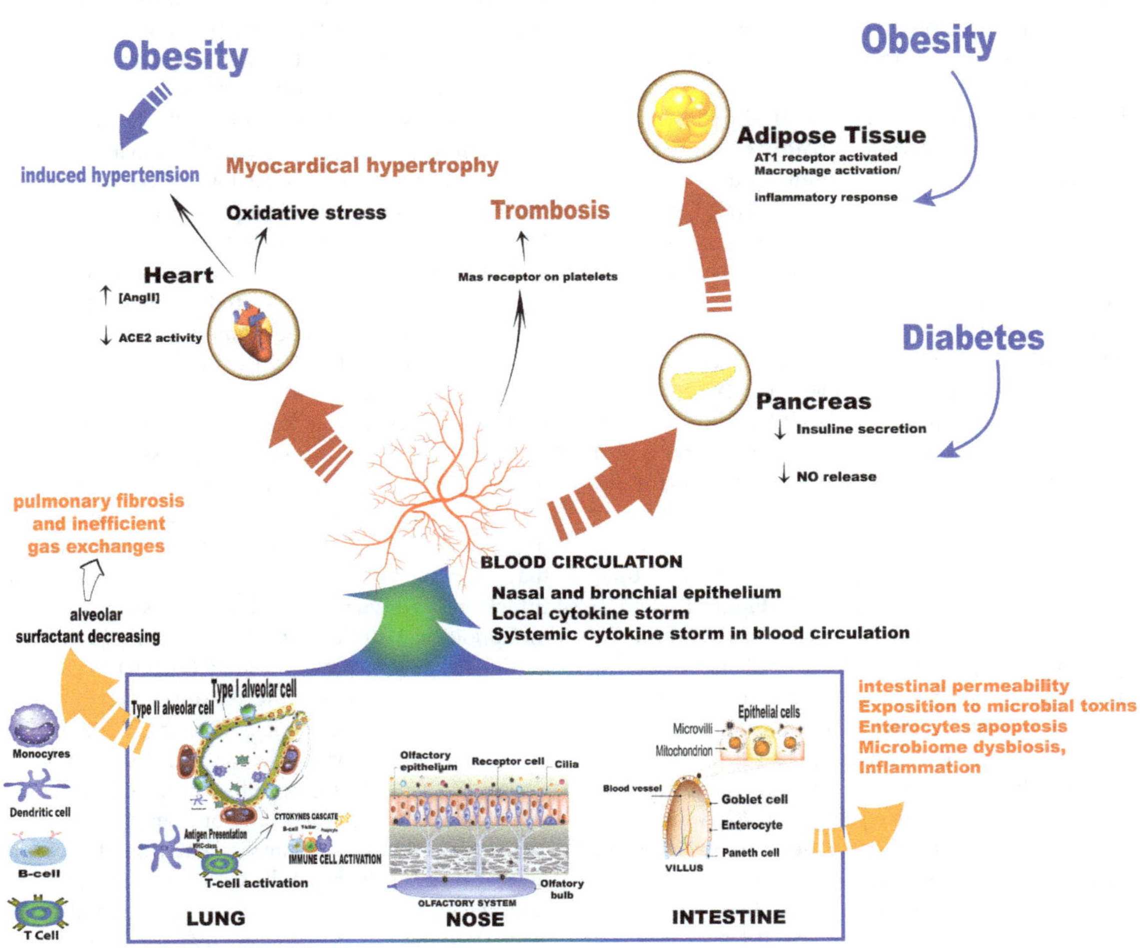

FIGURE 2 | Summary of the main events as a result of the SARS-Cov-2 virus entry into the body. Once in contact with the cells the virus triggers mechanisms that increase the production of cytokines, which in turn trigger an immune cascade.

Therefore, the respiratory and gastrointestinal tracts represent the most frequent routes of virus access to the body. A structural study showed that, in addition to showing high levels of expression in the small intestine, ACE2 also has significant expression in the testicles, kidneys, heart, thyroid, and adipose tissue, with lower expression in the spleen, bone marrow, brain, blood cells, blood vessels, and muscles (Li et al., 2020a).

Initially, SARS-CoV-2 mediated infection is dependent on the viral S1 domain binding to ACE2 and their cleavage by the transmembrane serine protease 2 (TMPRSS2), whereas the viral S2 domain is responsible for conformational changes that drive the fusion process between viral and host cell membranes (Brest et al., 2020; Wang et al., 2020a). Those events are followed by virus entry and its replication in the cells (Devaux et al., 2020; Wang et al., 2020a). However, other molecular factors have been implicated as essential not only for viral entry but mainly for infection progressive cellular effects, such as the membrane anchored metalloproteinase domain-containing protein 17 (ADAM 17), which evokes the ACE2 shedding mechanism (Brest et al., 2020; Gheblawi et al., 2020).

Virus binding induces ACE2 deficiency, amplifying the dysregulation between the ACE-Ang II-AT1 (type 1 receptor for angiotensin II) receptor and the ACE2-Ang 1-7-Mas receptor axis since there is a reduction in ACE2 catalytic properties favoring the ACE-Ang II-AT1 receptor pathway. Moreover, the renin–angiotensin–aldosterone system imbalance evokes pronounced detrimental effects in all COVID-19 stages, since multiple organ failure and a hyperinflammatory response are the main clinical findings in severe cases (Mahmudpour et al., 2020).

The dysregulation of the ACE2/Ang II/AT1R axis, attenuation of the ACE2/Mas receptor axis, and increase in the activation of the ACE2/bradykinin B1R/DABK pathway and their complementary cascades are the main molecular interactions that support the cytokine storm (Hirano and Murakami, 2020; Mahmudpour et al., 2020). Once the virus binds to ACE2, this enzyme does not convert Ang II into Ang 1-7, making it impossible to activate MasR and form the complex to control inflammation. In the absence of Ang 1-7, there is also an increase in the expression of p38 MAPK and NFk-β pathways and inflammatory factors, as well as the binding of Ang II to the AT1R receptor, triggering pro-inflammatory responses and, as a result, pulmonary deterioration (Gheblawi et al., 2020; Mahmudpour et al., 2020; South et al., 2020) (**Figure 3**).

The increase in Ang II and the consequent activation of its AT1R receptor also hyperactivate the complement system cascade, causing even more inflammatory responses, inducing vasoconstriction, increasing oxidative stress, and promoting inflammation and fibrosis (Risitano et al., 2020; South et al., 2020). In addition, there is an increase in the activity of the inflammatory lung factor [des-Arg9]-BK (DABK), which also causes the exacerbated release of cytokines (Tolouian et al., 2020). These events justify the relationship between a high viral load, severe lung damage, and Ang II levels in serum samples from patients infected with SARS-CoV-2 (Liu et al., 2020).

Lymphopenia is one of the immunological responses characteristic of severe cases of COVID-19 accompanied by a marked decrease in the absolute number of circulating CD4+ cells, CD8+ cells, B cells, and natural killer cells (NK) (Zhou et al., 2010; Tan et al., 2020a), as well as a decrease in other cell types and increased levels of pro-inflammatory cytokines (Moore and June, 2020; Verdecchia et al., 2020). The binding of SARS-CoV-2 with the ACE-2 receptor and the consequent change in the ACE-cascade triggers several molecular processes that lead to the overproduction of cytokines and hyperinflammation, and the activation of some cells that play a role in the immune system (Dhochak et al., 2020; Mahmudpour et al., 2020).

AN EXPLOSIVE RESPONSE

The dysregulation of the immune system triggers the evolution of COVID-19 to its severe form in some patients (Giamarellos-Bourboulis et al., 2020; Huang et al., 2020), and respiratory failure is generally associated with this characteristic and not necessarily with increased viral load (Risitano et al., 2020). The simultaneous activation of both innate and adaptative immune systems through the binding of SARS-CoV-2 to the cell receptor makes the immune system reaction more damaging to the cells than the virus itself. In this way, the events following infection lead to severe inflammatory disorders with a possible progression to death (Du et al., 2020; Zhang et al., 2020a).

A study by Tan et al. (2020b) concluded that a stronger antibody response is associated with delayed viral clearance and consequently more severe symptoms of the disease. Patients with COVID-19 and lower IgG titers experienced faster viral clearance when compared to patients with COVID-19 and higher IgG titers. Another study showed that asymptomatic individuals had lower IgG titers compared to those that were symptomatic ($p=0.005$) 3–4 weeks after exposure to SARS-CoV-2, and this difference remained during the convalescent phase ($p=0.02$), 8 weeks after hospital discharge (Long et al., 2020). This imbalance in immune response may occur due to a mechanism known as antibody-dependent enhancement (ADE), where there is an increase in pathogenicity in the presence of sub-neutralizing and non-neutralizing antibodies that facilitate viral entry into cells, triggering an increase in infection and virulence (Bournazos et al., 2020). Other immunological studies on SARS-CoV suggest that anti-SARS-CoV-2 antibodies may intensify COVID-19 symptoms through the ADE mechanism, increasing infection or triggering detrimental immunopathology (Lee et al., 2020).

According to Arvin et al. (2020), this phenomenon occurs when non-neutralizing or sub-neutralizing antibodies bind to viral antigens without blocking or eliminating infection and, in an unexpected way, facilitate viral entry into the cells through the interaction with crystallizable fragments or receptors' complements. Even if there is no active viral replication, the facilitated viral entry into cells can lead to the activation of macrophages, monocytes, and B cells and the production of

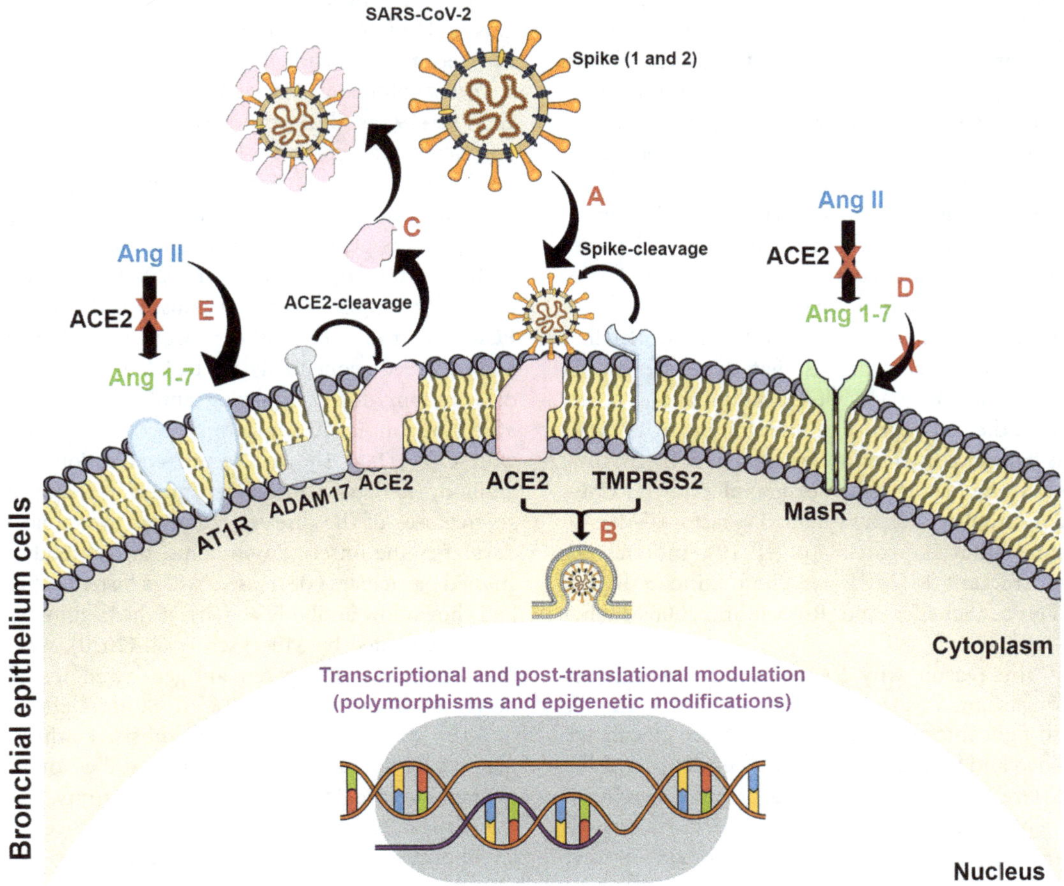

FIGURE 3 | Schematic representation of SARS-CoV-2 infection in target cells and its consequences on ACE2 signaling pathways. **(A)** SARS-CoV-2 spike proteins bind to ACE2 with their consequent cleavage by ACE2 and TMPRSS2; **(B)** viral fusion, internalization and release of viral genetic material; **(C)** ACE2 cleavage by ADAM17 forming a plasm-soluble ACE2 isoform and its binding on viral particle at non-target tissues; **(D)** The conversion of Ang II to Ang 1-7 is blocked with subsequent decrease on Mas receptor protective axis; **(E)** Ang II interacts with AT1 receptor and triggers detrimental pathways evoking inflammatory processes.

tumor necrosis factor alpha (TNFα) and interleukins 6 and 10 (IL-6 and IL-10), affecting disease prognosis, an approach previously observed by Taylor et al. (2015). This event may be responsible for the increase in the number of immune cells observed in patients with a poor prognosis.

The ADE mechanism is mediated by immunoglobulin receptor Fc(R), which has a pivotal role in immune response, controlling innate and humoral immunities that are essential for responses against infections and the prevention of chronic inflammation and autoimmune diseases. In addition, these immunoregulatory processes may play a role in the pathogenesis of the disease, triggering responses such as the release of cytokines and phagocytosis. Notably, these receptors have a large genetic polymorphism, with a variation in the immune response according to the presented gene (Hargreaves et al., 2015; Bournazos and Ravetch, 2017), which may contribute to a larger or smaller immune response regarding infection by SARS-CoV-2.

A study by Sun et al. (2020) reported that changes in peripheral blood inflammatory cells may signal the severity and spread of COVID-19. In this study, patients with severe infection showed a decrease in the number of lymphocytes, eosinophils, basophils, and an increase in neutrophil count. A decrease was observed in the total count of T lymphocytes (T CD4+, T CD8+), as well as NK cells 2 weeks after the treatment of patients who posteriorly died. Although there is a decrease in CD4 and CD8 lymphocyte cells and NK cells in the most severe cases of COVID-19, hyperactive circulating monocytes continue to produce proinflammatory cytokines, such as TNFα and IL-6. The hyperactivation of monocytes, decrease of lymphocytes, and high IL-6 release causes low expression of the cell surface receptor encoded by the human leukocyte complex (HLA-DR). As a result, there may be a failure in antigen presentation preventing the action of the immune system against the virus, followed by hyperinflammation due to the high production of pro-inflammatory cytokines (Giamarellos-Bourboulis et al., 2020).

In the study performed by Qin et al. (2020), most patients with severe COVID-19 symptoms showed an increase in cytokine and chemokine serum levels, in addition to high production of neutrophils and low production of lymphocytes, indicating that the hyperinflammatory response was responsible for the severity of the disease. The impaired immune system, with damaged T lymphocytes, may cause greater susceptibility to secondary pulmonary bacterial infections, which justifies the use of some antibiotics as an adjunctive pharmacological therapy.

Thus, a cytokine storm is one of the main characteristics of severe cases of SARS-CoV-2 infection, being associated with the severity of the disease and mortality (Giamarellos-Bourboulis et al., 2020; Lu et al., 2020b). It involves the uncontrolled release of a large amount of pro-inflammatory cytokines, such as TNFα, IL-6, and IL-1β, in a systemic way (Roshanravan et al., 2020). This reaction is formed by complex interconnected networks that interact in different ways, showing us that there are several molecular mechanisms to be unveiled (Mahmudpour et al., 2020). In summary, the consequence of infection by SARS-CoV-2 is that patients have increased serum levels of IL-6, IL-1β, IL-2, IL-8, IL-17, colony stimulating factor of granulocytes (G-CSF), granulocyte and macrophage colony stimulating factor (GMCSF), interferon gamma-induced protein 10 (IP-10), monocyte-1 protein-chemoattractant-1 (MCP-1), chemokine 3 ligand (CCL3), and TNFα (Scheller and Rose-John, 2006; Mehta et al., 2020).

In this way, the reason why SARS-CoV-2 differentially changes the organism's response and which strategies organisms use to fight infection are questions to be elucidated. According to Ulhaq and Soraya (2020), there is evidence that the circulating IL-6 levels are intricately linked to the severity of infection in patients with COVID-19, especially in those with lung injury. IL-6 is a pleiotropic multifunctional cytokine that plays an important role in human metabolism (Hunter and Jones, 2015). Its action is mainly linked to lymphocyte proliferation, antibody production and multiplication, and differentiation of hematopoietic cells, targeting B cells, T cells, neutrophils, eosinophils, and basophils. IL-6 is associated with diseases including leukemia, hypertension, atherosclerosis, and different types of malignant tumors. The greatest production of this cytokine occurs in T cells, endothelial cells, fibroblasts, macrophages, and monocytes (Brennan and Foey, 2002). An increase of pro-inflammatory cytokines was detected in the serum of patients infected by coronaviruses SARS-CoV and MERS-CoV, being related to inflammation and lung damage (Wong et al., 2004; Mahallawi et al., 2018).

UNDERSTANDING THE COURSE OF THE IMMUNE RESPONSE

As previously discussed, in addition to respiratory failure due to pulmonary inflammation, patients with severe COVID-19 symptoms may have systemic inflammation that causes damage to multiple organs, with distinct immune reactions among individuals. A current study, named ENE-COVID, which is being performed by the Spanish Ministry of Health and the Carlos III Institute of Public Health, showed that the majority of Spain's population, one of the European populations most affected by COVID-19, had negative serology for SARS-CoV-2. Only 5% of more than 61,000 participants in the study had serum prevalence for IgG antibodies, of which one third were asymptomatic. Among the patients with positive results for COVID-19 as determined by qRT-PCR, 90% of serum prevalence was observed 14 days after diagnosis. From these results, it was concluded that herd immunity cannot be achieved without major side effects and a high mortality rate in the susceptible population (Pollán et al., 2020).

In a study by Seow et al. (2020), serum samples were collected from 65 patients diagnosed with COVID-19 by qRT-PCR and from 31 healthcare workers with positive serology and analyzed sequentially up to 94 days after the appearance of symptoms for neutralizing antibody responses. Eight days after the onset of symptoms, 95% of patients diagnosed with COVID-19 showed serum conversion and neutralizing antibody activity, with greater antibody responses in the most severe cases of the disease. However, over time, more than 60 days after the onset of symptoms, the antibody levels of most studied participants decreased, with a faster decline in those who had shown low antibody activity at the beginning. This fact was also investigated by Muecksch et al. (2020), who reported that the sensibility of a given antigen-based test for N protein decreased from >95% to 85%, 61–80 days after diagnosis, and to 71%, 81–100 days after diagnosis, confirming that it is inadequate for serum prevalence studies or for individuals who show long-term chronic symptoms. Other immune mechanisms, such as long-term memory T-cell responses, play an important role in protecting against serious infections or diseases (Grifoni et al., 2020; Le Bert et al., 2020), however, the detailed analysis of responses of T cells is currently not viable in a high-performance clinical environment (Muecksch et al., 2020).

Knowing the mechanisms and long-term kinetics of antibody titers, as well as the effectiveness of serological assays, is essential for a precise interpretation of disease progression (Andersson et al., 2020; GeurtsvanKessel et al., 2020; Rosado et al., 2020); however, specific IgM and IgG antibodies are mostly investigated for the peak surface glycoprotein (S) and nucleocapsid protein (N) (Carter et al., 2020). In the future, it may be difficult to both verify seropositive individuals and study the immunization time of individuals and populations (herd immunization). In this way, new studies are developed in an attempt to improve the evaluation of the immune response through the identification of more specific regions for both early and late responses, such as ORF8 and ORF3b regions (Hachim et al., 2020; Wang et al., 2020b).

Regarding herd immunity, Britton et al. (2020) developed a mathematical model in which they evaluated how far preventive measures can lead to herd immunity for SARS-CoV-2. They applied the model in four different hypothetical populations, considering variations in age and activity levels, with the implementation of preventive measures. It was observed that the population heterogeneity, mainly related to variations in social activity, reduced the acquisition of herd immunity from

60% to 43%, considering the classic level for homogeneous populations. In the current scenario, considering the wide heterogeneity among populations, it is possible to predict the unattainability of herd immunity.

PREDICTING THE FUTURE: THE GENOTYPE AS AN INDICATOR OF SUSCEPTIBILITY

Several factors cause variations in individuals' responses to SARS-CoV-2, including viral load, genetic susceptibility, and concomitant pathological conditions (Le Bert et al., 2020). The fact that some individuals have exacerbated inflammatory reactions and others do not gives rise to different phenotypes of the disease that are linked to genetic factors (Tisoncik et al., 2012). According to Radzikowska et al. (2020), there are different receptors that are potentially involved with SARS-CoV-2 infection in epithelial barriers and immune cells, and their differential expression, depending on age, gender, presence of other characteristics, such as obesity, smoking, and polymorphisms, and the state of the disease, can contribute to the patterns of morbidity and severity of COVID-19 symptoms.

Therefore, we must remember that individuals are genetically distinct, which can contribute to the identification of different levels of disease severity. In addition to the comprehension of the molecular mechanisms involved in SARS-CoV-2 infection, it is necessary to understand the host organism's reaction to infection.

This raised the question: are individual differences responsible for the lethality of the disease? An initial investigation carried out by some researchers in relation to gender and age showed that there is no difference between males and females or between people of different ages in terms of infection and transmission (Scully et al., 2020; Stokes et al., 2020), which makes us believe that the individual responses after infection have great importance in determining the development of the disease (Jin et al., 2020; Mauvais-Jarvis et al., 2020; Stokes et al., 2020).

This has led researchers to several questions. Is it possible to predict a genetic composition that is less able to fight infection? Are we in a genomic era where genetic screening can identify the most resistant and the most susceptible individuals to new diseases? Could these results contribute to a more specific clinical assessment of infected individuals? To discuss these issues, the study of virus entry factors, expression profiles, polymorphisms, and epigenetic modifications may be important tools to detect susceptible individuals, which could facilitate control of COVID-19 outcomes (Anastassopoulou et al., 2020).

Since studies do not show difference between individuals in terms of transmission and infection by the SARS-CoV-2 virus, it is essential to assess individual responses and how they can be differentiated.

Almost 1 year since the start of COVID-19 pandemic, reports have shown that most patients who needed hospitalization, intensive care, intubation, and eventually died were male, with numbers 1.5- to 2-fold higher when compared to females (Mauvais-Jarvis et al., 2020). Another study showed that in relation to the studied COVID-19 cases, men showed greater complications with more severe symptoms than women ($p=0.035$). In the public data set, the number of men who died of COVID-19 was 2.4-fold greater than that of women (70.3% *vs.* 29.7%, $p=0.016$) (Jin et al., 2020).

In the United States, where the test to diagnose SARS-CoV-2 infection was prioritized for people with symptoms, the diagnostic rates were similar for both genders, but the male mortality rate was 1.5-fold higher than that of females (Stokes et al., 2020). There are reports that females have more effective innate and adaptative immunity responses to antigenic challenges (Klein, 2012; Klein and Flanagan, 2016). In addition, women respond better to different types of vaccines (Fink and Klein, 2015; vom Steeg and Klein, 2016; Fink et al., 2018).

According to Li et al. (2020b), the relationship between deaths from COVID-19 and the gender of patients may provide clues in the search for solutions to control the disease. Differences in chromosomes, genes, and hormones are influenced according to the individual's gender which causes varied responses to several diseases, including COVID-19. Gender may be considered when analyzing clinical trials in relation to SARS-CoV-2 infection, as gender differences may reveal different approaches that are necessary for the treatment of patients with COVID-19, such as estrogen-related compounds and androgen receptor antagonists (Li et al., 2020b).

Thus, the possible polymorphisms or loss of heterozygosity of some genes in males can interfere in the response to the virus, since the fact that females have two X chromosomes could be considered an advantage. Even with the inactivation of one X chromosome, this advantage is maintained since the process occurs randomly, allowing heterozygosity, a fact that is impossible in males due to the presence of a single X chromosome. The X chromosome has the ACE-2 gene, as well as genes related to the immune system responsible for innate and adaptive immune responses (Gemmati et al., 2020). The androgen receptor (AR), toll-like receptor 7 (TLR7), toll-like receptor 8 (TLR8), kinase 1 associated with the interleukin-1 receptor (IRAK1), beta chain of cytochrome B-245 (CYBB), fork head box P3 (FOXP3), and CD40 ligand (CD40L) are among X chromosome genes involved in innate and adaptive immunity (Schurz et al., 2019).

The AR gene is responsible for the synthesis of a signal transduction protein and transcription factor, necessary for the development and expression of male phenotypes. In addition, signaling of this gene leads to several chemical activations and deactivations in the immune system, such as the inhibition of antibody production, cell differentiation *via* granulocytes, regulation of the chemotactic capacity of macrophages, regulation of T and B cell function, activation of the immune response of T cells by Th1, and inactivation of type I interferon (IFN type I) signaling pathways (Olsen and Kovacs, 2001; Lai et al., 2012; Kissick et al., 2014).

The main hormones that bind to AR are dihydrotestosterone (DHT), testosterone, androstenedione, and dehydroepiandro sterone (DHEA), which are synthesized from cholesterol. Of these four androgens, only DHT cannot be converted to estrogen, so studies using DHT are more easily interpreted. It is interesting to remember that testosterone is present in greater quantity in adult males, which can lead to a response stimulation *via* Th1. Remarkably, the AR gene has polymorphs that influence the intensity of androgen signaling, and it affects both men and women (Kissick et al., 2014). Many differences in immune cells result from exposure to androgens, showing that there is a relationship between immunity and the gender of individuals. The suppression of immune reactivity and androgen-mediated inflammation raises the threshold for the development of autoimmunity; however, further studies are still needed to elucidate these mechanisms (Bupp and Jorgensen, 2018).

The TLR7 and TLR8 genes, together with TLR4, which is on chromosome 4, mediate part of the innate immune response because they are in one of the three classes of pattern recognition receptors, the toll-like receptors (TLRs). They specifically regulate the production of type 1 IFN and other cytokines so that sexual dimorphism may be observed during antiviral responses (Meier et al., 2009). Studies carried out using female lymphocytes reported that T and B cells showed biallelic expression of TLR7 and increased transcription of immune related genes linked to the X chromosome (Souyris et al., 2018). It would explain the 10-fold higher expression of TLR in females when compared to male cells (Klein and Pekosz, 2014), as well as the lower production of INF- α. Male peripheral blood mononuclear cells produced lower levels of IFN-α after stimulation by the ligand TLR7 and higher levels of the immunosuppressive cytokine IL-10 after stimulation by ligands TLR8 and TLR9 (Torcia et al., 2012).

The IRAK1 gene is the key encoder of the intracellular signaling pathway of TLR/IL-1R and assists the recognition of viruses by TLR7/8 and the production of IFN- α, being one of the main genes that contribute to the divergence of responses related to gender after trauma and sepsis (Gottipati et al., 2008; Sperry et al., 2014). The IRAK1 haplotype contributes to differentiated immunomodulation between the genders in all ethnic groups in relation to inflammatory responses. It probably occurs due to polymorphisms in the gene (Spolarics et al., 2017).

The CYBB gene was identified as possibly responsible for the innate immune response, contributing to the activation of an intracellular oxidative explosion for the production of superoxide in phagocytes, encoding catalytic subunits of NADPH oxidase and, consequently, causing the death of microorganisms by phagocytosis (Spolarics et al., 2017; Jaillon et al., 2019).

The FOXP3 and CD40L genes cooperate in the adaptive immune response (Jaillon et al., 2019). The protein synthesized by the FOXP3 gene is a key regulator of T cell activation, more specifically Treg (regulatory T cells) that prevent autoimmunity (Mercer and Unutmaz, 2009). The protein synthesized by CD40L is responsible for transmembrane signaling involved in the activation of platelet, endothelial, and immunological cells. It acts in antigen presentation, in the activation of B cells, and in the differentiation of T cells (Elgueta et al., 2009; Spolarics et al., 2017), which could be involved in the differential development of disseminated intravascular coagulation in some patients.

In addition to those genes, several genetic factors, such as inactivation of the X chromosome and cell mosaicism, may be responsible for the hyperresponsiveness of the female immune system (Pessach and Notarangelo, 2009; Libert et al., 2010; Rainville et al., 2018). An interesting factor regarding the different mediation of the immune response in men and women is that the immune response mediated by antibodies in women is stimulated predominantly by type 2 T helper cells (Th2), whereas in men, type 1 T helper cells (Th1) are predominant (Billi et al., 2019).

The gender-bias in response to immunological problems has already been shown by Lambert (2019), considering rheumatic diseases, where it was shown that, in addition to the heterozygosity that occurs in females, different genders go through different situations since birth, with molding of the epigenome and microchimerism. The author showed that men and women are genetically, epigenetically, hormonally, and chemically different, which has an influence on the health and success of long-term treatment. A better understanding and exploration of these differences is necessary to progress in the treatment and management of all patients. There is evidence that targeting candidate genes or reversing epigenetic dysregulation according to gender may be more effective and beneficial than current therapies (Lambert, 2019). Broadening the discussion of the topic, genetic, and epigenetic differences can be parameters to assess, in response to the presence of the virus, as they can be crucial in viral recognition and individual immune response, influencing the severity of SARS-CoV-2 infection. An example of epigenetic interference is the low susceptibility of children to SARS-CoV-2 infection, which can be explained, among several factors, by the high expression of ACE-2, which in spite of being the viral receptor, ends up having a protective effect on the lungs. The high expression of ACE2 enables the binding of the receptor to Ang II (**Figure 3**) even in the presence of the virus, without altering the signaling cascade activated after the coupling of viral particles. In addition, children have a more effective innate immune system, with the ability to fight infection immediately upon infection, showing high regeneration of the alveolar epithelium (Dhochak et al., 2020). Additionally, it was found that children's nasal epithelium, the first region of SARS-CoV-2 contact with the organism, presents low expression of ACE2, hampering virus binding (Bunyavanich et al., 2020).

In this context, other essential factors to be considered are the relationships between the levels of expression, polymorphisms, and epigenetic alterations, specifically for the viral entry factors ACE2, ADAM17, and TMPRSS2, since they are implicated in both susceptibility to viral infection in target cells and COVID-19 progressive symptoms (Hoffmann et al., 2020; Ortiz-Fernández and Sawalha, 2020).

For small bowel infections, the ACE2-TMPRSS2 and four serine protease axes also exert an essential role, being responsible for virus attachment and its internalization, explaining the gastrointestinal viral tropism (Wong et al., 2020; Zhang et al., 2020b). However, the presence of other elements on enterocytes, such as furin and B0AT1, an aminoacid transporter, can influence viral infection and its consequences. Intestinal viral infection includes the initial Spike cleavage by TMPRSS2 and furin, in segments 1 and 2, followed by S1 coupling with ACE2, while S2 mediates the membrane fusion. One of the main steps during SARS-CoV-2 bowel infection is the relationship between ACE2 and B0AT1, since B0AT1 function is regulated by the ACE2-like protein, viral coupling to ACE2 also blocks amino acid transporter activity. These effects lead to pathological conditions, similar to colitis, due to amino acid transport depletion, especially tryptophan, towards enterocytes' apical membrane with successive activation of the mTOR pathway, evoking the inflammatory process (Mönkemüller et al., 2020). Notably, its consequences on intestinal permeability and tissue exposition to other microbial toxins, enterocytes' apoptosis, and microbiome dysbiosis amplifies inflammation from local to systemic coverage (Vodnar et al., 2020). Then, in the presence of diabetes, inflammatory bowel diseases, and obesity as preexistent conditions, microbiome dysbiosis is markedly one of the main elements for enhancing the inflammatory consequences of viral infection.

Recent studies reported polymorphisms in the ACE2 gene in Chinese (Luo et al., 2019), Canadian (Malard et al., 2013), Indian (Patnaik et al., 2014), and Brazilian (Pinheiro et al., 2019) populations. Cao et al. (2020) conducted a study with database analysis and observed that the ACE2 gene has 1,700 variants, of which 11 variants were associated with increased expression of ACE2 in tissues, which can lead to differentiated infectivity by SARS-CoV-2. Different ACE2 variants related to hypertension manifestations were detected and low ACE2 mRNA expression levels were associated with hypertension, dyslipidemia, and heart failure, influencing SARS-CoV-2 infection susceptibility (Cao et al., 2020). In a complementary way, the expression of ACE2 was downregulated in infected cells (Devaux et al., 2020).

Other epidemiological investigations discussed the differential incidence of ACE insertion (I)/deletion (D) polymorphisms among populations and its correlations with viral infection, mortality rate, and recovered clinical cases. In fact, the highest ACE levels were attributed to the dominant allele of ACE I/D polymorphism, revealing a positive correlation between its frequency and infected people in Asian populations. This finding was associated with the presence of comorbidities (hypertension, type-2 diabetes, hyperlipidemia, for example), but no relationships were observed for ACE I/D polymorphisms and the recovery rate of infected patients (Pati et al., 2020). In a complementary way, a clinical study in Spain observed that ACE I/D polymorphisms were related to viral infection, depending on clinical hypertension severity (Gómez et al., 2020), indicating that both genetic and clinical factors are simultaneously implicated in COVID-19 outcomes.

In other analyses, it was reported that ACE2 expression was associated with differences in minor allele frequencies among populations, since Asian people express higher ACE2 levels than Caucasians. Additionally, single nucleotide polymorphisms (SNPs) were investigated for ADAM17 and TMPRSS2, indicating that some TMPRSS2 genotypes are more susceptible to other viral infections, such as H1N1, while ADAM17 expression quantitative trait loci are related to the modulation of the ACE2 shedding process (Brest et al., 2020). This could be explained by the suppression of the ACE2 shedding barrier and the production of soluble form of ACE2 in the presence of a high viral load, which enables infection. Other polymorphisms with effects on COVID-19 progression were also observed in non-coding sequences for cathepsin L, monocyte chemoattractant protein-1 (CCL2), and neutrophil elastase genes, enhancing virus infection and inflammation (Ghafouri-Fard et al., 2020; Vargas-Alarcón et al., 2020).

In addition to expression levels and polymorphisms, ACE2 is extensively regulated by post-translational mechanisms. Those epigenetic modifications include glycosylation, phosphorylation, and shedding processes. In conditions of cellular stress, such as during inflammation, NAD-dependent deacetylase SIRT1 is linked to the ACE2 promoter, favoring its transcription. However, DNA methylation in the ACE2 promoter was lower in lung epithelial cells when compared to other target cells, indicating its high transcription levels in lung tissue, which allows viral infection (Saponaro et al., 2020; Sen et al., 2021).

Taken together, those factors belong to a complex mechanism involving mutations affecting the essential molecular components for viral entry (ACE2, ADAM17, and TMPRSS2); changes in their mRNA expression and post-translational regulation, implicated the severity of clinical symptoms observed in the presence or absence of patients' comorbidities.

Asselta et al. (2020) compared variations of the TMPRSS2 gene between populations in Italy and other Europeans and Asians. The study indicated that the TMPRSS2 gene and its genetic variants may be promising for disease modulation, suggesting that ACE2 may not be the only target of the virus. In the same way, other genes may be responsible for presenting alterations that may interfere in the individual response to the virus (**Table 1**).

Human leukocyte antigen (HLA) genes, HLA-A, -B, and -C, among others, are located on chromosome 6 (6p21.34) and encode proteins involved in the processing and presentation of antigens, as well as a wide range of other immunological functions (Parham and Moffett, 2013). The connection of these genes with coronavirus infection was mentioned by Lin et al. (2003), who showed that the smallest binding peptides for SARS-CoV-1 were found for HLA-B * 46: 01. Furthermore, Nguyen et al. (2020) performed an in silico analysis covering the binding affinity of the viral peptide-MHC class I in 145 HLA-A, -B, and -C genotypes and found that HLA-B * 46: 01 also occurred for SARS-CoV-2, suggesting that this allelic variant leads to vulnerability to the disease. However, the HLA B * 15: 03 variant was linked with the ability to present SARS-CoV-2 peptides, suggesting cross-protection with immunity based on T cells. However, Wang et al. (2020c) presented preliminary results, where HLA-A * 11: 01, -B * 51: 01, and -C * 14: 02 alleles showed connection with worse clinical outcomes in patients with COVID-19.

TABLE 1 | Location and description of genetic polymorphisms that may be involved with a higher probability of COVID-19 severity.

Locus	Gene	Localization/Function of protein	Polymorphisms + SARS-CoV-2	References
Xp22.2	**ACE2**	SARS-CoV-2 receptor, Heart, lungs, nervous system, liver, and kidney cells	**Arg514-Gly** Cardiovascular and pulmonary conditions due to alteration of the AGT-ACE2 pathway **Ser19-Pro** **Glu329-Gly** Low binding affinity and lack of some of the key residues in the complex formation with the Spike SARS-CoV-2 protein	Hou et al. (2020) Hussain et al. (2020)
2p25.1	**ADAM17**	Release of ACE2 into the extracellular space Endothelial cell, astrocytes, and neurons	Evaluations of SNPs showed susceptible variations	Li et al. (2014)
2q24.2	**DPP4**	SARS-CoV-2 co-receptor Blood circulation and endothelial cells, including capillaries that surround endocrine and intestinal organs	–	Li et al. (2020c)
15q26.1	**PCSK3**	Viral pre-activation Pulmonary epithelium and fibroblasts	**Arg298Gln** Influence on the recognition of the target RxxR sequence within the SARS-CoV-2 spike protein	Latini et al. (2020)
19q13.32	**ApoE**	Co-expressed where the ACE2 receptor is highly expressed Alveolar type II cells, lung	**e^4 allele** **Cys112Arg** Serious disease, regardless of pre-existing dementia, cardiovascular disease, and type 2 diabetes	Kuo et al. (2020)
Xp22.2	**TLR7**	Essential component of innate immunity intracellularly, in the endosomes	**Val795Phe** Serious disease Allele homozygosis may have an adverse impact on the natural history and prognosis of COVID-19 in males	van der Made et al. (2020)
4q35.1	**TLR3**	NF-kappa-B activation, IRF3 nuclear translocation, cytokine secretion, and inflammatory response Endoplasmic reticulum membrane	Ser339fs/WT Pro554Ser/WT Trp769*/WT Met870Val/WT Rare loss-of-function variants	Zhang et al. (2020c)
11p15.5	**IRF7**	Key transcriptional regulator of immune responses dependent on interferon type I (IFN) which plays a critical role in the innate immune response against DNA and RNA viruses. It regulates the transcription of IFN type I genes (IFN-alpha and IFN-beta) and genes stimulated by IFN (ISG) by binding to an interferon-stimulated response element (ISRE) in their promoters.	Pro364fs/ Pro364fs Rare loss-of-function variants **Met371Val/** **Asp117Asn** Rare loss-of-function variants	

The Severe Covid-19 GWAS Group (2020) performed a meta-analysis of broad genomic association in which they analyzed SNPs in patients with severe acute respiratory syndrome by SARS-CoV-2 and control individuals in Italy and Spain. Two loci associated with respiratory failure in COVID-19 were found, one of which was the GA-G insertion-deletion variant in locus 3p21.31 that is composed of six genes (SLC6A20, LZTFL1, CCR9, FYCO1, CXCR6, and XCR1). Some of these genes are associated with greater severity of COVID-19 symptoms. The SLC6A20 gene synthesizes the SIT1 protein, which together with LZTFL1, interacts with ACE2 cell receptors. The other genes encode chemokine receptors of the C-C and CXC families, which control cell migration associated with immune surveillance by trafficking effector cells to sites of infection and inflammation. According to Zeberg and Pääbo (2020), this genomic sequence, a 49.4 kb haplotype, previously identified by The Severe Covid-19 GWAS Group (2020), was inherited from a Neanderthal who lived in Croatia 50,000 years ago and has a frequency of 30% in the South Asians, 8% in Europeans, and 4% in the American population. Despite the variations in the frequency of this genomic sequence, there are no differences in disease severity around the world due to several non-genetic factors, such as multiple comorbidities, advanced age, physical inactivity, and smoking, among others, which also contribute to respiratory failure.

The other region studied by The Severe Covid-19 GWAS Group (2020) regarding SARS-CoV-2 infection was the SNP A or C at locus 9q34.2, which is related to the ABO blood system, and showed the highest susceptibility of individuals in group A and the lowest susceptibility of individuals in group O. Other studies investigated patients in relation to blood groups and showed that patients in blood group O, regardless of Rh, had a lower incidence of SARS-CoV-2 infection, with individuals in group A being more sensitive and prone to disease, presenting a higher frequency among patients with COVID-19, in addition to being the most serious cases (Göker et al., 2020). The authors suggested that the biological mechanisms included in these results may be related to other biological effects of the identified variant, including stabilization of the von Willebrand factor or the development of neutralizing antibodies against protein-bound N-glycans (The Severe Covid-19 GWAS Group, 2020; Zhao et al., 2020).

Other studies have shown evidence of the increased probability of individuals in blood group A to have COVID-19 (Zietz et al., 2020). A possible explanation for this would be the fact that anti-A antibodies could inhibit the interaction of the Spike protein with the ACE-2 receptor (Guillon et al., 2008).

Therefore, blood group O appears to be protective, while group A may be more susceptible to the disease. In this way, patients in group A deserve greater attention when infected by SARS-CoV-2, and further molecular studies are also needed to obtain answers regarding the real protective role of the O antigen (Göker et al., 2020).

Another hypothesis is that susceptibility to SARS-CoV-2 may also be related to the composition of the intestinal microbiota. Based on the proteomic profile of patients with COVID-19, Gou et al. (2020) conducted a study in which they observed the direct relationship between the characteristics of the intestinal microbiota of some healthy individuals, generally older, and the abnormal activation of pro-inflammatory cytokines, which can determine the predisposition to the severe form of COVID-19.

PERSPECTIVES IN THE DIAGNOSIS AND TREATMENT OF COVID-19: THE CONTRIBUTION OF GENETIC ANALYSIS

Knowledge of the patients' immune phenotype/genotype is necessary to understand the complexity of COVID-19 (Mangalmurti and Hunter, 2020). Knowing the changes in the signaling pathways caused by the infection can also contribute to the elucidation of the molecular cascades that trigger infection and the severity of the clinical symptoms. So, it is necessary to find molecular targets and alternatives to prevent the progression of COVID-19 (Catanzaro et al., 2020).

Given the information collected since the pandemic began, it is almost certain that the organism's success in overcoming COVID-19 is linked to the genetics of each individual, their polymorphisms, their patterns of gene expression, and possibly the diversity of intestinal microbiota. However, there are still no parameters to assess genetic markers in individuals. According to Brest et al. (2020), in view of the multifactorial genetic impact for the risk of SARS-CoV-2 infection and disease severity, there is the possibility of assessing SNP profiles of the ACE2, ADAM17, and TMPRSS2 genes in an attempt to identify vulnerable populations, creating a risk score.

A study that is being conducted at the Center for Human Genome and Stem Cell Studies at the University of São Paulo (Brazil) aims to investigate the genome of super-resistant individuals and individuals susceptible to SARS-CoV-2. It is seeking to understand the factors associated with cases of nonagenarians with diabetes and hypertension that have recovered from the disease and young people with no history of chronic diseases that have died. According to the researchers, individuals who develop severe forms may have so-called "risk genes", while the infected group that does not develop the severe form of the disease, has "protective genes" (Alisson, 2020). An international consortium, the COVID Human Genetic Effort, is currently focused on investigating naturally resistant individuals and healthy young patients who developed severe symptoms. This group of researchers considers these studies a promising tool to understand the genetic determinants of COVID-19 (Casanova et al., 2020).

In this context, the need for genomic analysis and its application in diagnostic medicine is emphasized, since the identification of some genetic patterns can contribute to the clinical evaluation of patients and the amplification of choices for the treatment of each individual. As in other events related to infectious diseases throughout history, this new stage features the possibility to develop new skills and use different tools to guide and assist health professionals in different phases of the treatment and diagnosis of COVID- 19.

AUTHOR CONTRIBUTIONS

All authors contributed to the article and approved the submitted version. All the authors contributed equally to this work.

ACKNOWLEDGMENTS

The authors are grateful to University of Sorocaba/UNISO for supporting the publication charges.

REFERENCES

Alisson, E. (2020).Pesquisadores investigam fatores genéticos de resistência ou suscetibilidade à COVID-19. In: *FAPESP*. Available at: https://agencia.fapesp.br/pesquisadores-investigam-fatores-geneticos-de-resistencia-ou-suscetibilidade-a-covid-19/33593/ (Accessed August 22, 2020).

Anastassopoulou, C., Gkizarioti, Z., Patrinos, G. P., and Tsakris, A. (2020). Human genetic factors associated with susceptibility to SARS-CoV-2 infection and COVID-19 disease severity. *Hum. Genomics* 14, 1–8. doi: 10.1186/s40246-020-00290-4

Andersson, M., Low, N., French, N., Greenhalgh, T., Jeffery, K., Brent, A., et al. (2020). Rapid roll out of SARS-CoV-2 antibody testing-a concern. *BMJ* 369, e m2420. doi: 10.1136/bmj.m2420

Arvin, A. M., Fink, K., Schmid, M. A., Cathcart, A., Spreafico, R., Havenar-Daughton, C., et al. (2020). Perspective on Potential Antibody-Dependent Enhancement of SARS-CoV-2. *Nature* 584, 353–363. doi: 10.1038/s41586-020-2538-8

Asselta, R., Paraboschi, E. M., Mantovani, A., and Duga, S. (2020). ACE2 and TMPRSS2 variants and expression as candidates to sex and country differences in COVID-19 severity in Italy. *Aging* 12, 10087–10098. doi: 10.18632/aging.103415

Billi, A. C., Kahlenberg, J. M., and Gudjonsson, J. E. (2019). Sex bias in autoimmunity. *Curr. Opin. Rheumatol.* 31, 53–61. doi: 10.1097/BOR.0000000000000564

Bournazos, S., and Ravetch, J. V. (2017). Anti-retroviral antibody FcγR-mediated effector functions. *Immunol. Rev.* 275, 285–295. doi: 10.1111/imr.12482

Bournazos, S., Gupta, A., and Ravetch, J. V. (2020). The role of IgG Fc receptors in antibody-dependent enhancement. *Nat. Rev. Immunol.* 20, 633–643. doi: 10.1038/s41577-020-00410-0

Brennan, M. F., and Foey, A. D. (2002). Cytokine Regulation in RA Synovial Tissue: Role of T Cell/Macrophage Contact-Dependent Interactions. *Arthritis Res.* 4, 177–182. doi: 10.1186/ar556

Brest, P., Refae, S., Mograbi, B., Hofman, P., and Milano, G. (2020). Host Polymorphisms May Impact SARS-CoV-2 Infectivity. *Trends Genet.* 36, 813–815. doi: 10.1016/j.tig.2020.08.003

Britton, T., Ball, F., and Trapman, P. (2020). A mathematical model reveals the influence of population heterogeneity on herd immunity to SARS-CoV-2. *Science* 369, 846–849. doi: 10.1126/science.abc6810

Bunyavanich, S., Do, A., and Vicencio, A. (2020). Nasal Gene Expression of Angiotensin-Converting Enzyme 2 in Children and Adults. *JAMA* 323, 2427. doi: 10.1001/jama.2020.8707

Bupp, M. R. G., and Jorgensen, T. N. (2018). Androgen-induced immunosuppression. *Front. Immunol.* 9:794. doi: 10.3389/fimmu.2018.00794

Cao, Y., Li, L., Feng, Z., Wan, S., Huang, P., Sun, X., et al. (2020). Comparative genetic analysis of the novel coronavirus, (2019-nCoV/SARS-CoV-2) receptor ACE2 in different populations. *Cell Discov.* 6, 1–4. doi: 10.1038/s41421-020-0147-1

Carter, L. J., Garner, L. V., Smoot, J. W., Li, Y., Zhou, Q., Saveson, C. J., et al. (2020). Assay Techniques and Test Development for COVID-19 Diagnosis. *ACS Cent. Sci.* 6, 591–605. doi: 10.1021/acscentsci.0c00501

Casanova, J. L., Su, H. C.the COVID Human Genetic Effort (2020). A Global Effort to Define the Human Genetics of Protective Immunity to SARS-CoV-2 Infection. *Cell* 181, 1194–1199. doi: 10.1016/2Fj.cell.2020.05.016

Catanzaro, M., Fagiani, F., Racchi, M., Corsini, E., Govoni, S., and Lanni, C. (2020). Immune response in COVID-19: addressing a pharmacological challenge by targeting pathways triggered by SARS-CoV-2. *Signal Transduct. Target. Ther.* 5, 1–10. doi: 10.1038/s41392-020-0191-1

Chua, R. L., Lukassen, S., Trump, S., Hennig, B. P., Wendisch, D., Pott, F., et al. (2020). COVID-19 severity correlates with airway epithelium–immune cell interactions identified by single-cell analysis. *Nat. Biotechnol.* 38, 970–979. doi: 10.1038/s41587-020-0602-4

Devaux, C. A., Rolain, J. M., and Raoult, D. (2020). ACE2 receptor polymorphism: Susceptibility to SARS-CoV-2, hypertension, multi-organ failure, and COVID-19 disease outcome. *J. Microbiol. Immunol. Infect.* 53, 425–435. doi: 10.1016/j.jmii.2020.04.015

Dhochak, N., Singhal, S., Kabra, S. K., and Lodha, R. (2020). Pathophysiology of COVID-19: Why Children Fare Better than Adults? *Indian J. Pediatr.* 14, 1–10. doi: 10.1007/s12098-020-03322-y

Du, Y., Tu, L., Zhu, P., Mu, M., Wang, R., Yang, P., et al. (2020). Clinical Features of 85 Fatal Cases of COVID-19 from Wuhan: A Retrospective Observational Study. *Am. J. Respir. Care Med.* 201, 1372–1379. doi: 10.1164/rccm.202003-0543OC

Elgueta, R., Benson, M. J., De Vries, V. C., Wasiuk, A., Guo, Y., and Noelle, R. J. (2009). Molecular mechanism and function of CD40/CD40L engagement in the immune system. *Immunol. Rev.* 229, 152–172. doi: 10.1111/j.1600-065X.2009.00782.x

Fink, A. L., and Klein, S. L. (2015). Sex and gender impact immune responses to vaccines among the elderly. *Physiology* 30, 408–416. doi: 10.1152/physiol.00035.2015

Fink, A. L., Engle, K., Ursin, R. L., Tang, W. Y., and Klein, S. L. (2018). Biological sex affects vaccine efficacy and protection against influenza in mice. *PNAS* 115, 12477–12482. doi: 10.1073/pnas.1805268115

Gemmati, D., Bramanti, B., Serino, M. L., Secchiero, P., Zauli, G., and Tisato, V. (2020). COVID-19 and individual genetic susceptibility/receptivity: Role of ACE1/ACE2 genes, immunity, inflammation and coagulation. might the double x-chromosome in females be protective against SARS-COV-2 compared to the single x-chromosome in males? *Int. J. Mol. Sci.* 21, 1–23. doi: 10.3390/ijms21103474

GeurtsvanKessel, C. H., Okba, N. M. A., Igloi, Z., Bogers, S., Embregts, C. W. E., Laksono, B. M., et al. (2020). An evaluation of COVID-19 serological assays informs future diagnostics and exposure assessment. *Nat. Commun.* 11, e3436. doi: 10.1038/s41467-020-17317-y

Ghafouri-Fard, S., Noroozi, R., Vafaee, R., Branicki, W., Pospiech, E., Pyrc, K., et al. (2020). Effects of host genetic variations on response to, susceptibility and severity of respiratory infections. *Biomed. Pharmacother.* 128:110296. doi: 10.1016/j.biopha.2020.110296

Gheblawi, M., Wang, K., Viveiros, A., Nguyen, Q., Zhong, J. C., Turner, A. J., et al. (2020). Angiotensin-Converting Enzyme 2: SARS-CoV-2 Receptor and Regulator of the Renin-Angiotensin System: Celebrating the 20th Anniversary of the Discovery of ACE2. *Circ. Res.* 126, 1456–1474. doi: 10.1161/CIRCRESAHA.120.317015

Giamarellos-Bourboulis, E. J., Netea, M. G., Rovina, N., Akinosoglou, K., Antoniadou, A., Antonakos, N., et al. (2020). Complex Immune Dysregulation in COVID-19 Patients with Severe Respiratory Failure. *Cell Host Microbe* 27, 992–1000. doi: 10.1016/j.chom.2020.04.009

Gkogkou, E., Barnasas, G., Vougas, K., and Trougakos, I. P. (2020). Expression profiling meta-analysis of ACE2 and TMPRSS2, the putative anti-inflammatory receptor and priming protease of SARS-CoV-2 in human cells, and identification of putative modulators. *Redox Biol.* 36, e101615. doi: 10.1016/j.redox.2020.101615

Göker, H., Aladağ-Karakulak, E., Demiroğlu, H., Ayaz, C. M., Büyükaşik, Y., İnkaya, A. C., et al. (2020). The effects of blood group types on the risk of COVID-19 infection and its clinical outcome. *Turk. J. Med. Sci.* 50, 679–683. doi: 10.3906/sag-2005-395

Gómez, J., Albaiceta, G. M., García-Clemente, M., López-Larrea, C., Amado-Rodríguez, L., Lopez-Alonso, I., et al. (2020). Angiotensin-converting enzymes (ACE, ACE2) gene variants and COVID-19 outcome. *Gene* 762, 145102. doi: 10.1016/j.gene.2020.145102

Gottipati, S., Rao, N. L., and Fung-Leung, W. P. (2008). IRAK1: A critical signaling mediator of innate immunity. *Cell. Signal.* 20, 269–276. doi: 10.1016/j.cellsig.2007.08.009

Gou, W., Fu, Y., Yue, L., Chen, G., Cai, X., Shuai, M., et al. (2020). Gut microbiota may underlie the predisposition of healthy individuals to COVID-19. *medRxiv*. doi: 10.21203/rs.3.rs-45991/v1

Grifoni, A., Weiskopf, D., Ramirez, S. I., Mateus, J., Dan, J. M., Moderbacher, C. R., et al. (2020). Targets of T Cell Responses to SARS-CoV-2 Coronavirus in Humans with COVID-19 Disease and Unexposed Individuals. *Cell* 181, 1489–1501. doi: 10.1016/j.cell.2020.05.015

Guillon, P., Clément, M., Sébille, V., Rivain, J. G., Chou, C. F., Ruvoën-Clouet, N., et al. (2008). Inhibition of the interaction between the SARS-CoV Spike protein and its cellular receptor by anti-histo-blood group antibodies. *Glycobiology* 18, 1085–1093. doi: 10.1093/glycob/cwn093

Hachim, A., Kavian, N., Cohen, C. A., Chin, A. W. H., Chu, D. K. W., Mok, C. K. P., et al. (2020). ORF8 and ORF3b antibodies are accurate serological markers of early and late SARS-CoV-2 infection. *Nat. Immunol.* 21, 1293–1301. doi: 10.1038/s41590-020-0773-7

Hamming, I., Timens, W., Bulthuis, M. L. C., Lely, A. T., Navis, G. J., and Van Goor, H. (2004). Tissue Distribution of ACE2 Protein, the Functional Receptor for SARS Coronavirus. A First Step in Understanding SARS Pathogenesis. *J. Pathol.* 203, 631–637. doi: 10.1002/path.1570

Hargreaves, C. E., Rose-Zerilli, M. J., Machado, L. R., Iriyama, C., Hollox, E. J., Cragg, M. S., et al. (2015). Fcgamma receptors: genetic variation, function, and disease. *Immunol. Rev.* 2015) 268, 6–24. doi: 10.1111/imr.12341

Hirano, T., and Murakami, M. (2020). COVID-19: A New Virus, but a Familiar Receptor and Cytokine Release Syndrome. *Immunity* 52, 731–733. doi: 10.1016/j.immuni.2020.04.003

Hoffmann, M., Kleine-Weber, H., Schroeder, S., Krüger, N., Herrler, T., Erichsen, S., et al. (2020). SARS-CoV-2 Cell Entry Depends on ACE2 and TMPRSS2 and Is Blocked by a Clinically Proven Protease Inhibitor. *Cell* 181, 271–280. doi: 10.1016/j.cell.2020.02.052

Hou, Y., Zhao, J., Martin, W., Kallianpur, A., Chung, M. K., Jehi, L., et al. (2020). New insights into genetic susceptibility of COVID-19: An ACE2 and TMPRSS2 polymorphism analysis. *BMC Med.* 18, 216. doi: 10.1186/s12916-020-01673-z

Huang, C., Wang, Y., Li, X., Ren, L., Zhao, J., Hu, Y., et al. (2020). Clinical Features of Patients Infected with 2019 Novel Coronavirus in Wuhan, China. *Lancet* 395, 497–506. doi: 10.1016/S0140-6736(20)30183-5

Hunter, C. A., and Jones, S. A. (2015). IL-6 as a Keystone Cytokine in Health and Disease. *Nat. Immunol.* 16, 448–457. doi: 10.1038/ni.3153

Hussain, M., Jabeen, N., Raza, F., Shabbir, S., Baig, A. A., Amanullah, A., et al. (2020). Structural variations in human ACE2 may influence its binding with SARS-CoV-2 spike protein. *J. Med. Virol.* 92, 1580–1586. doi: 10.1002/jmv.25832

Jaillon, S., Berthenet, K., and Garlanda, C. (2019). Sexual Dimorphism in Innate Immunity. *Clin. Rev. Allergy Immunol.* 56, 308–321. doi: 10.1007/s12016-017-8648-x

Jin, J. M., Bai, P., He, W., Wu, F., Liu, X. F., Han, D. M., et al. (2020). Gender Differences in Patients With COVID-19: Focus on Severity and Mortality. *Front. Public Heal.* 8:152. doi: 10.3389/fpubh.2020.00152

Kissick, H. T., Sanda, M. G., Dunn, L. K., Pellegrini, K. L., On, S. T., Noel, J. K., et al. (2014). Androgens alter T-cell immunity by inhibiting T-helper 1 differentiation. *PNAS* 111, 9887–9892. doi: 10.1073/pnas.1402468111

Klein, S. L., and Flanagan, K. L. (2016). Sex differences in immune responses. *Nat. Rev. Immunol.* 16, 626–638. doi: 10.1038/nri.2016.90

Klein, S. L., and Pekosz, A. (2014). Sex-based biology and the rational design of influenza vaccination strategies. *J. Infect. Dis.* 209, 114–119. doi: 10.1093/infdis/jiu066

Klein, A. (2012). Slipping Racism into the Mainstream: A Theory of Information Laundering. *Commun. Theory* 22, 427–448. doi: 10.1111/j.1468-2885.2012.01415.x

Kuo, C. L., Pilling, L. C., Atkins, J. L., Masoli, J. A. H., Delgado, J., Kuchel, G. A., et al. (2020). APOE e4 genotype predicts severe COVID-19 in the UK biobank community cohort. *J. Gerontol. A Biol. Sci. Med. Sci.* 75, 2231–2232. doi: 10.1093/gerona/glaa131

Lai, J. J., Lai, K. P., Zeng, W., Chuang, K. H., Altuwaijri, S., and Chang, C. (2012). Androgen receptor influences on body defense system via modulation of innate and adaptive immune systems: Lessons from conditional AR knockout mice. *Am. J. Pathol.* 181, 1504–1512. doi: 10.1016/j.ajpath.2012.07.008

Lambert, N. C. (2019). Nonendocrine mechanisms of sex bias in rheumatic diseases. *Nat. Rev. Rheumatol.* 15, 673–686. doi: 10.1038/s41584-019-0307-6

Latini, A., Agolini, E., Novelli, A., Borgiani, P., Giannini, R., Gravina, P., et al. (2020). COVID-19 and Genetic Variants of Protein Involved in the SARS-CoV-2 Entry into the Host Cells. *Genes* 11, 1–8. doi: 10.3390/genes11091010

Le Bert, N., Tan, A. T., Kunasegaran, K., Tham, C. Y. L., Hafezi, M., and Chia, A. (2020). SARS-CoV-2-Specific T Cell Immunity in Cases of COVID-19 and SARS, and Uninfected Controls. *Nature* 584, 457–462. doi: 10.1038/s41586-020-2550-z

Lee, W. S., Wheatley, A. K., Kent, S. J., and Dekosky, B. J. (2020). Antibody-dependent enhancement and SARS-CoV-2 vaccines and therapies. *Nat. Microbiol.* 5, 1185–1191. doi: 10.1038/s41564-020-00789-5

Li, Y., Cui, L. L., Li, Q. Q., Ma, G. D., Cai, Y. J., Chen, Y. Y., et al. (2014). Association between ADAM17 promoter polymorphisms and ischemic stroke in a Chinese population. *J. Atheroscler. Thromb.* 21, 878–893. doi: 10.5551/jat.22400

Li, M. Y., Li, L., Zhang, Y., and Wang, X. S. (2020a). Expression of the SARS-CoV-2 Cell Receptor Gene ACE2 in a Wide Variety of Human Tissues. *Infect. Dis. Poverty.* 9, 1–7. doi: 10.1186/s40249-020-00662-x

Li, Y., Jerkic, M., Slutsky, A. S., and Zhang, H. (2020b). Molecular mechanisms of sex bias differences in COVID-19 mortality. *Crit. Care* 24, 405. doi: 10.1186/s13054-020-03118-8

Li, Y., Zhang, Z., Yang, L., Lian, X., Xie, Y., Li, S., et al. (2020c). The MERS-CoV Receptor DPP4 as a Candidate Binding Target of the SARS-CoV-2 Spike. *iScience* 23, 1–8. doi: 10.1016/j.isci.2020.101160

Libert, C., Dejager, L., and Pinheiro, I. (2010). The X chromosome in immune functions: When a chromosome makes the difference. *Nat. Rev. Immunol.* 10, 594–604. doi: 10.1038/nri2815

Lin, M., Tseng, H. K., Trejaut, J. A., Lee, H. L., Loo, J. H., Chu, C. C., et al. (2003). Association of HLA class I with severe acute respiratory syndrome coronavirus infection. *BMC Med. Genet.* 4, 1–7. doi: 10.1186/1471-2350-4-9

Liu, M. Y., Zheng, B., Zhang, Y., and Li, J. P. (2020). Role and mechanism of angiotensin-converting enzyme 2 in acute lung injury in coronavirus disease 2019. *Chronic Dis. Transl. Med.* 6, 98–105. doi: 10.1016/j.cdtm.2020.05.003

Long, Q. X., Tang, X. J., Shi, Q. L., Li, Q., Deng, H. J., YUAN, J., et al. (2020). Clinical and Immunological Assessment of Asymptomatic SARS-CoV-2 Infections. *Nat. Med.* 26, 1200–1204. doi: 10.1038/s41591-020-0965-6

Lu, R., Zhao, X., Li, J., Niu, P., Yang, B., Wu, H., et al. (2020a). Genomic Characterisation and Epidemiology of 2019 Novel Coronavirus: Implications for Virus Origins and Receptor Binding. *Lancet* 395, 565–574. doi: 10.1016/S0140-6736(20)30251-8

Lu, L., Zhang, H., Zhan, M., Jiang, J., Yin, H., Dauphars, D. J., et al. (2020b). Preventing Mortality in COVID-19 Patients: Which Cytokine to Target in a Raging Storm? *Front. Cell Dev. Biol.* 8:677. doi: 10.3389/fcell.2020.00677

Luo, Y., Liu, C., Guan, T., Li, Y., Lai, Y., Li, F., et al. (2019). Association of ACE2 genetic polymorphisms with hypertension-related target organ damages in south Xinjiang. *Hypertens. Res.* 42, 681–689. doi: 10.1038/s41440-018-0166-6

Mahallawi, W. H., Khabour, O. F., Zhang, Q., Makhdoum, H. M., and Suliman, B. A. (2018). MERS-CoV Infection in Humans Is Associated with a pro-Inflammatory Th1 and Th17 Cytokine Profile. *Cytokine* 104, 8–13. doi: 10.1016/j.cyto.2018.01.025

Mahmoudabadi, G., and Phillips, R. (2018). A Comprehensive and Quantitative Exploration of Thousands of Viral Genomes. *ELife* 7, 1–16. doi: 10.7554/eLife.31955

Mahmudpour, M., Roozbeh, J., Keshavarz, M., Farrokhi, S., and Nabipour, I. (2020). COVID-19 Cytokine Storm: The Anger of Inflammation. *Cytokine* 133, e155151. doi: 10.1016/j.cyto.2020.155151

Malard, L., Kakinami, L., O'Loughlin, J., Roy-Gagnon, M. H., Labbe, A., Pilote, L., et al. (2013). The association between the angiotensin-converting enzyme-2 gene and blood pressure in a cohort study of adolescents. *BMC Med. Genet.* 14, e117. doi: 10.1186/1471-2350-14-117

Mangalmurti, N., and Hunter, C. A. (2020). Cytokine Storms: Understanding COVID-19. *Immunity.* 53, 19–25. doi: 10.1016/j.immuni.2020.06.017

Mauvais-Jarvis, F., Bairey Merz, N., Barnes, P. J., Brinton, R. D., Carrero, J. J., DeMeo, D. L., et al. (2020). Sex and gender: modifiers of health, disease, and medicine. *Lancet* 396, 565–582. doi: 10.1016/S0140-6736(20)31561-0

Mehta, P., McAuley, D., Brown, M., Sanchez, E., Tattersall, R. S., and Manson, J. J. (2020). COVID-19: Consider Cytokine Storm Syndromes and Immunosuppression. *Lancet* 395, 1033–1034. doi: 10.1016/S0140-6736(20)30628-0

Meier, A., Chang, J. J., Chan, E. S., Pollard, R. B., Sidhu, H. K., Kulkarni, S., et al. (2009). Sex differences in the Toll-like receptor-mediated response of plasmacytoid dendritic cells to HIV-1. *Nat. Med.* 15, 955–959. doi: 10.1038/nm.2004

Mercer, F., and Unutmaz, D. (2009). The biology of FoxP3: AKey player in immune suppression during infections, autoimmune diseases and cancer. *Adv. Exp. Med. Biol.* 665, 47–59. doi: 10.1007/978-1-4419-1599-3_4

Mönkemüller, K., Fry, L. C., and Rickes, S. (2020). Covid-19, Coronavirus, SARS-CoV-2 and the small bowel. *Rev. Esp. Enferm. Dig.* 112, 383–388. doi: 10.17235/reed.2020.7137/2019

Moore, J. B., and June, C. H. (2020). Cytokine Release Syndrome in Severe COVID-19. *Science* 368, 473–474. doi: 10.1126/science.abb8925

Muecksch, F., Wise, H., Batchelor, B., Squires, M., Semple, E., Richardson, C., et al. (2020). Longitudinal Analysis of Clinical Serology Assay Performance and Neutralising Antibody Levels in COVID19 Convalescents. *J. Infect. Dis.* 223, 389–398. doi: 10.1093/infdis/jiaa659

Nguyen, A., David, J. K., Maden, S. K., Wood, M. A., Weeder, B. R., Nellore, A., et al. (2020). Human Leukocyte Antigen Susceptibility Map for Severe Acute Respiratory Syndrome Coronavirus 2. *J. Virol.* 94, 1–12. doi: 10.1128/JVI.00510-20

Olsen, N. J., and Kovacs, W. J. (2001). Effects of androgens on T and B lymphocyte development. *Immunol. Res.* 23, 281–288. doi: 10.1385/IR:23:2-3:281

Ortiz-Fernández, L., and Sawalha, A. H. (2020). Genetic variability in the expression of the SARS-CoV-2 host cell entry factors across populations. *Genes Immun.* 21, 269–272. doi: 10.1038/s41435-020-0107-7

Parham, P., and Moffett, A. (2013). Variable NK cell receptors and their MHC class i ligands in immunity, reproduction and human evolution. *Nat. Rev. Immunol.* 13, 133–144. doi: 10.1038/nri3370

Pati, A., Mahto, H., Padhi, S., and Panda, A. K. (2020). ACE deletion allele is associated with susceptibility to SARS-CoV-2 infection and mortality rate: An epidemiological study in the Asian population. *Clin. Chim. Acta* 510, 455–458. doi: 10.1016/j.cca.2020.08.008

Patnaik, M., Pati, P., Swain, S. N., Mohapatra, M. K., Dwibedi, B., Kar, S. K., et al. (2014). Association of angiotensin-converting enzyme and angiotensin-converting enzyme-2 gene polymorphisms with essential hypertension in the population of Odisha, India. *Ann. Hum. Biol.* 41, 145–152. doi: 10.3109/03014460.2013.837195

Pessach, I. M., and Notarangelo, L. D. (2009). X-linked primary immunodeficiencies as a bridge to better understandingX-chromosome related autoimmunity. *J. Autoimmun.* 33, 17–24. doi: 10.1016/j.jaut.2009.03.003

Pinheiro, D. S., Santos, R. S., Veiga Jardim, P. C. B., Silva, E. G., Reis, A. A. S., Pedrino, G. R., et al. (2019). The combination of ACE I/D and ACE2 G8790A polymorphisms revels susceptibility to hypertension: A genetic association study in Brazilian patients. *PloS One* 14, e0221248. doi: 10.1371/journal.pone.0221248

Pollán, M., Pérez-Gómez, B., Pastor-Barriuso, R., Oteo, J., Hernán, M. A., Pérez-Olmeda, M., et al. (2020). Prevalence of SARS-CoV-2 in Spain (ENE-COVID): A Nationwide, Population-Based Seroepidemiological Study. *Lancet* 396, 535,544. doi: 10.1016/S0140-6736(20)31483-5

Qin, C., Zhou, L., Hu, Z., Zhang, S., Yang, S., Tao, Y., et al. (2020). Dysregulation of Immune Response in Patients with COVID-19 in Wuhan, China. *Clin. Infect. Dis.* 71, 762–768. doi: 10.1093/cid/ciaa248

Radzikowska, U., Ding, M., Tan, G., Zhakparov, D., Peng, Y., Wawrzyniak, P., et al. (2020). Distribution of ACE2, CD147, CD26, and other SARS-CoV-2 associated molecules in tissues and immune cells in health and in asthma, COPD, obesity, hypertension, and COVID-19 risk factors. *Allergy* 75, 2829–2845. doi: 10.1111/all.14429

Rainville, J. R., Tsyglakova, M., and Hodes, G. E. (2018). Deciphering sex differences in the immune system and depression. *Front. Neuroendocrinol.* 50, 67–90. doi: 10.1016/j.yfrne.2017.12.004

Ren, L. L., Wang, Y. M., Wu, Z. Q., Xiang, Z. C., Guo, L., Xu, T., et al. (2020). Identification of a Novel Coronavirus Causing Severe Pneumonia in Human: A Descriptive Study. *Chin. Med. J.* 133, 1015–1024. doi: 10.1097/CM9.0000000000000722

Risitano, A. M., Mastellos, D. C., Huber-Lang, M., Yancopoulou, D., Garlanda, C., Ciceri, F., et al. (2020). Complement as a Target in COVID-19? *Nat. Rev. Immunol.* 20, 342–344. doi: 10.1038/s41577-020-0320-7

Rosado, J., Pelleau, S., Cockram, C., Merkling, S. H., Nekkab, N., Demeret, C., et al. (2020). Multiplex assays for the identification of serological signatures of SARS-CoV-2 infection: an antibody-based diagnostic and machine learning study. *Lancet Microbe.* 2, e60–e69. doi: 10.1016/S2666-5247(20)30197-X

Roshanravan, N., Ghaffari, S., and Hedayati, M. (2020). Angiotensin Converting Enzyme-2 as Therapeutic Target in COVID-19. *Diabetes Metab. Syndr.* 14, 637–639. doi: 10.1016/j.dsx.2020.05.022

Roy, S., Mazumder, T., and Banik, S. (2020). The Association of Cardiovascular Diseases and Diabetes Mellitus with COVID-19 (SARS-CoV-2) and Their Possible Mechanisms. *SN Compr. Clin. Med.* 2, 1077–1082. doi: 10.1007/s42399-020-00376-z

Saponaro, F., Rutigliano, G., Sestito, S., Bandini, L., Storti, B., Bizzarri, R., et al. (2020). ACE2 in the Era of SARS-CoV-2: Controversies and Novel Perspectives. *Front. Mol. Biosci.* 7:588618. doi: 10.3389/fmolb.2020.588618

Scheller, J., and Rose-John, S. (2006). Interleukin-6 and Its Receptor: From Bench to Bedside. *Med. Microbiol. Immunol.* 195, 173–183. doi: 10.1007/s00430-006-0019-9

Schurz, H., Salie, M., Tromp, G., Hoal, E. G., Kinnear, C. J., and Möller, M. (2019). The X chromosome and sex-specific effects in infectious disease susceptibility. *Hum. Genomics* 13, 1–12. doi: 10.1186/s40246-018-0185-z

Scully, E. P., Haverfield, J., Ursin, R. L., Tannenbaum, C., and Klein, S. L. (2020). Considering how biological sex impacts immune responses and COVID-19 outcomes. *Nat. Rev. Immunol.* 20, 442–447. doi: 10.1038/s41577-020-0348-8

Sen, R., Garbati, M. R., Bryant, K., and Lu, Y. (2021). Epigenetic Mechanisms Influencing COVID-19. *Genome*, 1–38. doi: 10.1139/gen-2020-0135

Seow, J., Graham, C., Merrick, B., Acors, S., Pickering, S., Steel, K. J. A., et al. (2020). Longitudinal Evaluation and Decline of Antibody Responses in SARS-CoV-2 Infection. *Nat. Microbiol.* 5, 1598–1607. doi: 10.1038/s41564-020-00813-8

South, A. M., Tomlinson, T., Edmonston, D., Hiremath, S., and Sparks, M. A. (2020). Controversies of Renin–Angiotensin System Inhibition during the COVID-19 Pandemic. *Nat. Rev. Nephrol.* 16, 305–307. doi: 10.1038/s41581-020-0279-4

Souyris, M., Cenac, C., Azar, P., Daviaud, D., Canivet, A., Grunenwald, S., et al. (2018). TLR7 escapes X chromosome inactivation in immune cells. *Sci. Immunol.* 3, eaap8855. doi: 10.1126/sciimmunol.aap8855

Sperry, J. L., Zolin, S., Zuckerbraun, B. S., Vodovotz, Y., Namas, R., Neal, M. D., et al. (2014). X chromosome-linked IRAK-1 polymorphism is a strong predictor of multiple organ failure and mortality postinjury. *Ann. Surg.* 260, 698–705. doi: 10.1097/2FSLA.0000000000000918

Spolarics, Z., Peña, G., Qin, Y., Donnelly, R. J., and Livingston, D. H. (2017). Inherent X-linked genetic variability and cellular mosaicism unique to females contribute to sex-related differences in the innate immune response. *Front. Immunol.* 8:1455. doi: 10.3389/fimmu.2017.01455

Stokes, E. K., Zambrano, L. D., Anderson, K. N., Marder, E. P., Raz, K. M., El Burai Felix, S., et al. (2020). Coronavirus Disease 2019 Case Surveillance — United States, January 22–May 30, 2020. *MMWR* 69, 759–765. doi: 10.15585/mmwr.mm6924e2

Sun, D., Zhang, D., Tian, R., Li, Y., Wang, Y., Cao, J., et al. (2020). The Underlying Changes and Predicting Role of Peripheral Blood Inflammatory Cells in Severe COVID-19 Patients: A Sentinel? *Clin. Chim. Acta* 508, 122–129. doi: 10.1016/j.cca.2020.05.027

Tan, M., Liu, Y., Zhou, R., Deng, X., Li, F., Liang, K., et al. (2020a). Immunopathological Characteristics of Coronavirus Disease 2019 Cases in Guangzhou, China. *Immunology* 160, 261–268. doi: 10.1101/2020.03.12.20034736

Tan, W., Lu, Y., Zhang, J., Wang, J., Dan, Y., Tan, Z., et al. (2020b). Viral Kinetics and Antibody Responses in Patients with COVID-19. *MedRxiv.* doi: 10.1101/2020.03.24.20042382

Taylor, A., Foo, S. S., Bruzzone, R., Dinh, L. V., King, N. J. C., and Mahalingam, S. (2015). Fc Receptors in Antibody-Dependent Enhancement of Viral Infections. *Immunol. Rev.* 268, 340–364. doi: 10.1111/imr.12367

The Severe Covid-19 GWAS Group (2020). Genomewide Association Study of Severe Covid-19 with Respiratory Failure. *N. Engl. J. Med.* 383, 1522–1534. doi: 10.1056/NEJMoa2020283

Tisoncik, J. R., Korth, M. J., Simmons, C. P., Farrar, J., Martin, T. R., and Katze, M. G. (2012). Into the Eye of the Cytokine Storm. *Microbiol. Mol. Biol. Rev.* 76, 16–32. doi: 10.1128/mmbr.05015-11

Tolouian, R., Vahed, S. Z., Ghiyasvand, S., Tolouian, A., and Ardalan, M. (2020). COVID-19 Interactions with Angiotensin-Converting Enzyme 2 (ACE2) and the Kinin System; Looking at a Potential Treatment. *J. Renal Inj. Prev.* 9, e19. doi: 10.34172/jrip.2020.19

Torcia, M. G., Nencioni, L., Clemente, A. M., Civitelli, L., Celestino, I., Limongi, D., et al. (2012). Sex Differences in the Response to Viral Infections: TLR8 and TLR9 Ligand Stimulation Induce Higher IL10 Production in Males. *PloS One* 7, e39853. doi: 10.1371/journal.pone.0039853

Ulhaq, Z. S., and Soraya, G. V. (2020). Interleukin-6 Is a Potential Biomarker of COVID-19 Progression: Evidence from a Meta-Analysis. *Med. Mal. Infect.* 50, 381–383. doi: 10.2139/ssrn.3562887

Valencia, I., Peiró, C., Lorenzo, O., Sánchez-Ferrer, C. F., Eckel, J., and Romacho, T. (2020). DPP4 and ACE2 in Diabetes and COVID-19: Therapeutic Targets for Cardiovascular Complications? *Front. Pharmacol.* 11. doi: 10.3389/2Ffphar.2020.01161

van der Made, C. I., Simons, A., Schuurs-Hoeijmakers, J., Van Den Heuvel, G., Mantere, T., Kersten, S., et al. (2020). Presence of Genetic Variants among Young Men with Severe COVID-19. *JAMA* 324, 663–673. doi: 10.1001/jama.2020.13719

Vargas-Alarcón, G., Posadas-Sánchez, R., and Ramírez-Bello, J. (2020). Variability in genes related to SARS-CoV-2 entry into host cells (ACE2, TMPRSS2, TMPRSS11A, ELANE, and CTSL) and its potential use in association studies. *Life Sci.* 260:118313. doi: 10.1016/j.lfs.2020.118313

Verdecchia, P., Cavallini, C., Spanevello, A., and Angeli, F. (2020). The Pivotal Link between ACE2 Deficiency and SARS-CoV-2 Infection. *Eur. J. Intern. Med.* 76, 14–20. doi: 10.1016/j.ejim.2020.04.037

ViralZone (2020). Coronaviridae. Available at: https://viralzone.expasy.org/30 (Accessed January 30, 2021).

Vodnar, D. C., Mitrea, L., Teleky, B. E., Szabo, K., Călinoiu, L. F., Nemeş, S. A., et al. (2020). Coronavirus Disease (COVID-19) Caused by (SARS-CoV-2) Infections: A Real Challenge for Human Gut Microbiota. *Front. Cell. Infect. Microbiol.* 10:575559. doi: 10.3389/fcimb.2020.575559

vom Steeg, L. G., and Klein, S. L. (2016). SeXX Matters in Infectious Disease Pathogenesis. *PLoS Pathog.* 12, e1005374. doi: 10.1371/journal.ppat.1005374

Wang, Q., Zhang, Y., Wu, L., Niu, S., Song, C., Zhang, Z., et al. (2020a). Structural and Functional Basis of SARS-CoV-2 Entry by Using Human ACE2. *Cell* 181, 894–904. doi: 10.1016/j.cell.2020.03.045

Wang, X., Lam, J. Y., Wong, W. M., Yuen, C. K., Cai, J. P., Wing-Ngor Au, S., et al. (2020b). Accurate diagnosis of covid-19 by a novel immunogenic secreted sars-cov-2 orf8 protein. *mBio* 11, e02431–e02420. doi: 10.1128/mBio.02431-20

Wang, F., Huang, S., Gao, R., Zhou, Y., Lai, C., Li, Z., et al. (2020c). Initial whole-genome sequencing and analysis of the host genetic contribution to COVID-19 severity and susceptibility. *Cell Discov.* 6, 83. doi: 10.1038/s41421-020-00231-4

WHO (2020). Situation report - 1: Novel Coronavirus, (2019-nCoV).

WHO (2021). WHO Coronavirus Disease (COVID-19) Dashboard. https://covid19.who.int/.

Wong, C. K., Lam, C. W. K. A., Wu, A. K. L., Ip, W. K., Lee, N. L. S., Chan, I. H. S., et al. (2004). Plasma Inflammatory Cytokines and Chemokines in Severe Acute Respiratory Syndrome. *Clin. Exp. Immunol.* 136, 95–103. doi: 10.1111/j.1365-2249.2004.02415.x

Wong, S. H., Lui, R. N. S., and Sung, J. J. Y. (2020). Covid-19 and the digestive system. *J. Gastroenterol. Hepatol.* 35, 744–748. doi: 10.1111/jgh.15047

Wrapp, D., Wang, N., Corbett, K. S., Goldsmith, J. A., Hsieh, C. L., Abiona, O., et al. (2020). Cryo-EM Structure of the 2019-NCoV Spike in the Prefusion Conformation. *Science* 367, 1260–1263. doi: 10.1101/2020.02.11.944462

Xu, H., Zhong, L., Deng, J., Peng, J., Dan, H., Zeng, X., et al. (2020). High Expression of ACE2 Receptor of 2019-NCoV on the Epithelial Cells of Oral Mucosa. *Int. J. Oral. Sci.* 12, 1–5. doi: 10.1038/s41368-020-0074-x

Yan, R., Zhang, Y., Li, Y., Xia, L., Guo, Y., and Zhou, Q. (2020). Structural Basis for the Recognition of SARS-CoV-2 by Full-Length Human ACE2. *Science* 367, 1444–1448. doi: 10.1126/science.abb2762

Yi, C., Sun, X., Ye, J., Deng, L., Liu, M., Yang, Z., et al. (2020). Key residues of the receptor binding motif in the spike protein of SARS-CoV-2 that interact with ACE2 and neutralizing antibodies. *Cell Mol. Immunol.* 17, 621–630. doi: 10.1038/s41423-020-0458-z

Zeberg, H., and Pääbo, S. (2020). The major genetic risk factor for severe COVID-19 is inherited from Neandertals Authors. *Nature* 587, 610–612. doi: 10.1101/2020.07.03.186296

Zhang, B., Zhou, X., Qiu, Y., Song, Y., Feng, F., Feng, J., et al. (2020a). Clinical Characteristics of 82 Death Cases with COVID-19. *PLoS One* 15, e0235458. doi: 10.1371/journal.pone.0235458

Zhang, H., Kang, Z., Gong, H., Xu, D., Wang, J., Li, Z., et al. (2020b). Digestive system is a potential route of COVID-19: an analysis of single-cell coexpression pattern of key proteins in viral entry process. *Gut* 69, 1010–1018. doi: 10.1136/gutjnl-2020-320953

Zhang, Q., Bastard, P., Liu, Z., Le Pen, J., Moncada-Velez, M., Chen, J., et al. (2020c). Inborn errors of type I IFN immunity in patients with life-threatening COVID19. *Science* 370, eabd4570. doi: 10.1126/science.abd4570

Zhao, Y., Zhao, Z., Wang, Y., Zhou, Y., Ma, Y., and Zuo, W. (2020). Single-Cell RNA Expression Profiling of ACE2, the Receptor of SARS-CoV-2. *Am. J. Respir. Crit. Care Med.* 202, 756–759. doi: 10.1164/rccm.202001-0179LE

Zheng, J. (2020). SARS-CoV-2: An Emerging Coronavirus That Causes a Global Threat. *Int. J. Biol. Sci.* 16, 1678–1685. doi: 10.7150/ijbs.45053

Zhou, X., Yu, S., Zhao, D. M., Harty, J. T., Badovinac, V. P., and Xue, H. H. (2010). Differentiation and Persistence of Memory CD8+ T Cells Depend on T Cell Factor 1. *Immunity* 33, 229–240. doi: 10.1016/j.immuni.2010.08.002

Zhou, P., Yang, X. L., Wang, X. G., Hu, B., Zhang, L., Zhang, W., et al. (2020). A Pneumonia Outbreak Associated with a New Coronavirus of Probable Bat Origin. *Nature* 579, 270–273. doi: 10.1038/s41586-020-2012-7

Ziegler, C. G. K., Allon, S. J., Nyquist, S. K., Mbano, I. M., Miao, V. N., Tzouanas, C. N., et al. (2020). SARS-CoV-2 Receptor ACE2 Is an Interferon-Stimulated Gene in Human Airway Epithelial Cells and Is Detected in Specific Cell Subsets across Tissues. *Cell* 181, 1016–1035. doi: 10.1016/2Fj.cell.2020.04.035

Zietz, M., Zucker, J., and Tatonetti, N. (2020). Associations between blood type and COVID-19 infection, intubation, and death. *Nat Comm.* 11, 1–6.

2

Is the "Common Cold" Our Greatest Ally in the Battle Against SARS-CoV-2?

Manu N. Capoor[1,2], Fahad S. Ahmed[3], Andrew McDowell[4] and Ondrej Slaby[5,6]*

[1] Laboratory of Bacterial Pathogenesis and Immunology, Rockefeller University, New York, NY, United States, [2] Executive Office, MMF Systems, Inc., New York, NY, United States, [3] Data Science and Engineering, MyMedicalFiles (MMF) Systems, Inc., New York, NY, United States, [4] Nutrition Innovation Centre for Food and Health (NICHE), School of Biomedical Sciences, Ulster University, Coleraine, United Kingdom, [5] Central European Institute of Technology (CEITEC), Masaryk University, Brno, Czechia, [6] Department of Biology, Faculty of Medicine, Masaryk University, Brno, Czechia

Correspondence:
Manu N. Capoor
mcapoor@mail.rockefeller.edu

The discovery of T-cell responses to SARS-CoV-2 in non-infected individuals indicates cross-reactive immune memory from prior exposure to human coronaviruses (HCoV) that cause the common cold. This raises the possibility that "immunity" could exist within populations at rates that may be higher than serology studies estimate. Besides specialized research labs, however, there is limited ability to measure HCoV CD4+ and CD8+ T-cell responses to SARS-CoV-2 infection, which currently impedes interpretation of any potential correlation between COVID-19 disease pathogenesis and the calibration of pandemic control measures. Given this limited testing ability, an alternative approach would be to exploit the large cohort of currently available data from which statistically significant associations may be generated. This would necessitate the merging of several public databases including patient and contact tracing, which could be created by relevant public health organizations. Including data from both symptomatic and asymptomatic patients in SARS-CoV-2 databases and surveillance systems could provide the necessary information to allow for more informed decisions.

Keywords: SARS-CoV-2, COVID-19, T-cell, human coronaviruses, immunity, contact tracing, children

INTRODUCTION—ASYMPTOMATIC INFECTION IN DENSE POPULATIONS

It is most curious that the majority of poor, highly populated countries have seen fewer deaths per million during the current pandemic than most advanced Western nations. In contrast, during the 1918 influenza pandemic, which had a global death rate approaching 3%, less-developed countries saw noticeably higher rates (Spreeuwenberg et al., 2018). The large variation in SARS-CoV-2 deaths per million people between countries, and even states and counties within the U.S., are on the surface confusing and difficult to explain. It seems counterintuitive that countries with both limited health resources and sick, aging populations have reported far fewer mortalities due to SARS-CoV-2 than countries with advanced healthcare resources, relatively healthy populations and greater lock-down measures (Worldometer; Contributors W; Engineering JHUCfSSa, 2020) (**Table 1**).

TABLE 1 | Covid-19 Deaths/Million – 40 most populous countries and United States counties.

Country/ Territory	Populace July '20	Rank	% World July '20	Covid-19 Deaths Nov. '20	Deaths/ Million	Rank	USA County	State	Populace July 2018	Rank	% US Populace July '18	Covid-19 Deaths Nov. '20	Deaths/ Million	Rank
Spain	46,754,778	30	0.6%	43,131	922.5	1	Bronx	NY	1,432,132	28	0.4%	5,033	3514.3	1
Italy	60,461,826	23	0.8%	50,453	834.5	2	Queens	NY	2,278,906	11	0.7%	7,338	3220.0	2
UK	67,886,011	21	0.9%	55,327	815.0	3	Kings	NY	2,582,830	9	0.8%	7,481	2896.4	3
Argentina	45,741,007	31	0.6%	37,002	808.9	4	New York	NY	1,628,701	21	0.5%	3,219	1976.4	4
Brazil	212,559,417	6	2.7%	169,183	795.9	5	Wayne	MI	1,753,893	19	0.5%	3,154	1798.3	5
Mexico	128,932,753	10	1.7%	101,676	788.6	6	Nassau	NY	1,358,343	29	0.4%	2,240	1649.1	6
USA	331,002,651	3	4.2%	257,072	776.6	7	Middlesex	MA	1,614,714	22	0.5%	2,385	1477.0	7
France	65,273,511	22	0.8%	49,307	755.4	8	Suffolk	NY	1,481,093	26	0.5%	2,032	1372.0	8
Colombia	50,882,891	29	0.7%	35,287	693.5	9	Miami-Dade	FL	2,761,581	7	0.8%	3,766	1363.7	9
Iran	83,783,942	19	1.1%	45,255	540.1	10	Philadelphia	PA	1,584,138	23	0.5%	1,952	1232.2	10
Poland	37,846,611	38	0.5%	13,774	363.9	11	Cook	IL	5,180,493	2	1.6%	6,303	1216.7	11
South Africa	59,734,218	24	0.8%	20,903	349.9	12	Palm Beach	FL	1,485,941	25	0.5%	1,648	1109.1	12
Canada	37,742,154	39	0.5%	11,535	305.6	13	Oakland	MI	1,259,201	33	0.4%	1,310	1040.3	13
Iraq	40,222,493	36	0.5%	11,996	298.2	14	Maricopa	AZ	4,410,824	4	1.3%	3,896	883.3	14
Ukraine	43,851,044	33	0.6%	11,423	260.5	15	Hennepin	MN	1,259,428	32	0.4%	1,080	857.5	15
Russia	145,934,462	9	1.9%	36,192	248.0	16	Broward	FL	1,951,260	17	0.6%	1,626	833.3	16
Germany	84,339,067	17	1.1%	14,277	169.3	17	Clark	NV	2,231,647	13	0.7%	1,690	757.3	17
Turkey	83,992,949	18	1.1%	12,511	149.0	18	Bexar	TX	1,986,049	16	0.6%	1,473	741.7	18
Morocco	36,910,560	40	0.5%	5,396	146.2	19	Los Angeles	CA	10,105,518	1	3.1%	7,438	736.0	19
India	1,380,004,385	2	17.7%	133,738	96.9	20	Harris	TX	4,698,619	3	1.4%	2,965	631.0	20
Philippines	109,581,078	13	1.4%	8,173	74.6	21	Hillsborough	FL	1,436,888	27	0.4%	884	615.2	21
Egypt	102,334,404	14	1.3%	6,548	64.0	22	Cuyahoga	OH	1,243,857	35	0.4%	734	590.1	22
Indonesia	273,523,615	4	3.5%	16,002	58.5	23	Riverside	CA	2,450,758	10	0.7%	1,400	571.3	23
Algeria	43,849,260	34	0.6%	2,294	52.3	24	Dallas	TX	2,637,772	8	0.8%	1,492	565.6	24
Afghanistan	38,928,346	37	0.5%	1,695	43.5	25	Fairfax	VA	1,150,795	38	0.4%	614	533.5	25
Bangladesh	164,689,383	8	2.1%	6,416	39.0	26	San Bernardino	CA	2,171,603	14	0.7%	1,127	519.0	26
Pakistan	220,892,340	5	2.8%	7,696	34.8	27	Franklin	OH	1,310,300	31	0.4%	664	506.8	27
Myanmar	54,409,800	26	0.7%	1,765	32.4	28	Orange	CA	3,185,968	6	1.0%	1,551	486.8	28
Sudan	43,733,762	35	0.6%	1,197	27.4	29	Tarrant	TX	2,084,931	15	0.6%	982	471.0	29
Kenya	53,771,296	27	0.7%	1,392	25.9	30	Orange	FL	1,348,975	30	0.4%	625	463.3	30
Japan	126,476,461	11	1.6%	1,949	15.4	31	Mecklenburg	SC	1,093,901	40	0.3%	429	392.2	31
Ethiopia	114,963,588	12	1.5%	1,651	14.4	32	Allegheny	PA	1,218,452	36	0.4%	475	389.8	32
South Korea	51,269,185	28	0.7%	509	9.9	33	Travis	TX	1,248,743	34	0.4%	476	381.2	33
Nigeria	206,139,589	7	2.6%	1,167	5.7	34	King	WA	2,233,163	12	0.7%	847	379.3	34
Uganda	45,195,774	32	0.6%	172	3.8	35	Sacramento	CA	1,540,975	24	0.5%	546	354.3	35
DR Congo	89,561,403	16	1.1%	329	3.7	36	Salt Lake	UT	1,152,633	37	0.4%	377	327.1	36
China	1,439,323,776	1	18.5%	4,742	3.3	37	Alameda	CA	1,666,753	20	0.5%	499	299.4	37
Thailand	69,799,978	20	0.9%	60	0.9	38	San Diego	CA	3,343,364	5	1.0%	966	288.9	38
Vietnam	97,338,579	15	1.2%	35	0.4	39	Santa Clara	CA	1,937,570	18	0.6%	463	239.0	39
Tanzania	59,308,690	25	0.8%	21	0.4	40	Contra Costa	CA	1,150,215	39	0.4%	257	223.4	40
Totals:	6,448,947,037		82.7%	1,179,251					88,652,927		27.1%	83,437		

While a number of factors may explain this anomaly, including differences in age, co-morbidities, socio-economic status, and testing capacity, it should not be overlooked that individuals in these poorer countries, who often reside in crowded multi-generational family groups with shared facilities, may have experienced increased and possibly sustained, exposure to human coronaviruses (HCoVs) that cause the "common cold". This elevated exposure, which may lead to greater levels of cross-immunity to SARS-CoV-2, may help explain why:

- A serology study of slums in three wards of Mumbai showed that residents there had 3·5 times the SARS-CoV-2 infection rate of those in housing societies (57% versus 16%), but lower fatality rates (0·05%–0·10%) (Malani et al., 2020). None of the people included in the study had been tested for active SARS-CoV-2 infection using an RT-qPCR assay, suggesting either asymptomatic infection or very mild symptoms.
- A study of the United States state prison systems in Arkansas, North Carolina, Ohio, and Virginia revealed a 70% infection rate amongst the 4,693 inmates tested, of whom 96% were asymptomatic. A significant number of these prisoners were older and, therefore, presumed to be more prone to complications, but this was not the case (So and Smith, 2020).
- Approximately 90% of 147 homeless shelter residents in Boston who were infected with SARS-CoV-2 exhibited no symptoms, even though the shelter's living space was shared by all residents. Similarly, 95% of the 481 infected workers at a Tyson Foods poultry plant in Springdale, Arkansas were asymptomatic (Cha, 2020).

ASYMPTOMATIC INFECTION IN SCHOOL CHILDREN

Schools are densely populated environments, so their reopening has left many people anxious about the role they may play in spreading SARS-CoV-2 within homes and the wider community.

Data has consistently shown that children who become infected with SARS-CoV-2 typically experience mild or no symptoms. There may be multiple reasons for this clinical outcome, including the lack of comorbidities and/or age-related immune system characteristics. However, an intriguing possibility is that cross-reactive T-cells generated in response to HCoV-related colds may be present at a higher prevalence within the younger population due to exposure in school environments (Arroll, 2011; Steinman et al., 2020). It may be possible that these "circulating" cross-reactive T-cells could suppress the development of clinical symptoms, despite a recent study demonstrating that viral nucleic acid loads in 5- to 17-year-olds match or exceed (for those less than 5 years old) those found in adults (Heald-Sargent et al., 2020). It is also unclear to what extent infected children shed SARS-CoV-2 or are vectors for its spread, especially those who are symptom-free. Studies to date have suggested that children, especially those in primary or elementary schools, are at low risk of contracting the disease, may be the initial source of infection in only a very small number of cases, and are unlikely to pass it on *via* child-to-child or child-to-adult transmission (Armann et al., 2020, Davies et al., 2020; Munro and Faust, 2020; Posfay-Barbe et al., 2020).

T-CELL RESPONSES TO SARS-COV-2 IN NON-INFECTED AND ASYMPTOMATIC INDIVIDUALS

While T-cell responses to SARS-CoV-2 in infected individuals have now been reported, the emerging descriptions of pre-existing SARS-CoV-2 cross-reactive $CD4^+$ and $CD8^+$ T-cells amongst individuals who have not been infected are of particular interest (Corman et al., 2018; Braun et al., 2020; Grifoni et al., 2020; Sette and Crotty, 2020). The presence of these cross-reactive T-cells appears to be explained by prior exposure to HCoVs, such as HCoV-HKU1, HCoV-OC43H, CoV-NL63, and HCoV-229E, that generate T-cells capable of recognizing SARS-CoV-2 antigens (Mateus et al., 2020). Though involving different viruses, a similar situation is reminiscent in the historical findings of physician Edward Jenner, who discovered that milkmaids rarely succumbed to smallpox and correctly deduced that exposure to cowpox, a related virus causing a much milder illness, protected them. Similarly, during the 2009 swine flu pandemic caused by H1N1/09, the majority of people over the age of 60 displayed levels of pre-existing immunity resulting from exposure to similar flu viruses earlier in life, while young individuals had very little immunity and were, in contrast to the current situation, at greater risk (Xu et al., 2010).

Immunocompetent children and adults with respiratory infections (the common cold) often present as asymptomatic, or develop mild respiratory tract illnesses. More than 200 viral strains have been implicated as causal factors of the common cold. Rhinoviruses are responsible for ~35% of upper respiratory infections; HCoVs, often asymptomatic, cause 15-25% of cases, while influenza, adenoviruses, and other viral types account for the rest. Adults average two to three common colds each year, while children get six to eight, of which one or two are caused by HCoVs (Simasek and Blandino, 2007). Accordingly, it was found in a study of 100 subjects that most individuals had evidence of serum antibodies to all four HCoV strains (Gorse et al., 2010). We envisage one potential study resulting from a synthesis of these observations could be to investigate whether levels of longer-lasting "immunity" to SARS-CoV-2 could be higher than serology tests indicate. A positive result would be welcome news from a public health perspective.

Our ability to measure HCoV CD4+ and CD8+ T-cell responses to SARS-CoV-2 infection is limited due to the specialized nature of the tests. This major knowledge gap makes the interpretation of COVID-19 disease pathogenesis more difficult and clouds our ability to quantify the usefulness of pandemic control measures, such as social distancing.

CURRENT DATABASES DO NOT CAPTURE SEVERITY OF SYMPTOMS AND COHABITATION DATA

Searches of relevant publicly available databases, including the Johns Hopkins Coronavirus Resource Centre, National Institutes of Health Open-Access Data and Computational Resources to Address COVID-19, CDC World Dataset, The Covid-19 Tracking Project, Florida Department of Health, New York City Department of Health and Mental Hygiene, 1Point3Acres, and others, revealed a lack of information relating to the severity of symptoms (symptomatic vs. asymptomatic), possibly related to lower testing rates in highly populated or developing countries for individuals who are asymptomatic. More importantly, information pertaining to cohabitation and contact tracing was not included. A retrospective analysis that combines information from SARS-CoV-2 patient and contact tracing databases might be useful in determining whether individuals infected with SARS-CoV-2 who reside with school-age children are more likely to be asymptomatic. Such an analysis could be used to test the hypothesis that exposure to HCoV in densely populated environments leads to greater levels of cross-immunity to SARS-CoV-2.

THE NEED TO INCLUDE ASYMPTOMATIC INDIVIDUALS IN SURVEILLANCE STUDIES

Surveillance studies of respiratory virus circulation in the United States (and globally) are typically limited to data collected by clinical labs from symptomatic individuals. This approach does not capture the impact of respiratory infections that are asymptomatic or associated with mild respiratory tract illness in immunocompetent children and adults. The largest such surveillance study of symptomatic HCoV patients, which was conducted in the U.S. from 1st July, 2014 through 30th June, 2017, contained the results of 854,575 HCoV rRT-PCR tests performed by 117 laboratories in 42 states. Overall, 2·2% were positive for HCoV-OC43, 1·0% for HCoV-NL63, 0·8% for HCoV-229E, and

0·6% for HCoV-HKU1 (Killerby et al., 2018). These data suggest that less than about 5% of symptomatic HCoV infections (colds) are likely to help build cross-immunity to SARS-CoV-2.

For a different perspective we turn to a unique, cross-sectional longitudinal study of individuals, both symptomatic and asymptomatic, that sought to identify changes in respiratory virus colonization before and after the 2013 Hajj, a 5- to 6-day religious pilgrimage to Mecca, Saudi Arabia (attended by more than 2 million people) (Memish et al., 2015). Pre- and post-Hajj nasal specimens were prospectively obtained from a paired cohort (692 pilgrims) and from nonpaired cohorts (514 arriving and 470 departing pilgrims) from 13 countries including the United States (8·4%) and countries in Africa (44·2%), Asia (40·2%), and Europe (7·2%). Nasal specimens were tested for 34 respiratory pathogens using RT-PCR. The prevalence of viruses increased from 7·4% before the Hajj to 45·4% after the Hajj, due to the acquisition of rhinoviruses, coronaviruses (229E, HKU1, OC43), and influenza A H1N1. Among the paired cohort, HCoV 229E infections increased from six to 101 (0·9%–14·6%; $p < 0{\cdot}001$). Among the non-paired cohort, HCoV 229E infections increased from five to 48 (1·0%–10·2%; $p < 0{\cdot}001$). These data, taken from both symptomatic and asymptomatic adults, show that HCoV 229E can, given the right conditions, spread extremely quickly in a short period of time. This supports the hypothesis that children, and potentially the adults with whom they live, are likely to have been exposed to HCoV strains that can elicit T-cells cross-reactive to SARS-CoV-2, perhaps leading to a clinically relevant easing of symptoms. However, acquiring the information needed to truly test the hypothesis, and make more informed decisions, necessitates the inclusion of data from both asymptomatic and symptomatic patients, SARS-CoV-2 databases, and surveillance systems.

CONCLUSION

It may be the case that seasonal HCoV colds have actually been, and will continue to be, one of our greatest allies in the fight against the current SARS-CoV-2 pandemic and possibly SARS-CoV-1 which surfaced in November 2002 (Feng et al., 2009).

Given other HCoVs are likely to provide levels of protection against SARS-CoV-2 *via* cross-reactive immune memory, it is important to maintain levels of immunity to the broader spectrum of HCoVs in the current environment. If the spread of other mild respiratory and HCoV-related infections in school is reduced from normal levels, what impact will this have on the normal transmission of the "common cold" between children and those with whom they reside, as well as the wider community? Could this lead to a reduction in the temporary buildup of cross-reactive T-cell responses to SARS-CoV-2 that could provide some vital protection in an older, higher risk population, particularly given the reduced level of T-cell diversity and loss of immunity to previous HCoV infections as individuals age? While speculative at this stage, it is possible that differential spread of respiratory viruses other than SARS-CoV-2 within the younger population could be beneficial for their older relatives.

Besides specialized research labs there is a limited ability to measure HCoV CD4+ and CD8+ T-cell responses to SARS-CoV-2 infection. This major knowledge gap currently impedes interpretation of COVID-19 disease pathogenesis, and the calibration of pandemic control measures including social distancing. Unfortunately, the data needed to demonstrate this is not available because current SARS-CoV-2 databases and surveillance systems do not include information about the people who might be benefitting from cross-reactive immune memory ie., those who are asymptomatic. Inclusion of this data could help paint a more accurate picture of the clinical course of the SARS-CoV-2 pandemic and enable better decision making.

AUTHOR CONTRIBUTIONS

MC conceived the idea for the manuscript and wrote the first draft. MC, FA, AM, and OS participated in rewriting, editing, and conducting literature search. All authors contributed to the article and approved the submitted version.

ACKNOWLEDGMENTS

The authors would like to thank Dr. Vincent A. Fischetti and John C. Baird for their insight and support.

REFERENCES

Armann, J. P., Unrath, M., Kirsten, C., Lueck, C., Dalpke, A., and Berner, R. (2020). Anti-SARS-CoV-2 IgG antibodies in adolescent students and their teachers in Saxony, Germany (SchoolCoviDD19): very low seropraevalence and transmission rates. doi: 10.1101/2020.07.16.20155143

Arroll, B. (2011). Common cold. *Am. Fam. Physician* 84 (12), 1390–1391.

Braun, J., Loyal, L., Frentsch, M., Wendisch, D., Georg, P., Kurth, F., et al. (2020). SARS-CoV-2-reactive T cells in healthy donors and patients with COVID-19. *Nature.* doi: 10.1038/s41586-020-2598-9

Cha, A. E. (2020). Forty percent of people with coronavirus infections have no symptoms. Might they be the key to ending the pandemic? *Washington Post* 2020.

Contributors W. *List of the most populous counties in the United States. Wikipedia, The Free Encyclopedia.* Available at: https://en.wikipedia.org/w/index.php?title=List_of_the_most_populous_counties_in_the_United_States&oldid=967385264 (Accessed 28 July 2020).

Corman, V. M., Muth, D., Niemeyer, D., and Drosten, C. (2018). Hosts and Sources of Endemic Human Coronaviruses. *Adv. Virus Res.* 100, 163–188. doi: 10.1016/bs.aivir.2018.01.001

Davies, N. G., Klepac, P., Liu, Y., Prem, K., Jit, M., Group, C. C.-W., et al. (2020). Age-dependent effects in the transmission and control of COVID-19 epidemics. *Nat. Med.* 26, 1205–1211. doi: 10.1101/2020.03.24.20043018

Engineering JHUCfSSa. (2020). *Coronavirus Resource Center* (Johns Hopkins University). Available at: https://coronavirus.jhu.edu/ (Accessed July 27, 2020)

Feng, D., de Vlas, S. J., Fang, L. Q., Han, X. N., Zhao, W. J., Sheng, S., et al. (2009). The SARS epidemic in mainland China: bringing together all epidemiological data. *Trop. Med. Int. Health* 14 (Suppl 1), 4–13. doi: 10.1111/j.1365-3156.2008.02145.x

Gorse, G. J., Patel, G. B., Vitale, J. N., and O'Connor, T. Z. (2010). Prevalence of antibodies to four human coronaviruses is lower in nasal secretions than in serum. *Clin. Vaccine Immunol.* 17 (12), 1875–1880. doi: 10.1128/CVI.00278-10

Grifoni, A., Weiskopf, D., Ramirez, S. I., Mateus, J., Dan, J. M., Moderbacher, C. R., et al. (2020). Targets of T Cell Responses to SARS-CoV-2 Coronavirus in Humans with COVID-19 Disease and Unexposed Individuals. *Cell* 181 (7), 1489–1501.e1415.

Heald-Sargent, T., Muller, W. J., Zheng, X., Rippe, J., Patel, A. B., and Kociolek, L. K. (2020). Age-Related Differences in Nasopharyngeal Severe Acute Respiratory Syndrome Coronavirus 2 (SARS-CoV-2) Levels in Patients With Mild to Moderate Coronavirus Disease 2019 (COVID-19). *JAMA Pediatr.* 174, 902–903. doi: 10.1001/jamapediatrics.2020.3651

Killerby, M. E., Biggs, H. M., Haynes, A., Dahl, R. M., Mustaquim, D., Gerber, S. I., et al. (2018). Human coronavirus circulation in the United States 2014-2017. *J. Clin. Virol.* 101, 52–56. doi: 10.1016/j.jcv.2018.01.019

Malani, A., Shah, D., Kang, G., Lobo, G. N., Shastri, J., Mohanan, M., et al. (2020). Seroprevalence of SARS-CoV-2 in slums versus non-slums in Mumbai, India. *Lancet Glob. Health.*

Mateus, J., Grifoni, A., Tarke, A., Sidney, J., Ramirez, S. I., Dan, J. M., et al. (2020). Selective and cross-reactive SARS-CoV-2 T cell epitopes in unexposed humans. *Science* 370, 89–94. doi: 10.1126/science.abd3871

Memish, Z. A., Assiri, A., Turkestani, A., Yezli, S., Al Masri, M., Charrel, R., et al. (2015). Mass gathering and globalization of respiratory pathogens during the 2013 Hajj. *Clin. Microbiol. Infect.* 21 (6), 571.e571–578. doi: 10.1016/j.cmi.2015.02.008

Munro, A. P. S., and Faust, S. N. (2020). Children are not COVID-19 super spreaders: time to go back to school. *Arch. Dis. Child.* 105 (7), 618–619. doi: 10.1136/archdischild-2020-319474

Posfay-Barbe, K. M., Wagner, N., Gauthey, M., Moussaoui, D., Loevy, N., Diana, A., et al. (2020). COVID-19 in Children and the Dynamics of Infection in Families. *Pediatrics* 146, e20201576. doi: 10.1542/peds.2020-1576

Sette, A., and Crotty, S. (2020). Pre-existing immunity to SARS-CoV-2: the knowns and unknowns. *Nat. Rev. Immunol.* 20, 457–458.

Simasek, M., and Blandino, D. A. (2007). Treatment of the common cold. *Am. Fam. Physician* 75 (4), 515–520.

So, L., and Smith, G. (2020). In four U.S. state prisons, nearly 3,300 inmates test positive for coronavirus - 96% without symptoms. *Reuters* 2020.

Spreeuwenberg, P., Kroneman, M., and Paget, J. (2018). Reassessing the Global Mortality Burden of the 1918 Influenza Pandemic. *Am. J. Epidemiol.* 187 (12), 2561–2567.

Steinman, J. B., Lum, F. M., Ho, P. P., Kaminski, N., and Steinman, L. (2020). Reduced development of COVID-19 in children reveals molecular checkpoints gating pathogenesis illuminating potential therapeutics. *Proc. Natl. Acad. Sci. U. S. A.* 117, 24620–24626.

Worldometer. *Countries in the world by population.* Available at: https://www.worldometers.info/world-population/population-by-country/ (Accessed July 27, 2020).

Xu, R., Ekiert, D. C., Krause, J. C., Hai, R., Crowe, J. E. Jr., and Wilson, I. A. (2010). Structural basis of preexisting immunity to the 2009 H1N1 pandemic influenza virus. *Science* 328 (5976), 357–360.

3

No Evidence for Human Monocyte-Derived Macrophage Infection and Antibody-Mediated Enhancement of SARS-CoV-2 Infection

Obdulio García-Nicolás [1,2], Philip V'kovski [1,2], Ferdinand Zettl [1], Gert Zimmer [1,2], Volker Thiel [1,2] and Artur Summerfield [1,2]*

[1] Institute of Virology and Immunology (IVI), Bern, Switzerland, [2] Department of Infectious Diseases and Pathobiology, Vetsuisse Faculty, University of Bern, Bern, Switzerland

***Correspondence:**
Obdulio García-Nicolás
obdulio.garcia-nicolas@ivi.admin.ch

Vaccines are essential to control the spread of severe acute respiratory syndrome coronavirus-2 (SARS-CoV-2) and to protect the vulnerable population. However, one safety concern of vaccination is the possible development of antibody-dependent enhancement (ADE) of SARS-CoV-2 infection. The potential infection of Fc receptor bearing cells such as macrophages, would support continued virus replication and inflammatory responses, and thereby potentially worsen the clinical outcome of COVID-19. Here we demonstrate that SARS-CoV-2 and SARS-CoV neither infect human monocyte-derived macrophages (hMDM) nor induce inflammatory cytokines in these cells, in sharp contrast to Middle East respiratory syndrome (MERS) coronavirus and the common cold human coronavirus 229E. Furthermore, serum from convalescent COVID-19 patients neither induced enhancement of SARS-CoV-2 infection nor innate immune response in hMDM. Although, hMDM expressed angiotensin-converting enzyme 2, no or very low levels of transmembrane protease serine 2 were found. These results support the view that ADE may not be involved in the immunopathological processes associated with COVID-19, however, more studies are necessary to understand the potential contribution of antibodies-virus complexes with other cells expressing FcR receptors.

Keywords: human coronaviruses, SARS-CoV-2, COVID-19 convalescent sera, ADE, human monocyte-derived macrophages

INTRODUCTION

Since the emergence of the severe acute respiratory syndrome coronavirus-2 (SARS-CoV-2) in December 2019 in the Chinese city of Wuhan, the virus has spread globally causing the coronavirus disease 2019 (COVID-19) pandemic. The high morbidity and severity of COVID-19 in some of the affected patients have jeopardized the public health system of affected countries. In addition, the public health measures that have been implemented to control the pandemic have affected the life and economy of millions of people around the world.

In the current situation, the lack of neutralizing antibodies against SARS-CoV-2, allows the virus to spread rapidly in the human population. A global vaccination campaign may have the potential to finally control the pandemic and vaccination programs have started recently. However, a concern is the possibility that vaccination could promote antibody-dependent enhancement (ADE) of SARS-CoV-2 infection which could be associated with enhancement of the disease (Lee et al., 2020).

The underlying mechanism of ADE of infection is based on the interaction between virion-antibody complexes and Fc gamma receptors (FcγR) that are expressed by cells of the immune system such as macrophages. The binding of virion-antibody complexes to Fc receptors could result in their uptake into the cells by receptor-mediated endocytosis leading to potential infection of the cells (Taylor et al., 2015). Despite speculation and alarming about this possibility at the time of initiation of our work, no data were published specifically addressing ADE of SARS-CoV-2 (Lee et al., 2020; Rogers et al., 2020). With this in mind, the present study aimed to investigate whether immune sera from convalescent COVID-19 patients would enhance SARS-CoV-2 infection and promote secretion of pro-inflammatory cytokines production by human macrophages. To this end we performed a comparative study on the susceptibility of human macrophages to infection with human coronavirus 229E (HCoV-229E), Middle East respiratory syndrome coronavirus (MERS-CoV), SARS-CoV and SARS-CoV-2 and the inflammatory cytokine response of these cells. Potential ADE of infections by SARS-CoV and SARS-CoV-2 were studied using immune sera from convalescent COVID-19 patients.

MATERIAL AND METHODS

Ethics Statement

Buffy coats from anonymous healthy blood donors were obtained from the regional transfusion blood service of the Swiss Red Cross (SRC) (Bern, Switzerland). The use of buffy coats was approved by the SRC review board. All serum samples employed in this study were collected following the guidance of the Act on Medical Devices (MPG guideline 98/79/EC) for the collection of human residual material to evaluate suitability of an *in vitro* diagnostic medical device (§24). For this study an informed consent and ethical approval was not needed because only leftovers of serum samples for diagnostic laboratory procedures were used.

Cells

Vero cells (E6 and B4 lineages, African Green monkey kidney epithelial cells) and Huh-7 cells (human hepatocellular carcinoma cells) were cultured in Dulbecco's minimal essential medium (DMEM; Life Technologies), supplemented with 10% fetal bovine serum (FBS), non-essential amino acids (Life Technologies), penicillin-streptomycin (Gibco) and HEPES (Gibco). A549 (adenocarcinomic human alveolar basal epithelial cells) stably transfected with angiotensin-converting enzyme 2 (ACE2) and transmembrane protease serine 2 (TMPRSS2) were purchased from Invivogen (Toulouse, France) and cultured in minimal essential medium (MEM) supplemented with 10% FBS, 0.5 μg/ml of puromycin (Invivogen) and 300 μg/ml of hygromycin B (Invivogen). *A. albopictus* C6/36 cells (ATCC® CRL-1660™) were cultured in MEM (Gibco) supplemented with 100 mM of sodium pyruvate (Gibco), non-essential amino acids and 10% FBS

For the production of human monocyte derived macrophages (hMDM), peripheral blood mononuclear cells (PBMCs) were isolated from buffy coats by density gradient centrifugation on Ficoll-Paque™ PLUS (1.077 g/L; GE healthcare). Then, monocytes were sorted using anti-CD14 beads as proposed by the manufacturer (Miltenyi Biotech GmbH), and seeded in 24 well plates at 2.5 x 10^5 cells/well in 500 μl of Roswell Park Memorial Institute (RPMI) 1640 medium (Gibco) and kept at 37°C and 5% CO_2 atmosphere for one hour. Non-adherent cells were removed and 500 μl of RPMI 1640 supplemented with 10% of FBS (Gibco), GlutaMAX (Gibco), penicillin-streptomycin (Gibco) and human M-CSF (100 ng/ml; Miltenyi Biotec) were added. The cells were cultured for six days at 37 °C and 5% CO_2. The full medium complemented with M-CSF was replaced every 48 to 72 hours.

Viruses

A collection of different coronaviruses was employed for the experiments of the present study including the human coronavirus 229E [HCoV-299E; (Thiel et al., 2001)], Middle East respiratory syndrome coronavirus [MERS-CoV, strain EMC/2012; (van Boheemen et al., 2012)], SARS-CoV [Frankfurt-1; (Thiel et al., 2003)] and SARS-CoV-2 (SARS-CoV-2/München-1.1/2020/929) kindly provided by Daniela Niemeyer, Marcel Müller, and Christian Drosten (Charité, Berlin, Germany). HCoV-299E was propagated in Huh-7 cells in DMEM supplemented with 5% of FBS and non-essential amino acids at 33°C. MERS-CoV was propagated in Vero B4 cells in MEM supplemented with 2% of FBS and non-essential amino acids at 37°C. For the propagation of SARS-CoV and SARS-CoV-2 Vero E6 cells in MEM supplemented with 2% of FBS and non-essential amino acids at 37°C was employed. All coronavirus titrations were performed by end point dilution (ten-fold serial dilutions of viral supernatants) taking advantage of the virus-induced cytopathic effect that was apparent 56 to 72 hours post infection (hpi). Virus titers were expressed as 50% tissue culture infective dose per ml ($TCID_{50}$/ml). As a positive control for ADE of infection, we used Japanese encephalitis virus (JEV) (Laos strain; GenBank CNS769_Laos_2009; kindly provided by Prof. Remi Charrel, Aix-Marseille Université, Marseille, France) with immune sera previously described (Garcia-Nicolas et al., 2017).

Infection With Coronaviruses

Vero E6 cells or hMDM were incubated for 1.5 h at 39°C or 37°C with the respective virus using a multiplicity of infection (MOI) of 1 $TCID_{50}$ per cell, including mock control. Subsequently, the virus inoculum was removed, the cells washed three times with warm phosphate buffered saline (PBS), and RPMI medium supplemented with 2% FBS was added to the cells. As a positive control for the induction of pro-inflammatory cytokines either 1 μg/ml of lipopolysaccharide (LPS; Sigma-Aldrich) or 10 μg/ml of polyinosinic-polycytidytic acid (poly I:C, Sigma-Aldrich) were added to the cell culture medium. As indicated for each experiment, after 24, 48 or 72 h, supernatants were collected and stored at -70°C.

ACE2/TMPRSS2 Determination

Human macrophages and A549 cells stably transfected with human ACE2 and human TMPRSS2 were harvested using TrypLETMSelect (Gibco) for 20 min at room temperature and washed with CellWash solution (Becton Dickinson). Subsequently, the cells were stained for 20 min with anti-human TMPRSS2 monoclonal antibody (P5H9-A3, Santa Cruz biotechnology) and anti-human ACE2 antibody (A20069, BioLegend) in CellWash. After a washing the cells with CellWash, they were incubated for 10 min with anti-rat Alexa 488 fluorochrome conjugate (ThermoFisher Scientific) and Alexa Fluor 647 conjugated anti-mouse IgG1 (ThermoFisher Scientific). Finally, cells were analyzed by flow cytometry using a FACSCantoII (Becton Dickinson). Data analysis was performed with Flowjo V.9.1 software (Treestars, Inc.). Dead cells were excluded by electronic gating in forward/side scatter plots, followed by exclusion of doublets.

Antibody-Dependent Enhancement of Infection

A collection of sera from COVID-19 convalescent patients from a previously published work was employed for the present study (Zettl et al., 2020). This included sera with a broad range of neutralization titers against SARS-CoV-2 (ND_{50} <1:10; 1:20; 1:160; 1:240 and 1:2560). In order to test the ADE potential of these sera, different serum dilutions (1:10; 1:100; 1:1000 and 1:10000) were incubated for 30 min at 37°C with an equal volume of viral suspension (SARS-CoV or SARS-CoV-2) corresponding to a MOI of 1 $TCID_{50}$/cell. Thereafter, the virus/serum mixtures were added to human macrophages or Vero E6 cells and incubated for 30 min at 37°C and 5% CO_2 atmosphere. The cells were washed three times with PBS before fresh medium was added. As a control for ADE of infection, we employed a serum from immunized pigs known to have a high capacity of inducing ADE of infection for JEV in macrophages (Garcia-Nicolas et al., 2017). The serum (ND_{50} of 1:160 for JEV Laos) was serially diluted (1:10; 1:100; 1:1000 and 1:10000) and incubated at 37°C for 30 min with JEV Laos at a MOI of 1 $TCID_{50}$/cell. Porcine naïve serum was included as control. After that, virus/serum mixtures were added on hMDM and incubated for 30 min at 37°C, washed off and fresh medium was added. After 24 h of incubation at 37°C viral infectivity was determined by means of flow cytometry as described below.

Determination of Infected Cells

For immunofluorescence microscopy, cells were fixed with 4% formaldehyde for 10 min at room temperature, washed with PBS, and permeabilized with 0.3% saponin (PanReac AppliChem). The permeabilization procedure was performed for 20 min on ice in the presence of J2 monoclonal antibody directed to dsRNA (English and Scientific Consulting), or some experiments a rabbit antibody directed to the SARS-CoV nucleocapsid (N) protein (Rockland-inc) was included in this step. Subsequently, the cells were washed with 0.1% saponin, and cells were incubated for 20 min on ice with Alexa Fluor 488 conjugated anti-mouse IgG2a (ThermoFisher Scientific) or with Alexa Fluor 546 conjugated anti-rabbit (ThermoFisher Scientific) in 0.3% saponin. Cells were washed once with PBS prior to incubation with 4′,6-diamidino-2-phenylindole (DAPI; Sigma) for 5 min at 37 °C. Finally, the percentage of infected cells was determined by enumerating the dsRNA positive cells in 10 fields/well using an Axio Observer Z1 inverted microscope equipped with a Zeiss Colibri Illuminator (CarlZeiss) and digital imaging Zeiss software (AxioVision, v4). All generated images were analyzed using ImageJ software.

For the determination of infected cells by flow cytometry, macrophages and Vero E6 cells were harvested using TrypLETMSelect (Gibco) for 20 min at room temperature and fixed with 4% (w/v) formaldehyde. Thereafter, the cells were permeabilized/stained for 20 min on ice with 0.3% (*w*/*v*) saponin in PBS in the presence of a rabbit antibody directed to the SARS-CoV N protein (Rockland-inc). For some experiments we used an anti-dsRNA monoclonal antibody (J2, English and Scientific Consulting). For the determination of JEV infected cells anti-flavivirus E protein mAb 4G2 (IgG2a) was employed as primary antibody. The cells were subsequently washed, incubated for 10 min with anti-rabbit Alexa 488 or Alexa Fluor 647-conjugated anti-mouse IgG2a (ThermoFisher Scientific) and analyzed by flow cytometry (FACSCantoII, Becton Dickinson). For analysis, Flowjo V.9.1 software (Treestars, Inc.) was used. Dead cells were excluded by electronic gating in forward/side scatter plots, followed by exclusion of doublets.

Determination of Cytokines

Cell culture supernatants were analyzed for the presence of the following cytokines: Tumor necrosis factor (TNF), interferon beta (IFN-β), interleukin 6 (IL-6) and IL-1β were quantified by ELISA (R&D Systems) following the manufacturer's instructions. Detection limits were 30 pg/ml for TNF, 10 pg/ml for IFN-β, 4 pg/ml for IL-1β and 9 pg/ml for IL-6.

Statistics

For the generation of figures and data analyses the GraphPad Prism 8 Software (GraphPad Software, Inc.) was employed. All experiments were independently performed 3 to 6 times with cells from different donors, and each experiment was run in triplicates. For viral titrations, differences between groups were assessed using a Kruskal–Wallis test, and for individual differences the Mann–Whitney *U*-test with Bonferroni correction as *post hoc* was employed. For group differences in the percentages of infected cells and levels of cytokines expression comparisons, a one-way ANOVA test with Bonferroni correction as *post hoc* was performed. Correlation analysis between infected cells, viral titers, and expressed cytokines were calculated by Spearman's Rho analysis; a correlation between two different factors was considered relevant with R^2 >0.5. A *p* value lower than 0.05 was considered statistically significant for every analyzed data. In figure 1, different superscript letters indicate a significant difference ($p < 0.05$) between the conditions. For the table 2 * indicates p <0.05, **p ≤0.002, ***p ≤0.001 and ****p ≤0.0001.

RESULTS

Visualization of Coronavirus Replication by Immunolabeling of dsRNA

Taking into account that dsRNA is a replication intermediate located in double-membrane vesicles during coronavirus replication (Wolff et al., 2020), coronavirus-infected cells may be specifically detected by antibodies to dsRNA rather than by antibodies directed to viral proteins. In order to evaluate the suitability of dsRNA immunolabeling for this purpose, Vero E6 cells infected with either SARS-CoV or SARS-CoV-2 at MOI of 1 $TCID_{50}$/ml, were double-stained for dsRNA and N protein, and analyzed by immunofluorescence microscopy or flow cytometry (**Figure 1**). While dsRNA staining allowed us to identify infected cells by immunofluorescence microscopy to a similar degree as N protein labeling (**Figures 1A, B**), flow cytometry only worked when the N protein was labeled (**Figure 1A**). This experiment demonstrated that immunolabeling of dsRNA allows the identification of cells infected with different coronaviruses by immunofluorescence microscopy in the absence of antibodies specifically recognizing viral proteins. On the other hand, the labeling of N protein in combination with flow cytometry is an efficient way of detecting cells infected by SARS-CoV or SARS-CoV-2.

Human Coronaviruses Differ in Their Ability to Infect hMDM

Infection of hMDM with HCoV-299E, MERS-CoV, SARS-CoV and SARS-CoV-2 at MOI of 1 $TCID_{50}$/cell demonstrated high susceptibility to infection with the common cold virus HCoV-229E, low susceptibility to infection with the highly pathogenic coronavirus MERS-CoV, and resistance to infection by SARS-CoV and SARS-CoV-2, in terms of dsRNA immunostaining (**Figures 2A, B**). Quantification of the number of infectious virus particles in the cell culture supernatants showed that only HCoV-229E and MERS-CoV replicated efficiently in hMDM (**Figure 2C**). Although HCoV-229E showed higher percentages of infected

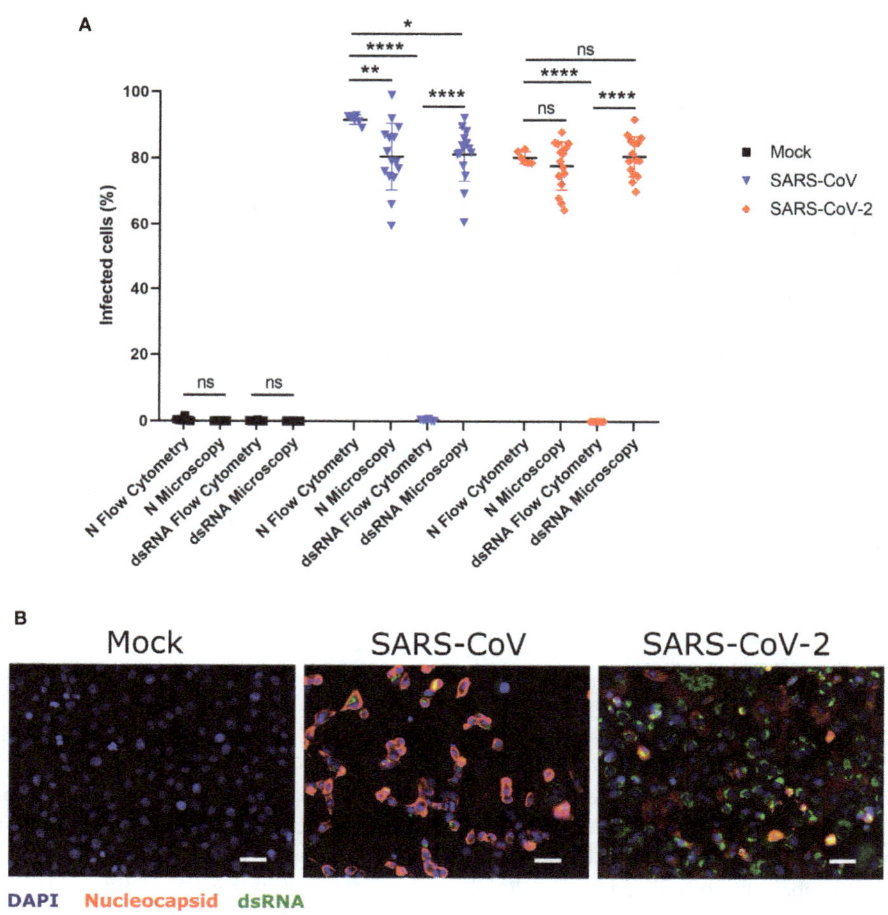

FIGURE 1 | Determination of SARS-CoV and SARS-CoV-2 infected hMDM by immunolabeling for dsRNA and N protein. Vere E6 cells were infected with SARS-CoV and SARS-CoV-2 at MOI 1 $TCID_{50}$/cell, and after 24 hpi dsRNA and N protein were labeled with specific antibodies. The nuclei were stained with DAPI. Then positive cells for dsRNA and N were quantified either by flow cytometry or immunofluorescence microscopy **(A)**. In **(B)** example of representative images acquired by fluorescence microscopy is shown. The scale bar represent 40 μm. The data are from three independent experiments. Statistically significant differences between the conditions are indicated by asterisks (ns indicates non-statistical differences, $^*p < 0.05$, $^{**}p \leq 0.002$ and $^{****}p \leq 0.0001$).

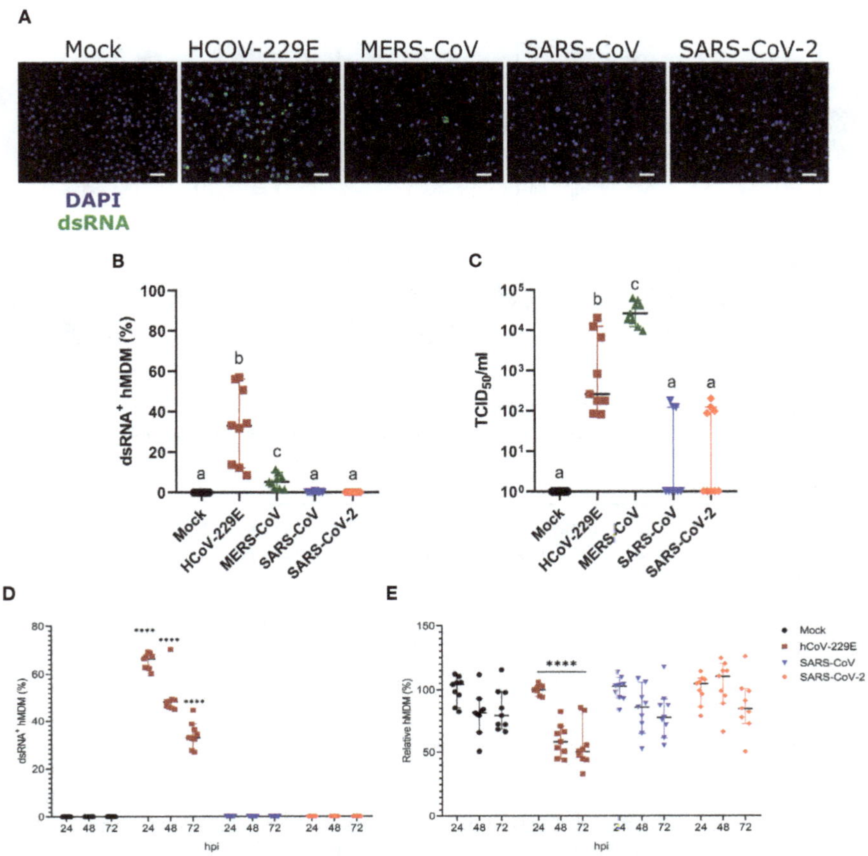

FIGURE 2 | Susceptibility of hMDM to different human coronaviruses. Human MDM were inoculated with different coronaviruses (hCoV-229E, MERS-CoV, SARS-CoV-1 and SARS-CoV-2) using an MOI of 1 $TCID_{50}$/cell. Mock-infected cells were included as controls. After incubating the cells for 1.5 hours, the inoculum was removed, the cells washed, and fresh medium added. At 24 hpi, dsRNA in the cells was detected with a specific antibody and nuclei were stained with DAPI; the scale bar represents 40 µm. **(A)** The percentage of dsRNA-positive hMDM was calculated for 10 fields per condition **(B)**. In **(C)** virus titers are shown. The same experiment was repeated with hCoV-229E, SARS-CoV-1 and SARS-CoV-2, and infected cells were quantified at 24, 48 and 72 hpi **(D)**. The relative number of total hMDM per well was calculated taking as reference the number of cells at 24 hpi **(E)**. The data from three independent experiments run in triplicates are shown in each panel. Statistically significant differences between the conditions are indicated by different superscript letters in **(B, C)** ($p < 0.05$), and by asterisks in **(D, E)** (****$p \leq 0.0001$).

hMDM (32.79% ± 18.79 SD) the highest virus titers were found in the cell culture supernatant of macrophages infected with MERS-CoV (**Figure 2C**). Nevertheless, it has to be taken into consideration that all experiments were performed at 37°C although the optimal temperature for HCoV-229E is 33°C (Dijkman et al., 2013). Viral titers of SARS-CoV and SARS-CoV-2 were not statistically significantly different compared to the mock control. The background signal detected for some wells might be due to remaining viral particles from the inoculum that stayed bound to the hMDM surface and were not removed by washing the cells.

We also tested infectivity of hMDM to SARS-CoV or SARS-CoV-2 at later time points, including 48 and 72 hpi. While HCoV-229E efficiently infected hMDM neither SARS-CoV nor SARS-CoV-2 were able to infect hMDM at any of the time points (**Figure 2D**). Moreover, only HCoV-299E but not SARS-CoV and SARS-CoV-2-infected hMDM showed a significant decrease of the number of cells, indicating a virus-induced cytopathogenic effect (**Figure 2E**).

Human MDM Produce Cytokines Following Infection With HCoV-229E

Human MDM infected by HCoV-229E, but not by MERS-CoV, SARS-CoV or SARS-CoV-2, secreted TNF, and low levels of both IFN-β and IL-6 (**Figure 3**). None of the tested coronaviruses induced secretion of IL-1β. Taking into consideration that viral RNA might induce innate immune responses, we tested the correlation between the percentage of dsRNA positive cells, viral titers and level of secreted cytokines. The results found a clear association between the percentage of infected cells and secreted cytokine levels but not with viral titers (**Table 1**).

Human MDM Express SARS-CoV-2 Receptor ACE2 but No or Low Levels of TMPRSS2

First, as hMDM were resistant to infection by SARS-CoV-2, we assessed the expression levels of the viral cell receptor ACE2, as well as TMPRSS2, a serine protease involved in the proteolytic activation

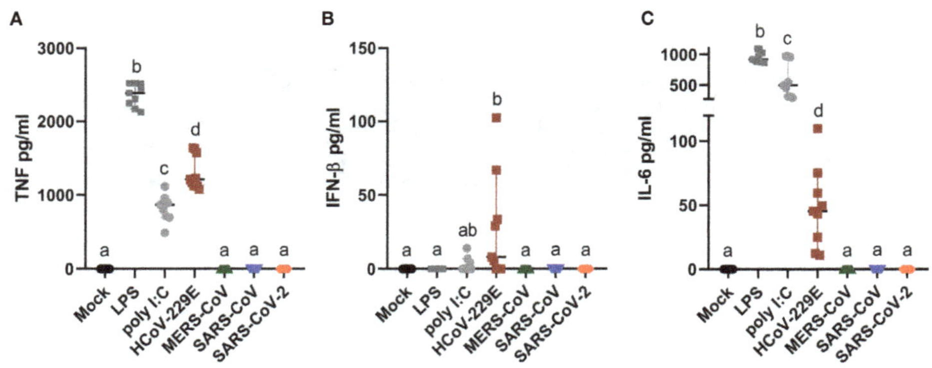

FIGURE 3 | Human MDM immune response after coronavirus infection. Human MDM were inoculated with different coronaviruses (hCoV-229E, MERS-CoV, SARS-CoV-1 and SARS-CoV-2) as described before. Mock-infected cells or cells treated with LPS or poly I:C served as controls. After 24 hpi TNF **(A)** IFN-β **(B)** and IL-6 **(C)** were determined in the cell culture supernatants. The data from three independent experiments run in triplicates are shown. Different superscript letters indicate a significant difference ($p < 0.05$) between the conditions.

TABLE 1 | Correlation analysis between dsRNA positive hMDM, infectious virus titers and pro-inflammatory cytokines.

R^2	Viral titer	TNF	IFN-β	IL-6
dsRNA	0.015	0.821****	0.682****	0.892****
Viral titer	–	0.004	0.006	0.001
TNF		–	0.490****	0.795****
IFN-β			–	0.729****

*****p ≤ 0.0001.*

of the spike protein (Hoffmann et al., 2020; Shang et al., 2020). For that, double immunolabeling of cell ACE2 and TMPRSS2 was performed in hMDM after differentiation, and their expression was assessed by flow cytometry (**Figure 4**); A549 cells transfected with ACE2 and TMPRSS2 were used as positive control. This experiment showed that hMDM express high levels of ACE2 (33.3% ± 8.25SD; **Figure 4A**) comparable to the A549 cells transfected with ACE2 and TMPRSS2 (29.8% ± 3.55SD; **Figure 4A**). On the other hand, the percentage of TMPRSS2 positive hMDM was very low (3.03% ± 2.17SD; **Figure 4A**) when compared to the A549 cells transfected with ACE2 and TMPRSS2 (25.3% ± 2.66SD; **Figure 4A**). These results indicate that although hMDM express the SARS-CoV-2 receptor ACE2, the lack of expression of TMPRSS2 might prevent infection.

Antibodies From Convalescent COVID-19 Patients Neither Induce Antibody-Dependent Enhancement of Infection of hMDM With SARS-COV-2 Nor Promote Cytokine Responses

First, as a positive control for ADE in hMDM, sera from immunized pig that were previously demonstrated to induce a high ADE of JEV in porcine MDM (Garcia-Nicolas et al., 2017) were used. Despite the low binding of porcine IgGs to human FcR (Antonsson and Johansson, 2001), this experiment showed that such JEV immune complexes can enhance the infection of hMDM (**Supplementary Figure 1**) compared with both the JEV Laos control for the infection and the same dilution for the naïve porcine serum. This experiment showed the validity of the methodology to test ADE of infection in hMDM.

Next, selected COVID-19 sera with a neutralization titer below 1:10 and with a neutralization titer of 1:240, were diluted serially from 1:10 to 1:1000, mixed with SARS-CoV and SARS-CoV-2, and then added to Vero E6 cells. Both sera demonstrated a dilution-dependent inhibition of SARS-CoV-2 infection. In addition, a cross-reactivity of COVID-19 convalescent patient sera with SARS-CoV-1 was observed, confirming previous reports (Zettl et al., 2020) (**Table 2**).

Using the same approach, a larger collection of sera from COVID-19 convalescent patients with neutralization titers ranging from <10 to 1:2560 was incubated at different concentrations with SARS-CoV and SARS-CoV-2 and added to hMDM. Importantly, with none of the tested serum dilutions which went up to 1:10000 infection of hMDM was observed. Moreover, hMDM exposed to virus-antibodies complexes did not secrete any detectable pro-inflammatory cytokines (**Table 2**). These results indicate that the potential uptake of SARS-CoV and SARS-CoV-2 *via* FcR does not result in infection and activation of human macrophages.

DISCUSSION

A first observation of the present study was that in contrast to the common cold virus hCoV-229E and MERS-CoV, SARS-CoV and SARS-CoV-2 were unable to infect hMDM. The receptor for SARS-

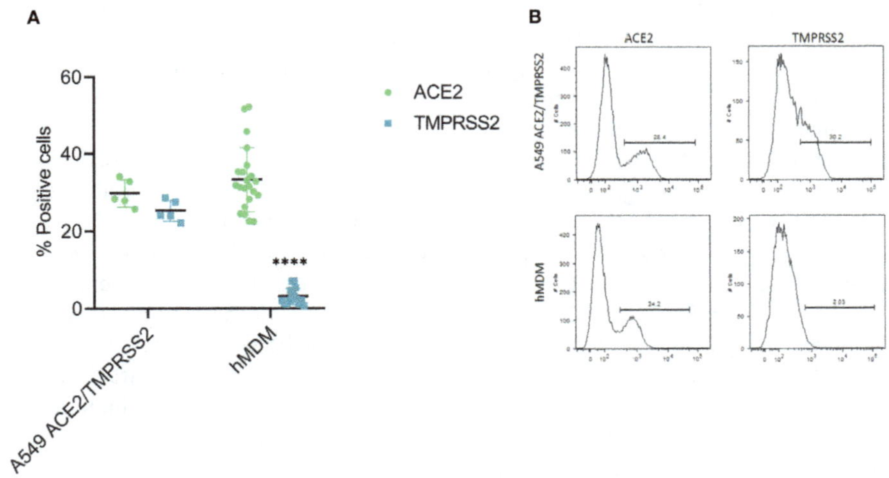

FIGURE 4 | ACE2 and TMPRSS2 expression in hMDM. After 6 days of differentiation ACE2 and TMPRSS2 were immunolabeled with specific antibodies and positive cells were assessed by flow cytometry. A549 cells transfected with ACE2 and TMPRSS2 were used as control **(A)**. Representative histograms for each marker in the analyzed cells are shown **(B)**. The data from 5 different human donor hMDM run in triplicates are shown. Statistically significant differences in the expression of each marker between both cell types are marked by asterisks (****p ≤ 0.0001).

TABLE 2 | Summary data for virus neutralization on Vero E6 cells and antibody-dependent enhancement of infection or cytokine response by hMDM for SARS-CoV and SARS-CoV-2-antibody complexes"+" detected; "-" not detected; "NT" not tested.

			Neutralization (% N⁺ Vero E6 cells n = 3)		**ADE (% N⁺ hMDM n = 6)**		**Cytokine response (hMDM n = 6)**	
			SARS-CoV	**SARS-CoV-2**	**SARS-CoV**	**SARS-CoV-2**	**TNF (pg/ml)**	**IFN-β (pg/ml)**
		Infection CTRL (%)	34 (± 1.5)	22.17 (± 2.11)	–	–	–	–
Immune serum	**Neutralizing titer**	Serum dilution						
A	< 1:10	1:10	10.41 (± 0.86)****	7.07 (± 0.23)****	–	–	–	–
		1:100	29.67 (± 3.99)	15.26 (± 1.92)****	–	–	–	–
		1:1000	36.57 (± 2.59)	23.40 (± 2.55)	–	–	–	–
		1:10000	34.23 (± 2.41)	32.93 (± 0.25)	–	–	–	–
B	1:20	1:10	NT	NT	NT	–	–	–
		1:100	NT	NT	NT	–	–	–
		1:1000	NT	NT	NT	–	–	–
		1:10000	NT	NT	NT	–	–	–
C	1:160	1:10	NT	NT	NT	–	–	–
		1:100	NT	NT	NT	–	–	–
		1:1000	NT	NT	NT	–	–	–
		1:10000	NT	NT	NT	–	–	–
D	1:240	1:10	10.08 (± 1.06)****	0.25 (± 0.26)****	–	–	–	–
		1:100	25.63 (± 1.63)***	2.25 (± 0.34)****	–	–	–	–
		1:1000	31.6 (± 0.72)	12.07 (± 0.58)****	–	–	–	–
		1:10000	32.93 (± 0.25)	18.73 (± 1.19)*	–	–	–	–
E	1:2560	1:10	NT	NT	NT	–	–	–
		1:100	NT	NT	NT	–	–	–
		1:1000	NT	NT	NT	–	–	–
		1:10000	NT	NT	NT	–	–	–

*Statistically significant differences compared to the control are indicated as: * for $p < 0.05$, *** for $p \leq 0.001$ and **** for $p \leq 0.0001$.*

CoV-2 is angiotensin-converting enzyme 2 (ACE2) typically expressed on ciliated epithelial cells, goblet cells, type II alveolar pneumocytes as well as other cells from different organs as enterocytes (Sungnak et al., 2020). However, there are conflicting reports on the infection of human macrophages by SARS-CoV. While one study described very limited ACE2 expression by macrophages (Sungnak et al., 2020), another report postulated that the receptor is expressed on tissue resident macrophages (Song et al., 2020). Although we showed in the present study that about 30% of the hMDM express ACE2 under the described culture/differentiation conditions, hMDM were not permissive to SARS-CoV or SARS-CoV-2. Of note, the expression of a truncated

ACE2 isoform (dAEC2) has been demonstrated upon IFN stimulation or viral infection (Onabajo et al., 2020). While remaining biologically active, dAEC2 does not facilitate SARS-CoV-2 spike binding and does not serve as an entry receptor. Whether hMDM express dACE2 remains to be formally determined. Following attachment of virions to the cell surface, the spike protein may be proteolytically activated and is able to trigger membrane fusion and release of the viral genome into the cytosol of the host cell. The proteolytic cleavage by TMPRSS2 or related enzymes normally takes place at the cell surface as well as the subsequent membrane fusion (Hoffmann et al., 2020). In the absence of TMPRSS2, SARS-CoV and SARS-CoV-2 may be proteolytically activated following receptor-mediated endocytosis by cathepsin B/L (Hoffmann et al., 2020; Shang et al., 2020). The present study shows that TMPRSS2 is expressed at very low levels in hMDM, which is in line with a previous publication describing very limited expression of TMPRSS2 expression in human macrophages (Sungnak et al., 2020). Therefore, we speculate that this might be an important limiting factor for the viral entry in macrophages. Moreover, recently it has been described that the p41 invariant chain of CD74 (major histocompatibility complex class II) can inhibit the cathepsin-mediated cleavage of viral envelope proteins (Bruchez et al., 2020). As macrophages constitutively express CD74 (Cho and Roche, 2013) the presence of the p41 invariant chain might block the activity of cathepsin B/L contributing to the resistance of hMDM to the infection by SARS-CoV and SARS-CoV-2. In COVID-19 patients, the viral nucleoprotein N has been detected in macrophages from lymphoid organs of COVID-19 patients (Park, 2020), but it is not clear whether this was caused by direct infection or as a consequence of phagocytosis of infected cells.

The infection of hMDM by HCoV-229E is in line with the expression by these cells of aminopeptidase N (CD13), the cellular receptor for HCoV-229E (Yeager et al., 1992). It is also in agreement with previous reports describing the infection of alveolar macrophages by HCoV-229E (Funk et al., 2012). The cellular receptor for MERS-CoV dipeptidyl peptidase-IV (DPP4 also known as CD26) is expressed at low levels by human monocytes and macrophages of healthy donors (Wang et al., 2013; Zhong et al., 2013; Rao et al., 2018; Rao et al., 2019), which could explain MERS-CoV infection of hMDM in our experiments.

Our results are also in line with a previous report demonstrating that following infection with HCoV-229E human macrophages strongly secrete TNF, but also produce IL-6 and some IFN-β (Funk et al., 2012). Finally, we also noticed a poor innate immune response of macrophages following infection with MERS-CoV, confirming a previous report that showed similar results (Zhou et al., 2014).

While writing the present manuscript contradictory data were published claiming that SARS-CoV-2 induces an immune activation of hMDM (Zheng et al., 2020). These conflicting results might be the consequence of different methodologies used. While we employed purified monocytes to generate macrophages in six days, Zheng and collaborators kept PBMC with M-CSF for four days and then for another 10 days when the cells became adherent (Zheng et al., 2020). Another important methodological difference is that our study used ELISA to detect cytokines while Zheng and collaborators analyzed mRNA by RT-PCR. As the levels of mRNA induction found were rather low (fold change increase below 0.3), it is possible that protein detection by ELISA would have been below the detection limit as well. We are therefore proposing that hMDM generated from pure monocytes are not permissive to SARS-CoV-2 infection and do not mount inflammatory responses. This is in contrast to HCoV-229E and the TLR ligand controls. While future studies expanding to tissue macrophages are important, our results indicate that proinflammatory responses observed during COVID-19 may not be the result of macrophage infection but rather originate from other innate immune cells or a complex interaction between different immune cells which could include macrophages. Therefore, to understand these events more immune cells such as plasmacytoid dendritic cells that are at the frontline of the antiviral cytokine responses should be investigated.

In view of a potential link between ADE and inflammation during COVID-19 in the presence of antibodies, we tested this hypothesis using hMDM. With the selected sera from convalescent COVID-19 patients and the described conditions, even at very high serum dilutions and with sera that had low levels of neutralizing antibodies, we did not find evidence for antibody mediated enhancement of macrophage infection or pro-inflammatory cytokine responses. Interestingly, sera of COVID-19 convalescent patients showed cross-reactivity to SARS-CoV (Zettl et al., 2020), despite that the sera did not enhance infection of hMDM by this virus. This is in line with a previous report showing that the presence of cross-reacting antibodies against SARS-CoV-2, originating from previous endemic coronavirus infections, were not linked with more severe COVID-19 (Ng et al., 2020). Furthermore, in vaccination/challenge experiments carried out in macaques no signs of enhanced disease were detected (Gao et al., 2020; Yu et al., 2020). Finally, COVID-19 patients treated with plasma transfusion from convalescent patients did not show signs of disease aggravation (Casadevall and Pirofski, 2020; Joyner et al., 2020). Altogether, these data are in line with our findings, demonstrating that hMDM are not infected or activated by SARS-CoV-2 neither by direct contact nor mediated by antibodies from convalescent COVID-19 patients. Although the lack of hMDM infection by SARS-CoV and SARS-CoV-2 provides evidence of a lack of ADE, our study cannot exclude ADE effects on other FcR-expressing cells as well as a possible role of the complement system or T-cell mediated inflammation.

AUTHOR CONTRIBUTIONS

OG-N, PV'K, and AS: conceptualization. OG-N, PV'K, FZ, GZ, VT and AS: methodology. OG-N, PV'K and FZ: investigation. OG-N, PV'K, FZ and AS: formal analysis. AS: supervision. OG-N and AS: writing–original draft. OG-N, PV'K, FZ, GZ, VT and AS: writing–review and editing. All authors contributed to the article and approved the submitted version.

ACKNOWLEDGMENTS

We would like to thank all members of the IVI and for their support and helpful discussions. We are grateful to Daniela Niemeyer, Marcel Müller, and Christian Drosten (Charité, Berlin, Germany) for providing the viruses and to the Swiss Transfusion SRC (Swiss Red Cross) Inc. (Regional transfusion blood service, Bern, Switzerland) for providing human buffy coats. OGN was supported by the Swiss National Foundation grant 310030_192498.

SUPPLEMENTARY MATERIAL

Supplementary Figure 1 | Positive control experiment for ADE with hMDM. Serum from pig vaccinated with an experimental JEV vaccine (red) and naïve serum (black) were ten-fold diluted (from 1:10 to 1:10000) and incubated with JEV Laos at MOI of 1 TCID50/ml for 30, then immune complexes were incubated with hMDM for another 30 min, after wash and incubation for 24 h, infected cells were quantified by flow cytometry. Data from four independent experiments run in triplicates are shown. Each symbol represents the average value of infection in hMDM from a different donor. Statistically significant differences are indicated by asterisks (*$p < 0.05$, **$p \leq 0.002$, and ***$p \leq 0.001$).

REFERENCES

Antonsson, A., and Johansson, P. J. H. (2001). Binding of human and animal immunoglobulins to the IgG Fc receptor induced by human cytomegalovirus. *J. Gen. Virol.* 82 (Pt 5), 1137–1145. doi: 10.1099/0022-1317-82-5-1137

Bruchez, A., Sha, K., Johnson, J., Chen, L., Stefani, C., McConnell, H., et al. (2020). MHC class II transactivator CIITA induces cell resistance to Ebola virus and SARS-like coronaviruses. *Science* 370 (6513), 241–247. doi: 10.1126/science.abb3753

Casadevall, A., and Pirofski, L. A. (2020). The convalescent sera option for containing COVID-19. *J. Clin. Invest.* 130 (4), 1545–1548. doi: 10.1172/JCI138003

Cho, K. J., and Roche, P. A. (2013). Regulation of MHC Class II-Peptide Complex Expression by Ubiquitination. *Front. Immunol.* 4, 69. doi: 10.3389/fimmu.2013.00369

Dijkman, R., Jebbink, M. F., Koekkoek, S. M., Deijs, M., Jonsdottir, H. R., Molenkamp, R., et al. (2013). Isolation and characterization of current human coronavirus strains in primary human epithelial cell cultures reveal differences in target cell tropism. *J. Virol.* 87 (11), 6081–6090. doi: 10.1128/JVI.03368-12

Funk, C. J., Wang, J., Ito, Y., Travanty, E. A., Voelker, D. R., Holmes, K. V., et al. (2012). Infection of human alveolar macrophages by human coronavirus strain 229E. *J. Gen. Virol.* 93 (Pt 3), 494–503. doi: 10.1099/vir.0.038414-0

Gao, Q., Bao, L., Mao, H., Wang, L., Xu, K., Yang, M., et al. (2020). Development of an inactivated vaccine candidate for SARS-CoV-2. *Science* 369 (6499), 77–81. doi: 10.1126/science.abc1932

Garcia-Nicolas, O., Ricklin, M. E., Liniger, M., Vielle, N. J., Python, S., Souque, P., et al. (2017). A Japanese Encephalitis Virus Vaccine Inducing Antibodies Strongly Enhancing In Vitro Infection Is Protective in Pigs. *Viruses* 9 (5). doi: 10.3390/v9050124

Hoffmann, M., Kleine-Weber, H., Schroeder, S., Kruger, N., Herrler, T., Erichsen, S., et al. (2020). SARS-CoV-2 Cell Entry Depends on ACE2 and TMPRSS2 and Is Blocked by a Clinically Proven Protease Inhibitor. *Cell* 181 (2), 271–280.e278. doi: 10.1016/j.cell.2020.02.052

Joyner, M. J., Wright, R. S., Fairweather, D., Senefeld, J. W., Bruno, K. A., Klassen, S. A., et al. (2020). Early safety indicators of COVID-19 convalescent plasma in 5000 patients. *J. Clin. Invest.* 130 (9), 4791–4797. doi: 10.1172/JCI140200

Lee, W. S., Wheatley, A. K., Kent, S. J., and DeKosky, B. J. (2020). Antibody-dependent enhancement and SARS-CoV-2 vaccines and therapies. *Nat. Microbiol.* 5 (10), 1185–1191. doi: 10.1038/s41564-020-00789-5

Ng, K. W., Faulkner, N., Cornish, G. H., Rosa, A., Harvey, R., Hussain, S., et al. (2020). Preexisting and de novo humoral immunity to SARS-CoV-2 in humans. *Science* 370 (6522), 1339–1343. doi: 10.1126/science.abe1107

Onabajo, O. O., Banday, A. R., Stanifer, M. L., Yan, W., Obajemu, A., Santer, D. M., et al. (2020). Interferons and viruses induce a novel truncated ACE2 isoform and not the full-length SARS-CoV-2 receptor. *Nat. Genet.* 52 (12), 1283–1293. doi: 10.1038/s41588-020-00731-9

Park, M. D. (2020). Macrophages: a Trojan horse in COVID-19? *Nat. Rev. Immunol.* 20 (6), 351. doi: 10.1038/s41577-020-0317-2

Rao, X., Deiuliis, J. A., Mihai, G., Varghese, J., Xia, C., Frieman, M. B., et al. (2018). Monocyte DPP4 Expression in Human Atherosclerosis Is Associated With Obesity and Dyslipidemia. *Diabetes Care* 41 (1), e1–e3. doi: 10.2337/dc17-0672

Rao, X., Zhao, S., Braunstein, Z., Mao, H., Razavi, M., Duan, L., et al. (2019). Oxidized LDL upregulates macrophage DPP4 expression via TLR4/TRIF/CD36 pathways. *EBioMedicine* 41, 50–61. doi: 10.1016/j.ebiom.2019.01.065

Rogers, T. F., Zhao, F., Huang, D., Beutler, N., Burns, A., He, W. T., et al. (2020). Isolation of potent SARS-CoV-2 neutralizing antibodies and protection from disease in a small animal model. *Science* 369 (6506), 956–963. doi: 10.1126/science.abc7520

Shang, J., Ye, G., Shi, K., Wan, Y., Luo, C., Aihara, H., et al. (2020). Structural basis of receptor recognition by SARS-CoV-2. *Nature* 581 (7807), 221–224. doi: 10.1038/s41586-020-2179-y

Song, X., Hu, W., Yu, H., Zhao, L., Zhao, Y., Zhao, X., et al. (2020). Little to no expression of angiotensin-converting enzyme-2 (ACE2) on most human peripheral blood immune cells but highly expressed on tissue macrophages. *Cytometry* 20, 1–10. doi: 10.1002/cyto.a.24285

Sungnak, W., Huang, N., Becavin, C., Berg, M., Queen, R., Litvinukova, M., et al. (2020). SARS-CoV-2 entry factors are highly expressed in nasal epithelial cells together with innate immune genes. *Nat. Med.* 26 (5), 681–687. doi: 10.1038/s41591-020-0868-6

Taylor, A., Foo, S. S., Bruzzone, R., Dinh, L. V., King, N. J., and Mahalingam, S. (2015). Fc receptors in antibody-dependent enhancement of viral infections. *Immunol. Rev.* 268 (1), 340–364. doi: 10.1111/imr.12367

Thiel, V., Herold, J., Schelle, B., and Siddell, S. G. (2001). Infectious RNA transcribed in vitro from a cDNA copy of the human coronavirus genome cloned in vaccinia virus. *J. Gen. Virol.* 82 (Pt 6), 1273–1281. doi: 10.1099/0022-1317-82-6-1273

Thiel, V., Ivanov, K. A., Putics, A., Hertzig, T., Schelle, B., Bayer, S., et al. (2003). Mechanisms and enzymes involved in SARS coronavirus genome expression. *J. Gen. Virol.* 84 (Pt 9), 2305–2315. doi: 10.1099/vir.0.19424-0

van Boheemen, S., de Graaf, M., Lauber, C., Bestebroer, T. M., Raj, V. S., Zaki, A. M., et al. (2012). Genomic characterization of a newly discovered coronavirus associated with acute respiratory distress syndrome in humans. *mBio* 3 (6). doi: 10.1128/mBio.00473-12

Wang, N., Shi, X., Jiang, L., Zhang, S., Wang, D., Tong, P., et al. (2013). Structure of MERS-CoV spike receptor-binding domain complexed with human receptor DPP4. *Cell Res.* 23 (8), 986–993. doi: 10.1038/cr.2013.92

Wolff, G., Limpens, R., Zevenhoven-Dobbe, J. C., Laugks, U., Zheng, S., de Jong, A. W. M., et al. (2020). A molecular pore spans the double membrane of the coronavirus replication organelle. *Science* 369 (6509), 1395–1398. doi: 10.1126/science.abd3629

Yeager, C. L., Ashmun, R. A., Williams, R. K., Cardellichio, C. B., Shapiro, L. H., Look, A. T., et al. (1992). Human aminopeptidase N is a receptor for human coronavirus 229E. *Nature* 357 (6377), 420–422. doi: 10.1038/357420a0

Yu, J., Tostanoski, L. H., Peter, L., Mercado, N. B., McMahan, K., Mahrokhian, S. H., et al. (2020). DNA vaccine protection against SARS-CoV-2 in rhesus macaques. *Science* 369 (6505), 806–811. doi: 10.1126/science.abc6284

Zettl, F., Meister, T. L., Vollmer, T., Fischer, B., Steinmann, J., Krawczyk, A., et al. (2020). Rapid Quantification of SARS-CoV-2-Neutralizing Antibodies Using Propagation-Defective Vesicular Stomatitis Virus Pseudotypes. *Vaccines (Basel)* 8 (3). doi: 10.3390/vaccines8030386

Zheng, J., Wang, Y., Li, K., Meyerholz, D. K., Allamargot, C., and Perlman, S. (2020). SARS-CoV-2-induced immune activation and death of monocyte-derived human macrophages and dendritic cells. *J. Infect. Dis.* 223 (5), 785–795. doi: 10.1093/infdis/jiaa753

Zhong, J., Rao, X., Deiuliis, J., Braunstein, Z., Narula, V., Hazey, J., et al. (2013). A potential role for dendritic cell/macrophage-expressing DPP4 in obesity-induced visceral inflammation. *Diabetes* 62 (1), 149–157. doi: 10.2337/db12-0230

Zhou, J., Chu, H., Li, C., Wong, B. H., Cheng, Z. S., Poon, V. K., et al. (2014). Active replication of Middle East respiratory syndrome coronavirus and aberrant induction of inflammatory cytokines and chemokines in human macrophages: implications for pathogenesis. *J. Infect. Dis.* 209 (9), 1331–1342. doi: 10.1093/infdis/jit504

4

The Unfolded Protein Response and Autophagy on the Crossroads of Coronaviruses Infections

Elisa B. Prestes[1], *Julia C. P. Bruno*[2], *Leonardo H. Travassos*[3] *and Leticia A. M. Carneiro*[2*]

[1] *Institut Necker Enfants Malades, Université Paris Descartes, Paris, France,* [2] *Laboratório de Inflamação e Imunidade, Instituto de Microbiologia Paulo de Goes, Universidade Federal do Rio de Janeiro, Rio de Janeiro, Brazil,* [3] *Laboratório de Imunoreceptores e Sinalização Celular, Instituto de Biofísica Carlos Chagas Filho, Universidade Federal do Rio de Janeiro, Rio de Janeiro, Brazil*

Correspondence:
Leticia A. M. Carneiro
leticiac@micro.ufrj.br

The ability to sense and adequately respond to variable environmental conditions is central for cellular and organismal homeostasis. Eukaryotic cells are equipped with highly conserved stress-response mechanisms that support cellular function when homeostasis is compromised, promoting survival. Two such mechanisms – the unfolded protein response (UPR) and autophagy – are involved in the cellular response to perturbations in the endoplasmic reticulum, in calcium homeostasis, in cellular energy or redox status. Each of them operates through conserved signaling pathways to promote cellular adaptations that include re-programming transcription of genes and translation of new proteins and degradation of cellular components. In addition to their specific functions, it is becoming increasingly clear that these pathways intersect in many ways in different contexts of cellular stress. Viral infections are a major cause of cellular stress as many cellular functions are coopted to support viral replication. Both UPR and autophagy are induced upon infection with many different viruses with varying outcomes – in some instances controlling infection while in others supporting viral replication and infection. The role of UPR and autophagy in response to coronavirus infection has been a matter of debate in the last decade. It has been suggested that CoV exploit components of autophagy machinery and UPR to generate double-membrane vesicles where it establishes its replicative niche and to control the balance between cell death and survival during infection. Even though the molecular mechanisms are not fully elucidated, it is clear that UPR and autophagy are intimately associated during CoV infections. The current SARS-CoV-2 pandemic has brought renewed interest to this topic as several drugs known to modulate autophagy – including chloroquine, niclosamide, valinomycin, and spermine – were proposed as therapeutic options. Their efficacy is still debatable, highlighting the need to better understand the molecular interactions between CoV, UPR and autophagy.

Keywords: coronavirus, autophagy, unfolded protein response, integrated stress response, host-pathogen interaction

INTRODUCTION

From single to multicellular, every living organism is frequently exposed to variable environmental conditions – including extremes of temperature, nutrient deprivation, irradiation, hypoxia, infections, and others – that can result in cell damage and/or dysfunction (Galluzzi et al., 2018). Eukaryotic cells have evolved mechanisms to cope with the stress generated by these conditions and support cellular functions, thereby maintaining microenvironmental and organismal homeostasis (Galluzzi et al., 2018). Such mechanisms include the DNA damage response (Jackson and Bartek, 2009), mitochondrial stress signaling (Chang et al., 2017), autophagy (Galluzzi et al., 2017) and the unfolded protein response (UPR), which is a component of the integrated stress response (Galluzzi et al., 2018) (ISR). The ISR is an evolutionarily conserved intracellular signaling network that can be initiated by several types of stress and converges to a common signaling hub – the phosphorylation of the α-subunit of the eukaryotic translation initiation factor 2, eIF2α (Costa-Mattioli and Walter, 2020). A family of four eIF2α-kinases is capable of sensing alterations in cellular homeostasis and respond by phosphorylating eIF2α: (i) double-stranded RNA (dsRNA)-dependent protein kinase (PKR) that is activated mainly by dsRNA during viral infection but also by oxidative and endoplasmic reticulum (ER) stress, growth factor deprivation, cytokines, bacterial infections, and ribotoxic stress (García et al., 2006); (ii) PKR-like ER protein kinase (PERK), which senses ER stress and also perturbations in calcium homeostasis, cellular energy or redox status (McQuiston and Diehl, 2017); (iii) heme-regulated eIF2α kinase (HRI), a sensor for low levels of intracellular heme as well as the formation of cytosolic protein aggregates, arsenite-induced oxidative stress, heat shock, nitric oxide, 26S proteasome inhibition, and osmotic stress (Girardin et al., 2020); and (iv) general control non-derepressible 2 (GCN2) that is activated in response to amino acid deprivation when it binds to deacylated transfer RNAs (tRNAs) *via* histidyl-tRNA synthetase-related domain (Battu et al., 2017). Not only do each of these pathways initiate crucial re-programming of the cell by modulating transcription of key genes and translation of new proteins, they also intersect with other stress-response pathways to restore homeostasis. Although ISR is primarily a homeostatic-preserving program by which cells adapt to survive, severe or long-lasting stress can induce cell death signaling by regulating autophagy or apoptosis.

The UPR is the cellular response to disturbances in the ER that ensues when its folding capacity is exceeded and unfolded proteins accumulate (Hetz, 2012). The ER is the primary site for the synthesis and folding of secreted and transmembrane proteins in eukaryotic cells. A myriad of environmental conditions (including nutrient deprivation, hypoxia, and loss of calcium homeostasis) can significantly alter the amount of proteins entering the ER, leading to UPR activation by one or more of three conserved ER-stress sensors: PERK, X-box-binding protein 1 (XBP-1) and activating transcriptional factor-6 (ATF-6) (Siqueira et al., 2018). These sensors display ER luminal domains capable of sensing modifications in the ER environment and cytosolic domains that trigger signaling pathways, resulting in reduced protein synthesis and increased ER folding capacity to ultimately preserve ER functions and cell viability. In addition, proteins that fail to correctly fold can be deployed to the ER distal secretory pathway, the ER-associated protein degradation (ERAD) pathway of the UPR (Hwang and Qi, 2018). In this case, misfolded proteins are retro-translocated from the ER back to the cytosol for degradation. Finally, in case of persistent stress, the UPR can initiate cell death programs.

Autophagy is another highly conserved process in which eukaryotic cells rely on to maintain cell homeostasis – in this case, by degrading and recycling cytoplasmic components, such as defective organelles or protein aggregates (Mizushima et al., 2008; Klionsky et al., 2014; Siqueira et al., 2018). The autophagosomes display a characteristic double-membrane structure that sequesters cytosolic targets, known as cargos, for degradation. Autophagy is carried out by at least 30 conserved ATG proteins divided into macromolecular complexes. Other hundreds of proteins have been shown to modulate this process in different contexts, including the master homeostatic regulator mechanistic target of rapamycin (mTOR). The formation of autophagosomes is divided into three successive stages: (i) initiation, which involves the ULK1-ATG13-FIP200 complex; (ii) membrane nucleation, that is dependent on the Beclin1 (BECN1)-ATG14-PI3K complex, and (iii) membrane elongation that requires ATG8/LC3 lipidation. LC3 lipidation is a hallmark of autophagy and is established by a covalent linkage of cytosolic LC3 to the lipid phosphatidylethanolamine on the surface of the autophagosome, which enables autophagosome elongation and recruitment of autophagy targets (Reggiori and Klionsky, 2005; Carneiro and Travassos, 2013). The entire process, which has been named autophagic flux, is completed when autophagosomes fuse with lysosomes and the cargo is degraded in autophagolysosomes.

There are many parallels between ISR/UPR and mTOR/autophagy pathways, as they are both highly conserved signaling modules that regulate essential metabolic circuits, both in homeostatic and stress conditions. Also, the ER and autophagosomes are intrinsically linked since the former seems to be an essential source of lipids for the formation of the latter, and also provides a site for ATG14 anchoring, which plays a crucial role in recruiting the BECN1-ATG14-PI3K complex from the cytosol to sites of autophagosome initiation in response to starvation (Diao et al., 2015; Tan et al., 2016). Besides, localized phosphorylation of lipids by PI3K generates ER domains called omegasomes enriched in phosphatidylinositol-3-phosphate (Ptdlns3P) that recruit Ptdlns3P-effector proteins to generate sites for autophagosome nucleation and expansion (Mercer et al., 2018). In the context of ER stress, autophagy can be accessory by participating in the degradation of protein aggregates through ERAD (II), which is an alternative to the classic ubiquitin-proteasome ERAD, designated ERAD (I), that clears most soluble misfolded proteins (Rashid et al., 2015).

Both UPR and autophagy are often observed during viral infections, in some cases as a host cell defense mechanism limiting viral replication and, in others, contributing to viral replication and establishment of infection (Blázquez et al., 2014; Chan, 2014; Xiao and Cai, 2020). Viral infections are a major cause of cellular stress as viruses are able to manipulate several cellular processes to complete their replicative cycle (Ríos-Ocampo et al., 2018). In particular, the ability to divert the cell protein translation machinery to produce massive amounts of viral proteins profoundly impacts ER physiology (Gale et al., 2000). Furthermore, plus-stranded RNA viruses can pose an additional challenge for ER homeostasis as they synthesize their genome in association with extensive virus-induced rearrangements of intracellular membranes - including ER, endosomes or mitochondria (Romero-Brey and Bartenschlager, 2014). Included in this group are many viruses that cause disease in animals and humans, such as flaviviruses (for example, Dengue virus, Zika virus, Yellow fever virus, and West Nile virus), alphaviruses (for example, Chikungunya virus and Mayaro virus), and coronaviruses (for example, SARS-CoV, MERS-CoV, and SARS-CoV-2) (Jheng et al., 2014; Lee et al., 2018; Mehrbod et al., 2019). In the following sections of this review, we will discuss how UPR signaling and autophagy intersect in homeostatic conditions and in circumstances of mild and severe cell stress. In the final sections, we will take this discussion to the context of coronaviruses infections and highlight how these stress response pathways interfere with their replicative cycle.

UPR AND AUTOPHAGY IN HOMEOSTATIC AND STRESS CONDITIONS

Initially, PERK, IRE1, and ATF6 were considered to be active only when protein misfolding was detected in the cell. However, the identification of novel binding partners for these proteins suggest they participate in protein complexes that are important for regulating mitochondrial bioenergetics, cytoskeleton dynamics and membrane contacts (Hetz and Papa, 2018). For example, both PERK and IRE1 are present in mitochondria-associated membranes (MAMs) and the latter mediates the transfer of Ca^{2+} from the ER to mitochondria, thus regulating mitochondrial bioenergetics and physiology (MAMs) (Vliet et al., 2017; Urra et al., 2018; Carreras-Sureda et al., 2019). The absence of IRE1 in MAMs led to AMP-activated protein kinase (AMPK) phosphorylation and activation of autophagy, as determined by increased basal levels of LC3B, a key component of the autophagosomal membrane (Carreras-Sureda et al., 2019). PERK and IRE1 also directly interact with components of the actin cytoskeleton. PERK regulates intracellular Ca^{2+} fluxes by forming dimers upon detection of increased cytosolic Ca^{2+} levels and then interacting with filamin A to reorganize the cytoskeleton and contact sites between the ER and the plasma membrane (Vliet et al., 2017). Likewise, the dimerization of IRE1 promotes its interaction with filamin A and controls cell migration (Urra et al., 2018). Together, these recent studies show that, in addition to their role in UPR, dimerization of PERK and IRE1 also participate in cell homeostatic pathways unrelated to ER stress.

In conditions where misfolded proteins accumulate in the ER lumen, chaperone binding immunoglobulin protein (BiP/GRP78) is recruited and thus detached from the luminal domains of the three ER sensors to which it was bound, releasing PERK and IRE1 from their inactive monomeric states and allowing ATF6 to transit to the Golgi (Smith and Wilkinson, 2017) (**Figure 1**). Activation of the UPR triggers two distinct events to mitigate protein misfolding: a quick reaction that involves phosphorylation of targets to immediately reduce protein synthesis and increase protein degradation; and a more durable response consisting of transcriptional upregulation of hundreds of target genes to restore proteostasis (Hetz and Papa, 2018).

An instantaneous reaction to ER stress is initiated by dimerized PERK, which phosphorylates eIF2α in the cytosol leading to global attenuation of protein synthesis by forming an inhibitory complex with eIF2B that restricts its ability to bind to Met-tRNA initiator (Adomavicius et al., 2019). Paradoxically, at the same time, it initiates the translation of specific mRNAs that contain internal ribosomal entry sites. These include ATF4, which induces genes involved in redox homeostasis, amino acid metabolism, protein synthesis, apoptosis, and autophagy (Hetz et al., 2020). Under hypoxia, ATF4 promotes upregulation of LC3B through direct binding to a cyclic AMP response element-binding site in the *LC3B* promoter (Rzymski et al., 2010). This process likely has a protective role for the cell, as inhibition of autophagy, under those circumstances, led to metabolic consequences of hypoxic stress (Rzymski et al., 2010). ATF4 also induces the expression of CHOP and, together, they transcriptionally activate genes involved in autophagy. These include genes encoding proteins involved in the formation and maturation of the autophagosome, such as *Becn1* (which encodes BECN1) and genes from the ubiquitin-like protein (Ubl) system, like *Atg12* and *Map1-lc3b* (for LC3B) (B'chir et al., 2013). Genes encoding the activating enzyme (*Atg7*), the target of ATG12 attachment (*Atg5*), as well as genes encoding cargo receptors that are involved in specific degradation of ubiquitinated substrates, like *p62*, are also upregulated by the eIF2α/ATF4/CHOP branch (B'chir et al., 2013). Finally, protein synthesis is restored when eIF2α is dephosphorylated by protein phosphatase 1 (PP1) regulatory subunit GADD34, which is also induced by ATF4 when ER stress is resolved (Hetz et al., 2020).

ER stress also results in dimerization of the transmembrane protein kinase/endoribonuclease IRE1, which autophosphorylates to switch on its RNase activity that consists of excising a short 26-nucleotide intron from the mRNA encoding transcription factor XBP1 (Hetz et al., 2020). This processing generates the spliced *Xbp1* mRNA, which is ultimately translated into the transcription factor XBP1s that upregulates genes involved in ER protein translocation, folding and secretion, as well as degradation of misfolded proteins mainly by ERAD (Hetz et al., 2020). IRE1 also induces a process known as regulated IRE1-dependent decay (RIDD), in which IRE1 cleaves and leads to the degradation of a small set of mRNAs or miRNAs (Hetz et al., 2020) (**Figure 1**). IRE1 activates autophagy in a more indirect manner, by interacting with adapter proteins like tumor necrosis factor (TNF) receptor- associated factor 2 (TRAF2) and apoptosis signal-regulating kinase 1 (ASK1), forming the IRE1/TRAF2/

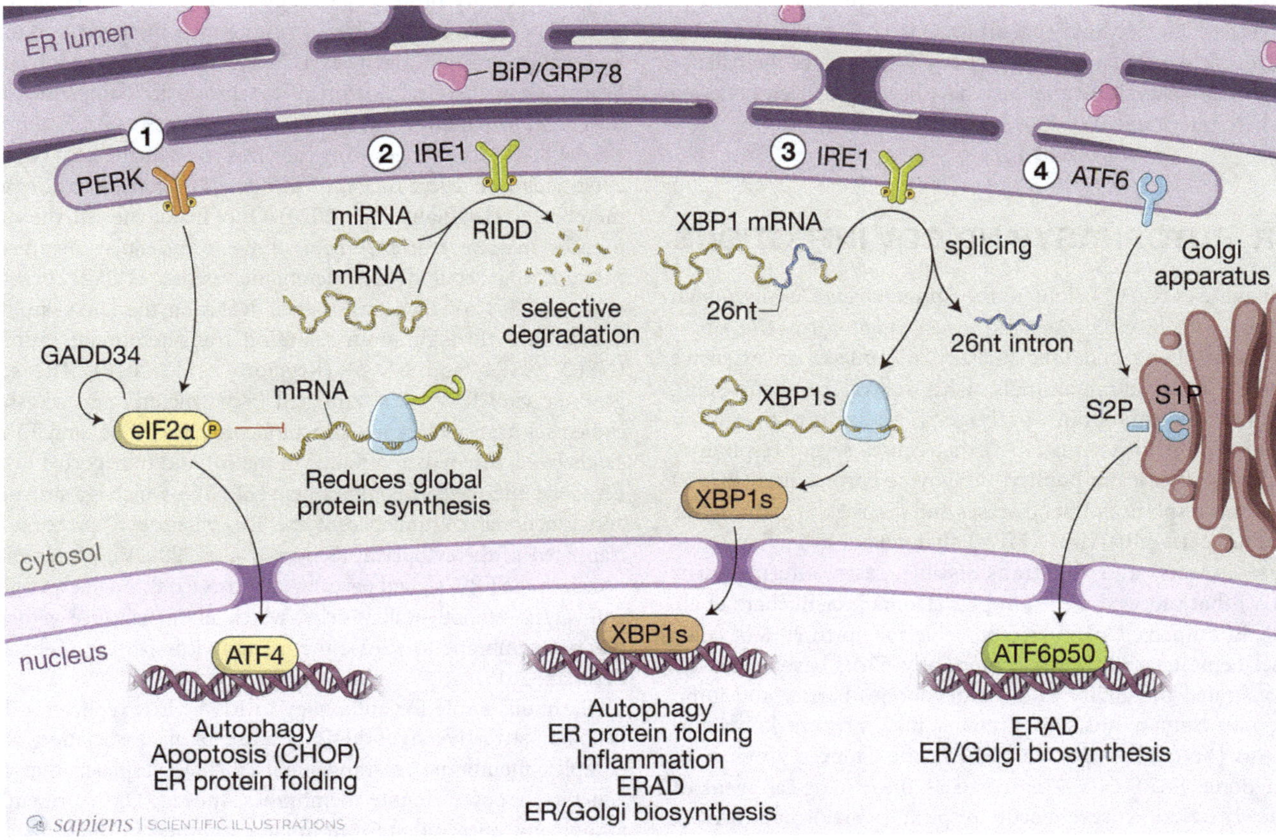

FIGURE 1 | The three branches of the unfolded protein response (UPR). When misfolded proteins accumulate in the endoplasmic reticulum (ER) lumen, chaperone binding immunoglobulin protein (BiP/GRP78) is detached from the luminal domains of the three ER sensors to which it was bound, allowing PKR-like ER protein kinase (PERK) and inositol-requiring protein-1 (IRE1) to form homodimers and activating transcriptional factor-6 (ATF6) to transit to the Golgi. (1) PERK phosphorylates the α-subunit of the eukaryotic translation initiation factor 2 (eIF2α), resulting in a global reduction of protein synthesis while still maintaining translation of a few key proteins, such as activating transcription factor 4 (ATF4), which induces expression of genes involved in redox homeostasis, amino acid metabolism, protein synthesis, autophagy and apoptosis, such as the transcription factor C/EBP homologous protein (CHOP). Protein synthesis is restored when eIF2α is dephosphorylated by protein phosphatase 1 (PP1) regulatory subunit GADD34, which is also induced by ATF4 when ER stress is resolved. (2) IRE1 autophosphorylates to switch on its RNase activity, inducing a process known as regulated IRE1-dependent decay (RIDD), in which IRE1 cleaves and leads to the selective degradation of a small set of mRNAs or miRNAs. (3) IRE1 also excises a short 26-nucleotide intron from the mRNA encoding transcription factor X-box-binding protein 1 (XBP1), generating the spliced *Xbp1* mRNA, which is ultimately translated into the transcription factor XBP1s that, like ATF4, upregulates genes involved in multiple cell signaling pathways, such as ER-associated protein degradation (ERAD). (4) Full length ATF6 translocates from the ER to the Golgi, where it is cleaved by site-1 protease (S1P) and site-2 protease (S2P). This releases a cytosolic fragment which then transits to the nucleus, transcription factor ATF6p50, which drives a transcriptional program to reestablish homeostasis.

ASK1 complex that activates c-Jun N-terminal kinase (JNK). JNK phosphorylates transcription factor c-Jun, which induces expression of *Becn1* (Senft and Ronai, 2015; Liu et al., 2020). Although activation of JNK by IRE1 promotes, at first, this protective autophagic pathway, during prolonged ER stress, it can turn into autophagy-dependent cell death (Liu et al., 2020; Lindner et al., 2020).

Upon sensing ER stress, full-length ATF6 (ATF6p90) translocates from the ER to the Golgi apparatus, where it is cleaved by site-1 protease (S1P) and site-2 protease (S2P) and releases a cytosolic fragment containing a basic leucine zipper (bZIP) transcription factor, ATF6p50, which then transits to the nucleus (Hetz et al., 2020) (**Figure 1**). ATF6p50 and XBP1s act simultaneously and may form heterodimers, driving specific gene expression programs that bring about chaperone activation and ER/Golgi biogenesis to increase the cell secretory capacity (Shoulders et al., 2013; Hetz et al., 2020).

As we have mentioned above, the type, intensity, and duration of circumstances that induce ER stress are critical in determining the cell fate upon UPR activation. Initially, the UPR attempts to resolve the misfolded protein build-up, but persistent and unresolved ER stress is bound to cause cell death by inducing apoptosis (Yao et al., 2020). For example, the different outcomes resulting from ATF4 activation make PERK and phosphorylated eIF2α crucial for determining the cell fate (Liu et al., 2020). Regarding the XBP-1 branch, while activation of *Xbp1* mRNA splicing is transient and attenuated after prolonged stimulation, the activity of RIDD can be sustained over time and eventually contribute to cell death (Hetz and Papa, 2018). It is important to note that although a variety of mechanisms by which UPR promotes apoptosis have been described, each UPR pathway contribution to this outcome is modest, suggesting the existence of cell-type specific networks that arbitrate the cell fate under severe ER stress. The mechanisms by which UPR regulates the balance between cell survival and apoptosis have been extensively reviewed elsewhere (Hetz and Papa, 2018; Hetz et al., 2020).

UPR, AUTOPHAGY AND COV INFECTIONS

Coronaviruses (CoV) belong to the *Coronaviridae* family, which together with *Roniviridae* and *Arteviridae* form the order Nidovirales (Fung and Liu, 2019a). CoV infects an extensive range of birds and mammals, with several of them being economically important pathogens, including the avian infectious bronchitis virus (IBV) that causes severe respiratory and kidney diseases in poultry; the bovine coronavirus (BCoV) that causes respiratory tract diseases and diarrhea in cattle; feline infectious peritonitis virus (FIPV) that causes a fatal systemic disease in cats; and the transmissible gastroenteritis virus (TGEV) that causes diarrhea in pigs (Domańska-Blicharz et al., 2020). In humans, CoV are responsible for up to 30% of colds (Mesel-Lemoine et al., 2012). Importantly, CoVs have repeatedly demonstrated the ability to cross the species barrier and jump from non-human hosts to humans in a process known as zoonosis (Ye et al., 2020). In 2003, in the Chinese province of Guangdong, SARS-CoV-2 emerged as the etiological agent of the newly described severe acute respiratory syndrome (SARS), with high mortality rate. It was suggested that SARS-CoV was originated from bats and likely jumped to humans *via* some intermediate host (probably, palm civets) (Cheng et al., 2007). Nine years later, another zoonosis, this time originating from dromedaries, was detected in Saudi Arabia and named Middle-East respiratory syndrome (MERS), caused by MERS-CoV (Mohd et al., 2016). In neither case, the fear of a pandemic was confirmed. More recently, however, another SARS-inducing CoV - now named SARS-CoV-2 – emerged in Wuhan (China) to cause a pandemic that, to date, has infected 135 million people and killed more than 2,92 million people around the world (https://github.com/CSSEGISandData/COVID-19).

COV REPLICATION: ER, AUTOPHAGY AND THE ORIGINS OF DMVs

CoVs are enveloped positive-sense RNA viruses (Chen et al., 2020). The first two-thirds of the genome consists of 2 large overlapping open reading frames, which encode 16 non-structural proteins (NSPs), including proteases, RNA-dependent RNA polymerase (prRdRp), RNA helicase, primase, and others, that form the viral replication and transcription complexes (RTCs), a platform to propagate viral mRNAs. The remaining portion of the genome includes interspersed open reading frames for the structural proteins – envelope (E), membrane (M), nucleocapsid (N), and the highly glycosylated spike (S) protein that projects from the viral envelope - as well as several accessory proteins generally nonessential for replication in tissue culture but capable of suppressing immune responses and enhancing pathogenesis (Ulferts et al., 2009). Infection begins when the viral S protein attaches to its complementary host receptor, angiotensin I converting enzyme 2 (ACE2) in the case of SARS-CoV-2, allowing the virus to enter the host cells by endocytosis or direct fusion of the viral envelope with the host membrane (Hoffmann et al., 2020). Once inside the cell, the virus induces massive rearrangement of the intracellular membrane network to generate double-membrane vesicles (DMVs) (Prentice et al., 2003). CoV then targets their RTCs on the DMV-limiting membranes through multi-spanning transmembrane proteins (NSP3, NSP4, and NSP6) (Reggiori et al., 2010). The sub-genomic viral RNAs are translated into structural and accessory proteins – transmembrane structural proteins (S, M, and E) are synthesized, inserted, and folded in the ER and transported to the ER-Golgi intermediate compartment (ERGIC), which is a structural and functional continuance of the ER, whereas N proteins are translated in the cytoplasm (Senger et al., 2020). Virion assembly occurs in the ERGIC, and particles are exported through a secretory pathway in smooth-wall vesicles, which ultimately fuse with the plasma membrane to release the mature virus particle (Fehr and Perlman, 2015).

Early on, a role for autophagy in RNA virus replication has been an attractive hypothesis because of its association with complex membrane rearrangements in the cytoplasm that can generate opposed double membranes. Indeed, DMVs resemble autophagosomes and are seen in large numbers in the cytosol of CoV-infected cells. In addition to DMVs, CoV replication complexes share other features of autophagosomes such as co-localization with multiple organelle markers and the acquisition of lysosomal markers throughout infection (Prentice et al., 2003). There have been different perspectives on the origin of CoV-induced DMVs – late endosomes, autophagosomes, and early secretory pathways have all been implicated as the membrane source of DMVs (Chen et al., 2020; V'kovski et al., 2020; Wolff et al., 2020). The major difficulty in solving this issue has been the lack or undetectable levels of marker proteins of subcellular organelles (Reggiori et al., 2011). Accumulating data now indicate that ER-derived membranes are the major source for DMVs formation: (i) several viral proteins, including proteins that are part of the RTCs such as NSP3 and NSP4, are glycosylated in the ER; (ii) also ectopically expressed NSP4 is found in the ER and moves to DMVs upon viral infection; (iii) blocking early steps of the secretory pathway abolishes CoV replication; (iv) electron tomography of cells infected with either SARS-CoV or mouse hepatitis virus (MHV) showed that DMVs are part of a reticulovesicular network of modified ER membranes with double-stranded RNA (dsRNA) inside; and, (v) the subunit of the ER translocon, Sec1α, is found on rearranged membranes during SARS-CoV infection (Knoops et al., 2008; Angelini et al., 2013). Finally, as we will discuss below, recent studies have suggested that DMVs biogenesis might be linked to ERAD tuning pathway. More recently, an effort to establish a compendium of host factors required for CoV infection, including SARS-CoV-2 and other seasonal CoV, identified an absolute requirement for the TMEM41B for infection with all the CoV tested. TMEM41B is a ER-transmembrane protein involved in autophagy, which, again, argues in favor of a role of the ER and components of the autophagy pathway in DMVs biogenesis (Schneider et al., 2021). Thus, CoV replication is structurally and functionally linked to the ER and autophagy.

AUTOPHAGY: IS IT REQUIRED OR A CONCOMITANT EVENT WITH COV REPLICATION?

Accumulated evidence has shown that CoVs interact differentially with components of the autophagic pathway with potential for both utilization of its components for replication and attenuation of autophagy but full understanding of their link to autophagy still awaits further investigation.

MHV is considered a prototype CoV and has been extensively used to investigate mechanistic details of the replication and assembly of CoV *in vitro* and *in vivo*. Early studies have shown that MHV induced the formation of DMVs derived from autophagosomes and that proteins known to localize to replication complexes (p22 and N) colocalize with LC3^{+} foci in infected cells throughout the entire course of infection. MHV-induced autophagy was impaired in murine embryonic stem cells lacking ATG5, resulting in decreased viral yield (Prentice et al., 2003). In addition, *atg5* knockout cells displayed a deranged morphology of the membranes, particularly hyper-swollen RER containing multiple vesicles, but no autophagosome formation suggesting that the RER might be the source of membranes for replication complexes. The reconstitution of the *atg5* knockout with an expression plasmid restored viral yields implying the autophagy is required for viral replication (Prentice et al., 2003). Even though the molecular mechanisms were not determined, the authors hypothesized that the formation of DMVs could serve to sequester and concentrate viral replicases that were translated in the ER and that MHV may have evolved to utilize a preexisting cellular process – autophagy – to maximize replication efficiency. In contrast, Zhao et al. (2007) showed that in bone-marrow derived macrophages (BMMs) or primary mouse embryonic fibroblasts (MEFs) neither ATG5 nor an intact autophagic flux were required for MHV replication or release (Zhao et al., 2007). Considering viruses tropism to different cell types and the different permissiveness for viral replication among these cell types, it is possible that these discrepancies could be, at least in part, related to the different experimental models used (**Figure 2**).

Following studies suggested that CoV might not require an intact autophagic flux to replicate but still exploit components of the autophagic pathway to enhance infection. In this sense, another gene essential for autophagy, *atg7*, was shown to be dispensable for the formation of MHV-induced DMVs and viral replication in MEFs (Reggiori et al., 2010). Nevertheless, it was observed that endogenous nonlipidated LC3 extensively colocalized with the DMV protein markers, NSP2 and NSP3, and that downregulation of LC3, but not inactivation of host cell autophagy, protected cells from CoV infection as a result of defects in DMVs biogenesis. Of note, ectopically expressed GFP-LC3, which is widely used to track autophagosomes, colocalized with neither NSP2 nor NSP3 but ectopically expressed C-terminally HA-tagged, nonlipidable LC3 did (Reggiori et al., 2010). This observation distinguishes DMVs from autophagosomes as LC3 lipidation, which is indispensable for autophagosome elongation, is not required for its association with DMVs. This feature is reminiscent of ERAD tuning vesicles known as EDEMosomes. Post-translational regulation of ERAD factors contained in the ER lumen by rapid and selective removal, which is critical for ER homeostasis, is known as ERAD tuning. In addition to chaperones and folding enzymes, ER also contains ERAD factors that recognize non-native proteins, extract them from the folding machinery and ensure their transport for proteasomal degradation. The ERAD regulators EDEM1, OS-9, and others are removed from the ER in vesicles that display LC3-I in their limiting membrane – the EDEMosomes - and degraded by endo-lysosomal enzymes. Based on this, the authors propose a mechanism by which MHV hijacks the ERAD tuning pathway to coopt cellular membranes for DMV formation and support viral RTCs. Indeed, MHV infection caused accumulation of EDEM1 and OS-9 in the DMVs, and this was independent of autophagy as *atg7* deletion did not affect the intracellular levels of EDEM1 as it did those of p62, an autophagy substrate. Importantly, viral-coopting of this cellular process blocks the normal clearance of these vesicles as illustrated by data showing that, in non-infected cells, EDEM1 has a half-life of about 1 hour but upon MHV infection, is still found after several hours of infection even with virus-induced host translational shutoff, indicating that there is actually defective clearance of EDEM1 in infected cells.

A screen using individual IBV non-structural proteins for their ability to induce autophagy showed that NSP6 was located to the ER and induced ER puncta containing DFCP1 and ATG5 (Cottam et al., 2011). NSP-6-induced autophagosomes required ATG5 and the recruitment of lipidated LC3-II, features of classic autophagosomes generated in the ER *via* omegasomes rather than EDEMosomes. Furthermore, class 3 PI3 kinase activity was also required, indicating PtdIns(3)P are generated from ER lipids to build phagophores. In the IBV model, the infection or ectopic expression of NSP6 induces a complete autophagic flux as the autophagosomes are fused with Lamp1-positive vesicles, which show their ability to deliver the cargo to the lysosomes. However, an intact autophagy flux is not required for viral replication as this was unaffected by pharmacological autophagy inhibitors or silencing of ATG5. NSP6 orthologs from other CoV (SARS-CoV and MHV) also localized to the ER, from where they generate autophagosomes *via* an omegasome intermediate. Targeting NSP6 to the ER resulted in partial XBP1 splicing and undetectable increase in CHOP expression, indicating that ER stress is limited and not mechanistically involved in autophagy induction (Cottam et al., 2014). It would be interesting to investigate other branches of the UPR since, as we mentioned

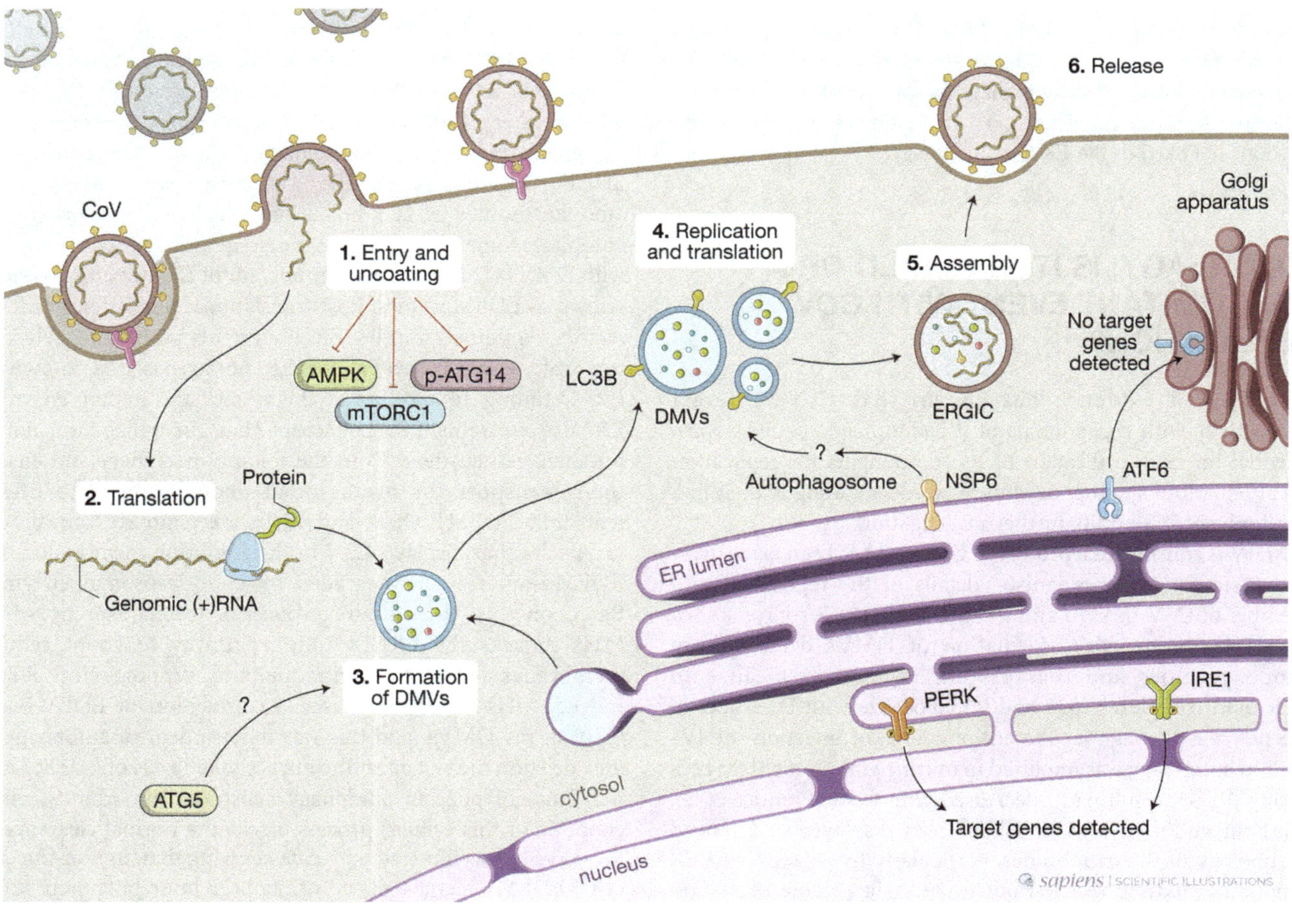

FIGURE 2 | Unfolded protein response (UPR), autophagy and coronavirus (CoV) infections. This figure represents data obtained by using different cell models infected by CoV viruses mouse hepatites virus (MHV), infectious bronchitis virus (IBV), SARS-CoV or SARS-CoV-2. CoV infection begins when the viral S protein attaches to its complementary host receptor, allowing the virus to enter the host cells by endocytosis or direct fusion of the viral envelop with the host membrane. The process of SARS-CoV2 virus entry and uncoating (1) downregulates AMPK and reduces phosphorylation of ATG14, disrupting the autophagy flux, while simultaneously inhibiting mTORC1, which promotes autophagy. Once inside the cell, the viral positive-sense RNA is translated (2) and the virus induces massive rearrangement of the intracellular membrane network to generate double membrane vesicles (DMVs) (3). CoV-induced DMVs may originate from late endosomes, autophagosomes or vesicles from the early secretory pathway. MHV-induced autophagy was impaired in cells lacking ATG5, which displayed a deranged morphology of the membranes and decreased viral yield. Nonlipidated LC3 extensively colocalizes with DMV protein markers and downregulation of LC3 protects cells from CoV infection as result of defects in DMVs biogenesis. CoV replication occurs within DMVs and transmembrane structural proteins (S, M and E) are synthesized in the ER (4). Non-structural protein NSP6 from IBV, MHV and SARS-CoV are localized in the ER and participate in autophagosome formation *via* omegasomes, which could be used for DMV formation. Finally, new viral particles are transported to the ER-Golgi intermediate compartment (ERGIC) for assembly (5) and exported through secretory pathway in smooth-wall vesicles, which ultimately fuse with the plasma membrane to release the mature virus (6). A high demand for membranes for DMV formation and virion exocytosis contributes to ER stress. MHV activates PERK/eIF2α and IRE1 and target genes from these two branches are detected upon infection. Cleavage of ATF6 can also be observed but no target genes are detected subsequently.

above, individual pathways might not represent the whole picture.

The same group investigated the characteristics of the autophagosomes induced by ectopic expression of NSP6 from several CoV (SARS-CoV, MHV or IBV) as well as IBV infection (Cottam et al., 2014). All of them induced the formation of a significant number of autophagosomes that were significantly smaller (< 0.5 μm diameter) than the ones induced by starvation (> 1.0 μm). Even with concomitant signals for autophagy activation, such as starvation or mTOR inhibition, IBV infection or IBV NSP6 ectopic expression limited expansion of omegasomes, thereby limiting the expansion of autophagosomes. The authors showed that mTOR was missing from the surface of lysosomes of cells expressing NSP6 even when cultured in nutrient media and suggested that NSP6 prevents mTOR association with lysosomes limiting the formation of large autophagosolysosomes. It still to be addressed if NSP6 acts by directly interacting with other proteins at the surface of lysosomes or indirectly by affecting other signaling pathways. Although smaller, NSP6-induced autophagosomes could still take up SQSTM1/p62 and deliver it to lysosomes. Additional work will be necessary to understand if limiting autophagosome expansion brings any advantage for CoV replication. Given that the size of DMVs is much smaller than what is observed in starvation-induced autophagosomes, the authors hypothesize that these smaller autophagosomes could be used to generate DMVs (Cottam et al., 2014).

In contrast to the studies above that suggest a positive correlation between the induction of autophagy and CoV replication, other studies have proposed an inhibitory effect of CoV on the autophagic process. For instance, MERS-CoV seems to establish a tug of war in which at the same time that autophagy limits viral propagation, the virus is able to impair autophagic flux by activation the E3-ligase S-phase kinase-associates protein 2 (SKP2) (Gassen et al., 2019). SPK2 acts *via* FKBP5, a stress-regulated protein involved in numerous pathways through scaffolding regulatory protein interactions and the involvement of AKT1 and PHLPP. Activated phosphorylated SPK2 polyubiquitinates the critical autophagy initiating protein BECN1 for proteasomal degradation. Conversely, pharmacological inhibition of SPK2 stabilizes BECN1, enhances autophagy, and restricts MERS-CoV propagation. Altogether these results indicate that autophagy is a relevant anti-MERS-CoV mechanism. Indeed, knocking down ATG5 resulted in a 52-fold increase in the formation of MERS-CoV particles (Gassen et al., 2019). More recently, the same authors have shown that similar to MERS-CoV, SARS-CoV-2 strongly reduced the autophagic flux in two different cell lines – the human bronchial epithelial cells NCI-H1299 and Vero cells (Gassen et al., 2020). This later study showed that the phosphorylated active forms of AMPK, AMPK substrates (LXRXX), AMPH downstream targets (TSC2 and ULK1) and mTORC1 were all downregulated upon SARS-CoV-2 infection. Concomitantly, increased levels of phosphorylated AKT1 were observed, leading to SKP2 activation and decreased BECN1 levels. This resulted in reduced ATG14 phosphorylation and oligomerization and subsequent lack of fusion of autophagosomes and lysosomes and disrupted autophagy flux. It had been previously suggested that the membrane-associated papain-like protease PLP2 (PLP2-TM) of SARS-CoV or MERS-CoV could be involved in blockage of autophagosomes-lysosomes fusion and suppression of the autophagic flux (Yang and Shen, 2020).

ER STRESS INDUCES DIFFERENT SIGNALING CIRCUITS IN RESPONSE TO COV INFECTION –

Despite the lack of consensus on the biogenesis of DMVs, it is clear that its membranes originate from the ER, whether it is through omegasomes/autophagosomes, EDEMosomes or both. Such high demand for membranes represents an additional burden to the ER that is also coopted to produce viral proteins. Indeed, during CoV replication, massive amounts of structural proteins are synthesized in the ER, and the production, folding and modification (in particular, extensive glycosylation of S protein) of these proteins increase the workload of the ER, eventually overloading its folding capacities and leading to UPR activation. Continuous depletion of the ER lipid content due to virion exocytosis also contributes to ER stress. Several pieces of evidence indicate that CoV infection induces ER stress: (i) genes and proteins involved in ER stress were shown to be upregulated in cells infected with SARS-CoV. Different studies showed that both the glucose-regulated protein 94 (GRP94) and GRP78/BiP are induced upon SARS-CoV infection in cell culture systems (Chan et al., 2006; Palmeira et al., 2020). In addition, infection with either MHV or SARS-CoV also results in up-regulation of homocysteine-inducible, ER-stress inducible, ubiquitin-like domain member 1 (HERPUD1), an ER stress marker (Fung and Liu, 2014).

Among the three branches of UPR, the PERK-eIF2α is the best characterized in CoV-infected cells. For example, MHV induces significant eIF2α phosphorylation and ATF4 upregulation in infected cells resulting in sustained translation repression. Even though there have been conflicting results in early studies on the role of the integrated stress response on CoV infections, it appears that both PERK and PKR, and subsequently eIF2α phosphorylation, occur at the early stages of CoV infections in cell cultures. In cells infected with SARS-CoV, PERK, PKR and eIF2α phosphorylation were detected as early as 8h post-infection (Krähling et al., 2009). Even though it significantly inhibited SARS-CoV-induced apoptosis, the knock-down of PKR did not affect eIF2α suggesting that this could be dependent on PERK activation. Supporting this is the previous observation that SARS-CoV accessory protein 3a induces PERK phosphorylation (Minakshi et al., 2009). Two complementary studies from the same group indicated that the PERK/PKR-eIF2α pathway is also activated at early stages of IBV infection *in vitro*, leading to ERK1/2 phosphorylation and promoting cell survival. After 8 h of infection, however, eIF2α is dephosphorylated as a feedback response due to the accumulation of GADD34, which is downstream of ATF4 and GADD153. Up-regulation of GADD153, which was partially blocked by silencing either PKR or PERK, also promoted apoptosis in IBV-infected cells (Wang et al., 2009; Liao et al., 2013). Altogether, these results highlight the delicate balance between cell survival and cell death upon UPR activation depending on the intensity and/or duration of stress.

The ORF3 protein of porcine epidemic diarrhea virus (PEDV), similar to SARS-CoV 3a protein or human pathogenic coronavirus NL63 (hCoV-NL63) ORF protein, localizes to the ER and triggers ER stress by upregulating GRP78 and activating the PERK-eIF2α pathway (Zou et al., 2019). This, in turn, results in induction of autophagy as shown by conversion of LC3-I into LC3-II. ORF3 protein is thought to function as an ion channel and to influence virus production and virulence (Wang et al., 2012).

Studies using MHV have demonstrated that the IRE1 axis also senses ER stress during infection, as shown by efficient splicing of XBP1 mRNA upon infection or overexpression of the S protein (Bechill et al., 2008). However, how this contributed to the cellular response was unclear since the protein product of the spliced XBP1 was not observed and genes known to be downstream of XBP1s – such as EDEM1, ER DNA J domain-containing protein 4 (ERdj4), and protein kinase inhibitor of 58 kDa ($p58^{IPK}$) – were not significantly up regulated following infection. It is possible that sustained eIF2α phosphorylation and translational repression observed during MHV infection interfere with the translation of the XBP1 protein. Another possibility is that IRE1 operates through alternative signaling pathways. It has been demonstrated that activation of IRE1 was essential for autophagy induction upon infection with another CoV, IBV (Fung and Liu, 2019b). Autophagosome formation and autophagic flux were also dependent on ATG5 but independent of BECN1. In this model, XBP1 splicing was dispensable, and IRE1 signaled through ERK1/2 to modulate autophagy induction in infected cells and protect them from apoptosis. A more recent study demonstrated that IBV can induce significant splicing of XBP1 mRNA and subsequent upregulation of EDEM1, ERdj4 and $p58^{IPK}$ in various cell lines (Fung et al., 2014). This was dependent on IRE1 activation as inhibiting or knocking down IRE1 effectively blocked IBV-induced XBP1 mRNA splicing and effector genes upregulation. In this context, the IRE1-XBP1 pathway seems to protect cells from apoptosis by modulating JNK and AKT phosphorylation. Altogether, these studies highlight how stress-related pathways intersect in different ways depending on cellular context and how different signaling circuits ultimately define cell fate. Also, it is important to evaluate the cell response as a whole, as it is not uncommon for RNA viruses to utilize only a subset of the components of stress response pathways that can signal through alternative pathways.

Similar to what was observed with IRE1, significant cleavage of ATF6 is observed following infection with MHV but the activation of target genes was not detected using luciferase reporter constructs under the control of ERSE promoters (Fung et al., 2014). In addition, ATF6 levels (full length and cleaved) significantly decrease at later time points of infection. The authors of this study suggest that global protein synthesis arrest following eIF2α phosphorylation impedes ATF6 accumulation and subsequent activation of target genes (Bechill et al., 2008).

ATF6 was implicated in the response to SARS-CoV. On the 2003 SARS-CoV outbreak, the accessory protein 8ab was found in animals and early human isolates. This protein was found to co-immunoprecipitate with and induce ATF6 cleavage and nuclear translocation (Sung et al., 2009). At the peak of the epidemic, human isolates presented a 29-nt deletion in the middle of ORF8, resulting in two smaller ORFs that encode the truncated polypeptides ORF8a and ORF8b. More recently, it was demonstrated that ORF8b forms insoluble intracellular aggregates leading to ER stress, lysosomal damage, and subsequent activation of the master regulator of the autophagy and lysosome machinery, transcription factor EB (TFEB), leading to increased autophagic flux. ORF8b aggregates are partially degraded by the autophagy-lysosome pathway. Depending on the cell type this may result in either cell death (as observed in epithelial cells) or a robust NLRP3 inflammasome activation by directly targeting its LRR domain with the release of inflammatory mediators (as observed in macrophages). In wild-type macrophages, ORF8b induces NLRP3-dependent pyroptosis while in NLRP3-deficient macrophages, cell death results from mitochondrial dysfunction (Shi et al., 2019).

MANIPULATION OF UPR AND AUTOPHAGY AS A STRATEGY TO LIMIT COV REPLICATION

As the current SARS-CoV-2 pandemic progressed, the repurposing of drugs already approved for human use could represent the fastest way to limit viral spread and/or severe disease, save lives, and prevent the collapse of health care systems. Drugs known to modulate both UPR (e.g. thapsigargin) (Al-Beltagi et al., 2021) and autophagy (e.g. hydroxichloroquine) (Senger et al., 2020) were shown to be broad-spectrum inhibitors for several respiratory viruses, including CoV, and emerged as candidates. Even though experimental findings have not yet been translated into efficient treatment and the use of these drugs remains controversial, the literature offers a rationale to target UPR and autophagy in the context of CoV infections. As we have described in this review, these two events are an integral part of the host cell-virus interactions and can be involved in different steps of the viral replicative cycle – from the establishment of replicative niches (DMVs) to regulating cell death. In particular, viral usage of double membranes vesicles resembling autophagosomes as a platform for replication, as a source of membrane for their envelope, as well as an intracellular shuttle for their exocytosis has been reported. Even though the precise mechanisms of DMVs biogenesis are still a matter of debate, components of the autophagic machinery and/or autophagic flux are often found to be necessary. Finally, all CoV identified so far have evolved to manipulate the autophagy pathway in some way, which once again argues that this pathway is essential for viral replication cycle.

One of the first proposed clinical trials in the wake of the COVID-19 pandemic draw huge worldwide attention to the putative benefits of hydroxychloroquine (HCQ) in the early treatment of patients infected with SARS-CoV-2 (Senger et al., 2020). Previously, HCQ had been shown to inhibit MERS-CoV replication *in vitro* in a screening of FDA-approved compound library (Touret et al., 2020). In experimental SARS-CoV infections, HCQ was able to limit inflammation markers even though it has not affected viral titers in the lungs of infected mice (Maisonnasse et al., 2020). The mechanisms proposed to explain the effects of HCQ on SARS-CoV-2 infection included the ability to interfere with ACE2 terminal glycosylation by raising the pH in the Golgi compartment thereby reducing the cell surface expression of SARS-CoV2 receptor (Kalra et al., 2020). In addition, by accumulating in the acidic organelles such as endosomes and lysosomes and neutralizing their pH, it can also disrupt fusion of viral endosomes with lysosomes or the activity of proteases preventing the cleavage of S protein blocking early steps in the viral life cycle (Chen and Geiger, 2020). Finally, HCQ is a well-known inhibitor of autophagy flux by impairing autophogasome fusion with lysosomes (Mauthe et al., 2018). After months of intense debate worldwide and follow-up studies, the efficacy of HCQ to treat COVID-19 was not confirmed, and its use has been discouraged by the FDA because of the risk of side effects. Nevertheless, one should not disregard autophagy as a potential pharmaceutical target because (i) it is a critical host process that controls all steps harnessed by SARS-CoV-2 and (ii) a collection of other drugs known to be autophagy modulators were shown to reduce or block SARS-CoV-2 infection *in vitro*. For instance, work from Gorshkov et al. (2020) identified 6 compounds known to be autophagy modulators that were able to reduce the cytopathic effects of SARS-CoV-2 *in vitro* with EC_{50} values ranging from 2.0 to 13 μM and selectivity indices ranging from 1.5 to >10-fold and their efficacy for inhibiting autophagy correlated with their ability to prevent SARS-CoV-2 cytopathic effects in various cell lines (Gorshkov et al., 2020).

As mentioned previously in this review, work from Gassen et al. (2019) showed that in their experimental conditions, MERS-CoV and SARS-CoV-2 impair autophagy by targeting BCL-1 for proteasomal degradation upon activation of SKP2. Blocking SKP2 with different compounds, including FDA-approved drugs, stabilized BECN1 limiting MERS-CoV and SARS-CoV-2 propagation which, in this case, contrary to HCQ that inhibits autophagy, indicates that boosting autophagy could be an efficient anti-CoV mechanism (Gassen et al., 2019). These authors tested a collection of known autophagy modulators such as spermidine, spermine, rapamycin, AKT1 inhibitors such as MK-2206, and the BCN1 stabilizing antihelmintic drug niclosamide and further advanced the idea that inducing autophagy can limit SARS-CoV infections (Gassen et al., 2020).

Manipulating the UPR has also been shown to be a potential strategy to treat infections with respiratory viruses. Al-Beltagi et al. showed that, *in vitro*, non-cytotoxic levels of thapsigargin (TG), an inhibitor of the ER-Ca ATPase pump, can block the replication of relevant human respiratory viruses such as CoV (including SARS-CoV-2), Respiratory Syncytial Virus and Influenza (Al-Beltagi et al., 2021). The effects of TG on CoV (hCoV-229E, MERS-CoV and SARS-CoV-2) replication have also been reported in another recent study (Shaban et al., 2020). The authors had previously shown that, in the case of CoV OC43 and RSV, TG-induced ER stress leading to UPR was a central innate immune driver that mediated several downstream host antiviral mechanisms that are particularly effective in blocking the replication of different RNA viruses, which include increased expression of ER stress genes (*DDIT3, HSPA5* and *HSP90B1*) and was accompanied by reduced viral transcription and viral protein expression (Goulding et al., 2020).

different ways, resulting in specific signaling circuits tailored to the cellular context. In this sense, it has been recently shown that there is a crosstalk between UPR and autophagy even in homeostatic conditions and it can be differentially modulated upon mild and severe or long-lasting stress. In the context of infections, stress-response mechanisms play multiple roles, including maintenance of homeostasis, fine-tuning of the immune response, and, in some cases, a direct anti-infectious role. The UPR/ISR and autophagy are known to limit the replication of several viruses. On the other hand, many RNA viruses, including CoV, take advantage of these responses to enhance their replication. There has been much debate on the biogenesis of CoV DMVs, which is a crucial step of the viral replicative cycle. Despite the lack of consensus, it is clear that its membranes originate from the ER, whether through omegasomes/autophagosomes, EDEMosomes or both. In addition, even though a complete autophagic flux seems to be dispensable, components of the autophagic machinery may be required in "alternative" pathways for CoV DMVs formation and replication. Similarly, ER stress induced upon CoV infection signals both through canonical UPR response as well as "alternative" signaling involving MAP kinases. There have been enough pieces added to the puzzle to establish a role for UPR and autophagy in CoV replication. However, the missing pieces will define the signaling circuits involved. This will be particularly important for the design of vaccines and therapeutic strategies to face the pandemic.

AUTHOR CONTRIBUTIONS

EP, JB, LT, and LC conceived and wrote the manuscript. LC revised the manuscript. All authors contributed to the article and approved the submitted version.

CONCLUDING REMARKS

As we understand cellular stress responses, it becomes clear that multiple pathways that are activated independently intersect in

REFERENCES

Adomavicius, T., Guaita, M., Zhou, Y., Jennings, M. D., Latif, Z., Roseman, A. M., et al. (2019). The Structural Basis of Translational Control by EIF2 Phosphorylation. *Nat. Commun.* 10, 2136. doi: 10.1038/s41467-019-10167-3

Al-Beltagi, S., Preda, C. A., Goulding, L. V., James, J., Pu, J., Skinner, P., et al. (2021). Thapsigargin is a Broad-Spectrum Inhibitor of Major Human Respiratory Viruses: Coronavirus, Respiratory Syncytial Virus and Influenza a Virus. *Viruses* 13, 234. doi: 10.3390/v13020234

Angelini, M. M., Akhlaghpour, M., Neuman, B. W., and Buchmeier, M. J. (2013). Severe Acute Respiratory Syndrome Coronavirus Nonstructural Proteins 3, 4, and 6 Induce Double-Membrane Vesicles. *Mbio* 4, e00524–e00513. doi: 10.1128/mbio.00524-13

Battu, S., Minhas, G., Mishra, A., and Khan, N. (2017). Amino Acid Sensing Via General Control Nonderepressible-2 Kinase and Immunological Programming. *Front. Immunol.* 8, 1719. doi: 10.3389/fimmu.2017.01719

B'chir, W., Maurin, A.-C. C., Carraro, V., Averous, J., Jousse, C., Muranishi, Y., et al. (2013). The EIF2α/Atf4 Pathway is Essential for Stress-Induced Autophagy Gene Expression. *Nucleic Acids Res.* 41, 7683–7699. doi: 10.1093/nar/gkt563

Bechill, J., Chen, Z., Brewer, J. W., and Baker, S. C. (2008). Coronavirus Infection Modulates the Unfolded Protein Response and Mediates Sustained Translational Repression∇. *J. Virol.* 82, 4492–4501. doi: 10.1128/jvi.00017-08

Blázquez, A.-B. B., Escribano-Romero, E., Merino-Ramos, T., Saiz, J.-C. C., and Martín-Acebes, M. A. (2014). Stress Responses in Flavivirus-Infected Cells: Activation of Unfolded Protein Response and Autophagy. *Front. Microbiol.* 5, 266. doi: 10.3389/fmicb.2014.00266

Carneiro, L. A., and Travassos, L. H. (2013). The Interplay Between Nlrs and Autophagy in Immunity and Inflammation. *Front. Immunol.* 4, 361. doi: 10.3389/fimmu.2013.00361

Carreras-Sureda, A., Jaña, F., Urra, H., Durand, S., Mortenson, D. E., Sagredo, A., et al. (2019). Non-Canonical Function of IRE1α Determines Mitochondria-Associated Endoplasmic Reticulum Composition to Control Calcium Transfer and Bioenergetics. *Nat. Cell Biol.* 21, 755–767. doi: 10.1038/s41556-019-0329-y

Chan, S.-W. (2014). The Unfolded Protein Response in Virus Infections. *Front. Microbiol.* 5, 518. doi: 10.3389/fmicb.2014.00518

Chang, H. H. Y., Pannunzio, N. R., Adachi, N., and Lieber, M. R. (2017). Non-Homologous DNA End Joining and Alternative Pathways to Double-Strand Break Repair. *Nat. Rev. Mol. Cell Bio* 18, 495–506. doi: 10.1038/nrm.2017.48

Chan, C.-P., Siu, K.-L., Chin, K.-T., Yuen, K.-Y., Zheng, B., and Jin, D.-Y. (2006). Modulation of the Unfolded Protein Response by the Severe Acute Respiratory Syndrome Coronavirus Spike Protein. *J. Virol.* 80, 9279–9287. doi: 10.1128/jvi.00659-06

Chen, X., and Geiger, J. D. (2020). Janus Sword Actions of Chloroquine and Hydroxychloroquine Against Covid-19. *Cell Signal* 73, 109706. doi: 10.1016/j.cellsig.2020.109706

Cheng, V. C. C., Lau, S. K. P., Woo, P. C. Y., and Yuen, K. Y. (2007). Severe Acute Respiratory Syndrome Coronavirus as an Agent of Emerging and Reemerging Infection. *Clin. Microbiol. Rev.* 20, 660–694. doi: 10.1128/cmr.00023-07

Chen, Y., Liu, Q., and Guo, D. (2020). Emerging Coronaviruses: Genome Structure, Replication, and Pathogenesis. *J. Med. Virol.* 92, 418–423. doi: 10.1002/jmv.25681

Costa-Mattioli, M., and Walter, P. (2020). The Integrated Stress Response: From Mechanism to Disease. *Sci. New York N. Y.* 368, 1–11. doi: 10.1126/science.aat5314

Cottam, E. M., Maier, H. J., Manifava, M., Vaux, L. C., Chandra-Schoenfelder, P., Gerner, W., et al. (2011). Coronavirus Nsp6 Proteins Generate Autophagosomes From the Endoplasmic Reticulum Via an Omegasome Intermediate. *Autophagy* 7, 1335–1347. doi: 10.4161/auto.7.11.16642

Cottam, E. M., Whelband, M. C., and Wileman, T. (2014). Coronavirus Nsp6 Restricts Autophagosome Expansion. *Autophagy* 10, 1426–1441. doi: 10.4161/auto.29309

Diao, J., Liu, R., Rong, Y., Zhao, M., Zhang, J., Lai, Y., et al. (2015). Atg14 Promotes Membrane Tethering and Fusion of Autophagosomes to Endolysosomes. *Nature* 520, 563–566. doi: 10.1038/nature14147

Domańska-Blicharz, K., Woźniakowski, G., Konopka, B., Niemczuk, K., Welz, M., Rola, J., Socha, W., et al. (2020). Animal Coronaviruses in the Light of COVID-19. *J. Vet. Res.* 64, 333–345. doi: 10.2478/jvetres-2020-0050

Fehr, A. R., and Perlman, S. (2015). Coronaviruses, Methods and Protocols. *Methods Mol. Biol. Clifton N J.* 1282, 1–23. doi: 10.1007/978-1-4939-2438-7_1

Fung, T. S., Huang, M., and Liu, D. X. (2014). Coronavirus-Induced ER Stress Response and Its Involvement in Regulation of Coronavirus–Host Interactions. *Virus Res.* 194, 110–123. doi: 10.1016/j.virusres.2014.09.016

Fung, T. S., Liao, Y., and Liu, D. X. (2014). The Endoplasmic Reticulum Stress Sensor Ire1α Protects Cells From Apoptosis Induced by the Coronavirus Infectious Bronchitis Virus. *J. Virol.* 88, 12752–12764. doi: 10.1128/jvi.02138-14

Fung, T. S., and Liu, D. X. (2014). Coronavirus Infection, Er Stress, Apoptosis and Innate Immunity. *Front. Microbiol.* 5, 296. doi: 10.3389/fmicb.2014.00296

Fung, T., and Liu, D. (2019a). Human Coronavirus: Host-Pathogen Interaction. *Annu. Rev. Microbiol.* 73, 529–557. doi: 10.1146/annurev-micro-020518-115759

Fung, T., and Liu, D. (2019b). The ER Stress Sensor IRE1 and MAP Kinase ERK Modulate Autophagy Induction in Cells Infected With Coronavirus Infectious Bronchitis Virus. *Virology* 533, 34–44. doi: 10.1016/j.virol.2019.05.002

Gale, M., Tan, S.-L., and Katze, M. G. (2000). Translational Control of Viral Gene Expression in Eukaryotes. *Microbiol. Mol. Biol. R* 64, 239–280. doi: 10.1128/mmbr.64.2.239-280.2000

Galluzzi, L., Pedro, J., Levine, B., Green, D. R., and Kroemer, G. (2017). Pharmacological Modulation of Autophagy: Therapeutic Potential and Persisting Obstacles. *Nat. Rev. Drug Discov.* 16, 487–511. doi: 10.1038/nrd.2017.22

Galluzzi, L., Yamazaki, T., and Kroemer, G. (2018). Linking Cellular Stress Responses to Systemic Homeostasis. *Nat. Rev. Mol. Cell Biol.* 19, 731–745. doi: 10.1038/s41580-018-0068-0

García, M. A., Gil, J., Ventoso, I., Guerra, S., Domingo, E., Rivas, C., et al. (2006). Impact of Protein Kinase PKR in Cell Biology: From Antiviral to Antiproliferative Action. *Microbiol. Mol. Biol. R* 70, 1032–1060. doi: 10.1128/mmbr.00027-06

Gassen, N. C., Niemeyer, D., Muth, D., Corman, V. M., Martinelli, S., Gassen, A., et al. (2019). Skp2 Attenuates Autophagy Through Beclin1-Ubiquitination and Its Inhibition Reduces Mers-Coronavirus Infection. *Nat. Commun.* 10, 5770. doi: 10.1038/s41467-019-13659-4

Gassen, N. C., Papies, J., Bajaj, T., Dethloff, F., Emanuel, J., Weckmann, K., et al. (2020). Analysis of SARS-Cov-2-Controlled Autophagy Reveals Spermidine, MK-2206, and Niclosamide as Putative Antiviral Therapeutics. *Biorxiv* 2020, 4.15.997254. doi: 10.1101/2020.04.15.997254

Girardin, S. E., Cuziol, C., Philpott, D. J., and Arnoult, D. (2020). The eIF2α kinase HRI in innate immunity, proteostasis and mitochondrial stress. *FEBS J.* doi: 10.1111/febs.15553

Gorshkov, K., Chen, C. Z., Bostwick, R., Rasmussen, L., Xu, M., Pradhan, M., et al. (2020). The SARS-Cov-2 Cytopathic Effect is Blocked With Autophagy Modulators. *bioRxiv.* doi: 10.1101/2020.05.16.091520

Goulding, L. V., Yang, J., Jiang, Z., Zhang, H., Lea, D., Emes, R. D., et al. (2020). Thapsigargin At non-Cytotoxic Levels Induces a Potent Host Antiviral Response That Blocks Influenza a Virus Replication. *Viruses* 12, 1093. doi: 10.3390/v12101093

Hetz, C. (2012). The Unfolded Protein Response: Controlling Cell Fate Decisions Under ER Stress and Beyond. *Nat. Rev. Mol. Cell Bio* 13, 89–102. doi: 10.1038/nrm3270

Hetz, C., and Papa, F. R. (2018). The Unfolded Protein Response and Cell Fate Control. *Mol. Cell* 69, 169–181. doi: 10.1016/j.molcel.2017.06.017

Hetz, C., Zhang, K., and Kaufman, R. J. (2020). Mechanisms, Regulation and Functions of the Unfolded Protein Response. *Nat. Rev. Mol. Cell Biol.* 21, 421–438. doi: 10.1038/s41580-020-0250-z

Hoffmann, M., Kleine-Weber, H., Schroeder, S., Krüger, N., Herrler, T., Erichsen, S., et al. (2020). Sars-Cov-2 Cell Entry Depends on ACE2 and TMPRSS2 and is Blocked by a Clinically Proven Protease Inhibitor. *Cell* 181, 271–280.e8. doi: 10.1016/j.cell.2020.02.052

Hwang, J., and Qi, L. (2018). Quality Control in the Endoplasmic Reticulum: Crosstalk Between ERAD and UPR Pathways. *Trends Biochem. Sci.* 43, 593–605. doi: 10.1016/j.tibs.2018.06.005

Jackson, S. P., and Bartek, J. (2009). The DNA-Damage Response in Human Biology and Disease. *Nature* 461, 1071–1078. doi: 10.1038/nature08467

Jheng, J.-R. R., Ho, J.-Y. Y., and Horng, J.-T. T. (2014). Er Stress, Autophagy, and RNA Viruses. *Front. Microbiol.* 5, 388. doi: 10.3389/fmicb.2014.00388

Kalra, R. S., Tomar, D., Meena, A. S., and Kandimalla, R. (2020). Sars-Cov-2, ACE2, and Hydroxychloroquine: Cardiovascular Complications, Therapeutics, and Clinical Readouts in the Current Settings. *Pathogens* 9, 546. doi: 10.3390/pathogens9070546

Klionsky, D. J., Eskelinen, E.-L., and Deretic, V. (2014). Autophagosomes, Phagosomes, Autolysosomes, Phagolysosomes, Autophagolysosomes... Wait, I'm Confused. *Autophagy* 10, 549–551. doi: 10.4161/auto.28448

Knoops, K., Kikkert, M., Worm, S. H. E. V. D., Zevenhoven-Dobbe, J. C., Meer, Y.V. d., Koster, A. J., et al. (2008). SARS-Coronavirus Replication is Supported by a Reticulovesicular Network of Modified Endoplasmic Reticulum. *PLoS Biol.* 6, e226. doi: 10.1371/journal.pbio.0060226

Krähling, V., Stein, D. A., Spiegel, M., Weber, F., and Mühlberger, E. (2009). Severe Acute Respiratory Syndrome Coronavirus Triggers Apoptosis Via Protein Kinase R But is Resistant to Its Antiviral Activity▿. *J. Virol.* 83, 2298–2309. doi: 10.1128/jvi.01245-08

Lee, Y.-R., Kuo, S.-H., Lin, C.-Y., Fu, P.-J., Lin, Y.-S., Yeh, T.-M., et al. (2018). Dengue Virus-Induced Er Stress is Required for Autophagy Activation, Viral Replication, and Pathogenesis Both in Vitro and In Vivo. *Sci. Rep-uk* 8, 489. doi: 10.1038/s41598-017-18909-3

Liao, Y., Fung, T. S., Huang, M., Fang, S. G., Zhong, Y., and Liu, D. X. (2013). Upregulation of CHOP/GADD153 During Coronavirus Infectious Bronchitis Virus Infection Modulates Apoptosis by Restricting Activation of the Extracellular Signal-Regulated Kinase Pathway. *J. Virol.* 87, 8124–8134. doi: 10.1128/jvi.00626-13

Lindner, P., Christensen, S. B. B., Nissen, P., Møller, J. V., and Engedal, N. (2020). Cell Death Induced by the ER Stressor Thapsigargin Involves Death Receptor 5, a Non-Autophagic Function of MAP1LC3B, and Distinct Contributions From Unfolded Protein Response Components. *Cell communication signaling : CCS* 18, 12. doi: 10.1186/s12964-019-0499-z

Liu, C., Yan, D.-Y. Y., Wang, C., Ma, Z., Deng, Y., Liu, W., et al. (2020). Ire1 Signaling Pathway Mediates Protective Autophagic Response Against Manganese-Induced Neuronal Apoptosis in Vivo and In Vitro. *Sci. Total Environ.* 712, 136480. doi: 10.1016/j.scitotenv.2019.136480

Maisonnasse, P., Guedj, J., Contreras, V., Behillil, S., Solas, C., Marlin, R., et al. (2020). Hydroxychloroquine Use Against SARS-Cov-2 Infection in Non-Human Primates. *Nature* 585, 584–587. doi: 10.1038/s41586-020-2558-4

Mauthe, M., Orhon, I., Rocchi, C., Zhou, X., Luhr, M., Hijlkema, K.-J., et al. (2018). Chloroquine Inhibits Autophagic Flux by Decreasing Autophagosome-Lysosome Fusion. *Autophagy* 14, 1435–1455. doi: 10.1080/15548627.2018.1474314

McQuiston, A., and Diehl, J. A. (2017). Recent Insights Into PERK-Dependent Signaling From the Stressed Endoplasmic Reticulum. *F1000research* 6, 1897. doi: 10.12688/f1000research.12138.1

Mehrbod, P., Ande, S. R., Alizadeh, J., Rahimizadeh, S., Shariati, A., Malek, H., et al. (2019). The Roles of Apoptosis, Autophagy and Unfolded Protein Response in Arbovirus, Influenza Virus, and HIV Infections. *Virulence* 10, 376–413. doi: 10.1080/21505594.2019.1605803

Mercer, T. J., Gubas, A., and Tooze, S. A. A. (2018). Molecular Perspective of Mammalian Autophagosome Biogenesis. *J. Biol. Chem.* 293, 5386–5395. doi: 10.1074/jbc.r117.810366

Mesel-Lemoine, M., Millet, J., Vidalain, P.-O., Law, H., Vabret, A., Lorin, V., et al. (2012). Human Coronavirus Responsible for the Common Cold Massively Kills Dendritic Cells But Not Monocytes. *J. Virol.* 86, 7577–7587. doi: 10.1128/jvi.00269-12

Minakshi, R., Padhan, K., Rani, M., Khan, N., Ahmad, F., and Jameel, S. (2009). The SARS Coronavirus 3a Protein Causes Endoplasmic Reticulum Stress and Induces Ligand-Independent Downregulation of the Type 1 Interferon Receptor. *PLoS One* 4, e8342. doi: 10.1371/journal.pone.0008342

Mizushima, N., Levine, B., Cuervo, A. M., and Klionsky, D. J. (2008). Autophagy Fights Disease Through Cellular Self-Digestion. *Nature* 451, 1069–1075. doi: 10.1038/nature06639

Mohd, H. A., Al-Tawfiq, J. A., and Memish, Z. A. (2016). Middle East Respiratory Syndrome Coronavirus (Mers-Cov) Origin and Animal Reservoir. *Virol. J.* 13, 87. doi: 10.1186/s12985-016-0544-0

Palmeira, A., Sousa, E., Köseler, A., Sabirli, R., Gören, T., Türkçüer, İ., et al. (2020). Preliminary Virtual Screening Studies to Identify Grp78 Inhibitors Which May Interfere With Sars-Cov-2 Infection. *Pharm* 13, 132. doi: 10.3390/ph13060132

Prentice, E., Jerome, G. W., Yoshimori, T., Mizushima, N., and Denison, M. R. (2003). Coronavirus Replication Complex Formation Utilizes Components of Cellular Autophagy. *J. Biol. Chem.* 279, 10136–10141. doi: 10.1074/jbc.m306124200

Rashid, H.-O., Yadav, R. K., Kim, H.-R., and Chae, H.-J. (2015). Er Stress: Autophagy Induction, Inhibition and Selection. *Autophagy* 11, 1956–1977. doi: 10.1080/15548627.2015.1091141

Reggiori, F., Haan, C. A. M. de, and Molinari, M. (2011). Unconventional Use of LC3 by Coronaviruses Through the Alleged Subversion of the ERAD Tuning Pathway. *Viruses* 3, 1610–1623. doi: 10.3390/v3091610

Reggiori, F., and Klionsky, D. J. (2005). Autophagosomes: Biogenesis From Scratch? *Curr. Opin. Cell Biol.* 17, 415–422. doi: 10.1016/j.ceb.2005.06.007

Reggiori, F., Monastyrska, I., Verheije, M. H., Calì, T., Ulasli, M., Bianchi, S., et al. (2010). Coronaviruses Hijack the LC3-I-Positive Edemosomes, ER-Derived Vesicles Exporting Short-Lived ERAD Regulators, for Replication. *Cell Host Microbe* 7, 500–508. doi: 10.1016/j.chom.2010.05.013

Ríos-Ocampo, W. A., Navas, M.-C., Faber, K. N., Daemen, T., and Moshage, H. (2018). The Cellular Stress Response in Hepatitis C Virus Infection: A Balancing Act to Promote Viral Persistence and Host Cell Survival. *Virus Res.* 263, 1–8. doi: 10.1016/j.virusres.2018.12.013

Romero-Brey, I., and Bartenschlager, R. (2014). Membranous Replication Factories Induced by Plus-Strand Rna Viruses. *Viruses* 6, 2826–2857. doi: 10.3390/v6072826

Rzymski, T., Milani, M., Pike, L., Buffa, F., Mellor, H. R., Winchester, L., et al. (2010). Regulation of Autophagy by ATF4 in Response to Severe Hypoxia. *Oncogene* 29, 4424–4435. doi: 10.1038/onc.2010.191

Schneider, W. M., Luna, J. M., Hoffmann, H.-H., Sánchez-Rivera, F. J., Leal, A. A., Ashbrook, A. W., et al. (2021). Genome-Scale Identification of SARS-Cov-2 and Pan-Coronavirus Host Factor Networks. *Cell* 184, 120–132.e14. doi: 10.1016/j.cell.2020.12.006

Senft, D., and Ronai, Z. A. (2015). Upr, Autophagy, and Mitochondria Crosstalk Underlies the ER Stress Response. *Trends Biochem. Sci.* 40, 141–148. doi: 10.1016/j.tibs.2015.01.002

Senger, M. R., Evangelista, T. C. S., Dantas, R. F., Santana, M. V. da S., Gonçalves, L. C. S., Neto, L. R. de S., et al. (2020). Covid-19: Molecular Targets, Drug Repurposing and New Avenues for Drug Discovery. *Memórias Instituto Oswaldo Cruz* 115, e200254. doi: 10.1590/0074-02760200254

Shaban, M. S., Müller, C., Mayr-Buro, C., Weiser, H., Albert, B. V., Weber, A., et al. (2020). Inhibiting Coronavirus Replication in Cultured Cells by Chemical Er Stress. *Biorxiv* 2020, 0826.266304. doi: 10.1101/2020.08.26.266304

Shi, C.-S., Nabar, N. R., Huang, N.-N., and Kehrl, J. H. (2019). Sars-Coronavirus Open Reading Frame-8b Triggers Intracellular Stress Pathways and Activates Nlrp3 Inflammasomes. *Cell Death Discov.* 5, 101. doi: 10.1038/s41420-019-0181-7

Shoulders, M. D., Ryno, L. M., Genereux, J. C., Moresco, J. J., Tu, P. G., Wu, C., et al. (2013). Stress-Independent Activation of XBP1s and/or ATF6 Reveals Three Functionally Diverse Er Proteostasis Environments. *Cell Rep.* 3, 1279–1292. doi: 10.1016/j.celrep.2013.03.024

Siqueira, M., Ribeiro, R., and Travassos, L. H. (2018). Autophagy and Its Interaction With Intracellular Bacterial Pathogens. *Front. Immunol.* 9, 935. doi: 10.3389/fimmu.2018.00935

Smith, M., and Wilkinson, S. (2017). Er Homeostasis and Autophagy. *Essays Biochem.* 61, 625–635. doi: 10.1042/EBC20170092

Sung, S.-C., Chao, C.-Y., Jeng, K.-S., Yang, J.-Y., and Lai, M. M. C. (2009). The 8ab Protein of SARS-Cov is a Luminal Er Membrane-Associated Protein and Induces the Activation of ATF6. *Virology* 387, 402–413. doi: 10.1016/j.virol.2009.02.021

Tan, X., Thapa, N., Liao, Y., Choi, S., and Anderson, R. A. (2016). Ptdins(4,5)P2 Signaling Regulates ATG14 and Autophagy. *Proc. Natl. Acad. Sci. U. S. A.* 113, 10896–10901. doi: 10.1073/pnas.1523145113

Touret, F., Gilles, M., Barral, K., Nougairède, A., Helden, J.v., Decroly, E., et al. (2020). In Vitro Screening of a FDA Approved Chemical Library Reveals Potential Inhibitors of SARS-Cov-2 Replication. *Sci. Rep-uk* 10, 13093. doi: 10.1038/s41598-020-70143-6

Ulferts, R., Imbert, I., Canard, B., and Ziebuhr, J. (2009). Expression and Functions of SARS Coronavirus Replicative Proteins. *Molecular Biology of the SARS-Coronavirus* 75–98. doi: 10.1007/978-3-642-03683-5_6

Urra, H., Henriquez, D. R., Cánovas, J., Villarroel-Campos, D., Carreras-Sureda, A., Pulgar, E., et al. (2018). Ire1α Governs Cytoskeleton Remodelling and Cell Migration Through a Direct Interaction With Filamin a. *Nat. Cell Biol.* 20, 942–953. doi: 10.1038/s41556-018-0141-0

V'kovski, P., Kratzel, A., Steiner, S., Stalder, H., and Thiel, V. (2020). Coronavirus Biology and Replication: Implications for SARS-Cov-2. *Nat. Rev. Microbiol.* 19, 1–16. doi: 10.1038/s41579-020-00468-6

Vliet, A. R. v., Giordano, F., Gerlo, S., Segura, I., Eygen, S. V., Molenberghs, G., et al. (2017). the Er Stress Sensor Perk Coordinates Er-Plasma Membrane Contact Site Formation Through Interaction With Filamin-a and F-Actin Remodeling. *Mol. Cell* 65, 885–899.e6. doi: 10.1016/j.molcel.2017.01.020

Wang, X., Liao, Y., Yap, P. L., Png, K. J., Tam, J. P., and Liu, D. X. (2009). Inhibition of Protein Kinase R Activation and Upregulation of GADD34 Expression Play a Synergistic Role in Facilitating Coronavirus Replication by Maintaining De Novo Protein Synthesis in Virus-Infected Cellsv. *J. Virol.* 83, 12462–12472. doi: 10.1128/jvi.01546-09

Wang, K., Lu, W., Chen, J., Xie, S., Shi, H., Hsu, H., et al. (2012). Pedv ORF3 Encodes an Ion Channel Protein and Regulates Virus Production. *FEBS Lett.* 586, 384–391. doi: 10.1016/j.febslet.2012.01.005

Wolff, G., Melia, C. E., Snijder, E. J., and Bárcena, M. (2020). Double-Membrane Vesicles as Platforms for Viral Replication. *Trends Microbiol.* 28, 1022–1033. doi: 10.1016/j.tim.2020.05.009

Xiao, Y., and Cai, W. (2020). Autophagy and Viral Infection. *Adv. Exp. Med. Biol.* 1207, 425–432. doi: 10.1007/978-981-15-4272-5_30

Yang, N., and Shen, H.-M. (2020). Targeting the Endocytic Pathway and Autophagy Process as a Novel Therapeutic Strategy in COVID-19. *Int. J. Biol. Sci.* 16, 1724–1731. doi: 10.7150/ijbs.45498

Yao, R.-Q. Q., Ren, C., Xia, Z.-F. F., and Yao, Y.-M. M. (2021). Organelle-Specific Autophagy in Inflammatory Diseases: A Potential Therapeutic Target Underlying the Quality Control of Multiple Organelles. *Autophagy* 17 (2), 385–401. doi: 10.1080/15548627.2020.1725377

Ye, Z.-W., Yuan, S., Yuen, K.-S., Fung, S.-Y., Chan, C.-P., and Jin, D.-Y. (2020). Zoonotic Origins of Human Coronaviruses. *Int. J. Biol. Sci.* 16, 1686–1697. doi: 10.7150/ijbs.45472

Zhao, Z., Thackray, L. B., Miller, B. C., Lynn, T. M., Becker, M. M., Ward, E., et al. (2007). Coronavirus Replication Does Not Require the Autophagy Gene Atg5. *Autophagy* 3, 581–585. doi: 10.4161/auto.4782

Zou, D., Xu, J., Duan, X., Xu, X., Li, P., Cheng, L., et al. (2019). Porcine Epidemic Diarrhea Virus Orf3 Protein Causes Endoplasmic Reticulum Stress to Facilitate Autophagy. *Vet. Microbiol.* 235, 209–219. doi: 10.1016/j.vetmic.2019.07.005

5

Identification of Immune Activation Markers in the Early Onset of COVID-19 Infection

Johannes J. Kovarik[1], Anna K. Kämpf[1], Fabian Gasser[1], Anna N. Herdina[2], Monika Breuer[2], Christopher C. Kaltenecker[3], Markus Wahrmann[1], Susanne Haindl[1], Florian Mayer[4], Ludwig Traby[5], Veronique Touzeau-Roemer[6], Katharina Grabmeier-Pfistershammer[6,7], Manuel Kussmann[5], Oliver Robak[5], Harald Willschke[8], Care Ay[8], Marcus D. Säemann[9,10], Klaus G. Schmetterer[4†] and Robert Strassl[2†]*

[1] *Department of Internal Medicine III, Division of Nephrology and Dialysis Medical University Vienna, Vienna, Austria,* [2] *Department of Laboratory Medicine, Institute of Clinical Virology, Medical University of Vienna, Vienna, Austria,* [3] *Department of Pathology, Medical University Vienna, Vienna, Austria,* [4] *Department of Laboratory Medicine, Medical University of Vienna, Vienna, Austria,* [5] *Department of Internal Medicine I, Medical University of Vienna, Vienna, Austria,* [6] *Department of Dermatology, Medical University Vienna, Vienna, Austria,* [7] *Institute of Immunology, Center for Pathophysiology, Infectiology and Immunology, Medical University Vienna, Vienna, Austria,* [8] *Department of Anaesthesia, Intensive Care Medicine and Pain Medicine, Medical University of Vienna, Vienna, Austria,* [9] *6th Medical Department With Nephrology and Dialysis, Wilhelminen Hospital, Vienna, Austria,* [10] *Sigmund Freud University, Vienna, Austria*

Correspondence:
Robert Strassl
robert.strassl@meduniwien.ac.at
These authors have contributed equally to this work

†

This study aimed to determine the specific cytokine profile in peripheral blood during the early onset of COVID-19 infection. This was a cross-sectional exploratory, single center study. A total of 55 plasma samples were studied. Serum samples of adults showing symptoms of COVID-19 infection who were tested positive for SARS-CoV-2 infection (CoV+, n=18) at the COVID-19 outpatient clinic of the Medical University of Vienna were screened for immune activation markers by Luminex technology. Additionally, age and gender-matched serum samples of patients displaying COVID-19 associated symptoms, but tested negative for SARS-CoV-2 (CoV-, n=16) as well as healthy controls (HC, n=21) were analyzed. COVID-19 positive (CoV+) patients showed a specific upregulation of BLC (141; 74-189 pg/mL), SCD30 (273; 207-576 pg/mL), MCP-2 (18; 12-30 pg/mL) and IP-10 (37; 23-96 pg/mL), compared to patients with COVID19-like symptoms but negative PCR test (CoV-), BLC (61; 22-100 pg/mL), sCD30L (161; 120-210 pg/mL), MCP-2 (8; 5-12 pg/mL) and IP-10 (9; 6-12 pg/mL) and healthy controls (HC) (BLC 22; 11-36 pg/mL, sCD30 74; 39-108 pg/mL, MCP-2 6; 3-9. pg/mL, IP-10 = 8; 5-13). The markers APRIL, sIL-2R, IL7, MIF, MIP-1b, SCF, SDF-1a, sTNF-RII were elevated in both CoV+ and CoV- patient groups compared to healthy controls. HGF, MDC and VEGF-A were elevated in CoV- but not CoV+ compared to healthy controls. BLC, sCD30, MCP-2 and IP-10 are specifically induced during early stages of COVID-19 infection and might constitute attractive targets for early diagnosis and treatment of this disease.

Keywords: COVID-19, SARS-CoV-2, cytokines, inflammatory markers, infection

INTRODUCTION

According to World Health Organization (WHO), the outbreak of a novel coronavirus strain termed severe acute respiratory syndrome coronavirus type 2, SARS-CoV-2 at the end of the year 2019 has led to an unprecedented global pandemic having infected an estimated more than 80 million people. First case descriptions have focused on the respiratory symptoms of the disease such as cough, shortness of breath and, in severe cases, low oxygenation requiring hospitalization and ventilation (Lescure et al., 2020). Furthermore, SARS-CoV-2 infection induces pathologies in multiple organs which contributes to the unusually high lethality (Becher and Frerichs, 2020). It is now agreed that one of the most severe clinical problems is a state of hyperinflammation induced by SARS-CoV-2 infection during early stages of the disease (de la Rica et al., 2020; Reddy et al., 2020). Inflammation is governed by the interaction of multiple different cell types such as granulocytes, macrophages, endothelial along with epithelial cells which interact with cells of the adaptive immune system. Many of these interactions are regulated by the early secretion of cytokines, chemokines, and other messenger substances resulting in an exacerbation of the inflammatory reaction, that can culminate in a systemic cytokine storm also activating inflammasomes affecting multiple compartments of the organism (Rodrigues et al., 2021). Accordingly, several studies have aimed to better define the inflammatory pattern induced by Coronavirus Disease (COVID)-19 infection. First reports in January 2020 from a Chinese cohort described high serum levels of inflammatory cytokines with the chemokine CXCL10/IP-10 showing the most pronounced increase and allowing stratification of risk patients (Huang et al., 2020) which was also corroborated in an Israelian cohort (Lev et al., 2021). Similarly, a more recent study analyzing 185 serum markers of inflammation and cardiovascular disease has identified several significantly up-regulated inflammatory markers in the peripheral blood of hospitalized SARS-CoV-2 patients (Sims et al., 2020). A broad up-regulation of inflammatory cytokines and chemokines has also been described in Chinese cohorts from the first wave as well (Chi et al., 2020; Zhao et al., 2020). Subsequently, numerous studies have further addressed COVID-19 induced hyperinflammation drawing a multi-faceted picture with different immunological processes contributing to immediate and late pathologies in SARS-CoV-2 infection (Buszko et al., 2021). Treatment strategies concomitantly focused on this cytokine storm and treatment options investigating approved anti-inflammatory agents such as the interleukin-(IL)-6 blocker tocilizumab (Guaraldi et al., 2020) and the IL-1 blocker anakinra have been explored (Cavalli et al., 2021). Most notably, recent trials using the broadly anti-inflammatory glucocorticoids showed promising results regarding mortality in critically ill patients (Horby et al., 2020). Surprisingly, though it has not been established yet whether the overall quality or quantity of the SARS-CoV-2 induced cytokine inflammatory response differs from that caused by other common respiratory infections. Better understanding of the underlying mechanisms of specific individuals, which may alter the propensity of individual patients to experience over exuberant inflammatory responses after viral infection is urgently needed (Forbester and Humphreys, 2020). Furthermore, a deeper knowledge of disease specific cytokine patterns especially at the early onset of the disease is necessary to specifically ameliorate clinical symptoms and to personalize treatment.

A detailed characterization of the cytokine pattern during the early onset of the COVID-19 infection in comparison to healthy controls and symptomatic but COVID negative persons is lacking so far. Hence in this study peripheral blood specimens from symptomatic patients at the COVID outpatient clinic of the Medical University of Vienna were stratified into patients tested COVID-19 negative and positive with age- and sex-matched healthy volunteers as control group.

METHODS

Ethics Statement

This exploratory study is in compliance with the Helsinki Declaration (Ethical Principles for Medical Research Involving Human Subjects) and was conducted in accordance with the guidelines of research boards at the study site. This single-center study was approved by the local ethics committee of the Medical University of Vienna (EC#1280/2020).

Patient Recruitment and Detection of SARS-CoV-2 by RT-PCR

Healthy volunteers were recruited at the Vienna General Hospital (AKH Wien) Medical University of Vienna. COVID-19 symptomatic patients were randomly included by order of appearance at the COVID-19 outpatient ward of the Medical University of Vienna. Onset of symptoms was anamnestically determined and for this study only patients with a symptom onset ≤2 days were included. At the time of presentation a serum blood draw was performed and samples were stored at -80°C and similarly respiratory swabs were taken once from the nasopharyngeal cavity of each patient to determine the SARS-CoV-2 status. RT-PCR was performed on the fully-automated Roche Cobas 6800 RT-PCR system (Roche Diagnostics GmbH, Rotkreuz, Switzerland) from respiratory swab samples agitated in 0,9% saline solution (NaCl). The cobas® SARS-CoV-2 assay was used according to the manufacturer's instructions for the detection of SARS-CoV-2 specific ribonucleic acid (RNA). According to clinical routine testing protocols, all analyses were performed within six hours after sample extraction. The control group was recruited from age- and sex-matched healthy volunteers from the General Hospital of Vienna between 2017 and the end of 2019. As this was prior to the COVID-19 pandemic, SARS-CoV-2 PCR was not performed in this group.

Analysis of Inflammatory Markers in Patient Serum

Undiluted blood serum samples were analyzed using the ProcartaPlex™ Multiplex Immunoassay (Human immune monitoring 65 Plex, Thermo Fisher Scientific, Reference

Number MAN0017980) according to manufacturer's instruction. Of the 65 analytes, 39 were below the lower limit of quantification in >95% of all samples (irrespective of group) and were therefore excluded from further analysis. Measurements and analysis of all Human ProcartaPlex Immunoassays were performed on a Luminex 200 instrument (Luminex Corp., Austin, Tx, USA) as described previously (Muhlbacher et al., 2020). In short, patient samples were adjusted to 10 mM EDTA to prevent the complement-mediated prozone effect. Then, 50 μL of the Magnetic Bead solution was added to each well of the provided 96-well flate bottom plate. After washing of magnetic beads, 25 μL of Universal Assay Buffer (1x) was added to each well, followed by 25 uL of patient sample, prepared standards or blank [Universal Assay Buffer (1x)]. The plate was incubated at RT in the dark on a plate shaker at 550 rpm for 60 min. After incubation, the plate was washed and incubated with pre-mixed Detection Antibody Mixture (25 μL/well) as above for 30 min. Subsequently, the beads were washed to remove unbound antibody, 50 μL of Streptavidin-PE (SAPE) solution was added to each well and the incubation step was repeated. As a final step, 120 μL of Reading Buffer was added to each well after washing and plates were processed on a Luminex 200 instrument.

Statistical Analysis

Each analyte was plotted separated by patient group to assess data distribution. Group differences between the three cohorts were tested using Kruskal-Wallis-test in conjunction with Dunn's multiple comparisons test using multiplicity adjusted calculation of p-values. Correlation analyses were calculated using a Spearman correlation algorithm. GraphPad Prism 6.05 (GraphPad Software, CA, USA) was used for statistical analysis and data presentation.

RESULTS

Patient Recruitment and Characteristics

A total of 34 patients who presented to the COVID-19 outpatient ward of the Medical University of Vienna between March 2020 and August 2020 with typical COVID-19 symptoms including cough, fever, sore throat, myalgia, loss of taste and/or smell, fatigue or dyspnoea were selected from the database for this cross-sectional analysis. Patients with anamnestic symptom onset within the last two days before presentation were included into the study. All patients were tested for the presence of SARS-CoV-2 RNA by routine PCR testing from nasopharyngeal swabs at the time of presentation and stratified into a symptomatic COVID-19 negative (CoV-; n=16) and a symptomatic COVID-19 positive (CoV+; n=18) group (PCR Ct-value: median 24.7 [interquartile range IQR 13.2-41.1]. At this time point also a venous blood draw for inflammatory marker determination was performed. 21 age and sex matched healthy volunteers were recruited and served as control group. Characteristics from all three groups are shown in **Table 1**.

TABLE 1 | Patient characteristics of healthy control (HC) volunteers, symptomatic, COVID-19 negative tested patients (CoV-) and symptomatic, COVID-19 positive tested patients (CoV+).

	HC (n = 21)	CoV- (n = 16)	CoV+ (n = 18)
female: male (%)	5 : 16	4 : 12	3 : 15
age (y; median, range)	42.0 (20-63)	35.0 (20-74)	42.0 (21-69)
cough	/	13 (0.81)	17 (0.94)
fever	/	12 (0.75)	6 (0.33)
sore throat	/	5 (0.31)	6 (0.33)
myalgia	/	3 (0.19)	6 (0.33)
loss of taste and/or smell	/	1 (0.06)	6 (0.33)
fatigue	/	2 (0.13)	4 (0.22)
dyspnea	/	9 (0.56)	3 (0.17)
hospitalization	/	3 (0.19)	7 (0.39)

Data are given in absolute numbers and in brackets relative to the whole group (100%). For age, the total range is given in brackets. Group comparison with ANOVA showed no significant differences between gender and age between the three study groups.

Assessment of Inflammatory Markers in Serum Specimens

Serum specimen from the three study groups were subjected to analysis using a commercially available 65 analyte multiplex immunoassay panel containing most relevant cytokines, chemokines and soluble receptors and growth factors typically found in inflammation (refer to **Supplementary Material 1** for the full list). Thereby, we aimed to analyze a broad range of factors produced by cells of the innate as well as the adaptive immune system, thus covering the breadth of the SARS-CoV-2 induced immune response. Out of the 65 assessed molecules, 39 were below the lower limit of quantification in >95% of all samples (irrespective of group) and were therefore excluded from further analysis (marked with an *asterisk in **Supplementary Material 1**). Of note, these excluded analytes also contained IFN-γ and IL-8 which were described as elevated in COVID-19 positive patients in other studies on hospitalized patients (Galani et al., 2021). Individual levels of analyzed proteins above the detection limit are shown in **Supplementary Material 2**. 10 analytes were observed at detectable levels in the sera of all three groups but showed no significant differences between the healthy control group and the specimens from either of the symptomatic groups. The respective analytes and their levels in all three groups are summarized in **Table 2**.

TABLE 2 | Median serum concentration, 25% quartile and 75% quartile in pg/mL of analytes showing no significant differences in specimen from healthy control (HC) volunteers, symptomatic, COVID-19 negative tested patients (CoV-) and symptomatic, COVID-19 positive tested patients (CoV+).

Analyte (pg/mL)	HC (n = 21)	CoV-(n = 16)	CoV+(n = 18)
CD40L	9 [5 ; 118]	68 [46 ; 118]	45 [24 ; 79]
ENA-78	227 [187 ; 277]	214 [102 ; 597]	150 [72 ; 1054]
Eotaxin	37 [23 ; 43]	54 [16 ; 63]	36 [25 ; 44]
Eotaxin-2	127 [74 ; 167]	193 [96 ; 285]	179 [84 ; 409]
IL-16	64 [33 ; 150]	13 [13 ; 127]	45 [13 ; 356]
IL-17A	32 [23 ; 83]	90 [23 ; 166]	32 [23 ; 401]
MCP-1	83 [41 ; 117]	129 [29 ; 173]	126 [74 ; 269]
MIP-1a	5 [2 ; 19]	8 [5 ; 22]	9 [3 ; 14]
MMP-1	20 [11 ; 48]	29 [5 ; 66]	63 [17 ; 134]
TWEAK	1133 [842 ; 1509]	1470 [1185 ; 2139]	1186 [918 ; 1652]

COVID-19 Infection Presents With a Distinct Inflammatory Pattern Compared to Other Common Respiratory Infections

In accordance with a general inflammatory response in respiratory infections, 7 analytes (APRIL, sIL-2R, MIF, MIP-1b, SCF, SDF-1a, sTNF-RII) showed a significant increase in serum levels in both the CoV- and CoV+ group compared to the healthy control cohort (**Figure 1** and **Supplementary Material 3**), while remaining statistically indifferent between CoV- and CoV+. These markers include the soluble form of TNFSF13 (tumor necrosis factor ligand superfamily member 13), also known as APRIL (A proliferation-inducing ligand), which nevertheless showed a clear trend towards higher serum levels in the CoV+ compared to the CoV- group (median; IQR25%-75% HC: CoV-: CoV+ = 44; 44-89 pg/mL: 290; 112-370 pg/mL: 598; 207-1055 pg/mL). All other markers showed a robust increase compared to the control cohort but no apparent differences between the CoV- and CoV+ symptomatic group. Thus, these proteins can be considered as general markers of respiratory inflammation. Additionally, IL-7 was significantly up-regulated in the CoV+ but not in the CoV- group compared to the control group while showing no significant difference between the two symptomatic groups. In this respect, IL-7 levels were generally very low with all sera analyzed showing values <10 pg/mL (**Figure 1** and **Supplementary Material 3**). Of note, four further analytes were significantly up-regulated in the symptomatic CoV- group but not in the CoV+ group. HGF (median, IQR25%-75% HC: CoV-: CoV+ = 89; 61-102 pg/mL: 212; 114-310 pg/mL: 126; 80-164 pg/mL), MDC (median, IQR25%-75% HC: CoV-: CoV+ = 131; 94-159 pg/mL: 224; 155-399 pg/mL: 178; 137-257 pg/mL) and VEGF-A (median, IQR25%-75% HC: CoV-: CoV+ = 115; 58-151 pg/mL: 207; 126-315 pg/mL: 189; 74-494 pg/mL) were significantly up-regulated in the symptomatic COV- group while the CoV+ group showed no significant difference compared to the control group (**Figure 2** and **Supplementary Material 3**). VEGF-A levels showed a high variance within the CoV+ group ranging from near baseline values to extremely high concentrations (total range: 5-17545 pg/mL) suggesting that this protein might be very heterogeneously affected by COVID-19 infection. Intriguingly, IL-18 was significantly down-regulated in the symptomatic CoV- group but remained at healthy control levels in the CoV+ group (median, IQR25%-75% HC: CoV-: CoV+ = 34; 23-61 pg/mL: 23; 20-33 pg/mL: 45; 27-63 pg/mL).

Of note, four analytes showed no differences between the healthy control and the symptomatic CoV- group but were significantly up-regulated in the CoV+ group. These were BCL/CXCL13, soluble (s)CD30, IP-10 and MCP-2/CCL8 (**Figure 3** and **Supplementary Material 3**). BLC (median,

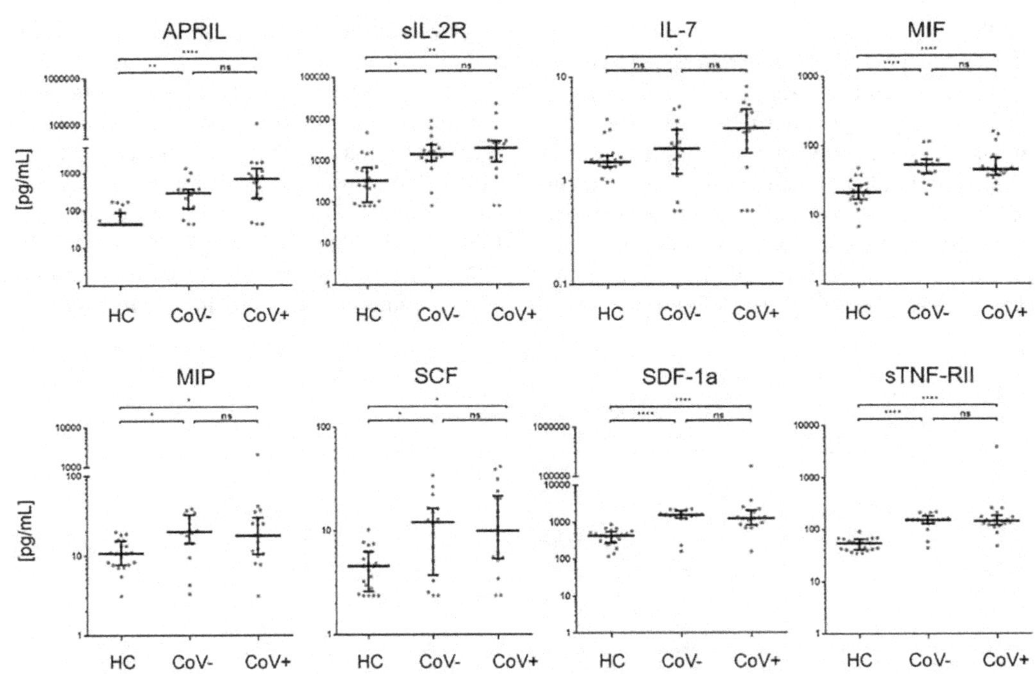

FIGURE 1 | Serum markers elevated in COVID-19- and COVID-19+ symptomatic patients compared to healthy controls. The indicated inflammatory markers were assessed by multiplex analysis from the serum of healthy control (HC) volunteers, symptomatic, COVID-19 negative tested patients (CoV-) and symptomatic, COVID-19 positive tested patients (CoV+). For each marker, individual results are depicted as dot plots. Each point represents the median of two technical replicates of each individual. Data are shown on a logarithmic scale for better visualization. Data are shown as median and interquartile range 25%-75%. $p > 0.05$ = ns not significant; *$p < 0.05$, **$p < 0.01$, ****$p < 0.0001$, Group differences between the three cohorts were tested using Kruskal-Wallis-test in conjunction with Dunn's multiple comparisons test using multiplicity adjusted calculation of p-values. (HC, n=21), (CoV-, n=16), (CoV+, n=18); APRIL, a proliferation-inducing ligand; sIL-2R-soluble interleukin 2 receptor; IL-7, interleukin 7; MIF, Macrophage migration inhibitory factor; MIP, macrophage inflammatory proteins; SCF, stem cell factor; SDF, 1a-stromal cell-derived factor 1; sTNF, RII-tumor necrosis factor receptor.

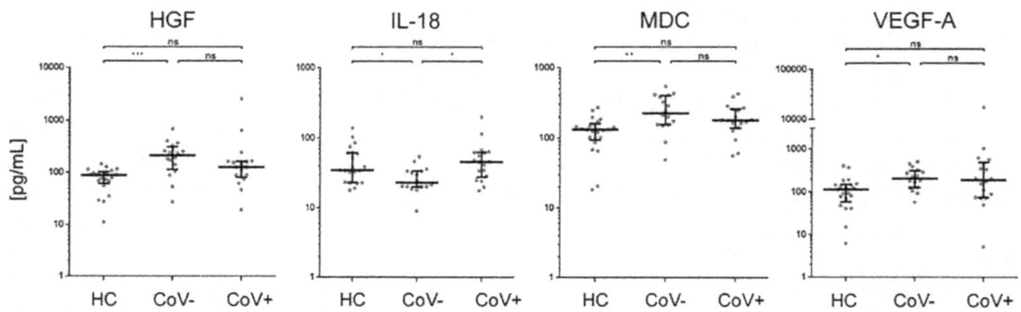

FIGURE 2 | Serum markers elevated or downregulated markers in COVID-19- patients compared to healthy controls and COVID-19+ patients. The indicated inflammatory markers were assessed by multiplex analysis from the serum of healthy control (HC) volunteers, symptomatic, COVID-19 negative tested patients (CoV-) and symptomatic, COVID-19 positive tested patients (CoV+). For each marker, individual results are depicted as dot plots. Each point represents the median of two technical replicates of each individual. Data are shown on a logarithmic scale for better visualization. Data are shown as median and interquartile range 25%-75%. p > 0.05 = ns not significant; *p < 0.05, **p < 0.01, ***p < 0.001, Group differences between the three cohorts were tested using Kruskal-Wallis-test in conjunction with Dunn's multiple comparisons test using multiplicity adjusted calculation of p-values. (HC, n=21), (CoV-, n=16), (CoV+, n=18). (HC, n=21)); HGF, hepatocyte growth factor; IL-18, interleukin-18; MDC, macrophage-derived chemokine; VEGF-A, vascular endothelial growth factor A.

IQR25%-75% HC: CoV-: CoV+ = 22; 11-36 pg/mL: 61; 22-100 pg/mL: 141; 74-189 pg/mL) and sCD30 (median, IQR25%-75% HC: CoV-: CoV+ = 74; 39-108 pg/mL: 161; 120-210 pg/mL: 273; 207-576 pg/mL) also showed a trend towards higher serum levels in symptomatic CoV- patients but were even further increased in the CoV+ group. For IP-10 (median, IQR25%-75% HC: CoV-: CoV+ = 8; 5-13 pg/mL: 10; 7-12 pg/mL: 37; 24-97 pg/mL) and MCP-2 (median, IQR25%-75% HC: CoV-: CoV+ = 6; 3-10 pg/mL: 8; 5-12 pg/mL: 18; 12-30 pg/mL) no differences between the healthy control and the symptomatic CoV- group were observable. Correlation analyses of these four parameters did not reveal robust correlation in any of the analyzed groups underscoring a highly individual inflammatory response in symptomatic SARS-CoV-2 negative and positive patients (**Supplementary Material 4**). Taken together, our analyses thus identify a unique COVID-19 specific inflammatory signature of four serum proteins in an early onset of disease setting.

DISCUSSION

By performing Luminex based Multiplex Immunoassay analysis in negative and positive tested cohorts with clinical signs of COVID-19 infection, we were able to identify an exclusive upregulation of BLC, sCD30, MCP-2 and IP-10 in patients early after onset of SARS-CoV-2 infection.

It has been shown previously that patients with severe COVID-19 infection display a hyperinflammatory milieu in the circulation with concomitant elevation of a variety of inflammatory cytokines and vascular endothelial damage markers and it has been now extensively discussed that the SARS-Cov-2 induced "cytokine storm" is a major source of complications but also provides promising therapeutic targets (Sinha et al., 2020; Chen and Quach, 2021; Mulchandani et al., 2021). Interestingly though, coronavirus infections trigger a very distinct immunological program, which is especially seen by the

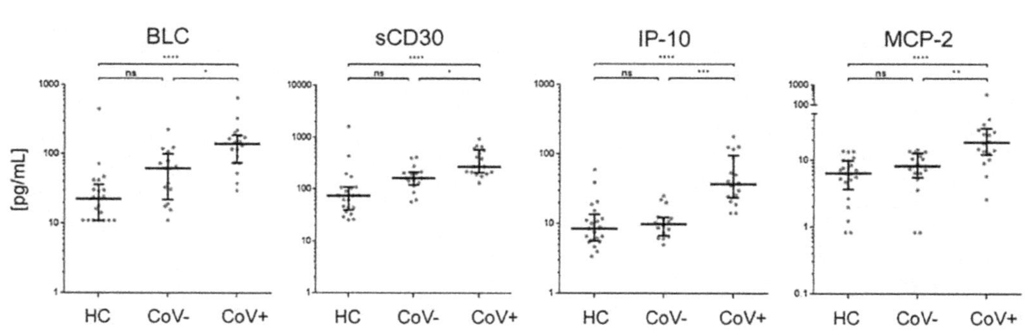

FIGURE 3 | Immune activation markers specifically elevated in the serum of COVID-19+ patients compared to COVID- patients and healthy controls. The indicated inflammatory markers were assessed by multiplex analysis from the serum of healthy control (HC) volunteers, symptomatic, COVID-19 negative tested patients (CoV-) and symptomatic, COVID-19 positive tested patients (CoV+). For each marker, individual results are depicted as dot plots. Each point represents the median of two technical replicates of each individual. Data are shown on a logarithmic scale for better visualization. Data are shown as median and interquartile range 25%-75%. p > 0.05 = ns not significant; *p < 0.05, **p < 0.01, ***p < 0.001, ****p < 0.0001, Group differences between the three cohorts were tested using Kruskal-Wallis-test in conjunction with Dunn's multiple comparisons test using multiplicity adjusted calculation of p-values. (HC, n=21), (CoV-, n=16), (CoV+, n=18); BLC, chemokine B lymphocyte chemoattractant; sCD30, soluble CD30; IP-10, interferon-gamma induced protein 10; MCP-2, monocyte chemotactic protein-2.

lack or delayed onset of a type I interferon response (Blanco-Melo et al., 2020; Hadjadj et al., 2020).

Dampening the excessive inflammation induced by SARS-CoV-2 infection has been the focus of clinical management. Accordingly, recent data on the ratio of the pro-inflammatory cytokine IL-6 and the anti-inflammatory cytokine IL-10 suggested that serum cytokines may be used for risk stratification in hospitalized COVID-19 patients (McElvaney et al., 2020). These observations were based on increased levels of multiple cytokines most prominently IL-6. Yet, the data were obtained from critically ill patients potentially also suffering from multiple co-morbidities (Tang et al., 2020).

Our study dissected the systemic cytokine response in symptomatic COVID-19 patients at the time of first hospital contact at the COVID outpatient clinic and compared results of COVID-positive and -negative tested individuals to each other and to healthy controls. We focused on the early inflammatory response of the COVID-19 infection and not on aged, hospitalized and often polymorbid patients.

In line with our results, it has been shown previously, that IP-10, a marker that induces T-cells and is therefore important for antiviral defense, is upregulated in hospitalized COVID-19 positive patients (Huang et al., 2020). Serum concentrations of IP-10 were higher in ICU patients compared to non-ICU patients. It has been shown that serum IP-10 levels are highly associated with disease severity and predict the progression of COVID-19 (Yang et al., 2020; Lev et al., 2021). Typically, IP-10 is associated as downstream chemokine of an IFN-γ response, although it can also be induced by other stimuli such as LPS or stressors such as heat shock or UV light *in vitro* [reviewed in (Vazirinejad et al., 2014)]. Along those lines, it is now discussed whether IFN-γ and IP-10 levels are independently affected by SARS-CoV-2 (Buszko et al., 2021). In contrast to previous studies, IFN-γ serum levels in all our cohorts were below the detection limit. This could be due to our recruitment strategy focusing on patients early after onset of symptoms. Thus, it could be hypothesized that an early IP-10 response in SARS-CoV-2 infection is followed by a later induction of IFN-γ which in turn further enhances IP-10 production. In this regard, it will be interesting to observe the results of the ongoing trial with the IFN-γ blocking antibody Emapalumab (trial NCT04324021) and how this affects the inflammatory situation in COVID-19 patients and the overall clinical outcome.

In our study, patients with severe COVID-19 infection display high levels of the monocyte chemoattractant MCP-2 (Sims et al., 2020), a chemokine that utilizes multiple cellular receptors to attract and activate different immune cells (Proost et al., 1996). Transcriptional analyses of respiratory cell populations and serum analysis in response to SARS-CoV-2 infection show strong upregulation of MCP-2 (Blanco-Melo et al., 2020; Zizzo and Cohen, 2020).

Therefore, anti-CCL8/MCP-2 antibodies might offer a novel point of intervention in the management of patients with COVID-19 induced hyperinflammation. Yet, our analyses also identified a significant upregulation of sCD30, a marker implicated in T-cell response and BLC/CXCL13 in CoV+ compared to symptomatic yet CoV- patients. sCD30 is a member of the tumor-necrosis-factor receptor superfamily. Low serum levels of sCD30 were found in healthy humans, whereas increased sCD30 concentrations were measured in autoimmune diseases such as systemic lupus erythematosus, rheumatoid arthritis, certain viral infections and adult T cell leukemia/lymphoma (van der Weyden et al., 2017).

A limited number of studies assessed the physiological role of CD30/CD30 ligand interactions in control of infection and it has been shown that after Epstein-Barr (EBV) infection, large numbers of CD30+ cells are generated (Zhou et al., 2017). However, the regulation of this factor early after COVID-19 infection has not been elucidated in detail so far.

BLC/CXCL13 on the other hand, is a small homeostatic CXC family chemokine that is highly expressed in the pleural cavity and critically involved in B-cell recruitment during infection (Ansel et al., 2002). A recent study has identified BLC as novel biomarker for lethal SARS-Cov-2 infection (Horspool et al., 2021). The authors, also found a correlation between BLC levels and antibody production. From these observations and the known biological role, it might be deduced that BLC is crucial in mediating the adaptive immune response e.g. in follicular B helper cells after COVID-19 infection and promotes antibody production. Interestingly, contrary, to previously published results in critically ill patients (Guaraldi et al., 2020), we could not detect IL-6, IL-8 and IFN-γ in our tested cohorts. However, in accordance with a previous study, an explanation might be the very early onset of infection at the time of blood withdrawal in our analysis (Zhang et al., 2020). Of note, correlation analyses of the four COVID-19 specific parameters only revealed low correlations between individuals. This indicates that patients show highly individual inflammatory responses to COVID-19 infection. Therefore, for potential diagnostic or therapeutic settings, all four parameters have to be considered in parallel.

We further demonstrated an upregulation of the chemokines APRIL, sIL-2R, IL-7, MIF, MIP-1b, SCF, SDF-1a, sTNF-RII in CoV+ patients, which was not specific for SARS-CoV-2 infection but also found in the COV- group. Still, these findings support the general finding that SARS-CoV-2 induces a broad cytokine storm. Several of these markers have been associated with distinct features of SARS-CoV-2 infection. Recently, a potential contribution of increased soluble IL-2R to lymphopenia in COVID-19 patients has been indicated (Zhang et al., 2020). IL-7 is a pleiotropic cytokine (Laterre et al., 2020), currently studied in clinical trials for oncologic and infectious disorders (Mackall et al., 2011). An upregulation of this cytokine early after COVID-19 infection might be an important immunomodulatory step of the host immunity in response to the infection.

MIF is an important regulator of innate immunity (Calandra and Roger, 2003). Previous studies showed decreased MIF levels and selective modulation after coronavirus infection (Frieman et al., 2008). MIP serum levels were found to be elevated in patients with COVID-19, requiring ICU admission (Huang et al., 2020). Similarly, serum SCF concentrations were significantly higher in fatal than severe or mild COVID-19 cases (Xu et al., 2020). sTNF-RII inhibit the TNF-alpha biological effects and thus may constitute a negative regulatory mechanism in acute inflammation. However, we did not find a significant upregulation of IL-18, a cytokine participating in host defense against infection, in early COVID-19 infection. This discrepancy might be due to different expression kinetics in the course of SARS-CoV-2 infection. In accordance to previous studies which indicate severe dysregulation of type I interferon responses in COVID-19, where these central mediators of the immune response seem actually to be blunted, we did not measure any interferon levels in our analysis (Acharya et al., 2020; Meffre and Iwasaki, 2020).

Some limitations should be addressed for our analysis. First, clinical data were only available from one center. Due to the exploratory study design, the number of analysed patients is relatively small and should be confirmed by larger longitudinal multi-center trials. Second, no detailed follow up of the investigated subpopulations could be provided within the scope of this study, hence, the viral genesis of disease of CoV- persons could not be ultimately confirmed. In this respect, especially a stratification of symptomatic SARS-CoV-2 negative patients according to the underlying pathogen (e.g. other endemic human coronaviruses, influenza A/B, etc.) would further add to the understanding of respiratory viral infections. Third the clinical assessment of COVID-19 symptoms was subjective according to the clinician at the COVID-19 triage at the outpatient clinic. Fourth, although restricted to a maximum of two days, the individual duration of disease symptoms varied between the persons before appearance at the outpatient clinic.

In conclusion, our study demonstrates that BLC/CXCL13, sCD30, MCP-2/CCL8 and IP-10/CXCL10 are specifically and individually upregulated in symptomatic COVID-19-positive patients but not in patients suffering from other respiratory infections with similar symptoms. Thus, our study might help to gain novel insights into the specific systemic immune response of the host, early after COVID-19 infection and ultimately might help to develop innovative therapeutic strategies against COVID-19 infection.

AUTHOR CONTRIBUTIONS

JK, KS, and RS conceived the study and wrote the first draft. AH and MB helped with sample processing. AK, SH, and MW carried out the Luminex analysis. CK and FG provided support for statistical analysis. FM, LT, VT-R, KG-P, and MK provided support in recruiting and analysis of the study populations. MS read and edited the draft. All authors contributed to the article and approved the submitted version.

ACKNOWLEDGMENTS

We gratefully acknowledge the contribution of the COVID outpatient clinic team of the Medical University of Vienna.

SUPPLEMENTARY MATERIAL

Supplementary Material 1 | Full list of 65 analytes. Analytes marked with an asterisk were below the limit of quantification.

Supplementary Material 2 | Levels of analyzed proteins from individual donors/ patients from the three groups.

Supplementary Material 3 | Median serum concentration, 25% quartile and 75% quartile in pg/mL of analytes showing differential levels in specimen from at least one group of healthy control (HC) volunteers, symptomatic, COVID-19 negative tested patients (CoV-) and symptomatic, COVID-19 positive tested patients (CoV+).

Supplementary Material 4 | Heat map of correlation of BLC, sCD30, IP-10 and MCP-2 in the three study groups. Healthy control (HC) volunteers, symptomatic, COVID-19 negative tested patients (CoV-) and symptomatic, COVID-19 positive tested patients (CoV+). Numbers indicate the respective Spearman r correlation coefficient.

REFERENCES

Acharya, D., Liu, G., and Gack, M. U. (2020). Dysregulation of Type I Interferon Responses in COVID-19. *Nat. Rev. Immunol.* 20 (7), 397–398. doi: 10.1038/s41577-020-0346-x

Ansel, K. M., Harris, R. B., and Cyster, J. G. (2002). CXCL13 Is Required for B1 Cell Homing, Natural Antibody Production, and Body Cavity Immunity. *Immunity* 16 (1), 67–76. doi: 10.1016/S1074-7613(01)00257-6

Becher, T., and Frerichs, I. (2020). Mortality in COVID-19 Is Not Merely a Question of Resource Availability. *Lancet Respir. Med.* 8 (9), 832–833. doi: 10.1016/S2213-2600(20)30312-X

Blanco-Melo, D., Nilsson-Payant, B. E., Liu, W. C., Uhl, S., Hoagland, D., Moller, R., et al. (2020). Imbalanced Host Response to SARS-CoV-2 Drives Development of COVID-19. *Cell* 181 (5), 1036–1045.e9. doi: 10.1016/j.cell.2020.04.026

Buszko, M., Nita-Lazar, A., Park, J. H., Schwartzberg, P. L., Verthelyi, D., Young, H. A., et al. (2021). Lessons Learned: New Insights on the Role of Cytokines in COVID-19. *Nat. Immunol.* 22 (4), 404–411. doi: 10.1038/s41590-021-00901-9

Calandra, T., and Roger, T. (2003). Macrophage Migration Inhibitory Factor: A Regulator of Innate Immunity. *Nat. Rev. Immunol.* 3 (10), 791–800. doi: 10.1038/nri1200

Cavalli, G., Larcher, A., Tomelleri, A., Campochiaro, C., Della-Torre, E., De Luca, G., et al. (2021). Interleukin-1 and Interleukin-6 Inhibition Compared With Standard Management in Patients With COVID-19 and Hyperinflammation: A Cohort Study. *Lancet Rheumatol* 3 (4), e253–ee61. doi: 10.1016/S2665-9913(21)00012-6

Chen, L. Y. C., and Quach, T. T. T. (2021). COVID-19 Cytokine Storm Syndrome: A Threshold Concept. *Lancet Microbe* 2 (2), e49–e50. doi: 10.1016/S2666-5247(20)30223-8

Chi, Y., Ge, Y., Wu, B., Zhang, W., Wu, T., Wen, T., et al. (2020). Serum Cytokine and Chemokine Profile in Relation to the Severity of Coronavirus Disease 2019 in China. *J. Infect. Dis.* 222 (5), 746–754. doi: 10.1093/infdis/jiaa363

de la Rica, R., Borges, M., and Gonzalez-Freire, M. (2020). COVID-19: In the Eye of the Cytokine Storm. *Front. Immunol.* 11, 558898. doi: 10.3389/fimmu.2020.558898

Forbester, J. L., and Humphreys, I. R. (2020). Genetic Influences on Viral-Induced Cytokine Responses in the Lung. *Mucosal Immunol.* 14, 14–25. doi: 10.1038/s41385-020-00355-6

Frieman, M., Heise, M., and Baric, R. (2008). SARS Coronavirus and Innate Immunity. *Virus Res.* 133 (1), 101–112. doi: 10.1016/j.virusres.2007.03.015

Galani, I. E., Rovina, N., Lampropoulou, V., Triantafyllia, V., Manioudaki, M., Pavlos, E., et al. (2021). Untuned Antiviral Immunity in COVID-19 Revealed by Temporal Type I/III Interferon Patterns and Flu Comparison. *Nat. Immunol.* 22 (1), 32–40. doi: 10.1038/s41590-020-00840-x

Guaraldi, G., Milic, J., Cozzi-Lepri, A., Pea, F., and Mussini, C. (2020). Tocilizumab in COVID-19: Finding the Optimal Route and Dose - Authors' Reply. *Lancet Rheumatol.* 2 (12), e739–ee40. doi: 10.1016/S2665-9913(20)30333-7

Hadjadj, J., Yatim, N., Barnabei, L., Corneau, A., Boussier, J., Smith, N., et al. (2020). Impaired Type I Interferon Activity and Inflammatory Responses in Severe

COVID-19 Patients. *Science* 369 (6504), 718–724. doi: 10.1126/science.abc6027

Horby, P., Lim, W. S., Emberson, J. R., Mafham, M., Bell, J. L., Linsell, L., et al. (2020). Dexamethasone in Hospitalized Patients With Covid-19 - Preliminary Report. *N. Engl. J. Med.* 384 (8), 693–704. doi: 10.1101/2020.06.22.20137273

Horspool, A. M., Kieffer, T., Russ, B. P., DeJong, M. A., Wolf, M. A., Karakiozis, J. M., et al. (2021). Interplay of Antibody and Cytokine Production Reveals CXCL13 as a Potential Novel Biomarker of Lethal SARS-CoV-2 Infection. *mSphere* 6 (1), e01324-20. doi: 10.1128/mSphere.01324-20

Huang, C., Wang, Y., Li, X., Ren, L., Zhao, J., Hu, Y., et al. (2020). Clinical Features of Patients Infected With 2019 Novel Coronavirus in Wuhan, China. *Lancet* 395 (10223), 497–506. doi: 10.1016/S0140-6736(20)30183-5

Laterre, P. F., Francois, B., Collienne, C., Hantson, P., Jeannet, R., Remy, K. E., et al. (2020). Association of Interleukin 7 Immunotherapy With Lymphocyte Counts Among Patients With Severe Coronavirus Disease 2019 (COVID-19). *JAMA Netw. Open* 3 (7), e2016485. doi: 10.1001/jamanetworkopen.2020.16485

Lescure, F. X., Bouadma, L., Nguyen, D., Parisey, M., Wicky, P. H., Behillil, S., et al. (2020). Clinical and Virological Data of the First Cases of COVID-19 in Europe: A Case Series. *Lancet Infect. Dis.* 20 (6), 697–706. doi: 10.1016/S1473-3099(20)30200-0

Lev, S., Gottesman, T., Sahaf Levin, G., Lederfein, D., Berkov, E., Diker, D., et al. (2021). Observational Cohort Study of IP-10's Potential as a Biomarker to Aid in Inflammation Regulation Within a Clinical Decision Support Protocol for Patients With Severe COVID-19. *PloS One* 16 (1), e0245296. doi: 10.1371/journal.pone.0245296

Mackall, C. L., Fry, T. J., and Gress, R. E. (2011). Harnessing the Biology of IL-7 for Therapeutic Application. *Nat. Rev. Immunol.* 11 (5), 330–342. doi: 10.1038/nri2970

McElvaney, O. J., Hobbs, B. D., Qiao, D., McElvaney, O. F., Moll, M., McEvoy, N. L., et al. (2020). A Linear Prognostic Score Based on the Ratio of Interleukin-6 to Interleukin-10 Predicts Outcomes in COVID-19. *EBioMedicine* 61, 103026. doi: 10.1016/j.ebiom.2020.103026

Meffre, E., and Iwasaki, A. (2020). Interferon Deficiency can Lead to Severe COVID. *Nature* 587 (7834), 374–376. doi: 10.1038/d41586-020-03070-1

Muhlbacher, J., Doberer, K., Kozakowski, N., Regele, H., Camovic, S., Haindl, S., et al. (2020). Non-Invasive Chemokine Detection: Improved Prediction of Antibody-Mediated Rejection in Donor-Specific Antibody-Positive Renal Allograft Recipients. *Front. Med. (Lausanne)* 7, 114. doi: 10.3389/fmed.2020.00114

Mulchandani, R., Lyngdoh, T., and Kakkar, A. K. (2021). Deciphering the COVID-19 Cytokine Storm: Systematic Review and Meta-Analysis. *Eur. J. Clin. Invest.* 51 (1), e13429. doi: 10.1111/eci.13429

Proost, P., Wuyts, A., and Van Damme, J. (1996). Human Monocyte Chemotactic Proteins-2 and -3: Structural and Functional Comparison With MCP-1. *J. Leukoc. Biol.* 59 (1), 67–74. doi: 10.1002/jlb.59.1.67

Reddy, K., Rogers, A. J., and McAuley, D. F. (2020). Delving Beneath the Surface of Hyperinflammation in COVID-19. *Lancet Rheumatol.* 2 (10), e578–e5e9. doi: 10.1016/S2665-9913(20)30304-0

Rodrigues, T. S., de Sá, K. S. G., Ishimoto, A. Y., Becerra, A., Oliveira, S., Almeida, L., et al. (2021). Inflammasomes Are Activated in Response to SARS-Cov-2 Infection and are Associated With COVID-19 Severity in Patients. *J. Exp. Med.* 218 (3), e20201707. doi: 10.1084/jem.20201707

Sims, J. T., Krishnan, V., Chang, C. Y., Engle, S. M., Casalini, G., Rodgers, G. H., et al. (2020). Characterization of the Cytokine Storm Reflects Hyperinflammatory Endothelial Dysfunction in COVID-19. *J. Allergy Clin. Immunol.* 147 (1), 107–111. doi: 10.1016/j.jaci.2020.08.031

Sinha, P., Matthay, M. A., and Calfee, C. S. (2020). Is a "Cytokine Storm" Relevant to COVID-19? *JAMA Intern. Med.* 180 (9), 1152–1154. doi: 10.1001/jamainternmed.2020.3313

Tang, Y., Liu, J., Zhang, D., Xu, Z., Ji, J., and Wen, C. (2020). Cytokine Storm in COVID-19: The Current Evidence and Treatment Strategies. *Front. Immunol.* 11, 1708. doi: 10.3389/fimmu.2020.01708

van der Weyden, C. A., Pileri, S. A., Feldman, A. L., Whisstock, J., and Prince, H. M. (2017). Understanding CD30 Biology and Therapeutic Targeting: A Historical Perspective Providing Insight Into Future Directions. *Blood Cancer J.* 7 (9), e603. doi: 10.1038/bcj.2017.85

Vazirinejad, R., Ahmadi, Z., Kazemi Arababadi, M., Hassanshahi, G., and Kennedy, D. (2014). The Biological Functions, Structure and Sources of CXCL10 and Its Outstanding Part in the Pathophysiology of Multiple Sclerosis. *Neuroimmunomodulation* 21 (6), 322–330. doi: 10.1159/000357780

Xu, Z. S., Shu, T., Kang, L., Wu, D., Zhou, X., Liao, B. W., et al. (2020). Temporal Profiling of Plasma Cytokines, Chemokines and Growth Factors From Mild, Severe and Fatal COVID-19 Patients. *Signal Transduct Target Ther.* 5 (1), 100. doi: 10.1038/s41392-020-0211-1

Yang, Y., Shen, C., Li, J., Yuan, J., Wei, J., Huang, F., et al. (2020). Plasma IP-10 and MCP-3 Levels are Highly Associated With Disease Severity and Predict the Progression of COVID-19. *J. Allergy Clin. Immunol.* 146 (1), 119–1127.e4. doi: 10.1016/j.jaci.2020.04.027

Zhang, J., Hao, Y., Ou, W., Ming, F., Liang, G., Qian, Y., et al. (2020). Serum Interleukin-6 Is an Indicator for Severity in 901 Patients With SARS-CoV-2 Infection: A Cohort Study. *J. Transl. Med.* 18 (1), 406. doi: 10.1038/s41423-020-0484-x

Zhang, Y., Wang, X., Li, X., Xi, D., Mao, R., Wu, X., et al. (2020). Potential Contribution of Increased Soluble IL-2R to Lymphopenia in COVID-19 Patients. *Cell Mol. Immunol.* 17 (8), 878–880. doi: 10.1038/s41423-020-0484-x

Zhao, Y., Qin, L., Zhang, P., Li, K., Liang, L., Sun, J., et al. (2020). Longitudinal COVID-19 Profiling Associates IL-1RA and IL-10 With Disease Severity and RANTES With Mild Disease. *JCI Insight* 5 (13), e139834. doi: 10.1172/jci.insight.139834

Zhou, A. C., Snell, L. M., Wortzman, M. E., and Watts, T. H. (2017). CD30 is Dispensable for T-Cell Responses to Influenza Virus and Lymphocytic Choriomeningitis Virus Clone 13 But Contributes to Age-Associated T-Cell Expansion in Mice. *Front. Immunol.* 8, 1156. doi: 10.3389/fimmu.2017.01156

Zizzo, G., and Cohen, P. L. (2020). Imperfect Storm: Is Interleukin-33 the Achilles Heel of COVID-19? *Lancet Rheumatol* 2 (12), e779–ee90. doi: 10.1016/S2665-9913(20)30340-4

6

Clinical Predictors of COVID-19 Severity and Mortality

Jitender Sharma[1], Roopali Rajput[2], Manika Bhatia[3], Pooja Arora[3] and Vikas Sood[2*]*

[1] Department of Biochemistry, All India Institute of Medical Sciences, Bathinda, India, [2] Department of Biochemistry, School of Chemical and Life Sciences, Jamia Hamdard, New Delhi, India, [3] Department of Zoology, Hansraj College, University of Delhi, Delhi, India

The COVID-19 pandemic has caused huge socio-economic losses and continues to threat humans worldwide. With more than 4.5 million deaths and more than 221 million confirmed COVID-19 cases, the impact on physical, mental, social and economic resources is immeasurable. During any novel disease outbreak, one of the primary requirements for effective mitigation is the knowledge of clinical manifestations of the disease. However, in absence of any unique identifying characteristics, diagnosis/prognosis becomes difficult. It intensifies misperception and leads to delay in containment of disease spread. Numerous clinical research studies, systematic reviews and meta-analyses have generated considerable data on the same. However, identification of some of the distinct clinical signs and symptoms, disease progression biomarkers and the risk factors leading to adverse COVID-19 outcomes warrant in-depth understanding. In view of this, we assessed 20 systematic reviews and meta-analyses with an intent to understand some of the potential independent predictors/biomarkers/risk factors of COVID-19 severity and mortality.

Keywords: SARS-CoV-2, prognosis, biomarkers, risk factors, obesity, diabetes, radiological, sleep

Correspondence:
Jitender Sharma
jitendersharma.clinchem@gmail.com
Vikas Sood
v.sood@jamiahamdard.ac.in;
vikas1101@gmail.com

INTRODUCTION

Coronaviruses belong to Coronaviridae family of viruses. The degree of disease caused by coronaviruses can vary from mild like common cold to severe like severe acute respiratory syndrome (SARS) and the middle east respiratory syndrome (MERS). These viruses have been successful in crossing inter-species barriers. SARS-coronavirus jumped from civet cats to humans while MERS-coronavirus got transmitted to humans from camels (Woo et al., 2012). The recent emergence of the novel SARS Coronavirus 2 (SARS-CoV-2) is another incidence of zoonotic transmission of coronaviruses. As per the genomic sequence analysis, the source of novel SARS-CoV-2 is speculated to be a previously identified bat coronavirus strain RaTG13 (96.2- 97.41% identity match) (Shi, 2021; Malaiyan et al., 2021) or pangolin-CoV (91.02- 92.22% genomic identity match) (Zhang T. et al., 2020; Malaiyan et al., 2021). However, the origin of the SARS-CoV-2 is still unclear due to the lack of definitive evidence. Further investigations are being undertaken in this regard (WHO News release, 2021).

Since the first case reported late in 2019, SARS-CoV-2 has taken more than 4.5 million human lives (as of September 08, 2021) and continues to spread worldwide with more than 221 million confirmed cases (WHO, 2021). The case fatality rate of the disease caused by the SARS-CoV-2 (3.26- 4.16% in Latin America; 5.8% in the United States) (Undurraga et al., 2021; Loomba et al., 2021) is way less as compared to the previous coronavirus outbreaks (Zhu et al., 2020). Nevertheless, the fatality caused by Coronavirus Disease 2019 (COVID-19) has surpassed that of the SARS and MERS combined (Song et al., 2019). The COVID-19 pandemic has also resulted in huge economic losses (speculated to be trillions of dollars) around the world (Emem, 2020).

COVID-19 initially emerged as novel pneumonia of unknown etiology with majorly non-specific symptoms and quite quickly engulfed the entire globe. During the initial months of the pandemic, lack of specific diagnostic modalities, the variable intensity of the disease surveillance, changing case definitions, asymptomatic period of infection and overwhelmed health care facilities largely contributed to the rapid spread of the virus, resulting in the global outbreak. Also, the novel COVID-19 in a way bridged the gap between the developing and developed world, bringing all on the same footing. With more than 85 million confirmed cases, the Americas are the worst affected, followed by Europe (> 66 million), South-East Asia (> 41 million), the East Mediterranean region (> 15 million), Western Pacific (> 7 million) and Africa (> 5 million) (WHO, 2021). A major breakthrough in the current pandemic period witnessed rapid development and administration of different vaccines against COVID-19. However, despite the massive vaccine roll-out programs, the emergence of virus variants sustains the challenge of controlling the pandemic and continues to spread in its wild-type and mutant forms across the globe.

Since the onset of the disease, several groups have published various systematic reviews and meta-analyses that aim to shed light on the disease prognosis. However, the evidence was limited and the data were mostly heterogenous. Further, due to ever-changing viral dynamics, multiple new symptoms have been witnessed. With the generation of more data, it is expected that the analysis will continue with a focus on identifying unique clinical manifestations, laboratory findings, radiological investigations, and therapy that could correlate with varying degree of COVID-19 or adverse outcomes, and fatality. However, the studies published earlier have highlighted the significance of some important biomarkers and clinical features in diagnosis, prognosis and management of mild to severe COVID-19.

METHODOLOGY

In the present work, we aim to identify key players of the disease and summarize important findings from already published studies on diverse clinical aspects of COVID-19. The search terms 'COVID-19', 'SARS-CoV-2', 'clinical predictors', 'signs and symptoms' were used individually or in appropriate combinations and only the 'systematic reviews and/or meta-analysis' articles that were published until February, 2021 were included for the present work. We carefully studied 20 systematic review/meta-analysis/meta-regression articles (**Table 1A**) that spanned the global population.

PROGNOSTIC FACTORS ASSOCIATED WITH SEVERE COVID-19

Clinical Manifestations

Since the start of the pandemic, COVID-19 displayed a wide spectrum of clinical signs and symptoms, which included: fever, cough, sore throat, nasal congestion, sputum, headache, diarrhea, fatigue, dyspnea, chest tightness, myalgia, nausea, rhinorrhea, dizziness or confusion, hemoptysis, anorexia, vomiting, chest and abdominal pain (Huang et al., 2020; Jutzeler et al., 2020; Mudatsir et al., 2020). The eagerness to know any unique/distinct features was evident even in the layman. Fever, cough, fatigue, dyspnea (Figliozzi et al., 2020; Israfil et al., 2021) and a loss of sense of taste and smell (Hannum et al., 2020) remained some of the most experienced and identifying symptoms. In a systematic review involving more than 12000 patients, fever was the most common clinical manifestation in adults (78.5%), pregnant women (71.4%), pediatric and neonatal (53.1%) patients. Other important clinical signs and symptoms were cough (53.8%) and fatigue (25%) in adults, cough (41.4%) and myalgia (33.3%) in pregnant women and cough (47.9%) and sputum (27.5%) in children and neonates (Jutzeler et al., 2020). Only about 5% of patients were asymptomatic. Another meta-analysis, involving early data from 3578 patients, identified relation of dyspnea [odds ratio (OR)= 3.28, 95% confidence interval (CI) 2.09- 5.15], anorexia (OR= 1.83, 95% CI 1.00- 3.34), fatigue (OR= 2.00, 95% CI 1.25- 3.20) and dizziness (OR= 2.67, 95% CI 1.18- 6.01) with COVID-19 severity (Mudatsir et al., 2020). The vastly experienced COVID-19 symptoms, viz., fever, cough and breathing problem have been associated with problems in having sound sleep (Ferrando et al., 2016; Singh et al., 2020). An interesting systematic review and meta-analysis attempted to understand the impact of COVID-19 pandemic on quality or quantity of sleep under different study groups: COVID-19 patients, healthcare workers and the general population (Jahrami et al., 2021). As expected, about 75% of the COVID-19 patients had disturbed sleep, which was the highest prevalence among the different study groups (Jahrami et al., 2021). Physical pain or side-effects of the treatments were also speculated to impact the sound sleep in COVID-19 patients (Shi et al., 2020). These findings suggest that monitoring of sleep problems must not be ignored during COVID-19.

Comorbidities as Risk Factors for Adverse Outcomes of COVID-19

In one of the early meta-analyses aimed at assessing the impact of comorbidities on the course and clinical outcome of COVID-19, it was found that about 31% of adult patients (2329/7608) had comorbidities, with hypertension being the most prevalent condition (20.93%, 1352/6460), followed by heart failure (10.5%, 37/354), diabetes mellitus (10.4%, 678/6535) and coronary heart disease (8.5%, 194/2388) (Jutzeler et al., 2020).

TABLE 1A | Overview of the methodology of the analyzed systematic reviews and meta-analysis in relation to severity, adverse prognosis and mortality of COVID-19.

S. No.	Reference	Date of publication (or acceptance for publication)	Methodology									
			Type of analysis	**Diseases compared**	**Features analyzed**	**Data sources**	**Data set**	**Records screened**	**Records selected**	**Period (up to)**	**Total patients studied**	**Region of study**
1.	Zhang JJY. et al., 2020	May 14, 2020	Systematic review, meta-analysis and meta-regression	COVID-19	Laboratory investigations as predictors of poor COVID-19 outcomes; and efficacy of therapies (involving experimental antiviral and immunomodulatory treatments)	Ovid MEDLINE, EMBASE, CENTRAL and PubMed	Heterogenous	1481	45	March 15, 2020	4203	China, Singapore, South Korea and Hong Kong
2.	Li et al., 2021	June 12, 2020	Systematic review and meta-analysis	COVID-19	Clinical features and outcome of severe and non -severe pneumonia patients	PubMed, EMBASE, Cochrane	Heterogenous	201	12	April 14, 2020	2445	China
3.	Földi et al., 2020	June 21, 2020	Systematic review, meta-analysis and meta-regression	COVID-19	Obesity as a risk factor	MEDLINE (via PubMed), EMBASE, CENTRAL, Scopus and Web of Science	Heterogenous	15168	24	May 11, 2020	Meta-analysis: 2,770 and 509 for ICU admission and IMV requirement, respectively Meta-regression: 2522	China, France, USA, Portugal, Netherlands, Italy and Qatar
4.	Lu et al., 2020	July 04, 2020	Systematic review and meta-analysis	COVID-19, SARS and MERS	Predictors of mortality	MEDLINE, Epistemonikos, COCHRANE, CKNI, WANFANG STATA and manual search	Heterogenous	712	28	April 11, 2020	16095 (COVID-19: 11818; SARS: 3292; MERS: 985)	COVID-19: China, Italy, South Korea and the United States SARS: Beijing, Guangdong, Shanxi, Hong Kong and Taiwan in China, and Toronto MERS: Saudi Arabia and South Korea
5.	Figliozzi et al., 2020	July 20, 2020	Systematic review and meta-analysis	COVID-19	Predictors of adverse prognosis	PubMed, MEDLINE, Scopus	Heterogenous	6843	49	April 24, 2020	20211	China, USA, France, Japan, Italy and Canada
6.	Henry et al., 2020	July 20, 2020	Systematic review and meta-analysis	COVID-19	Association of 'at admission lymphopenia and neutrophilia' with COVID-19 severity and mortality	PubMed, CNKI, CENTRAL	Heterogenous	53	22	May 06, 2020	4969	China, USA and Italy

(Continued)

TABLE 1A | Continued

S. No.	Reference	Date of publication (or acceptance for publication)	Methodology									
			Type of analysis	Diseases compared	Features analyzed	Data sources	Data set	Records screened	Records selected	Period (up to)	Total patients studied	Region of study
7.	Shao et al., 2020	July 22, 2020	Systematic review and meta-analysis	COVID-19	Association of AKI with severe COVID-19 and related mortality	PubMed, Web of Science, Science Direct, medRxiv	Heterogenous	878	40	June 20, 2020	24527	China, South Korea, Korea, Spain, New York, Kuwait and Turkey
8.	Li et al., 2020	July 28, 2020	Systematic review and meta-analysis	COVID-19	Association of cardiac injury and severity and mortality	PubMed, EMBASE, Cochrane, CNKI, medRxiv, ChinaXiv	Heterogenous	1331	23	March 30, 2020	4631	China
9.	Ghahramani et al., 2020	August 03, 2020	Systematic review and meta-analysis	COVID-19	Laboratory features of severe and non-severe patients	PubMed, Web of Science, Science, EMBASE, Scopus	Heterogenous	1988	22	March 03, 2020	3396	China and Singapore
10.	Jutzeler et al., 2020	August 04, 2020	Systematic review and meta-analysis	COVID-19	Risk ratio of comorbidities, clinical features, laboratory parameters, imaging features, treatment and complications with morbidity and mortality	PubMed, Web of Science, EMBASE, Scopus, manual search	Heterogenous	2605	148	March 28, 2020	12149	China, Italy, USA, South Korea, Taiwan, Germany, France, Scotland, Japan, Vietnam, Canada, Singapore, Belgium, Finland, Russia, Spain and Sweden
11.	Lippi et al., 2020	August 25, 2020	Systematic review and meta-analysis	COVID-19	RDW as predictor of severity	MEDLINE, Web of Science, Science, Scopus	Heterogenous	13	3	July, 2020	11445	China, USA
12.	Moutchia et al., 2020	October 01, 2020	Systematic review and meta-analysis	COVID-19	Clinical laboratory parameters of severe or critical COVID-19	MEDLINE, EMBASE, Web of Science, CINAHL and Google Scholar databases	Heterogenous	1722	45	April, 18, 2020	9508	China, USA, France, Germany, Japan and Singapore
13.	Jahrami et al., 2021	October 13, 2020	Systematic review and meta-analysis	COVID-19	Impact of COVID-19 pandemic on quantity or quality of sleep	PubMed, MEDLINE, Web of Science, Science, Scopus and others	Heterogenous	371	44	July 05, 2020	54231	China, Iraq, Germany, India, Italy, France, Mexico, Spain, Bahrain, Greece, Australia and Canada
14.	Mudatsir et al., 2020	November 02, 2020	Systematic review and meta-analysis	COVID-19	Clinical manifestations and laboratory findings of mild to severe COVID-19	PubMed, EMBASE, Cochrane, Web of science	Heterogenous	39	19	April 05, 2020	3578	China (cities-Wuhan, Shenzen, Fuyang and Chongqing)
15.	Mesas et al., 2020	November 03, 2020	Systematic review and meta-analysis	COVID-19	Predictors of in-hospital mortality	PubMed, MEDLINE, Web of Science, Science, Scopus	Heterogenous	12254	60	May 17, 2020	51225	China, Italy, Israel, Pakistan, Brazil, Spain, UK, Switzerland, France, USA, South Korea and Iran

(Continued)

TABLE 1A | Continued

S. No.	Reference	Date of publication (or acceptance for publication)	Methodology									
			Type of analysis	Diseases compared	Features analyzed	Data sources	Data set	Records screened	Records selected	Period (up to)	Total patients studied	Region of study
16.	Izcovich et al., 2020	November 17, 2020	Systematic review and meta-analysis	COVID-19	Prognostic factors for severity and mortality	PubMed, MEDLINE, EMBASE, CENTRAL	Heterogenous	569	207	April 28, 2020	57044	China, USA, Canada, Spain, France, Turkey, Korea, Japan, Italy, Germany, India and Singapore
17.	Del Zompo et al., 2020	December, 2020	Systematic review and meta-analysis	COVID-19	Prevalence of liver injury with COVID-19 severity and in-hospital fatality	PubMed, MEDLINE, PMC, EMBASE, Web of Science, clinical trial registries, publications from ArXiv, BioRxiv, Elsevier, MedRxiv, WHO sources and other databases searched for coronavirus family publications	Heterogenous	12484	36	August 03, 2020	20724	China, USA, Italy, South Korea, France and Germany
18.	Hannum et al., 2020	December 05, 2020	Systematic review and meta-analysis	COVID-19	Olfactory loss in COVID-19	PubMed, MEDLINE and Google Scholar	Heterogenous	43	34	April 30, 2020	19746	China, Italy, Sweden, Iran, Germany, Israel, Switzerland, UK, USA Taiwan, Korea, Belgium, Spain, France, Australia, Singapore and Iceland
19.	Israfil et al., 2021	January 11, 2021	Systematic review	COVID-19	Clinical characteristics	PubMed, Web of Science, Scopus, Science Direct, and Google Scholar	Heterogenous	557	34	May 07, 2020	10889	China, USA, Italy, Singapore, UK, France, Japan and Macau
20.	Poly et al., 2021	February 05, 2021	Systematic review and meta-analysis	COVID-19	Impact of obesity, associated comorbidities and other factors on risk of COVID-19 related mortality	PubMed, EMBASE, Google Scholar, Web of Science, and Scopus	Heterogenous	252	17	August 30, 2020	543399	China, Italy, Mexico, USA, France and UK

CENTRAL, Cochrane Central Register of Controlled Trials; CINAHL, Cumulative Index of Nursing and Allied Health Literature; CKNI, China National Knowledge Infrastructure; COVID-19, coronavirus disease 2019; EMBASE, Excerpta Medica database; MEDLINE, Medical Literature Analysis and Retrieval System Online; PMC, PubMed Central; UK, United Kingdom; USA, United States of America.

These pre-existing comorbidities were found to be linked with the severity of COVID-19 (relative risk, RR= 2.11, p= 0.046) (Jutzeler et al., 2020). Also, hypertension (RR= 2.15, p< 0.001), diabetes (RR= 2.56, p= 0.005), any heart condition (RR= 4.09, p< 0.001) and chronic obstructive pulmonary disease (COPD) (RR= 5.10, p< 0.001) were associated with adverse disease outcome. In addition, disease severity was more in male (RR= 1.11, p= 0.039) and old age patients (standardized mean difference, SMD= 0.68, p< 0.001) (Jutzeler et al., 2020). The meta-analysis revealed that older age (SMD= 1.25, 95% CI 0.78– 1.72, p< 0.001), male gender (RR= 1.32, 95% CI 1.13–1.54, p= 0.005) and pre-existing comorbidities (RR= 1.69, 95% CI 1.48– 1.94, p< 0.001) were associated with less survival. Furthermore, mechanical ventilation was also more frequently required for treatment of non-survivors as compared to survivors (RR= 6.05, 95% CI 1.41–26.05, p= 0.026); with more common administration of extracorporeal membrane oxygenation (RR= 4.39, 95% CI 1.64– 11.78, p= 0.014) in the non-survivors (Jutzeler et al., 2020). The risk of developing complications during the course of COVID-19 was higher in the non-survivors as compared to the survivors. The complications included, in particular, acute kidney injury (AKI) (RR= 20.77, 95% CI 2.43– 177.44, p= 0.017) and acute respiratory distress syndrome (ARDS) (RR= 4.24, 95% CI 1.30–13.83, p= 0.026) (Jutzeler et al., 2020).

Liver injury has been reported as another comorbidity being associated with the severity and in-hospital fatality of COVID-19 patients. In a meta-analysis of 20724 COVID-19 confirmed cases from 36 articles, pre-existing liver disease was present in up to 37.6% of cases (Del Zompo et al., 2020) at the time of hospital admission. The etiology of abnormal liver function was mentioned in only a few of the studies analyzed in the said meta-analysis. The authors recommended frequent testing of liver function test (LFT) markers as an additional tool for early stratification and monitoring of COVID-19 patients (Del Zompo et al., 2020). Further prospective cohort investigations are need-of-the-hour to validate the significance of LFT biochemistries in the management of COVID-19. Likewise, about 4.5% of COVID-19 patients displayed pre-known viral hepatitis in a study conducted by a different research group (Gu et al., 2020).

Another noteworthy comorbidity is AKI. In view of this, a systematic review and meta-analysis was conducted involving 24527 COVID-19 patients, where the overall rate of severe COVID-19 and COVID-19 related fatality was 26.4% and 20.3%, respectively (Shao et al., 2020). The robust meta-analysis revealed significant association of AKI with severity (OR= 8.11, 95% CI 5.01-13.13, p< 0.00001) and fatality (OR= 14.63, 95% CI 9.94- 21.51, p< 0.00001) in COVID-19 patients. Prevalence of severe COVID-19 and fatality due to COVID-19 was considerably high (55.6% and 63.1% respectively, p< 0.01) in patients with AKI as compared to those without AKI (17.7% and 12.9% respectively) (Shao et al., 2020). Cardiac impairment was a significant factor associated with severe COVID-19 outcomes (OR= 3.15, 95% CI 2.26- 4.41) and fatality (OR= 1.95, 95% CI 1.08- 3.54) (Figliozzi et al., 2020; Li et al., 2020). Smoking (OR= 2.24, 95% CI 1.40- 3.58), history of diabetes mellitus (OR= 2.34, 95% CI 1.64- 3.33), COPD (OR= 2.63, 95% CI 1.55- 4.44) or hypertension (OR= 2.25, 95% CI 1.80- 2.82) contributed to progression to adverse COVID-19 (Figliozzi et al., 2020). Diabetes mellitus (OR= 1.74, 95% CI 1.22- 2.48), cardiovascular disease (OR= 1.95, 95% CI 1.08- 3.54), COPD (OR= 2.98, 95% CI 1.38-6.44), or cerebrovascular disease (OR= 2.93, 95% CI 1.84- 4.26) indicated high mortality risk (Figliozzi et al., 2020).

Apart from the above-mentioned somewhat obvious comorbidities, obesity emerged as another major condition that would worsen the outcomes in COVID-19 patients (Földi et al., 2020; Poly et al., 2021). A meta-analysis involving 2770 patients revealed that obesity was a significant risk factor associated with admission to critical care units (OR= 1.21, 95% CI 1.002- 1.46) (Földi et al., 2020). Also, the requirement of invasive mechanical ventilation (IMV) was more (up to 78%) for obese patients as analyzed in 509 subjects. A body-mass-index (BMI) of ≥ 25 was a significant risk factor for IMV requirement (OR= 2.63, 95% CI 1.64-4.22) (Földi et al., 2020). Like obesity, psychiatric comorbidities (like anxiety and depression) must also be considered during COVID-19 management. Potential bi-directional associations between psychiatric comorbidities and sleep have been reported (Jahrami et al., 2021), amounting to sleep problems during COVID-19. This may impact the recovery from the disease.

Biochemical Biomarkers as Independent Predictors of Severity, Adverse Prognosis or Mortality of COVID-19

Recent evidence highlighted the relevance of various biochemical tests as independent or combined correlates for the determination of severity, poor prognosis or mortality related to COVID-19. Clinical laboratory tests encompassing biochemical, hematological, inflammatory and coagulation parameters were considered useful to recognize severe or critical COVID-19. Additionally, these parameters also provided valuable clinical information for effective monitoring of the clinical course of COVID-19. As per findings of a large meta-analysis of 45 studies across 6 countries, neutrophilia (meta-median difference, MMD= 1.23 x 10^9 cells/μl) and lymphopenia (MMD= -0.39 x 10^9 cells/μl) were associated with critical COVID-19 (Moutchia et al., 2020). Similar findings were also reported in another meta-analysis comprising 4969 patients (Henry et al., 2020). In this meta-analysis, reduced lymphocyte count and increased neutrophil count at the time of admission were significantly associated with progression to severe disease (OR= 4.20, 95% CI 3.46- 5.09 and OR= 7.99, 95% CI 1.77- 36.14, respectively), and mortality (OR= 3.71, 95% CI, 1.63- 8.44 and OR= 7.87, 95% CI 1.75- 35.35, respectively) (Henry et al., 2020). Inflammatory markers, namely, C-reactive protein (CRP), Interleukin 6 (IL-6), and erythrocyte sedimentation rate (ESR) (MMD= 36.97 mg/l, 17.37 pg/ml, 21.93 mm/hr, respectively) were raised in severe COVID-19 cases (Moutchia et al., 2020). Biochemical indices like alanine aminotransferase (ALT), aspartate aminotransferase (AST), blood urea nitrogen (BUN), creatinine (MMD= 6.89 u/l, 11.96 u/l, 1.04 mmol/l, 4.87 μmol/l) were significantly elevated in severe or critical cases in comparison to non-severe COVID-19 patients (Moutchia et al., 2020). A meta-regression analysis observed that higher leukocyte counts (p< 0.0001), elevated levels of ALT (p= 0.024), AST (p=

0.0040), lactate dehydrogenase (LDH) ($p< 0.0001$) and raised procalcitonin (PCT) ($p< 0.0001$) were note-worthy predictors of admission to intensive care unit (Zhang JJY. et al., 2020). Further, the researchers found that elevated LDH ($p< 0.0001$) and high leukocyte counts ($p= 0.0005$) were significantly associated with COVID-19 led mortality. Other laboratory parameters that were found to be significantly associated with critical disease were myocardial biomarkers, Troponin I (MMD= 0.01 ng/ml), and creatine kinase-MB (CK-MB) (MMD= 1.46 u/l), tissue damage marker, LDH (MMD= 124.26 u/l), platelet count (MMD= -21.48 x 10^9 cells/l) and D-dimer (MMD= 0.65 mg/ml) (Moutchia et al., 2020). These laboratory parameters indicated that innate immune response gets activated during COVID-19 as indicated by markedly raised neutrophil to lymphocyte ratio (NLR) and CRP. In contrast, adaptive immune response is unable to limit virus replication during severe COVID-19, as evidenced by reduced levels of lymphocytes and its subsets. Thus, routine testing for NLR, CRP, ESR, Troponin-I, BUN, creatinine, AST, ALT, CK-MB, LDH and D-dimer in severe COVID-19 is beneficial in monitoring clinical progression and can predict outcome of the disease. Anisocytosis, a condition that is characterized by heterogeneity in volumes of circulating red blood cells (RBCs), has also been linked to severe COVID-19. This low-cost parameter is expressed as RBC distribution width (RDW) and may be calculated as either RDW-standard deviation (SD) or coefficient of variation (CV). In this view, an analysis of RDW in 11445 COVID-19 patients was conducted and a 0.69% increase (95% CI 0.40- 0.98, $p< 0.001$) in absolute RDW-CV value of severe COVID-19 patients was found in comparison to mildly ill COVID-19 patients (Lippi et al., 2020). Hence, estimation of RDW may assist in risk stratification of adverse COVID-19 progression (Lippi et al., 2020).

Laboratory results were useful in differentiating severe from non-severe COVID-19 patients at the time of admission to the intensive care unit, as per the systematic review and meta–analysis conducted by Ghahramani et al. (Ghahramani et al., 2020). Results of routine tests like LFT, kidney function tests (KFT), glucose, albumin, electrolytes and complete blood count (CBC) were significantly altered in severe or critical COVID-19 patients belonging to the Asian population. In the same systematic review and meta-analysis, elevated PCT levels and higher neutrophil count were associated with bacterial co-infection in severe COVID-19 patients. Further, sensitivity analysis revealed significant differences in pooled effect size (p-ES) for NLR, lymphocyte to CRP ratio (LCR), PCT, AST, ALT, sodium, glucose, BUN, creatinine, ESR, myoglobin and D-dimer (Ghahramani et al., 2020). Laboratory parameters like decreased platelet count (p-ES= -1.7), low hemoglobin concentration (p-ES= -0.6), low albumin (p-ES= -3.1), raised IL-6 (p-ES = 2.4), elevated creatinine (p-ES = 2.4) and higher troponin-I (p-ES = 0.7) were markedly associated with in-hospital mortality (Mesas et al., 2020). As per another meta-analysis, low albumin levels (SMD= -1.13, 95% CI -1.41– -0.85, $p< 0.001$) and lymphocyte counts (SMD= -0.92, 95% CI -1.3– -0.55, $p< 0.001$) as well as high IL-6 levels (SMD= 1.21, 95% CI 0.93– 1.5, $p< 0.001$), leucocyte counts (SMD= 2.21, 95% CI 0.61– 3.64, $p= 0.06$), and prolonged prothrombin time (SMD= 7.99, 95% CI 4.64–11.34, $p< 0.01$) were found to be linked with COVID-19 related mortality (Jutzeler et al., 2020). Hence, abnormal indices of the above-mentioned parameters could be prognostic markers of adverse COVID-19 outcomes.

In another large-scale analysis, including more than 57000 COVID-19 patients, 49 parameters were identified as high/ moderate predictors of poor prognosis (Izcovich et al., 2020). The variable parameters included demographic factors: increasing age, male gender and smoking; comorbidities: diabetes, cerebrovascular disease, COPD, cardiovascular disease, cardiac arrhythmia, arterial hypertension, chronic kidney disease, cancer, dementia and dyslipidemia; physical examination factors: respiratory failure, fever, myalgia or arthralgia, fatigue, abdominal pain, tachycardia, hypoxemia, dyspnea, anorexia, tachypnoea, low blood pressure, hemoptysis; laboratory assessments: elevated PCT, myocardial injury markers, increased WBC counts, elevated blood lactate, reduced lymphocyte count, reduced platelet count, increased neutrophil count, raised plasma creatinine, elevated D-dimer, raised LDH, elevated CRP, raised AST levels, decreased albumin, elevated IL-6 levels, raised B-type natriuretic peptide (BNP), elevated BUN, raised ESR, elevated CK and raised bilirubin; radiological factors: pleural effusion and consolidative infiltrate; and high sequential organ failure assessment (SOFA) score (**Tables 1B**, **2**) (Izcovich et al., 2020).

A systematic review and meta-analysis of 36 studies involving more than 20000 patients demonstrated important findings (Del Zompo et al., 2020). With an intent to correlate liver injury with clinical outcomes in COVID-19 patients, the researchers found that nearly 47% of COVID-19 cases had abnormal LFT. They also found that the laboratory tested AST, ALT and total bilirubin were independent predictors of COVID-19 severity and in-hospital mortality (**Table 2**) (Del Zompo et al., 2020). However, there was insufficient information on the etiology of pre-existing liver injury in COVID-19 patients at the time of hospitalization. Hence, further prospective cohort studies would be essential to validate these findings.

Other noteworthy biochemical findings are elevated levels of BUN and serum creatinine (SCr) (Shao et al., 2020). A robust meta-analysis recorded significant ($p< 0.00001$) rise in levels of BUN and SCr in severe COVID-19 cases and non-survivors (**Table 1B**) (Shao et al., 2020). Increased SCr and BUN values were identified as independent biomarkers for COVID-19 related severity and in-hospital mortality early during the pandemic (Chen et al., 2020; Cheng et al., 2020). However, the rate of severe and fatal cases in the study by Shao et al. was quite high, which could be due to the fact that the studies analyzed represented majorly poor COVID-19 outcomes (Shao et al., 2020). Hence, over-estimation of severity and fatality rate may be a limitation to this otherwise crucial set of findings.

Radiological Investigations

Identification of viral pathogens is possible by careful examination of imaging patterns since the latter are associated with viral pathogenesis. Since, viruses belonging to a single viral family share a similar pathogenesis, computed tomography (CT) was considered a trusted technique to distinguish patterns and features of COVID-19 in immunocompetent patients (Chung

TABLE 1B | Summary of the major outcomes of the analyzed systematic reviews and meta-analyses.

S. No.	Reference	Outcome						Conclusion
		Demographics	Signs and symptoms	Comorbidities	Laboratory findings	Radiological (CT scan) findings	Therapies	
1.	Zhang JJY. et al., 2020	• Higher proportion of males (66.5%) vs. females (33.5%) suffered from COVID-19; • Pooled mean age: 45 years (95% CI, 35.5– 54.5 years; • ICU admission: 10.9%, patients analyzed= 2153; • Mortality: 4.3%, patients analyzed = 2921.	• Most common: fever (80.5%, patients analyzed= 3934), cough (58.3%, patients analyzed= 3718) and dyspnea; • (23.8%, patients analyzed= 2992); • Fever definition as: ≥ 37.3°C (7 studies) or ≥ 37.5°C (2 studies); • Pooled mean incubation period: 6.1 days (95% CI 5.0– 7.3 days); • Pooled mean time from onset of symptoms to hospital admission: 7.2 days (95% CI 5.5– 8.9 days).	• Most common: Hypertension (16.4%, patients analyzed= 2928), cardiovascular diseases (12.1%, patients analyzed= 1498) and diabetes mellitus (9.8%, patients analyzed= 3060).	• Most common: Increased levels of CRP (59.4%) and lactate dehydrogenase (LDH) (51.7%), low levels of albumin (58.6%) and lymphopenia (47.7%).	• Most common: Bilateral infiltrates (80.8%), ground-glass opacities (73.0%, patients analyzed= 2618), interlobular septal thickening (46.3%, patients analyzed= 522), subpleural lines (45.5%, patients analyzed= 245), and consolidation (41.6%, patients analyzed= 2395).	• Antivirals- Combinations of oseltamivir, ganciclovir, lopinavir, ritonavir, ribavirin, arbidol; • Antibiotics- Moxifloxacin, ceftriaxone, azithromycin.	• High counts of leukocytes, high levels of ALT, AST, LDH, and PCT are important laboratory markers that are associated with ICU admission, mortality and ARDS; • Use of corticosteroids is significantly associated with higher proportion of patients with ARDS; • Use of lopinavir and ritonavir is not distinctly related to lowering mortality due to COVID-19; • Further prospective studies are necessary to validate the findings.
2.	Li et al., 2021	• COVID-19 severity not significantly linked with gender (OR= 1.14, 95% CI 0.91- 1.43, I^2 = 0.0%, p= 0.267) or Wuhan exposure history (OR= 0.92, 95% CI 0.53-1.59, I^2 = 0.0%, p= 0.764); • Smoking significantly associated with	• Fever (OR= 1.67, 95% CI 1.15- 2.42, p= 0.007, I^2 = 38.8%) and dyspnea (OR= 4.17, 95% CI 2.04- 8.53, p< 0.001, I^2 = 71.3%) related to severe COVID-19.	• Severity or ICU admission related to diabetes (OR= 3.17, 95% CI 2.26- 4.45, p< 0.001, I^2 = 35.3%), COPD (OR= 5.08, 95% CI 2.68- 9.63, p< 0.001, I^2 = 0.0%), coronary heart disease (OR= 2.66, 95% CI 1.71- 4.15, p< 0.001, I^2 = 0.0%), hypertension (OR= 2.40, 95% CI 1.47-3.90, p< 0.001, I^2 = 51.5%), cerebrovascular diseases (OR= 2.68, 95% CI 1.29- 5.57, p= 0.008, I^2 = 41.8%), and malignancy (OR= 2.21, 95% CI 1.04- 4.72, p= 0.040, I^2 = 0.0%).	• Severity indicators: • Elevated leucocyte counts (OR= 3.46, 95% CI 1.06- 11.28, p= 0.040, I^2 = 75.1%), PCT (OR= 6.69, 95% CI 3.99- 11.20, p≤ 0.001, I^2 = 13.6%), CRP (OR= 4.02, 95% CI 2.80- 5.79, p≤ 0.001, I^2 = 11.1%), LDH (OR= 3.36, 95% CI 2.46- 4.58, p< 0.001, I^2 = 48.3%), AST (OR= 3.26, 95% CI 2.40- 4.42, p< 0.001, I^2 = 5.3%), ALT (OR= 1.95, 95% CI 1.35- 2.80, p< 0.001, I^2 = 39.6%), Creatinine (OR= 2.14, 95% CI 1.14- 4.01, p= 0.018, I^2 = 0.0%), CK (OR= 2.45, 95% CI 1.60 3.55, p< 0.001, I^2 = 46.7%); • Decreased platelets (OR= 2.82, 95% CI 2.07- 3.83, p< 0.001, I^2 = 0.0%) and lymphocytes (OR= 4.60, 95% CI 3.25- 6.51, p< 0.001, I^2 = 0.0%).	NA	• Severe COVID-19 or ICU admitted patients required more frequent use of: Antibiotics (OR= 3.58, 95% CI 1.29- 9.87, p= 0.014, I^2 = 84.1%), antivirals (OR= 1.79, 95% CI 1.35- 2.38, p< 0.001, I^2 = 0.0%), systemic corticosteroids (OR= 5.46, 95% CI 4.17- 7.14, p< 0.001, I^2 = 0.0%), mechanical ventilation including invasive and non-invasive ventilation (OR= 171.72, 95% CI 27.38- 1,077.21, p< 0.001, I^2 = 73.2%), ECMO (OR= 29.36, 95% CI 5.36- 160.68, p< 0.001, I^2 = 0.0%) and continuous renal replacement	• Significant differences in outcome of severe and non-severe pneumonia in terms of discharge and death were observed.

(Continued)

TABLE 1B | Continued

S. No.	Reference	Outcome						Conclusion
		Demographics	Signs and symptoms	Comorbidities	Laboratory findings	Radiological (CT scan) findings	Therapies	
		severe COVID-19 (OR = 1.70, 95% CI: 1.20- 2.41, I^2 = 43.4%, p= 0.003).					therapy (OR= 25.45, 95% CI 6.97- 92.89, p< 0.001, I^2 = 0.0%).	
3.	Földi et al., 2020	• A range of 9% to 43% (2,770 patients from 6 studies) patients required ICU admission; • A range of 58% to 78% (509 patients from 5 studies) required IMV.	NA	• Obesity significantly associated with higher risk for ICU admission (OR= 1.21, 95% CI 1.002- 1.46, I^2 = 0.0%); • Obesity associated with higher risk for IMV (OR= 2.05, 95% CI 1.16- 3.64, I^2 = 34.86%); • 6 times higher risk for ICU admission in patients with BMI≥ 35 as compared to BMI< 25 (OR= 6.16, 95% CI 1.42- 26.66).	NA	NA	• Significantly higher likelihood of IMV requirement in patients with BMI≥ 25 as compared to BMI< 25 (OR= 2.63, 95% CI 1.64- 4.22, I^2 = 0.0%).	• Obesity may serve as important clinical predictor of risk gradation for COVID-19, and related ICU admission, especially IMV requirement; • Higher BMI ranges carried significantly higher risk for IMV in contrast to lower BMI ranges; • Careful monitoring of obese patients is necessary to better manage COVID-19; • Early escalation of therapy may be needed in such patients to dodge unfavorable clinical outcomes; • High recommendation to improve guidelines for patients with obesity owing to the returning pandemic waves.
4.	Lu et al., 2020	• Higher mortality rates in elderly (total OR= 7.86, 95% CI 5.46– 11.29; COVID-19: OR= 6.45, 95%	• Respiratory rate was a sensitive indicator of mortality for COVID-19 (OR= 4.90, 95% CI 1.08– 22.24) and SARS (OR= 8.88, 95% CI 5.64– 13.97).	• Chronic lung disease, hypertension, diabetes, increasing age and male gender.	• Predictors of mortality for COVID-19 patients: Lower platelet count (OR= 0.33, 95% CI 0.24– 0.44), lower lymphocyte counts (OR= 0.21, 95% CI 0.12– 0.38), higher neutrophil (OR= 17.56, 95% CI 10.67– 28.90), raised WBC count (OR= 9.13, 95% CI 5.71– 14.59), decreased albumin levels (OR= 0.11,	• Similar pulmonary consolidation and bilateral GGO observed in SARS, MERS and COVID-19;	NA	• Mortality indicators for COVID-19 are similar to SARS and MERS.

(Continued)

TABLE 1B | Continued

S. No.	Reference	Outcome						Conclusion
		Demographics	Signs and symptoms	Comorbidities	Laboratory findings	Radiological (CT scan) findings	Therapies	
		CI 3.86– 10.77; SARS: OR= 11.97, 95% CI 8.82– 16.24; MERS: OR= 7.02, 95% CI 4.59–10.73); • Among the non-survivors, higher mortality rate observed in males (total OR= 1.82, 95% CI 1.56– 2.13; COVID-19: OR= 1.96, 95% CI 1.43– 2.69; SARS: OR= 1.81, 95% CI 1.43– 2.30; MERS: OR= 1.74, 95% CI 1.32- 2.30). Higher mortality rate observed in patients with comorbidities (total OR= 4.41, • 95% CI 3.18– 6.12; COVID-19: OR= 3.50, 95% CI 2.35– 5.20; SARS: • OR= 6.47, 95% CI 4.93– 8.50; MERS: OR= 3.08, 95% CI 0.35– 27.01.			95% CI 0.06– 0.19), raised LDH (OR= 37.52, 95% CI 24.68– 57.03), elevated CRP (OR= 12.11, 95% CI 5.24– 27.98) and elevated BUN (OR= 8.49, 95% CI 5.81– 12.40); • Mortality indicators for all 3 coronavirus diseases, i.e., SARS, MERS and COVID-19: LDH, neutrophils, CRP, BUN and albumin; • Higher variation among laboratory parameters in COVID-19 as compared to SARS and MERS.	• Majority of the COVID-19 patients with above-said abnormal imaging features died (consolidation: OR= 3.26, 95% CI 1.16– 9.13; GGO: OR= 1.45, 95% CI 0.47– 4.49).		
5.	Figliozzi et al., 2020	• Patients aged above 70 years had 13-fold higher odds of death than younger patients (OR=	• Non-productive cough and fever.	• Diabetes mellitus (OR= 1.74, 95% CI 1.22-2.48, n = 13), history of CVD (OR= 1.95, 95% CI 1.08- 3.54, n = 7) or cerebrovascular disease (OR= 2.93, 95% CI 1.84- 4.26, n= 5),	• Elevated CRP levels, D-dimer levels, and lymphocytopenia.	NA	• During acute phase: steroids, antibiotics and antivirals.	• High odds of mortality indicated by various comorbidities, laboratory findings and increasing age.

(Continued)

TABLE 1B | Continued

S. No.	Reference	Outcome						Conclusion
		Demographics	Signs and symptoms	Comorbidities	Laboratory findings	Radiological (CT scan) findings	Therapies	
		13.19, 95% CI 7.72- 22.55); • Males had higher risk of death (OR= 1.71, 95% CI 1.39- 2.09, p< 0.001).		hypertension (OR= 2.71, 95% CI 1.99- 3.69, n = 15) and COPD (OR= 2.98, 95% CI 1.38-6.44, n= 8) associated with higher risk of mortality; • Progressing age associated with worse prognosis (p- OR= 1.027 per year, 95% CI 1.00- 1.06, p= 0.069); • Hypertension identified as an overall link between increasing age and worse prognosis; • Male gender associated with higher risk of mortality; • Smoking not a predictor of mortality (OR= 3.14, 95% CI 0.48-20.56, n= 4), but only associated with greater likelihood of composite adverse outcome (OR= 2.24 per comparison to non-smokers, 95% CI 1.40- 3.58, p= 0.003, n= 11).				
6.	Henry et al., 2020	• Severe lymphopenia: Number of total patients ranged from 12 (6 severe) to 1099 (153 severe); females: 15% to 50%; age range of severe cases: 25 to 87 years; • Fatal lymphopenia: Number of total patients ranged from 108 (96 non-survivors) to 274 (113	NA	NA	• Admission lymphopenia significantly indicated more than 4-fold increased risk of developing severe COVID-19 (OR= 4.20, 95% CI 3.46- 5.09, p< 0.001; I^2 = 0.0%) and in-hospital mortality (OR= 3.71, 95% CI 1.63- 8.44, p= 0.002; I^2 = 88.4%); • Admission neutrophilia significantly linked to 8-fold increased odd of developing severe COVID-19 (OR= 7.99, 95% CI 1.77- 36.14, p=0.007, I^2 = 75.9) and mortality (OR= 7.87, 95% CI 1.75- 35.35, p= 0.007, I^2 = 89.3).	NA	NA	• Lymphopenia and neutrophilia at first visit should be included in risk stratification models; These are independent risk factors for adverse outcome.

(Continued)

TABLE 1B | Continued

S. No.	Reference	Outcome						Conclusion
		Demographics	Signs and symptoms	Comorbidities	Laboratory findings	Radiological (CT scan) findings	Therapies	
		non-survivors); females: 27% to 41%; Age range of fatal cases: 51 to 84 years; • Severe neutrophilia: Total patients ranged from 12 (6 severe) to 548 (267 severe); Females: 34.4% to 50%; Age range of severe cases: 38 to 72 years; • Fatal neutrophilia (2 studies): Total patients 144 (70 severe) and 274 (113 severe); Females: 35.7% and 27%; Age range of fatal cases: 62 to 84 years.						
7.	Shao et al., 2020	• Number of patients ranged from 41 to 5700; Mean/ median age: 45.4 ± 17.2 to 69 years; Males: 38.8% to 73%.	NA	• AKI in 10% (95% CI 8–13) COVID-19 patients (with statistical heterogeneity among the studies analyzed, I^2 = 98%); • AKI significantly associated with high mortality (OR = 14.63, 95% CI 9.94–21.51, p< 0.00001, I^2 = 77%, p< 0.01).	• Higher SCr levels (MD= 20.19 μmol/l, 95% CI 14.96– 25.42, p< 0.00001, I^2 = 55%, Cochran's Q, p= 0.03); • Higher BUN levels associated with severity and mortality.	NA	NA	• AKI significantly associated with fatality in COVID-19 patients; • Kidney damage monitoring crucial during early stage of COVID-19.
8.	Li et al., 2020	• Total subjects analyzed: 4631;	NA	NA	• Elevated TnI levels associated with severity (64.5%), ICU admission (56%) and mortality (59.3%);	NA	NA	• Combination of cardiac examination and

(Continued)

TABLE 1B | Continued

S. No.	Reference	Outcome						Conclusion
		Demographics	Signs and symptoms	Comorbidities	Laboratory findings	Radiological (CT scan) findings	Therapies	
		Among the studies analyzed sample size ranged from 41 to 1099 and was over 100 in 16 studies; Males: 42.5% to 73.2%; Mean/median age: 43.1 to 62 years.			• Mean NT-proBNP levels significantly higher in patients with elevated TnI levels (SMD= 1.63, 95% CI 1.02- 2.23, p< 0.001; I^2 = 86.6%) than the ones with non-elevated TnI; • Higher mean CK levels significantly associated with severity/ICU admission (SMD= 0.39, 95% CI 0.11- 0.67, p= 0.006; I^2 = 69.0%); • Elevated CK-MB levels more frequent in severe COVID-19/ICU-admitted patients (45.7%); • Higher CK-MB levels associated with higher risk of severe COVID-19 or ICU admission (RR= 3.24, 95% CI 1.66- 6.34, p= 0.001, I^2 = 79.8%); • Increased LDH levels in 60.1% of severe or ICU-admitted patients; • Higher LDH levels associated with increased risk of severity or ICU admission (RR= 2.20, 95% CI 1.55- 3.12, p< 0.001, I^2 = 79.7%); Elevated levels of IL-6 significantly associated with severity or ICU admission (SMD= 0.54, 95% CI 0.27- 0.81, p< 0.001, I^2 = 0.0%) and mortality (SMD= 1.28, 95% CI 1.00- 1.57, p< 0.001, I^2 = 13.7%); • Emerging arrythmia linked to higher risk of severity or ICU admission (RR= 13.09, 95% CI 7.00- 24.47, p< 0.001, I^2 = 42.0%).			biomarkers can improve accuracy of cardiac injury assessment; • Careful monitoring of cardiac injury biomarkers during acute phase of COVID-19 is recommended.
9.	Ghahramani et al., 2020	• A total of 3396 (range 12 to 1099) patients analyzed; • Severe: 720 and non-severe: 2676.	NA	NA	• Decreased levels of sodium, lymphocytes, monocytes, eosinophil, hemoglobin and platelets, albumin; • Increased levels of ALT, AST, total bilirubin, BUN, creatinine, CRP, LDH, PCT, ESR and glucose.	NA	NA	• Results of CBC, LFT, KFT, inflammatory markers, glucose and electrolytes significantly varied between severe and non-severe patients; • Further studies in other populations are recommended.
10.	Jutzeler et al., 2020	• Higher proportion of males vs. females suffered	• Most common in **adult** patients: Fever (78.5%, 6955/8859), cough (53.8%, 4778/	• Most common in **adult** patients: Hypertension (20.93%, 1352/6460), heart failure (10.5%, 37/	• **Adults**: Elevated levels of IL-6 [22 pg/ml (4.68–51.8)], erythrocyte sedimentation rate [32.5 mm/h (17.3–53.8)], D-dimer [0.5 µg/m (0.3–1.08)], fibrinogen [4.5 g/l (3.66–5.1)], and	• **Adults**: Pneumonia (unilateral or bilateral, 83.6%,	• **Adults**: Antivirals (73.8%, 4475/6068), oxygen therapy (69.4%, 1300/1872) and antibiotics (52.2%, 2518/	• Clinical signs and imaging features comparable

(Continued)

TABLE 1B | Continued

S. No.	Reference	Outcome						Conclusion
		Demographics	Signs and symptoms	Comorbidities	Laboratory findings	Radiological (CT scan) findings	Therapies	
		from COVID-19 across all single studies analyzed.	8885) and fatigue (25%, 1996/7980); • Most common in **pregnant women** patients: Fever (71.4%, 25/35), cough (41.4%, 12/29) and myalgia (33.3%, 3/9); • Most common in **pediatric and neonatal** patients: Fever (53.1%, 170/320), cough (47.9%, 149/311) and sputum (27.5%, 14/51 patients); • **Asymptomatic** patients: Overall (7.8%, 297/3′822) including 5.4% adult (148/2749) patients, 14% (149/1054) children and neonates.	354), diabetes mellitus (10.4%, 678/6535), coronary heart disease (8.5%, 194/2388); • Only 5 **pregnant women** patients had comorbidities, of which 2 were unidentified, while the other 3 were: Hypothyroidism, allergies or influenza; • None in **pediatric and neonatal** patients, except 2 children.	LDH [213 u/l (173–268)]; • **Pregnant women**: Increased levels of CRP [19.25 mg/l (12.35–25.7)], procalcitonin (0.187 ng/ml), neutrophil count (9.14 × 10^9/l) and lactate dehydrogenase (544 u/l); • **Pediatrics and neonates**: No generalized conclusions can be made as the normative values are age-dependent within this age-group.	6620/7917), including air bronchogram (50.5%, 264/523) and GGO with consolidation (47.4%, 153/323) and without (43.8%, 2446/5591); • **Pregnant women**: Pneumonia (unilateral or bilateral, 88.6%, 31/35), GGO (85.3%, 29/34) and consolidation (50%, 8/16); • **Pediatrics and neonates**: Pneumonia (65%, 194/298), GGO (38.9%, 108/278) and local patchy shadowing (23.3%, 52/223).	4825); **Pregnant women**: Antibiotics (100%, 14/14), antivirals (78.6%, 11/14) and oxygen therapy (high flow nasal cannula; 25%, 3/12); • **Pediatrics and neonates**: Antibiotics (72.1%, 31/43), oxygen therapy (high flow nasal cannula; 55.6%, 5/9) and alpha interferon aerosol inhalation therapy (59.6%, 31/52).	between survivors and non-survivors. Pre-existing comorbidities associated with increased disease severity; • Abnormal laboratory tested blood parameters are associated with disease severity.
11.	Lippi et al., 2020	• Only 3 studies with total 11445 (161 to 11095 range) samples and 2654 (23.2%) severe cases; Females: 41.3% to 48.9%; Mean age: 39 ± 13 to 65 ± 7 years.	NA	NA	• RDW-CV values are raised in severe illness; • Increased RDW at admission carried 2.5-fold risk of in-hospital mortality; • Incremental RDW values in hospitalized patients associated with increased mortality	NA	NA	• RDW is a low-cost parameter and can be used for assessing the risk of adverse clinical progression; • Further studies recommended to analyze if RDW is also useful to predict the post-recovery course of COVID-19.
12.	Moutchia et al., 2020	• Sample size ranged from 5 to 1582; Mean/	NA	• Patients had varied degrees of comorbidities:	• Severe or critical COVID-19 patients displayed significantly higher counts/levels of WBCs, neutrophils, CRP, IL-6, ESR, ALT,	NA	NA	• Severe COVID-19 displays increased levels of

(Continued)

TABLE 1B | Continued

S. No.	Reference	Outcome						Conclusion
		Demographics	Signs and symptoms	Comorbidities	Laboratory findings	Radiological (CT scan) findings	Therapies	
		median age: 35 to 68 years; Males: 33.3% to 81%.		hypertension, diabetes and cancer	AST, serum creatinine, D-dimer and LDH in comparison to non-severe COVID-19 patients			biomarkers of innate immune response, tissue damage and major organ failure; and decreased levels of biomarkers of adaptive immune response.
13.	Jahrami et al., 2021	• Total patients analyzed: 54231; Study population ranged from general public to healthcare workers; Age range: 18 to 60 years; Males: 0% to 91.5%.	• Global pooled prevalence rate of sleep problems among all populations: 35.7% (95% CI 29.4–42.4); • COVID-19 patients most affected with a pooled rate: 74.8% (95% CI 28.7–95.6); • Health care workers and general population: comparable rates: 36.0% (95% CI 21.1–54.2) and 32.3% (95% CI 25.3–40.2), respectively.	NA	NA	NA	NA	• High prevalence (40%) of sleep problems in patients and health-workers; • Sleep self-assessment questionnaires, like, PSQI (39.6%; 95% CI 29.6– 50.6) more sensitive to diagnose sleep problems associated with COVID-19; • Further longitudinal studies required to understand trajectories of sleep problems post-COVID in different populations.
14.	Mudatsir et al., 2020	• Sample size of severe patients ranged from 7 to 926, while that of mildly ill patients ranged from 10 to 283.	• Lower risk of severe COVID-19 due to dry cough vs. productive cough (OR= 0.66, 95% CI 0.44- 0.97) • Higher risk of severe COVID-19 due to: Dyspnea (OR= 3.28, 95% CI 2.09-5.15), fatigue (OR= 2.00, 95% CI 1.25-3.20), anorexia (OR= 1.83, 95% CI 1.00-3.34), elevated	• Higher risk of developing severe form of COVID-19 due to: Chronic respiratory disease (OR= 2.48, 95% CI 1.44- 4.27), cardiovascular disease (OR= 1.70, 95% CI 1.05-2.78), diabetes mellitus (OR= 2.10, 95% CI 1.33-3.34), and hypertension (OR= 2.33, 95% CI 1.42-3.81) were associated with a greater risk of severe COVID-19	• Lower risk of severe COVID-19: low leukocyte levels (OR= 0.59, 95% CI 0.41-0.87) and elevated lymphocyte (OR= 0.34, 95% CI 0.23- 0.50); • Higher risk of severe COVID-19 indicators: Elevated WBC count (OR= 4.92, 95% CI 2.12- 11.31), raised neutrophil count (OR= 5.45, 95% CI 2.04- 14.54), lymphocytopenia (OR= 3.19, 95% CI 1.14-7.07), reduced hemoglobin levels (OR= 0.76, 95%CI 0.58-1.00), elevated AST (OR= 4.91), elevated ALT (OR= 3.23), raised SCr (OR= 2.14), elevated BUN (OR= 6.15, 95% CI 3.05- 12.37), elevated Hs-troponin I (OR= 9.25, 95% CI	NA	NA	• COVID-19 exhibits an unknown pattern of disease development; • 34 factors associated with severe COVID-19 were identified in the systematic review and meta-analysis; • These factors may improve the

(Continued)

TABLE 1B | Continued

S. No.	Reference	Outcome						Conclusion
		Demographics	Signs and symptoms	Comorbidities	Laboratory findings	Radiological (CT scan) findings	Therapies	
			respiratory rate (OR= 2.85, 95% CI 1.28- 6.33), dizziness (OR= 2.67, 95% CI 1.18, 6.01), and increased systolic blood pressure (OR: 1.84, 95% CI 1.31- 2.60).		3.51- 24.37), raised CK (OR= 2.44, 95% CI 1.65- 3.62), high Hs-CRP (OR= 14.27, 95% CI 5.13- 39.71), high IL-6 (OR= 6.68, 95% CI 3.20- 13.94), raised D-dimer (OR= 6.19, 95% CI 4.22- 9.08), increased ferritin (OR= 1.96, 95% CI 1.06- 3.62), high LDH (OR= 8.28, 95% CI 4.75- 14.46), elevated PCT (OR= 6.62, 95% CI 3.32- 13.21), raised ESR (OR= 4.45, 95% CI 2.56- 7.76), and CRP >8 (OR= 8.34, 95% CI 1.85- 37.62).			understanding of the disease and allow upgradation of prediction models to enable better prognosis of COVID-19.
15.	Mesas et al., 2020	• Mean age of participants: 40 to 73 years; • Of the 51,225 patients, 24.3% were non-survivors.	• Indicators of mortality: Dyspnea (p-OR= 2.5) and smoking (p-OR= 1.6); • Lower risk of mortality: Headache (p-OR= 0.5), cough (p-OR= 0.7), vomiting (p-OR= 0.6), diarrhea (p-OR= 0.6) and fever (p-OR= 0.8).	• Kidney disease, CVD, Hypertension, Diabetes, Malignancy, Pulmonary disease.	• Decreased albumin and lymphocytes, increased CRP, BUN, IL-6, LDH, neutrophil, Ferritin, Cardiac TnI.	NA	NA	• Epidemiological data should be stratified by age, gender and baseline comorbidities for accurate determination of mortality predictors.
16.	Izcovich et al., 2020	• Total patients: 75607 with range of 10 to 8910 patients per study; • Increasing age identified as risk factor of poor prognosis and mortality.	• Prognostic factors of severity: Hemoptysis (OR= 4.39, 95% CI 2.18- 8.81), abdominal pain (OR= 1.95, 95% CI 1.36- 1.79), fatigue (OR= 1.41, 95% CI 1.19- 1.68), fever (OR= 1.84, 95% CI 1.54- 2.21) and myalgia or arthralgia (OR= 1.29, 95% CI 1.03- 1.61); • Prognostic factors of mortality: Respiratory failure (OR= 21.17, 95% CI 4.9- 91.3), low blood pressure (OR= 6.7, 95% CI 3.14- 14.33), hypoxemia (OR= 5.46, 95% CI 2.05- 14.53), tachycardia (OR= 2.61, 95% CI 1.62- 4.22), dyspnea (OR= 3.45, 95% CI 2.72- 4.38),	• Indicators of mortality: COPD (OR= 2.43, 95% CI 1.88- 3.14), CKD (OR= 2.27, 95% CI 1.69- 3.05), cerebrovascular disease (OR= 2.85, 95% CI 2.02- 4.01, CVD (OR= 2.12, 95% CI 1.77- 2.56), cardiac arrhythmia (OR= 2.13, 95% CI 1.72- 2.65), arterial hypertension (OR= 2.02, 95% CI 1.71- 2.38), diabetes (OR= 1.84, 95% CI 1.61- 2.1), dementia (OR= 1.54, 95% CI 1.31- 1.81), obesity (OR= 1.41, 95% CI 1.15- 1.74), cancer (OR= 1.35, 95% CI 1.17- 1.55) and dyslipidemia (OR= 1.26, 95% CI 1.06– 1.5).	• Severity indicators: High neutrophil count (OR= 5.66, 95% CI 3.71- 8.63), high BNP (OR= 4.99, 95% CI 3.2- 7.77), High BUN (OR= 3.66, 95% CI 2.82- 4.74), high CK (OR= 3.1, 95% CI 2.32- 4.16), high bilirubin (OR= 2.94, 95% CI 2.18- 3.97), high IL-6 (OR= 7.36, 95% CI 2.97- 18.27), elevated ESR (OR= 3.08, 95% CI 2.04- 4.65); • Mortality indicators: High procalcitonin (OR= 12.42, 95% CI 7.18- 21.5), myocardial injury markers (OR= 10.89, 95% CI 5.39- 22.04), high WBC counts (OR= 4.06, 95% CI 2.7- 6.12), high lactate (OR= 3.66, 95% CI 2.26- 5.94), low platelet count (OR= 5.43, 95% CI 2.55- 11.56), high D-dimer (OR= 4.81, 95% CI 3.15- 7.34), high LDH (OR= 4.09, 95% CI 1.18- 14.17), high CRP (OR= 6.6, 95% CI 3.36- 12.99), reduced lymphocyte counts (OR= 3.57, 95% CI 2- 6.67), elevated AST (OR= 3.5, 95% CI 1.59– 7.71), elevated albumin levels (OR= 1.53, 95% CI 1.32- 1.78) and increased creatinine (OR= 1.14, 95%CI 1.02- 1.28).	• Severity indicators: Consolidative infiltrate (OR= 2.46, 95% CI 1.54- 3.93) and pleural effusion (OR= 3.31, 95% CI 2.03- 5.38).	NA	• Risk of severe disease and mortality is higher in elderly patients, with previous comorbidities, raised lab biomarkers of inflammation; • Radiological features were not good predictors.

(Continued)

TABLE 1B | Continued

S. No.	Reference	Outcome						Conclusion
		Demographics	Signs and symptoms	Comorbidities	Laboratory findings	Radiological (CT scan) findings	Therapies	
			anorexia (OR= 2.16, 95% CI 1.14- 4.12) and tachypnea (OR= 1.21, 95% CI 1.12- 1.31).					
17.	Del Zompo et al., 2020	• Pre-known liver disease in 0% to 37.6% patients; • 46.9% prevalence of at least one abnormal LFT at admission (95% CI 37- 56.8, 2306 patients).	NA	• Presence of liver abnormality.	• Elevated AST, ALT, tBIL levels.	NA	NA	• Abnormal LFT findings were considered as hallmark of COVID-19, with association with disease severity and in-hospital mortality.
18.	Hannum et al., 2020	• Sample size ranged from 15 to 7178; Number of smell loss cases/article: 2 to 4668 (prevalence rate: 5% to 98.3%).	• Loss of smell- overall prevalence rate of 50.2%, 95% CI 38.9- 61.5; prevalence rate per study: 5- 88%; • Meta-analysis for pooled prevalence yielded Cochrane's Q= 5784.14, df= 33, $p< 0.001$, $I^2 = 99.4\%$.	NA	NA	NA	NA	• Longitudinal assessments of chemosensory function would be useful to identify patients with continued impairment who might require further treatment and olfactory training.
19.	Israfil et al., 2021	• Mean age: 50.6 years (range 0.5– 94 years); • Higher proportion of male patients: 60.3% (6567/ 10889) while female: 39.7% (4322/10889); • Ethnic origin: Asian, European and North American; • Smokers	• Most common symptoms: Cough/dry cough 59.6% (2146/ 3598), fever 46.9% (4342/9242), fatigue 27.8% (1000/3598), dyspnea/shortness of breath 20.23% (728/ 3598), muscle ache/ myalgia 12.64% (455/ 3598), diarrhea 11.95% (430/3598), headache 10.8% (389/3598), anorexia 9.9% (356/ 3598), sore throat 7.5% (270/3598), expectoration 7.48%	• Most common: Hypertension 35.9% (3909/10889), diabetes 20.17% (2196/10889), obesity 15.95% (1735/ 10889), cardiovascular disease 13.92% (1516/ 10889), asthma 4.42% (481/10889), COPD 4.31% (469/10889) and malignancy 3.99% (435/ 10889).	• Most common: lymphocytopenia 55.9% (4177/7470); • Other major findings: Elevated levels of CRP 61.9% (830/1340), AST 53.3% (3481/ 6537), ALT 35.64% (2318/6503), LDH 40.8% (392/973), ESR 72.99% (173/237), serum ferritin 63% (62/99), (IL-6) 52% (51/99), prothrombin time 35.47% (102/286) and D-dimer 28.06% (179/638).	• Most common abnormality: Bilateral lungs 71.1% (1581/ 2223); • Other major findings: GGO 48% (432/900), consolidation 21.88% (140/ 640), pleural effusion 20.6% (195/947), lung lesions 78.3% (180/230), enlarged lymph	NA	• Laboratory investigations and CT scan reports with clinical correlation can provide useful information to enable correct diagnosis and better management of COVID-19 patients.

(Continued)

TABLE 1B | Continued

S. No.	Reference	Outcome						Conclusion
		Demographics	Signs and symptoms	Comorbidities	Laboratory findings	Radiological (CT scan) findings	Therapies	
		(active): about 14.2% (641/ 4530); • Severe patients: 37.4% (2408/6446).	(269/3598), upper airway congestion 6.67% (240/3598) and rhinitis 5.86% (211/ 3598); • Asymptomatic case: 0.56% (20/3598).			nodes 50.7% (153/302), thickened bronchial walls 30.3% (80/264), thickened lung texture 84.9% (62/73) and thickened interlobular septa 47.1% (80/170).		
20.	Poly et al., 2021	• Total sample size of studies analyzed ranged from 58 to 177133; males: 43.3% to 80.2%; Mean/median age: 49.1 to 76 years.	• Obesity significantly associated with an increased risk of mortality (p-RR 1.42, 95% CI 1.24–1.63, p< 0.001); • Class III obesity patients observed a greater risk (p-RR= 1.92, 95% CI 1.50–2.47, p< 0.001, I^2 = 31.99).	Risk of mortality assessment in obese COVID-19 patients: Diabetes (p-RR= 1.19 (95% CI 1.07–1.32, p= 0.001), stroke (p-RR= 1.80 (95% CI 0.89– 3.64, p= 0.10), hypertension (p-RR= 1.07, 95% CI 0.92– 1.25, p= 0.35), CKD (p-RR= 1.57, 95% CI 1.57– 1.91, p< 0.001), COPD (p-RR= 1.34, 95% CI 1.18–1.52, p< 0.001).	NA	NA	NA	• Obesity is a risk factor for mortality in COVID-19; • Clinicians must quickly start medical interventions in obese COVID-19 patients; • Further investigations would urgently be required to understand the pathophysiological association between obesity and risk of COVID-19 related mortality.

NA- Data under the respective heading was either not analyzed or not reported for the entire number of patients in the respective article. ALT, alanine aminotransferase; AST, aspartate aminotransferase; BMI, body mass index; BNP, B-type natriuretic peptide; BUN, blood urea nitrogen; CBC, complete blood count; CI, confidence interval; CK, creatine kinase; CKD, chronic kidney disease; CK-MB, creatine kinase,myocardial band, an isoenzyme of creatine kinase; COPD, chronic obstructive pulmonary disease; COVID-19, coronavirus disease 2019; CRP, C-reactive protein; CT, computed tomography; CVD, cardiovascular disease; df, degree of freedom; ECMO, extracorporeal membrane oxygenation; ESR, erythrocyte sedimentation rate; GGO, ground glass opacity; ICU, intensive care unit; IL (interleukin); KFT, kidney function test; LDH, lactate dehydrogenase; LFT, liver function test; MERS, middle east respiratory syndrome; NT-proBNP, N-terminal pro-BNP; OR, odds ratio; PCT, procalcitonin; p-OR, pooled odds ratio; p-RR, pooled relative risk; PSQI, Pittsburgh sleep quality index; RBC, red blood cell; RDW, RBC distribution width; RDW-CV, RBC distribution width- coefficient of variation; RR, relative risk; SARS, severe acute respiratory syndrome; SCr, serum creatinine; TnI, troponin I; WBC, white blood cell.

TABLE 2 | Putative independent predictors of COVID-19 adverse prognosis, severity or mortality.

S. No.	Biomarkers	Article reference	Clinical outcome	Number of patients	Severity or Fatality estimate
PARAMETERS OF LIVER FUNCTION					
1.	Elevated AST	Del Zompo et al., 2020	Severe COVID-19	6263	OR= 3.17, 95% CI 2.10 - 4.77
			In-hospital fatality	2395	OR= 4.39, 95% CI 2.68 - 7.18
		Moutchia et al., 2020	Severe/critical COVID-19	2705	MPR= 2.14, 95% CI 1.80 - 2.54
		Jutzeler et al., 2020	Severe COVID-19	184	SMD: 0.85, 95% CI 0.61-1.09
		Zhang JJY. et al., 2020	ICU admission	2153	p= 0.0040
		Li et al., 2021	ICU admission	479*	OR= 3.26, 95% CI 2.40-4.42, p< 0.001, I^2 = 5.3%
		Izcovich et al., 2020	Severe COVID-19	9179	OR= 3.41, 95% CI 2.7– 4.3
			Fatality	2969	OR= 3.5, 95% CI 1.59– 7.71
2.	Elevated ALT	Del Zompo et al., 2020	Severe COVID-19	6249	OR= 1.54, 95% CI 1.17 - 2.03
			In-hospital fatality	2613	OR= 1.48, 95% CI 1.12 - 1.96
		Moutchia et al., 2020	Severe/critical COVID-19	2540	MPR= 1.59, 95% CI 1.36 - 1.87
		Zhang JJY. et al., 2020	ICU admission	2153	p=0.024
3.	Increased tBIL	Del Zompo et al., 2020	Severe COVID-19	5153	OR= 2.32, 95% CI 1.18- 4.58
			In-hospital fatality	2086	OR= 7.75, 95% CI 2.28- 26.40
		Izcovich et al., 2020	Severe COVID-19	5098	OR= 2.94, 95% CI 2.18–3.97
4.	Decreased albumin	Jutzeler et al., 2020	Severe COVID-19	131	SMD= -1.60, 95% CI -2.97- (– 0.24)
			Fatality	110	SMD= – 1.14, 95% CI -1.41 – (– 0.85)
		Lu et al., 2020	Fatality	615	OR= 0.11, 95% CI 0.06– 0.19
		Izcovich et al., 2020	Severe COVID-19	1266	OR= 1.11, 95% CI 1.01– 1.21
			Fatality	336	OR= 1.53, 95% CI 1.32– 1.78
PARAMETERS OF KIDNEY FUNCTION					
5.	Elevated SCr	Shao et al., 2020	Severe COVID-19	1968	MD= 7.78 µmol/l, 95% CI 4.43-11.14
			Fatality	2138	MD= 20.19 µmol/l, 95% CI 14.96- 25.42
		Moutchia et al., 2020	Severe/critical COVID-19	2019	MPR= 1.90, 95% CI 1.07- 3.36
		Izcovich et al., 2020	Severe COVID-19	1116	OR= 1.89, 95% CI 0.87– 4.10
			Fatality	1508	OR= 1.14, 95% CI 1.02– 1.28
		Li et al., 2021	ICU admission	479*	OR= 2.14, 95% CI 1.14-4.01, p= 0.018, I^2 = 0.0%
6.	Higher BUN	Shao et al., 2020	Severe COVID-19	1445	MD= 2.12 µmol/l, 95% CI 1.74 - 2.50
			Fatality	1458	MD= 4.07 µmol/l, 95% CI 3.33- 4.81
		Lu et al., 2020	Fatality	424	OR= 8.49, 95% CI 5.81–12.40
		Izcovich et al., 2020	Severe COVID-19	3890	OR= 3.66, 95% CI 2.82– 4.74
	Elevated blood urea	Moutchia et al., 2020		624	MPR= 3.63, 95% CI 1.73- 7.65
HAEMATOLOGICAL PARAMETERS					
7.	Absolute RDW-CV	Lippi et al., 2020	Severe COVID-19	2,654	Fold increase: 1.05, 95% CI 1.03- 1.08-fold
8.	Low hemoglobin	Jutzeler et al., 2020	Severe COVID-19	342	SMD= – 0.23, 95% CI -0.41- (– 0.06)
9.	Low platelet count	Jutzeler et al., 2020	Severe COVID-19	357	SMD= – 0.57, 95% CI -0.68-(-0.45)
		Lu et al., 2020	Fatality	615	OR= 0.33, 95% CI 0.24–0.44
		Li et al., 2021	ICU admission	479*	OR= 2.82, 95% CI 2.07-3.83, p< 0.001, I^2 = 0.0%
		Izcovich et al., 2020	Fatality	3676	OR= 5.43, 95% CI 2.55– 11.56
10.	Low lymphocyte count	Henry et al., 2020	Severe COVID-19	1140	OR= 4.20, 95% CI 3.46-5.09
			In-hospital fatality	800	OR= 3.71, 95% CI 1.63 - 8.44 Severe lymphopenia (< $0.5\times10x^9$/l) had 12-fold increased odds of in-hospital mortality.
			Severe COVID-19	198$	OR= 3.19, 1.14- 7.07, p< 0.0001

(Continued)

TABLE 2 | Continued

S. No.	Biomarkers	Article reference	Clinical outcome	Number of patients	Severity or Fatality estimate
		Mudatsir et al., 2020			
		Moutchia et al., 2020	Severe COVID-19	3875	MPR= 1.74, 95% CI 1.43, 2.12
		Jutzeler et al., 2020	Fatality	255	SMD = – 0.92, 95% CI -1.3 – (– 0.55)
		Li et al., 2021	ICU admission	479*	OR= 4.60, 95% CI 3.25-6.51, $p< 0.001$, $I^2 = 0.0\%$
		Lu et al., 2020	Fatality	615	OR= 0.21, 95% CI 0.12– 0.38
		Izcovich et al., 2020	Severe COVID-19 Fatality	1909 544	OR= 2.28, 95% CI 1.21– 4.30 OR= 3.57, 95% CI 2– 6.67
11.	Increased neutrophil count	Henry et al., 2020	Severe COVID-19 Fatality	313 183	OR= 7.99, 95% CI 1.77- 36.14 OR= 7.87, 95% CI 1.75- 35.35
		Moutchia et al., 2020	Severe COVID-19	1237	Severe COVID-19 with higher likelihood MPR= 4.29, 95% CI 1.74 - 10.64
		Lu et al., 2020	Fatality	274	OR= 17.56, 95% CI 10.67–28.90
		Izcovich et al., 2020	Severe COVID-19	4945	OR= 5.66, 95% CI 3.71–8.63
12.	Increased leukocyte count	Moutchia et al., 2020	Severe COVID-19	3455	Severe COVID-19 with higher likelihood MPR= 3.95, 95% CI 2.35- 6.65
		Jutzeler et al., 2020	Fatality	277	SMD = 2.21, 95% CI 0.61–3.64
		Lu et al., 2020	Fatality	615	OR= 9.13, 95% CI 5.71–14.59
		Zhang JJY. et al., 2020	ICU admission Fatality	2153	$p< 0.0001$ $p= 0.0005$
		Izcovich et al., 2020	Severe COVID-19 Fatality	9331 2870	OR= 4.67, 95% CI 3.17– 6.88 OR= 4.06, 95% CI 2.7– 6.12
		Mudatsir et al., 2020	Severe COVID-19	102[$]	OR= 5.38, 95% CI 3.36- 8.62
PARAMETERS OF INFLAMMATION/INFECTION					
13.	Elevated CRP	Moutchia et al., 2020	Severe/critical COVID-19	2740	MPR= 1.60, 95% CI 1.32- 1.93
		Jutzeler et al., 2020	Severe COVID-19	277	SMD= 1.47, 95% CI 0.88–2.07
		Lu et al., 2020	Fatality	424	OR= 12.11, 95% CI 5.24–27.98
		Izcovich et al., 2020	Severe COVID-19 Fatality	9094 2107	OR= 4.5, 95% CI 3.1– 6.23 OR= 6.6, 95% CI 3.36– 12.99
		Li et al., 2021	ICU admission	479*	OR= 4.02, 95% CI 2.80-5.79, $p\leq 0.001$, $I^2 = 11.1\%$
14.	Higher ESR	Moutchia et al., 2020	Severe/critical COVID-19	545	MPR= 1.67, 95% CI 0.67- 4.17
15.	Increased IL-6	Jutzeler et al., 2020	Fatality	110	SMD= 1.21, 95% CI 0.93–1.5
		Izcovich et al., 2020	Severe COVID-19	1211	OR= 7.36, 95% CI 2.97- 18.27
16.	Elevated PCT	Zhang JJY. et al., 2020	ICU admission	2153	$p< 0.0001$
		Li et al., 2021	ICU admission	479*	OR= 6.69, 95% CI 3.99-11.20, $p\leq 0.001$, $I^2 = 13.6\%$
		Izcovich et al., 2020	Fatality	4735	OR= 12.42, 95% CI 7.18– 21.5
OTHER BIOCHEMICAL PARAMETER					
17.	Elevated serum ferritin	Moutchia et al., 2020	Severe/critical COVID-19	412	MPR= 2.3, 95% CI 1.67- 3.17
COAGULATION PARAMETER					
18.	Elevated D-dimer	Moutchia et al., 2020	Severe/critical COVID-19	2030	MPR= 2.27, 95% CI 1.67- 3.09
		Figliozzi et al., 2020	Combined adverse outcome (ICU admission or IMV or fatality) Fatality	3270	OR= 4.39, 95% CI 1.85-10.41, $p= 0.003$ OR= 4.40, 95% CI 1.10-17.58, $p= 0.04$
		Izcovich et al., 2020	Severe COVID-19 Fatality	6356 4361	OR= 3.27, 95% CI 2.46– 4.36 OR= 4.81, 95% CI 3.15–7.34
19.	Prolonged PT	Jutzeler et al., 2020	Fatality	206	SMD = 7.99, 95% CI 4.64–11.34

(Continued)

TABLE 2 | Continued

S. No.	Biomarkers	Article reference	Clinical outcome	Number of patients	Severity or Fatality estimate
MARKER OF TISSUE DAMAGE					
20.	Elevated LDH	Moutchia et al., 2020	Severe/critical COVID-19	1893	MPR= 2.41, 95% CI 1.65- 3.51
		Jutzeler et al., 2020	Severe COVID-19	93	SMD = 1.71, 95% CI 1.08–2.34
		Lu et al., 2020	Fatality	465	OR= 37.52, 95% CI 24.68–57.03
		Zhang JJY. et al., 2020	ICU admission ARDS Fatality	2153	p< 0.0001 p< 0.0001 p< 0.0001
		Izcovich et al., 2020	Severe COVID-19 Fatality	7955 1440	OR= 4.48, 95% CI 3.21–6.25 OR= 4.09, 95% CI 1.18– 14.17
PARAMETERS OF CARDIAC INJURY					
21.	Increased TnI or myocardial injury	Izcovich et al., 2020	Severe COVID-19 Fatality	3627 3855	OR= 10, 95% CI 6.84–14.62 OR= 10.89, 95% CI 5.39–22.04
	Elevated TnI or TnT	Li et al., 2020	Fatality	1028	RR= 4.69, 95% CI 3.39- 6.48, p< 0.001, I^2 = 22.5%
22.	Elevated CK	Li et al., 2020	Severe COVID-19	2174	RR= 1.98, 95% CI 1.50- 2.61, p< 0.001, I^2 = 0.0%

*NA- The parameter value was not applicable or not mentioned or could not be ascertained with the given information. *- The number of patients as mentioned for ICU COVID-19 cases in overall results section. $- The number of severe and non-severe patients as per the table in the citation. May or may not be specific to the respective parameter. ALT, alanine aminotransferase; ARDS, acute respiratory distress syndrome; AST, aspartate aminotransferase; BUN, blood urea nitrogen; CRP, C-reactive protein; CK, creatine kinase; ESR, erythrocyte sedimentation rate; LDH, lactate dehydrogenase; MD, mean difference; MPR, meta-prevalence ratio; SMD, standardized mean difference; NA, not applicable; OR, odds ratio; PCT, procalcitonin; PT, prothrombin time; RDW-CV, red blood cell distribution width-coefficient of variation; RR, relative risk; SCr, serum creatinine; tBIL, total bilirubin; TnI, troponin I; TnT, troponin T.*

et al., 2020; Jin et al., 2020; Tao et al., 2020). The systematic review and meta-analysis conducted by Jutzeler et al. identified abnormal CT scans in nearly 90% (89.6% specifically) of the COVID-19 confirmed adult patients, 88.6% of the pregnant patients and 65% of the pediatric and neonatal patients (Jutzeler et al., 2020). The major finding in CT imaging was the occurrence of unilateral or bilateral pneumonia in 83.6% (6620/7917) adult patients, 88.6% (31/35) pregnant and 65% (194/298) pediatric and neonatal COVID-19 cases (Jutzeler et al., 2020). Other prominent abnormal CT features included air bronchogram (50.5%, 264/523) and ground-glass opacity (GGO) with consolidation (47.4%, 153/323) and without (43.8%, 2446/5591) in adult patients, GGO (85.3%, 29/34) and consolidation (50%, 8/16) in pregnant patients, and GGO (38.9%, 108/278) and local patchy shadowing (23.3%, 52/223) in pediatric and neonatal patients (Jutzeler et al., 2020).

CONCLUSIONS

Identification of high-risk clinical and laboratory features contribute to early prediction, diagnosis and efficient treatment of patients (Li et al., 2021). A fatality rate of 7.7% with about 8% of the COVID-19 patients being asymptomatic was observed during the early pandemic period (Jutzeler et al., 2020). Since, it is difficult to record the exact number of asymptomatic cases, owing to obvious reasons (like no hospital/clinic visit, hence no medical record; or lack of awareness that a potentially fatal disease can be asymptomatic in some patients) such value is deemed to be 6- to 10- fold higher (Jutzeler et al., 2020). Hence, more aggressive antigen detection, as well as serological surveillance of contacts of confirmed COVID-19 patients, is necessary to enable screening and identification of asymptomatic COVID-19 patients. Further, prospective well-planned cohort studies would be necessary to enable further characterization of the overall, gender-specific and/or geographical location-based risk factors.

It is imperative to categorize COVID-19 patients based on their comorbidities, like impaired kidney or liver functions or cardiac injury, etc. As discussed in the present work, AKI is a critical complication of COVID-19 and calls for immediate care and monitoring (Shao et al., 2020) to minimize the risk of severity and poor prognosis. Similarly, abnormal LFTs are important early predictors of COVID-19 severity and in-hospital mortality (Del Zompo et al., 2020). Also, pre-existing chronic liver disease, especially cirrhosis, is an indicator of a high risk of mortality. Hence, aggressive interventions for such cases must be exercised. This would enable better patient management and may improve the disease outcome. Measurement of anthropometric parameters, especially BMI, is also recommended for COVID-19 patient management, importantly for patients who are or above 65 years of age (Földi et al., 2020; Poly et al., 2021). Basic hematological screening that can be done with minimal resources can be a life-saver. The findings that lymphopenia and neutrophilia at the time of hospital admission indicate poor COVID-19 outcome call for routine hematological monitoring. It would enable an early careful intervention in such patients enabling better patient care. Such regular monitoring may also aid in the stratification and the management of risk associated with COVID-19 (Henry et al., 2020). Further, it is also important to stratify epidemiological data based on demographic characteristics and risk factors for adverse COVID-19 outcomes, to enable exact and aggressive patient care (Mesas et al., 2020). Based on the analysis in this work, we can conclude that careful monitoring of clinical data, risk factors and disease biomarkers (Israfil et al., 2021) may enable early determination of COVID-19-led severity. Such an early estimate would be helpful in efficient patient management and possibly minimize the related mortality.

AUTHOR CONTRIBUTIONS

JS conceptualized the study, retrieved the articles, analyzed the data and guided inclusion of specific information, drafted and proof-read the manuscript. RR reviewed the data, analyzed the information, tabulated findings, drafted and proof-read the manuscript. MB helped in information retrieval and inclusion of findings. PA provided intellectual inputs and proof-read the manuscript. VS conceived the study, provided intellectual inputs, guided the inclusion of information, proof-read and approved the final version of the manuscript. All authors contributed to the article and approved the submitted version.

REFERENCES

Coronavirus Could Cost the Global Economy Trillions on a Sars Baseline. Available at: https://www.ccn.com/coronavirus-could-cost-the-global-economy-trillions-on-a-sars-baseline/.

Cheng, Y., Luo, R., Wang, K., Zhang, M., Wang, Z., Dong, L., et al. (2020). Kidney Disease Is Associated With in-Hospital Death of Patients With COVID-19. *Kidney Int.* 97 (5), 829–838. doi: 10.1016/j.kint.2020.03.005

Chen, N., Zhou, M., Dong, X., Qu, J., Gong, F., Han, Y., et al. (2020). Epidemiological and Clinical Characteristics of 99 Cases of 2019 Novel Coronavirus Pneumonia in Wuhan, China: A Descriptive Study. *Lancet* 395 (10223), 507–513. doi: 10.1016/s0140-6736(20)30211-30217

Chung, M., Bernheim, A., Mei, X., Zhang, N., Huang, M., Zeng, X., et al. (2020). CT Imaging Features of 2019 Novel Coronavirus, (2019-Ncov). *Radiology* 295 (1), 202–207. doi: 10.1148/radiol.2020200230

Del Zompo, F., De Siena, M., Ianiro, G., Gasbarrini, A., Pompili, M., and Ponziani, F. R. (2020). Prevalence of Liver Injury and Correlation With Clinical Outcomes in Patients With COVID-19: Systematic Review With Meta-Analysis. *Eur. Rev. Med. Pharmacol. Sci.* 24 (24), 13072–13088. doi: 10.26355/eurrev_202012_24215

Emem, M. (2020) *Multi-Billion Dollar Coronavirus Vaccine Deal Could Save the Economy. CCN Headlines Opinion.* Available at: https://www.ccn.com/coronavirus-could-cost-the-global-economy-trillions-on-a-sars-baseline/.

Ferrando, M., Bagnasco, D., Roustan, V., Canonica, G. W., Braido, F., and Baiardini, I. (2016). Sleep Complaints and Sleep Breathing Disorders in Upper and Lower Obstructive Lung Diseases. *J. Thorac. Dis.* 8 (8), E716–E725. doi: 10.21037/jtd.2016.07.82

Figliozzi, S., Masci, P. G., Ahmadi, N., Tondi, L., Koutli, E., Aimo, A., et al. (2020). Predictors of Adverse Prognosis in COVID-19: A Systematic Review and Meta-Analysis. *Eur. J. Clin. Invest.* 50 (10), e13362. doi: 10.1111/eci.13362

Földi, M., Farkas, N., Kiss, S., Zádori, N., Váncsa, S., Szakó, L., et al. (2020). Obesity Is a Risk Factor for Developing Critical Condition in COVID-19 Patients: A Systematic Review and Meta-Analysis. *Obes. Rev.* 21 (10), e13095. doi: 10.1111/obr.13095

Ghahramani, S., Tabrizi, R., Lankarani, K. B., Kashani, S. M. A., Rezaei, S., Zeidi, N., et al. (2020). Laboratory Features of Severe vs. non-Severe COVID-19 Patients in Asian Populations: A Systematic Review and Meta-Analysis. *Eur. J. Med. Res.* 25 (1), 30. doi: 10.1186/s40001-020-00432-3

Gu, X., Li, X., An, X., Yang, S., Wu, S., Yang, X., et al. (2020). Elevated Serum Aspartate Aminotransferase Level Identifies Patients With Coronavirus Disease 2019 and Predicts the Length of Hospital Stay. *J. Clin. Lab. Anal.* 34, e23391. doi: 10.1002/jcla.23391

Hannum, M. E., Ramirez, V. A., Lipson, S. J., Herriman, R. D., Toskala, A. K., Lin, C., et al. (2020). Objective Sensory Testing Methods Reveal a Higher Prevalence of Olfactory Loss in COVID-19 Positive Patients Compared to Subjective Methods: A Systematic Review and Meta-Analysis. *Chem. Senses.* 45 (9), 865–874. doi: 10.1093/chemse/bjaa064

Henry, B., Cheruiyot, I., Vikse, J., Mutua, V., Kipkorir, V., Benoit, J., et al. (2020). Lymphopenia and Neutrophilia at Admission Predicts Severity and Mortality in Patients With COVID-19: A Meta-Analysis. *Acta BioMed.* 91 (3), e2020008. doi: 10.23750/abm.v91i3.10217

Huang, C., Wang, Y., Li, X., Ren, L., Zhao, J., Hu, Y., et al. (2020). Clinical Features of Patients Infected With 2019 Novel Coronavirus in Wuhan, China. *Lancet* 395, 497–506. doi: 10.1016/S0140-6736(20)30183-5

Israfil, S. M. H., Sarker, M. M. R., Rashid, P. T., Talukder, A. A., Kawsar, K. A., Khan, F., et al. (2021). Clinical Characteristics and Diagnostic Challenges of COVID-19: An Update From the Global Perspective. *Front. Public Health* 8, 567395. doi: 10.3389/fpubh.2020.567395

Izcovich, A., Ragusa, M. A., Tortosa, F., Lavena Marzio, M. A., Agnoletti, C., Bengolea, A., et al. (2020). Prognostic Factors for Severity and Mortality in Patients Infected With COVID-19: A Systematic Review. *PloS One* 15 (11), e0241955. doi: 10.1371/journal.pone.0241955

Jahrami, H., BaHammam, A. S., Bragazzi, N. L., Saif, Z., Faris, M., and Vitiello, M. V. (2021). Sleep Problems During the COVID-19 Pandemic by Population: A Systematic Review and Meta-Analysis. *J. Clin. Sleep Med.* 17 (2), 299–313. doi: 10.5664/jcsm.8930

Jin, Y.-H., Cai, L., Cheng, Z.-S., Cheng, H., Deng, T., Fan, Y.-P., et al. (2020). A Rapid Advice Guideline for the Diagnosis and Treatment of 2019 Novel Coronaviru-Ncov) Infected Pneumonia (Standard Version). *Mil. Med. Res.* 7 (1), 4. doi: 10.1186/s40779-020-0233-6

Jutzeler, C. R., Bourguignon, L., Weis, C. V., Tong, B., Wong, C., Rieck, B., et al. (2020). Comorbidities, Clinical Signs and Symptoms, Laboratory Findings, Imaging Features, Treatment Strategies, and Outcomes in Adult and Pediatric Patients With COVID-19: A Systematic Review and Meta-Analysis. *Travel Med. Infect. Dis.* 37, 101825. doi: 10.1016/j.tmaid.2020.101825

Li, J., He, X., Yuan, Y., Zhang, W., Li, X., Zhang, Y., et al. (2021). Meta-Analysis Investigating the Relationship Between Clinical Features, Outcomes, and Severity of Severe Acute Respiratory Syndrome Coronavirus 2 (SARS-Cov-2) Pneumonia. *Am. J. Infect. Control* 49 (1), 82–89. doi: 10.1016/j.ajic.2020.06.008

Li, X., Pan, X., Li, Y., An, N., Xing, Y., Yang, F., et al. (2020). Cardiac Injury Associated With Severe Disease or ICU Admission and Death in Hospitalized Patients With COVID-19: A Meta-Analysis and Systematic Review. *Crit. Care* 24, 468. doi: 10.1186/s13054-020-03183-z

Lippi, G., Henry, B. M., and Sanchis-Gomar, F. (2020). Red Blood Cell Distribution Is a Significant Predictor of Severe Illness in Coronavirus Disease 2019. *Acta Haematol.* 25, 1–5. doi: 10.1159/000510914

Loomba, R. S., Aggarwal, G., Aggarwal, S., Flores, S., Villarreal, E. G., Farias, J. S., et al. (2021). Disparities in Case Frequency and Mortality of Coronavirus Disease 2019 (COVID-19) Among Various States in the United States. *Ann. Med.* 53 (1), 151–159. doi: 10.1080/07853890.2020.1840620

Lu, L., Zhong, W., Bian, Z., Li, Z., Zhang, K., Liang, B., et al. (2020). A Comparison of Mortality-Related Risk Factors of COVID-19, SARS, and MERS: A Systematic Review and Meta-Analysis. *J. Infect.* 81 (4), e18–e25. doi: 10.1016/j.jinf.2020.07.002

Malaiyan, J., Arumugam, S., Mohan, K., and Radhakrishnan, G. (2021). An Update on the Origin of SARS-Cov-2: Despite Closest Identity, Bat (Ratg13) and Pangolin Derived Coronaviruses Varied in the Critical Binding Site and O-Linked Glycan Residues. *J. Med. Virol.* 93 (1), 499–505. doi: 10.1002/jmv.26261

Mesas, A. E., Cavero-Redondo, I., Álvarez-Bueno, C., Sarriá Cabrera, M. A., Maffei de Andrade, S., Sequí-Dominguez, I., et al. (2020). Predictors of in-Hospital COVID-19 Mortality: A Comprehensive Systematic Review and Meta-Analysis Exploring Differences by Age, Sex and Health Conditions. *PloS One* 15 (11), e0241742. doi: 10.1371/journal.pone.0241742

Moutchia, J., Pokharel, P., Kerri, A., McGaw, K., Uchai, S., Nji, M., et al. (2020). Clinical Laboratory Parameters Associated With Severe or Critical Novel Coronavirus Disease 2019 (COVID-19): A Systematic Review and Meta-Analysis. *PloS One* 15 (10), e0239802. doi: 10.1371/journal.pone.0239802

Mudatsir, M., Fajar, J. K., Wulandari, L., Soegiarto, G., Ilmawan, M., Purnamasari, Y., et al. (2020). Predictors of COVID-19 Severity: A Systematic Review and Meta-Analysis. *F1000Res* 9, 1107. doi: 10.12688/f1000research.26186.2

Poly, T. N., Islam, M. M., Yang, H. C., Lin, M. C., Jian, W. S., Hsu, M. H., et al. (2021). Obesity and Mortality Among Patients Diagnosed With COVID-19: A Systematic Review and Meta-Analysis. *Front. Med.* 8, 620044. doi: 10.3389/fmed.2021.620044

Shao, M., Li, X., Liu, F., Tian, T., Luo, J., and Yang, Y. (2020). Acute Kidney Injury Is Associated With Severe Infection and Fatality in Patients With COVID-19: A Systematic Review and Meta-Analysis of 40 Studies and 24,527 Patients. *Pharmacol. Res.* 161, 105107. doi: 10.1016/j.phrs.2020.105107

Shi, Z. L. (2021). Origins of SARS-Cov-2: Focusing on Science. *Infect. Dis. Immun.* 1 (1), 3–4. doi: 10.1097/ID9.0000000000000008

Shi, L., Lu, Z.-A., Que, J.-Y., Huang, X.-L., Lu, L., Ran, M.-S., et al. (2020). Prevalence of and Risk Factors Associated With Mental Health Symptoms Among the General Population in China During the Coronavirus Disease 2019 Pandemic. *JAMA Netw. Open* 3 (7), e2014053. doi: 10.1001/jamanetworkopen.2020.14053

Singh, D. P., Jamil, R. T., and Mahajan, K. (2020). "Nocturnal Cough," in *Statpearls*. Eds. M. Cascella, M. Rajnik, A. Cuomo, S. C. Dulebohn and R. S. Di Napoli (Treasure Island, FL: StatPearls Publishing).

Song, Z., Xu, Y., Bao, L., Zhang, L., Yu, P., Qu, Y., et al. (2019). From SARS to MERS, Thrusting Coronaviruses Into the Spotlight. *Viruses* 11 (1), 59. doi: 10.3390/v11010059

Tao, A., Zhenlu, Y., Hongyan, H., Chenao, Z., Chong, C., Wenzhi, L., et al. (2020). Correlation of Chest CT and RT-PCR Testing in Coronavirus Disease 2019 (COVID-19) in China: A Report of 1014 Cases. *Radiology* 296 (2), E32–E40. doi: 10.1148/radiol.2020200642

Undurraga, E. A., Chowell, G., and Mizumoto, K. (2021). COVID-19 Case Fatality Risk by Age and Gender in a High Testing Setting in Latin America: Chile, March–August 2020. *Infect. Dis. Poverty* 10, 11. doi: 10.1186/s40249-020-00785-1

WHO (2021) *WHO Coronavirus Disease (COVID-19) Dashboard. Updated on: 27 February 2021*. Available at: https://covid19.who.int/ (Accessed on: July 15, 2021).

WHO News release (2021) *WHO Calls for Further Studies, Data on Origin of SARS-Cov-2 Virus, Reiterates That All Hypotheses Remain Open*. Available at: https://www.who.int/news/item/30-03-2021-who-calls-for-further-studies-data-on-origin-of-sars-cov-2-virus-reiterates-that-all-hypotheses-remain-open.

Woo, P. C., Lau, S. K., Lam, C. S., Lau, C. C. Y., Tsang, A. K. L., Lau, J. H. N., et al. (2012). Discovery of Seven Novel Mammalian and Avian Coronaviruses in the Genus Deltacoronavirus Supports Bat Coronaviruses as the Gene Source of Alphacoronavirus and Betacoronavirus and Avian Coronaviruses as the Gene Source of Gammacoronavirus and Deltacoronavirus. *J. Virol.* 86, 3995–4008. doi: 10.1128/JVI.06540-11

Zhang, J. J. Y., Lee, K. S., Ang, L. W., Leo, Y. S., and Young, B. E. (2020). Risk Factors for Severe Disease and Efficacy of Treatment in Patients Infected With COVID-19: A Systematic Review, Meta-Analysis, and Meta-Regression Analysis. *Clin. Infect. Dis.* 71 (16), 2199–2206. doi: 10.1093/cid/ciaa576

Zhang, T., Wu, Q., and Zhang, Z. (2020). Probable Pangolin Origin of SARS-Cov-2 Associated With the COVID-19 Outbreak. *Curr. Biol.* 30 (8), 1578. doi: 10.1016/j.cub.2020.03.063

Zhu, Z., Lian, X., Su, X., Wu, W., Marraro, G. A., and Zeng, Y. (2020). From SARS and MERS to COVID-19: A Brief Summary and Comparison of Severe Acute Respiratory Infections Caused by Three Highly Pathogenic Human Coronaviruses. *Respir. Res.* 21 (1), 224. doi: 10.1186/s12931-020-01479-w

7

T-Helper Cell Subset Response is a Determining Factor in COVID-19 Progression

Francisco Javier Gil-Etayo[1], *Patricia Suàrez-Fernández*[2], *Oscar Cabrera-Marante*[1], *Daniel Arroyo*[1], *Sara Garcinuño*[2], *Laura Naranjo*[1], *Daniel E. Pleguezuelo*[1], *Luis M. Allende*[1,2], *Esther Mancebo*[1,2], *Antonio Lalueza*[2,3,4], *Raquel Díaz-Simón*[3], *Estela Paz-Artal*[1,2,5] *and Antonio Serrano*[1,2,6*]

[1] Department of Immunology, Hospital Universitario 12 de Octubre, Madrid, Spain, [2] Departamento de Inmunologá, Instituto de Investigación, Sanitaria Hospital 12 de Octubre (imas12), Madrid, Spain, [3] Department of Internal Medicine, Hospital Universitario 12 de Octubre, Madrid, Spain, [4] Departamento de Medicina, Facultad de Medicina, Universidad Complutense de Madrid, Madrid, Spain, [5] Departamento de Inmunología, Oftalmología y Otorrinolaringología, Facultad de Medicina, Universidad Complutense de Madrid, Madrid, Spain, [6] Department of Epidemiology, Biomedical Research Centre Network for Epidemiology and Public Health (CIBERESP), Madrid, Spain

***Correspondence:**
Antonio Serrano
aserrano@h12o.es

The immune response type organized against viral infection is determinant in the prognosis of some infections. This work has aimed to study Th polarization in acute COVID-19 and its possible association with the outcome through an observational prospective study. Fifty-eight COVID-19 patients were recruited in the Medicine Department of the hospital "12 de Octubre," 55 patients remaining after losses to follow-up. Four groups were established according to maximum degree of disease progression. T-helper cell percentages and phenotypes, analyzed by flow cytometer, and serum cytokines levels, analyzed by Luminex, were evaluated when the microbiological diagnosis (acute phase) of the disease was obtained. Our study found a significant reduction of %Th1 and %Th17 cells with higher activated %Th2 cells in the COVID-19 patients compared with reference population. A higher percent of senescent Th2 cells was found in the patients who died than in those who survived. Senescent Th2 cell percentage was an independent risk factor for death (OR: 13.88) accompanied by the numbers of total lymphocytes (OR: 0.15) with an AUC of 0.879. COVID-19 patients showed a profile of pro-inflammatory serum cytokines compared to controls, with higher levels of IL-2, IL-6, IL-15, and IP-10. IL-10 and IL-13 were also elevated in patients compared to controls. Patients who did not survive presented significantly higher levels of IL-15 than those who recovered. No significant differences were observed according to disease progression groups. The study has shown that increased levels of IL-15 and a high Th2 response are associated with a fatal outcome of the disease.

Keywords: COVID-19, SARS-Cov2, T-helper, immunity, cytokines

INTRODUCTION

Coronavirus disease 2019 (COVID-19) is an emergent condition caused by SARS-Cov2 infection that manifests with a wide spectrum of clinical profiles (Diao et al., 2020; Qin et al., 2020; Wang et al., 2020) and that presents a medical challenge due to its contagiousness rates (Guo et al., 2020; Rothan and Byrareddy, 2020). In general, COVID-19 begins as a mild disease with fever, cough, vomiting, myalgia, fatigue or diarrhea similar to those symptoms produced by a seasonally circulating common cold coronavirus. In many cases, the symptoms are so weak, even null, that the condition is not observed (Gao et al., 2020; Kim et al., 2020). However, some COVID-19 patients present lung involvement with severe pneumonia, pulmonary edema, acute distress respiratory syndrome (ARDS) and even death (2.5–7.2% of symptomatic patients) (Guan et al., 2020; Rothan and Byrareddy, 2020; Vardhana and Wolchok, 2020; Yang et al., 2020; Yuki et al., 2020). The disease severity has been associated with ageing and cardiovascular comorbidities (Huang W. et al., 2020; Hurwitz, 2020).

Among others parameters, mild and severe forms of the COVID-19 are characterized by a marked decrease in the total number of peripheral blood lymphocytes including T cells, both CD4+ and CD8+, B lymphocytes and Natural Killer (NK) cell (Song et al., 2020). It is interesting to note that T cells from severe patients present an effector, activated and senescent phenotype mainly associated with CD8+ cells (Vardhana and Wolchok, 2020). Furthermore, cytokine storm is the most life-threatening complication associated with COVID-19 (Schett et al., 2020; Buszko et al., 2020), characterized by a hyperactivated and pro-inflammatory state of the immune system. These features highlight the importance of the immune system response in the physiopathology of the disease (Chen and Wherry, 2020; Diao et al., 2020; Huang C. et al., 2020; Tan et al., 2020; Weiskopf et al., 2020; Vabret et al., 2020; Xu et al., 2020; Zheng et al., 2020; Zheng et al., 2020; Zhou et al., n.d).

The adaptive immune system, especially T cells, plays an important role against viral infections (Diao et al., 2020). T cell responses can mainly be polarized into effector cytotoxic cells (CTLs) and T helper (Th) cells (Mescher et al., 2006; Zhu et al., 2010). Th cells are subdivided into Th1, Th2, Th9, Th17 and follicular helper T cells (Tfh) subsets, each one having a characteristic function against infections (Alberts et al., 2002; Wan, 2010). Two major subtypes of Th cells coordinate responses to infection. One of them, the Th1 subset, coordinates the cell-mediated response, which is essential in macrophage, CTLs and NK activation *via* IL-2 and INF-gamma. Another one, the Th2 cells, which coordinates the humoral response, activates eosinophils, basophils and mast cells *via* IL4 and IL-6. In some infections, the type of Th lymphocytes that coordinates the immune response can condition the evolution of the clinical process. The polarization of the Th response will be determinant in the outcome of the disease (Mosmann and Sad, 1996; Infante-Duarte, 1999).

This phenomenon is well known in viral diseases such as lymphocytic choriomeningitis, where robust Th1 response is associated with a good prognosis (asymptomatic), whereas Th2 responses lead to anorexia and Wasting Syndrome (persistent viral load) (Kamperschroer et al., 2020). A similar situation is also observed in Human Immunodeficiency Virus (HIV) infection. Patients infected with HIV, who show a Th1 response, are seronegative and do not develop acquired immunodeficiency syndrome (AIDS), whereas Th2 patients become seropositive and evolve to AIDS (Clerici and Shearer, 1993; Mosmann and Sad, 1996; Calarota and Weiner, 2004).

The Th1/Th2 balance in COVID-19 has been associated with the outcome of the disease. When the viral infection is established, an appropriate immune response by Th1 is able to clear it discreetly. However, if this immune response is not well organized, an exacerbated reaction precedes the cytokine storm, priming Th2 cells that are linked to poor prognosis (Neidleman et al., 2020; Roncati et al., 2020). Thus, Th polarization seems to play an important role in determining COVID-19 severity, although it is still not totally understood.

This study has aimed to study the percentage and activation grade of Th subsets as well as the cytokine production in the acute moment of the COVID-19 and its association with outcomes.

MATERIALS AND METHODS

Study Design

A prospective observational study that enrolled patients in the initial stages of COVID-19 in a Spanish tertiary university hospital was conducted. Peripheral blood lymphocyte immunophenotypes and cytokines levels were evaluated at the time of diagnosis. Patients were followed-up until discharge or death.

Patients

A random sample of 58 patients with suspicion of COVID-19 were sequentially enrolled in the emergency department of the Hospital Universitario 12 de Octubre (Madrid, Spain) during 2020. Inclusion criteria were 1) Adult patients (>18 years) with symptoms of COVID-19 infection 2) Clinical characteristics or radiological findings that required hospital admission 3) Confirmed diagnosis by RT-PCR or serologic test at any moment of the disease.

As three subjects were lost to the follow-up, finally, 55 patients were included in the study. A reference group of 21 anonymous healthy blood donors representing the general population was established to compare the Th subset.

In tandem, 15 patients with symptoms consistent with COVID-19 initial infection (fever, headache, and cough), but who were SARS-Cov2 RT-PCR negative were recruited in order to compare peripheral blood lymphocyte immunophenotypes with confirmed COVID-19 patients. This group was named "COVID-Like." All the patients in this group had a benign evolution and none required admission to the Intensive Care Unit (ICU).

A new cytokine anonymous control group (obtained before the pandemic) was created with 94 blood donors (other than those in the reference group) in order to compare cytokine levels with the COVID-19 cohort.

The remaining 55 patients recruited in this study were divided into four groups according to their evolution and most critical event 1) Patients who died (Group-1, Death, N = 9), 2) Patients who were treated in ICU (Group-2, ICU, N = 7), 3) Patients with severe involvement who required immunomodulatory treatment (Group-3, Immunomodulators, N = 14) and 4) Patients with a benign course that did not require complex therapies (Group-4, Benign Course, N = 25) (**Figure 1**).

Patients were also classified according to the worst SpO_2/FiO_2 (blood oxygen saturation/fractional inspired oxygen) during their disease into 1) Ventilatory failure, SpO_2/FiO2<300. 2) Normal ventilation, SpO2/FiO2>300 (No ventilatory failure).

Diagnosis was made by RT-PCR in 73% of the patients using nasopharyngeal or oropharyngeal swabs as well as sputum samples. For those patients with a negative RT-PCR, the serologic diagnostic test against the spike and nucleocapsid protein was performed (27%) (Anti-SARS-Cov-2 ELISA (IgG/A) and Anti-NCP-SARS-Cov-2, (IgM/IgG) Euroimmun, Germany 2020, respectively).

Ethics Statement

This study was conducted in accordance with the principles of the Declaration of Helsinki and was approved by the Clinical Research Ethics Committee of the University Hospital 12 de Octubre (reference no. 20/167). Oral or written informed consent was obtained from all patients.

Study Definitions

COVID-19 case was defined as a person fulfilling both the clinical and laboratory criteria of COVID-19.

COVID-19 laboratory criteria were a positive result for severe acute respiratory syndrome coronavirus 2 (SARS-CoV-2) according to reverse transcription polymerase chain reaction (RT-PCR) or serological assays, performed by nasal swab sampling and sera or plasma, respectively.

Data Collection

An anonymized database containing the patient data, including demographic, clinical and laboratory data from the electronic medical record, was created. Laboratory parameters included D-dimer, lactate dehydrogenase (LDH), C reactive protein (CRP), ferritin and the number of lymphocytes (lymphopenia was defined as total lymphocyte count of less than 0.85×10^9/liter).

Samples

Sera and EDTA-treated blood samples were collected in the first 24 h after hospitalization with a median of 7 days from the beginning of the symptoms before treatment.

Flow Cytometry

Peripheral blood mononuclear cells (PBMCs) were isolated from EDTA-treated whole blood samples by density gradient centrifugation using Lymphoprep ™ (Fresenius Kabi, Oslo, Norway).

Peripheral blood lymphocytes (PBL) were isolated and stained with the following fluorochrome-conjugated monoclonal antibodies: CD4-APC-H7, CXCR3-PE, CCR6-BB515, PD-1-PE-Cy7 and ICOS-BV450 (all from BD biosciences, San José, CA, USA) (Mallett et al., 2019; Mousset et al., 2019). Acquisition of PBLs was performed with a FACS CANTO II flow cytometry (BDbiosciences) and analyzed with Flow-Jo software v10.6.2. Gating strategy is shown (**Figure S1**).

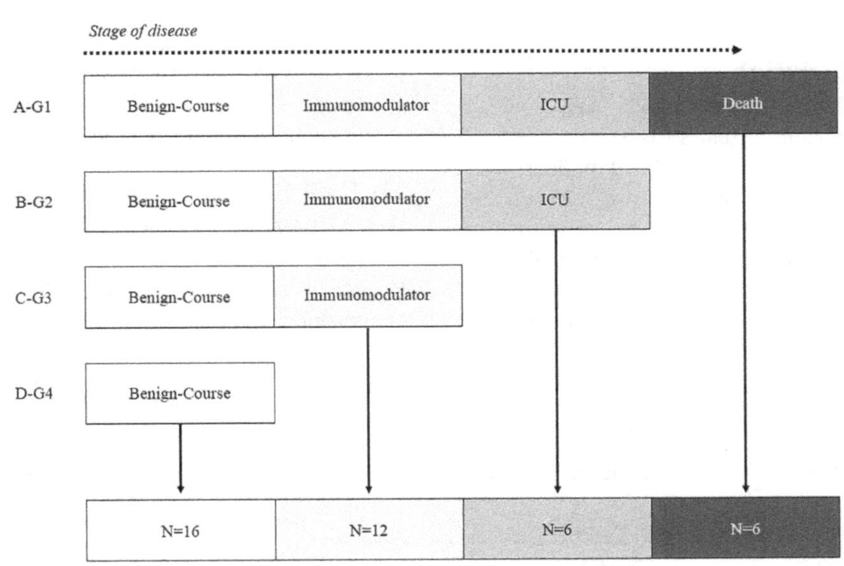

FIGURE 1 | Patient classification according to the most critical event during hospitalization. **(A)** G1-Hospitalized patients who died. **(B)** G2-Alive patients who ended up in ICU. **(C)** G3-Hospitalized patients with poor prognosis characteristics who needed immunomodulatory treatment. **(D)** G4-Hospitalized patients with mild symptoms who did not need immunomodulatory treatment.

Cells CXCR3+/CCR6- gated from CD4 were considered Th1 cells, CXCR3-/CCR6+ cells were considered as Th17 and CXCR3-/CCR6- as Th2. Regarding the activation grade, cells PD-1-/ICOS- were considered as quiescent Th cells, PD-1-/ICOS+ cells as early-activated cells, PD-1+/ICOS+ as late activation markers and PD-1+/ICOS- as exhausted or senescent cells (Mallett et al., 2019).

Cytokine Profile Assay

Serum cytokine Th profile was determined by Human Cytokine Magnetic Bead Panel Kit (EMD Millipore Corporation) using a LABScan™ 100 Luminex. The results were analyzed with Luminex xPONENT42 softwarev3.1. Cytokines included were IL-2, IL-4, IL-6, IL-10, IL-12p70, IL-13, IL-15, INF-gamma, IP-10, MCP-1, and VEGFα.

Statistical Analysis

Results of qualitative variables were expressed as absolute frequency and percentage. Results of the scaled variables were expressed as median with interquartile range. Comparison between qualitative variables was evaluated with Pearson's Chi-square test or Fisher's exact test, when appropriate.

Comparison between scaled variables with two categories were performed using Mann-Whitney's U test, whereas variables with more than two categories were analyzed using Kruskal-Wallis test.

The odds ratio was used to express the relative measure of an effect between a binary outcome variable and a predictor variable. Multivariate analysis was performed using logistic regression model. Significant results were considered with a p-value < 0.05.

Data were analyzed with MedCalc ® version 19.3 (MedCalc Software, Ostend, Belgium).

RESULTS

Patient's Characteristics

Median age of the COVID-19 cohort was 55 years (IQR: 44–75.25) with a higher proportion of males (67%). No significant age differences were found when COVID-19 patients were compared with the reference population (55 vs. 50, respectively, p = 0.195). Sex distribution was also analyzed between groups, no significant differences being found (**Table 1**).

COVID-19 patients were classified according to their most critical event during the evolution of the disease (**Figure 1**).

Deceased patients in COVID-19 group were significantly older than the reference population (p < 0.001) and COVID-19 survival patients (p < 0.001). No significant differences were observed in sex distribution (**Table 1**). Similarly, when laboratory parameters were compared among COVID-19 groups, the total number of lymphocytes were significantly depleted in deceased patients compared to survival patients (p = 0.014). The patients who died also presented a high rate of lymphopenia (p = 0.013) and higher D-dimer levels (p = 0.011). No significant differences were found regarding LDH concentration, CRP levels, ferritin, % RT-PCR or serology, and the development of ARDS (**Table 2**).

Differences in Th Subsets Between Reference Population and COVID-19 Patients

When analyzing the differences in the Th subsets between in COVID-19 patients and controls, it was found that the percentage of CD4+ T lymphocytes with Th1 and Th17 phenotype was significantly reduced in the cells of COVID-19 patients (2.99% vs. 6.68%, p < 0.001 for Th1; and 3.41% vs. 6.95%, p = 0.012 for Th17).

Quiescent Th cells were analyzed when between COVID-19 patients and healthy controls. The percentages of quiescent Th1 cells (6% vs. 9.76% in controls, p = 0.007). Percentage of Th17 and Th2 tends to be reduced in COIVD-19 patients (10.1% vs. 13.2%, p = 0.19 for Th17; 21.3% vs. 35.9%, p = 0.111 for Th2).

The percentage of early-activated cells in the Th1 and Th17 subsets were reduced compared with healthy controls (0.65% vs. 1.17%, p = 0.026 for Th1; 0.8% vs. 1.19%, p = 0.091 for Th17). The percentage of Th17 was significantly depleted in COVID-19 patients versus controls (0.58% vs. 1.44%, p = 0.007) regarding the late activity phenotype. The activated status was augmented in Th2 subset (17.6% in COVID-19 patients vs. 1.31% in healthy controls, p = 0.004).

COVID-19 patients presented a reduced percentage of senescent Th2 cells compared to controls (4.7% vs. 11.5%, p < 0.001)

No significant differences were shown in **Table S1**.

Th Cell Subsets Imbalance According to the Disease Progression

After examining the Th cell subsets differences between COVID-19 patients and healthy controls, the COVID-19 groups were compared according to disease evolution. No significant

TABLE 1 | Age and sex comparison between reference population and COVID-19 cohort.

Variables	Reference population N = 21	COVID-19 patients N = 55	p-value*	COVID-19 patients groups N = 55			
				Deceased; N = 9	Alive; N = 46	p-value**	p-value***
Age	50 (43.75–59.25)	55 (44–75.25)	0.195	87 (82.25–91.75)	53 (44–62)	<0.001	<0.001
Sex	–	–	–	–	–	–	–
Female	8 (38%)	18 (33%)	0.738	2 (22%)	16 (35%)	0.514	0.748
Male	13 (62%)	37(67%)		7 (78%)	30 (65%)		

*Reference population vs. COVID-19 cohort; **Reference population vs. Deceased COVID-19 patients; ***Alive COVID-19 patients vs. Death COVID-19 patients.*

TABLE 2 | Laboratory parameters compared among COVID-19 groups show median and IQR.

Variables	COVID-19 patients groups N = 55				p-value
	G1-Deceased; N = 9	G2-ICU; N = 7	G3-Immunomodulators; N = 14	G4-Benign Course; N = 25	
Biochemical Markers	–	–	–	–	–
D-Dimer	4196 (1105–14116)	1714 (1162–1886)	628 (554.25–822)	579.5 (298–959)	0.011
LDH	206.5 (287–338)	314.5 (271.5–370.5)	345 (255–411)	279 (226.25–362)	0.369
CRP	8.29(5.51–24.24)	4 (1.07–20.37)	6.05 (3.94–13.92)	4.49 (1.3–11.1)	0.169
Ferritin	963.4 (535.4–1569.5)	1268 (700.1–1837)	1014 (533.6–1574.9)	646.9 (283.75–1146.35)	0.319
Immunological Markers	–	–	–	–	–
Lymphocyte	650 (500–1,050)	1500 (800–2,600)	1550 (1400–2,000)	1300 (775–1,855)	0.014
Lymphopenia	5 (55.5%)	3 (43%)	0 (0%)	8 (32%)	0.013
Diagnosis	–	–	–	–	–
RT-PCR	8 (89%)	6 (86%)	9 (64%)	17 (68%)	0.463
Serology	1 (11%)	1 (14%)	5 (36%)	8 (32%)	0.392
ARDS	4 (44.5%)	4 (57%)	5 (36%)	7 (28%)	0.351

LDH, lactate dehydrogenase; CRP, C-reactive protein; RT-PCR, retrotranscriptase polymerase chain reaction; ARDS, acute respiratory distress syndrome; ICU, intensive care unit.

differences in the percentage of Th1, Th2 or Th17 and activation grade were observed in the COVID-19 patient groups.

Deceased COVID-19 patients showed a lower percentage of quiescent Th1 cells compared to COVID-19 patients with a benign course of the disease (p = 0.016). Increased percentage of senescent Th1 cells tends to be associated with a benign course of the disease. However, higher proportions of senescent Th2 were associated with death (p = 0.009).

There were no significant results regarding total proportion of Th, the grade activation and the senescent status (**Figure 2**).

Differences in Th Subsets Between COVID-Like and COVID-19 Patients

Comparing the Th subsets between COVID-Like and COVID-19 patients, no significant differences were found in the total proportion of Th1, Th17, and Th2.

COVID-19 patients presented a significantly higher percentage of late-activated Th2 cells than COVID-19 patients (17.6% vs. 0.76%, p = 0.006). The result of this comparation is shown in **Table S2**. As can be seen in **Figure 2**, when the COVID-Like patients were compared with the four subgroups of COVID-19 patients, their similarity with the COVID patients with good progression (groups 3 and 4) stands out.

Death-Associated Factors

Th subsets were evaluated in relationship with mortality (**Table 3**). The two factors that conferred risk in the univariate analysis, that is, the total number of lymphocytes (p = 0.018) and the senescent Th2 percent (p = 0.021), were included in a multivariate analysis. The total number of lymphocytes (OR 0.15, 95% CI: 0.02–0.81, p = 0.027) and the higher senescent percentage of Th2 cells (OR: 13.88, 95% CI: 1.33–143.88, p = 0.027) behaved like independent and significant risk factors for death with an area under the ROC curve of 0.879 (95% CI: 0.760–0.952) (**Table 3**).

Cytokine Profiling

The cytokine serum profile was compared between COVID-19 patients and healthy controls. An increased expression of IL-2 (p < 0.001) and INF-gamma (p = 0.024) and a reduction of IL-12p70 (p < 0.001) in COVID-19 patients were observed regarding the Th1 cytokines. Regarding Th2 cytokines, COVID-19 patients showed higher levels of IL-6, IL-10 and IL-13, but lower levels of IL-4 (p < 0.001, for all of them). Other cytokines like IL-15 and IP-10 presented significantly increased levels in COVID-19 compared to healthy donors (p < 0.001, in both cases). No significant differences were observed in relationship to MCP-1 and VEGFα (**Table S3**).

Cytokine levels were studied according to the worst event during hospitalization, without any significant results among groups (**Figure S3**).

Patients who died presented significantly higher levels of IL-15: 9.65 pg/ml, IQR: 7.5–15.3 vs. 5.06 pg/ml, IQR: 2–8.18; (p = 0.036). A marked trend was observed when MCP-1, IL-6 and IL-10 were analyzed to describe which ones of the higher levels were associated to poorer evolution of the disease, but these differences did not achieve statistical significance (**Table 4**).

DISCUSSION

We have demonstrated in this study that a Th1 coordinated immune response during the infection by SARS-CoV-2 associates with good prognosis and resolution of COVID-19. The type of Th response impacted the disease outcome, since 78% of patients who finally died had produced an overreactive Th2 response. The type of Th response has been demonstrated to be crucial for the resolution of the disease (Infante-Duarte, 1999; Spellberg and Edwards, 2001).

We have not been able to observe changes in activated cells because they are localized in tissues controlling the infection. On the other hand, those that have already ended their task abandon the tissue and migrate into the blood (Morris, 1998). The detection of senescent Th cells in blood could be an indicator of the type of the past immune response.

In intracellular *M. tuberculosis* infection, Bacillus Calmette-Guerin (BCG) vaccine promotes a Th1 response, protecting human beings from tuberculosis development. The utility of BCG vaccine has been studied in COVID-19 patients with very surprising results. Lower mortality and infective rates were

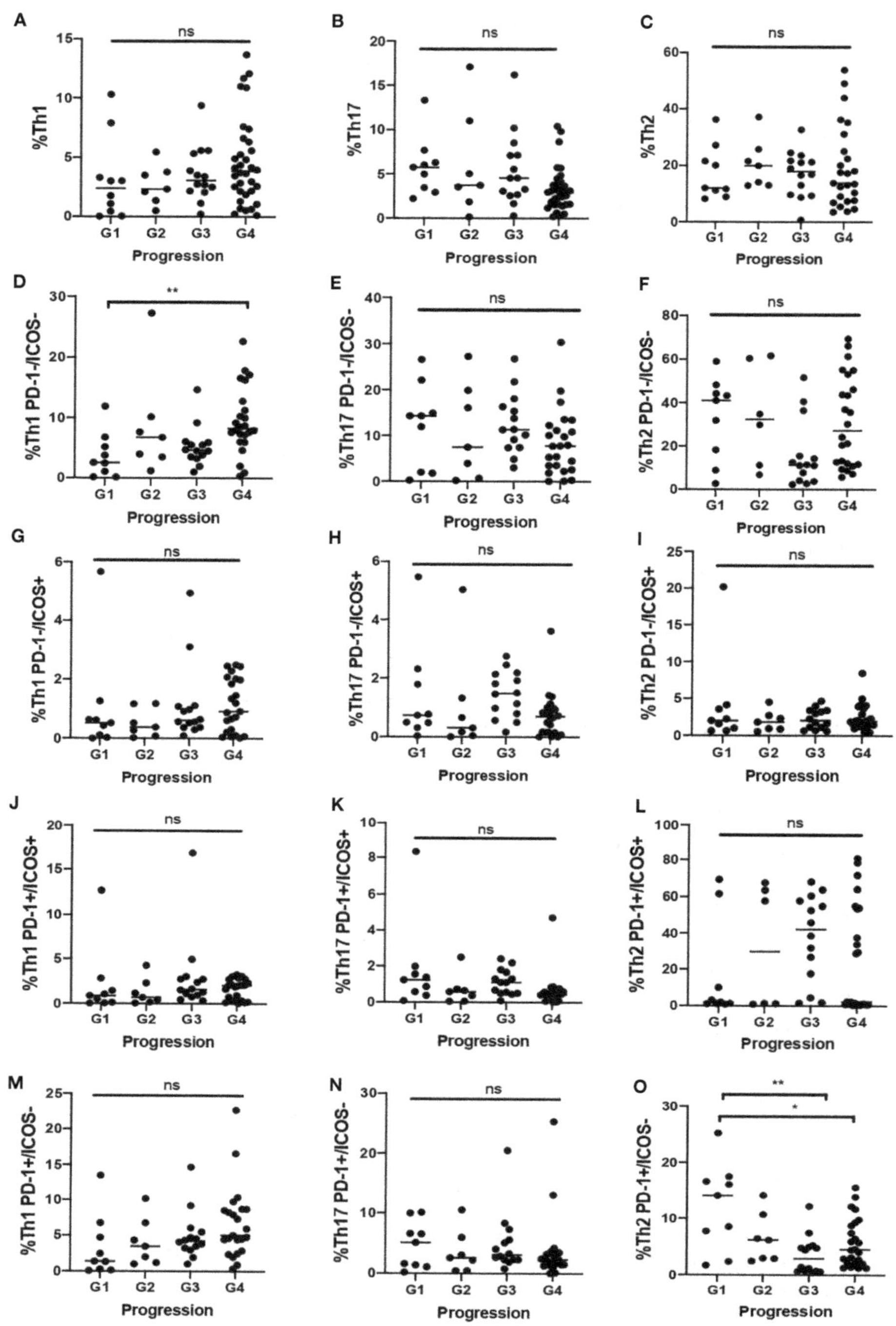

FIGURE 2 | Th distribution in COVID-19 patients according to the most critical event during disease. **A–C)** Total proportion of Th 1 **(A)**. Th17 **(B)** and Th2 **(C)**. **(D, F)** Proportion of quiescent Th1 **(D)**, Th17 **(E)** and Th2 **(F)**. **(G–I)** Proportion of early activated Th1 **(G)**. Th17 **(H)** and Th2 **(I)**. **(J–L)** Proportion of late activated Th1 **(J)**, Th17 **(K)**, and Th2 **(L)**. **(M–O)** Proportion of senescent Th1 **(M)**, Th17 **(N)**, and Th2 **(O)**. G1: Death; G2: Intensive Care Unit; G3: Immunomodulators; G4: Benign-Course. *. <0.05 **. <0.01 ns, not significant.

observed in vaccinated patients, who produced Th1 responses (Ozdemir et al., 2020). Our study has highlighted the importance of Th1 hypoactivation and Th2 overreaction, with subsequent exhaustion, associated with poorer prognosis. A possible hypothesis to explain the severe forms of COVID-19 is that the Th2 responses prevail in those patients, producing an ineffective response to intracellular pathogens like viruses. However, contrary to other studies, which propose that a higher % of Th2 cells is associated with critical care and poor prognosis (Wei et al., 2020), we did not observe any differences

TABLE 3 | Univariate and multivariate analyses associated to death risk with all significant variables.

VARIABLES	p-value	OR	OR 95% CI	AUC	AUC 95% CI	p-value	OR	OR 95% CI
Lymphocytes	0.018	0.2	0.05–0.076	0.77	0.634–0.873	0.027	0.15	0.02–0.81
% Th1	0.514	0.65	0.18–2.33	0.55	0.413–0.687	–	–	–
%Th17	0.085	3.8	0.83–17.37	0.63	0.495–0.761	–	–	–
% Th2	0.777	0.86	0.31–2.38	0.52	0.385–0.661	–	–	–
%Th1 PD-1-/ICOS–	0.067	0.28	0.07–10.9	0.68	0.545–0.803	–	–	–
%Th17 PD-1-/ICOS–	0.257	2.38	0.53–10.69	0.6	0.464–0.734	–	–	–
%Th2 PD-1-/ICOS–	0.259	27.778	0.47–16.35	0.618	0.451–0.766	–	–	–
% Th1 PD-1-/ICOS+	0.710	0.72	0.13–3.96	0.53	0.391–0.666	–	–	–
%Th17 PD-1-/ICOS+	0.574	1.53	0.34–6.31	0.55	0.411–0.685	–	–	–
%Th2 PD-1-/ICOS+	0.161	2.57	0.68–9.69	0.58	0.429–0.712	–	–	–
%Th1 PD-1+/ICOS+	0.631	1.79	0.14–19.46	0.52	0.384–0.659	–	–	–
%Th17 PD-1+/ICOS+	0.238	5.6	0.31–99.41	0.54	0.405–0.68	–	–	–
%Th2 PD-1+/ICOS +	0.09	0.24	0.04–1.28	0.66	0.52–0.783	–	–	–
%Th1 PD-1+/ICOS–	0.750	0.69	0.07–6.47	0.52	0.382–0.657	–	–	–
%Th17 PD-1+/ICOS–	0.073	3.86	0.87–16.97	0.656	0.514–0.780	–	–	–
%Th2 PD-1+/ICOS–	0.021	7.23	1.33–39.12	0.72	0.589–0.837	0.027	13.88	1.33–143.88
Area Under the Curve						0.879	0.760–952	

PD-1-/ICOS–, Quiescent; PD-1-/ICOS+, early-activated; PD-1+/ICOS+, late-activated; PD-1+/ICOS, senescent.

TABLE 4 | Cytokine profile differences in alive and deceased patients.

Cytokines	Alive; N = 28		Death; N = 6		p-value
	Median	**IQR**	**Median**	**IQR**	
IL-2	0.1	0.1–0.85	0.29	0.1–0.86	0.573
IL-4	1.4	1.4–5.56	1.4	1.4–381.12	0.827
IL-6	14.33	2.12–41.49	39.55	8.6–69.36	0.258
IL-10	8.78	3.2–18.28	17.19	00.18–26.84	0.113
IL-12p70	0.05	0.05–0.44	0.05	0.05–0.08	0.667
IL-13	0.5	0.5–1.61	0.55	0.5–16.04	0.46
IL-15	5.05	2–8.18	9.65	7.5–15.3	0.036
INFg	0.39	0.3–8.77	5.15	2.24–7.18	0.314
IP-10	1183.65	296.29–3151.72	1358.33	876.82–3858.76	0.588
MCP-1	527.91	358.96–889.92	1248.8	535.58–1999.45	0.064
VEGFα	92.73	17.45–297.8	75.84	16–93.99	0.401

when we analyzed the total % of Th1, Th2, and Th17 between the different clinical course of the disease. This finding could suggest that the activation grade could be a more important prognostic factor than the total percentage of each Th as we have observed that patients with a more benign course of the disease tend to present higher % of senescent Th1 cells as a consequence of their rapid activation. The absence of significance could be due to the small size of each group.

When we compared the patients with COVID-19 with the healthy controls, we found that the majority of the patients not only presented a general reduction in the total percentage of Th but also in their degree of activation. This clear reduction could be related to the common lymphopenia (Wang et al., 2020; Yang et al., 2020). We have observed that COVID-19 patients had an overactive Th2 response against the virus. Therefore, compared to COVID-like patients, COVID-19 patients also had an overactive Th2 response.

Observations from the COVID-Like group should be handled with caution. The World Health Organization has reported that in pandemic situations it is not possible to rule out that patients who have had symptoms similar to COVID and RT-PCR negative had the disease (WHO, 2020). It is possible that some patients in the COVID-Like group were seronegative COVID-19 patients with a mild form of the disease. In this way, it is worth highlighting the similarities observed between the patients in this group and the COVID-19 patients with good evolution.

The mortality rate described in COVID-19 is highly variable: from 2.2% to 15% in some studies (Cao et al., 2020; Chen et al., 2020; Huang C. et al., 2020; Rothan and Byrareddy, 2020; Wang et al., 2020). The factors associated with high mortality in COVID-19 are only partially known (obesity, age, previous illnesses, etc.) (Wolff et al., 2020; Zheng et al., 2020).

Our results have shown that total number of lymphocytes and higher exhausted Th2 are independent risk factors for death. Our findings are consistent with that previously described in SARS-Cov (Li et al., 2008; Vabret et al., 2020). Lymphopenia was an important finding as similar results were observed in SARS-Cov and MERS-Cov (Peiris et al., 2003; Wong et al., 2003; Erickson et al., 2013; Ko et al., 2016; Min et al., 2016). The presence of higher exhausted Th2 suggests an over-activation with the consequent exhaustion, a phenomenon that has been observed in CD8+ cell. All this activation is driven by rapid viral replication and its exposure to lymphocytes (Ko et al., 2016; Min et al., 2016). Th2 hyperactivation could explain why severe patients have higher antibody titers than mild or asymptomatic patients, as their cytokines stimulate antibody production (Spellberg and Edwards, 2001).

We have observed that the SARS-Cov2 infection is characterized by a pro-inflammatory environment with increased levels of IL-2, IL-6, IL-15, IP-10, and INF-gamma. As described previously, cytokines are important for the clearance of respiratory infections (Kimura et al., 2013).

Our results have shown that patients with a poor prognosis present a Th cytokine profile associated with changes in the inflammatory status, as previously described (Lucas et al., 2020), with a slight increase in the expression of IL-6, IL-10, MCP-1, and INF-gamma and a marked increase of IL-15.

High levels of these cytokines have been reported in publications to be related with a worse respiratory status (Vabret et al., 2020; Yao et al., 2020). It has also been described that critical respiratory manifestations have correlated with high levels of IL-6 and IL-15, this being an important predictor of disease progression (Leahy et al., 2016; Rocio et al., 2020). High levels of IL-6, MCP-1 and IL-15 correlated to poor prognosis in SARS-Cov and MERS-Cov infections, acting as hypercytokinemia and systemic syndrome predictors, have also been reported (Wang et al., 2004; Wong et al., 2004; Zhang et al., 2004; Li et al., 2020). Another factor which could help to understand Th imbalance in COVID-19 is IL-10, a potent inhibitor of IL-12 and Th1 response. The significance of the presence of IL10 in COVID-19 patients has been extensively described in the literature, this suggesting that IL-10 could discriminate disease progression (Gong et al., 2020; Zhou et al., 2020).

IL-15 is a cytokine secreted by different cell types like endothelial cells, respiratory epithelium or neurons. It matures in macrophages and dendritic cells and plays a pleiotropic role in innate and adaptive immunity. Similarly to IL-2, IL-15 is a very important molecule in NK and T lymphocyte activation and proliferation like IL-2 (Perera et al., 2012). Activated T cell recruitment and contraction in inflammatory tissues, enriched with antigenic molecules, is a crucial event in the immune response, which principally depends on antigenic presentation by endothelial cells from swollen vessels (Ward et al., 2017). IL-15 has been identified as an important mediator in T cell and NK migration to infected tissue, due to IL-15 improves LFA-1/ICAM-1 binding affinity in endothelial cells (Oppenheimer-marks et al., 1998). We hypothesize that its elevation is due to an additional effort of the immune system in T lymphocyte activation in an alternate way, as a compensatory mechanism to substitute an inefficient Th1 response.

Nowadays, there is extensive state of the art knowledge regarding the causes of lymphopenia. Some authors have stated that lymphopenia is caused by direct infection of lymphocyte, as they express ACE2 in their surface (Xu et al., 2020). Another hypothesis states that the immune system hyperactivation could lead to lymphocyte apoptosis by inflammatory cytokines (Liao et al., 2002; Sähr et al., 2015). On the other hand, other publications support the idea that immune system dysregulation in COVID-19 leads to a "cytokine storm," suggesting a polyclonal activation of T lymphocytes, possibly associated to superantigens (Cossarizza, 1997). Others have reported that the lymphopenia associated with COVID-19 could be a consequence of pulmonary recruitment and entrapment of lymphocytes, due to modification of adhesion molecules (CD44, LFA-1 and ICAM-1) (Morris, 1998; Bohn et al., 2020). Recently, Roncati et al. published that SARS-Cov2 is able to infect lymphocytes *via* dipeptidyl peptidase-4 (DPP-4) receptor, which is overexpressed in Th1 lymphocyte rather in Th2 (Willheim et al., 1997; Annunziato et al., 1998; Sakata-Kaneko et al., 2000). This finding could support our results as we have observed that COVID-19 patients have reduced total % Th1 compared with healthy controls. Moreover, the total %Th2 was slightly higher in COVID-19 patients.

When a Th effector response is polarized to Th2, antibody production is not only stimulated but the cell-mediated immunity is also suppressed (Kaiko et al., 2007). This fact is very important regarding the treatment that patients receive. In many cases, glucocorticoids are chosen as a treatment of choice in this novel condition, but they are a double-edged sword as they act as immunosuppressant reducing IL-2, which is essential for Th1 responses, where only Th2 are able to proliferate (Krakauer, 1995; Larsson and Linden, 1998; Ramírez et al., 1998; Vieira et al., 1998; Franchimont et al., 2000), this severely affecting the patients.

Recently, some authors have proposed that patients susceptible to severe lung pathology in COVID-19 may have the highest Th17. This response could be promoted by IL-6 and may be accompanied by eosinophilia. In our patients, Th17 was significantly reduced compared to controls, but no differences were found according to clinical presentations of the disease (Hotez et al., 2020; Wu and Yang, 2020).

Several limitations exist in this study. First of all, it is limited by the reduced sample size of our study so that these markers not only need to be evaluated in a larger cohort but also further independent studies are needed to validate our results. Secondly, in order to perform a multivariate analysis, due to the few events that were of interest in this study, the univariate and multivariate evaluation could not be carried out with raw data, thus requiring each variable to be transformed into ranges by histogram of frequency analysis (**Table S4**). Another limitation is that we studied the cytokine profile of each patient in sera but not in cell culture and we have not studied antibody titration to examine its association to prognosis. Finally, using blood donors is a disadvantage regarding age as severe forms of the disease usually affect patients older than 65 in whom blood donation is not recommended.

In summary, although Th1/Th2 imbalance related to poor prognosis is well known in infections of different etiology, much remains to be known in COVID-19 patients. At present, most of the effects are directed toward reducing an exacerbated inflammatory response. Therefore, the search for new therapies, which redirect Th2 responses to Th1, may tip the scale toward less severe forms of the disease.

AUTHOR CONTRIBUTIONS

AS and EP-A developed the theory. AS and FG-E designed the study and planned the experiments. PS-F, LN, DA, SG and FG-E carried out the experiments. AL, DP, and RD-S supported the clinical aspects of the study. FG-E analyzed the data and took the lead in writing the manuscript. AS, EP-A, EM, LA and OC-M reviewed the final manuscript. All authors provided critical feedback and helped shape the research, analysis and manuscript. All authors contributed to the article and approved the submitted version.

ACKNOWLEDGMENTS

We thank Barbara Shapiro for her exceptional work of translation and English revision of the article.

REFERENCES

Alberts, B., Johnson, A., Lewis, J., Raff, M., Roberts, K., and Walter, P. (2002). Molecular Biology of the Cell. *Helper T Cells and Lymphocyte Activation. 4th edition*, New York: Garland Science. Available at: https://www.ncbi.nlm.nih.gov/books/NBK26827/.

Annunziato, F., Galli, G., Cosmi, L., Romagnani, P., Manetti, R., Maggi, E., et al. (1998). Molecules Associated with Human Thl or Th2 Cells. *Eur. Cytokine Netw.* 9 (3 Suppl), 12–16.

Bohn, M. K., Hall, A., Sepiashvili, L., Jung, B., Steele, S., and Adeli, K. (2020). Pathophysiology of COVID-19 : Mechanisms Underlying Disease Severity and Progression. *Physiology (Bethesda)* 89, 288–301. doi: 10.1152/physiol.00019.2020

Buszko, M., Park, J. H., Verthelyi, D., Sen, R., Young, H. A., and Rosenberg, A. S. (2020). The Dynamic Changes in Cytokine Responses in COVID-19: A Snapshot of the Current State of Knowledge. *Nat. Immunol.* 21 (10), 1146–1151. doi: 10.1038/s41590-020-0779-1

Calarota, S. A., and Weiner, D. B. (2004). Enhancement of Human Immunodeficiency Virus Type 1-DNA Vaccine Potency through Incorporation of T-Helper 1 Molecular Adjuvants. *Immunol. Rev.* I (99), 84–99. doi: 10.1111/j.0105-2896.2004.00150.x

Cao, B., Wang, Y., Wen, D., Liu, W., Wang, J., Fan, G., et al. (2020). A Trial of Lopinavir–Ritonavir in Adults Hospitalized with Severe Covid-19. *New Engl. J. Med.* 382 (19), 1787–1799. doi: 10.1056/NEJMoa2001282

Chen, N., Zhou, M., Dong, X., Qu, J., Gong, F., Han, Y., et al. (2020). Epidemiological and Clinical Characteristics of 99 Cases of 2019 Novel Coronavirus Pneumonia in Wuhan, China: A Descriptive Study. *Lancet* 395 (10223), 507–513. doi: 10.1016/S0140-6736(20)30211-7

Chen, Z., and Wherry, E.J. (2020). T Cell Responses in Patients with COVID-19. *Nat. Rev. Immunol.* 20 (9), 529–536. doi: 10.1038/s41577-020-0402-6

Clerici, M., and Shearer, G. M. (1993). A TH1→TH2 Switch Is a Critical Step in the Etiology of HIV Infection. *Immunol. Today Immunol. Today* 14 (3), 107–111. doi: 10.1016/0167-5699(93)90208-3

Cossarizza, A. (1997). T-Cell Repertoire and HIV Infection. *AIDS* 11, 1075–1088. doi: 10.1097/00002030-199709000-00001

Diao, Bo., Wang, C., Tan, Y., Chen, X., Liu, Y., Ning, L., et al. (2020). Reduction and Functional Exhaustion of T Cells in Patients With Coronavirus Disease 2019 (COVID-19). *Front. Immunol.* 11, 827. doi: 10.3389/fimmu.2020.00827

Erickson, J. J., Gilchuk, P., Hastings, A. K., Tollefson, S. J., Johnson, M., Downing, M. B., et al. (2012). Viral Acute Lower Respiratory Infections Impair CD8 + T Cells through PD-1. *J. Clin. Invest.* 122 (8), 2967–2982. doi: 10.1172/JCI62860

Franchimont, D., Galon, J., Gadina, M., Visconti, R., Zhou, Y.-J., Aringer, M., et al. (2000). Inhibition of Thl Immune Response by Glucocorticoids: Dexamethasone Selectively Inhibits IL-12-Induced Stat4 Phosphorylation in T Lymphocytes. *J. Immunol.* 164 (4), 1768–1774. doi: 10.4049/jimmunol.164.4.1768

Gao, Z., Xu, Y., Sun, C., Wang, X., Guo, Y., Qiu, S., et al. (2020). A Systematic Review of Asymptomatic Infections with COVID-19. *J. Microbiol. Immunol. Infect.* doi: 10.1016/j.jmii.2020.05.001

Gong, J., Dong, H., Xia, S. Q., Huang, Y. Z., Wang, D., Zhao, Y., et al. (2020). Correlation Analysis Between Disease Severity and Inflammation-Related Parameters in Patients with COVID-19 Pneumonia. *BMC Infect. Dis* 20 (963), 2020.02.25.20025643. doi: 10.1101/2020.02.25.20025643

Guan, W. J., Ni, Z. Y., Hu, Y., Liang, W. H., Ou, C. Q., He, J. X., et al. (2020). Clinical Characteristics of Coronavirus Disease 2019 in China. *New Engl. J. Med.* 382 (18), 1708–1720. doi: 10.1056/NEJMoa2002032. April.

Guo, Y. R., Cao, Q. D., Hong, Z. S., Tan, Y. Y., Chen, S. D., Jin, H. J., et al. (2020). The Origin, Transmission and Clinical Therapies on Coronavirus Disease 2019 (COVID-19) Outbreak- A n Update on the Status. *Mil. Med. Res.* 7 (1), 11. doi: 10.1186/s40779-020-00240-0

Hotez, P. J., Bottazzi, M. E., and Corry, D. B. (2020). The Potential Role of Th17 Immune Responses in Coronavirus Immunopathology and Vaccine-Induced Immune Enhancement. *Microbes Infect.* 22 (4–5), 165–167. doi: 10.1016/j.micinf.2020.04.005

Huang, W., Berube, J., Mcnamara, M., Saksena, S., Hartman, M., Arshad, T., et al. (2020) Lymphocyte Subset Counts in COVID-19 Patients: A Meta-Analysis. Cytometry Part A. *Cytometry Part A* 97 (8), 772–776. doi: 10.1002/cytoa.24172

Huang, C., Wang, Y., Li, X., Ren, L., Zhao, J., Hu, Y., et al. (2020). Clinical Features of Patients Infected with 2019 Novel Coronavirus in Wuhan, China. *Lancet* 395 (10223), 497–506. doi: 10.1016/S0140-6736(20)30183-5

Hurwitz, J. L. (2020). B Cells, Viruses, and the SARS-COV-2/COVID-19 Pandemic of 2020. *Viral Immunol.* 33 (4), 251–252. doi: 10.1089/vim.2020.0055

Infante-Duarte, C. (1999). Thl/Th2 Balance in Infection., in *Springer Seminars in Immunopathology*. Germany: Springer Verlag. doi: 10.1007/BF00812260

Kaiko, G. E., Horvat, J. C., and Beagley, K. W. (2007). Immunological Decision-Making : How Does the Immune System Decide to Mount a Helper T-Cell Response? *Immunology* 123 (3), 326–338. doi: 10.1111/j.1365-2567.2007.02719.x

Kamperschroer, C., Quinn, D. G., Kamperschroer, C., and Quinn, D. G. (2020). The Role of Proinflammatory Cytokines in Wasting Disease During Lymphocytic Choriomeningitis Virus Infection. *J. Immunol.* 169 (1), 340–349. doi: 10.4049/jimmunol.169.1.340

Kim, G. U., Kim, M. J., Ra, S. H., Lee, J., Bae, S., Jung, J., et al. (2020). Clinical Characteristics of Asymptomatic and Symptomatic Patients with Mild COVID-19. *Clin. Microbiol. Infect.* 26 (7), 948.e1–948.e3. doi: 10.1016/j.cmi.2020.04.040

Kimura, H., Yoshizumi, M., Ishii, H., Oishi, K., and Ryo, A. (2013). Cytokine Production and Signaling Pathways in Respiratory Virus Infection. *Front. Microbiol.* 4, 2013.00276 (SEP). doi: 10.3389/fmicb.2013.00276

Ko, J. H., Park, G. E., Lee, J. Y., Lee, J. Y., Cho, S. Y., Ha, Y. E., et al. (2016). Predictive Factors for Pneumonia Development and Progression to Respiratory Failure in MERS-CoV Infected Patients. *J. Infect.* 73 (5), 468–475. doi: 10.1016/j.jinf.2016.08.005

Krakauer, T. (1995). Differential Inhibitory Effects of Interleukin-10, Interleukin-4 and Dexamethasone on Staphylococcal Enterotoxin-Induced Cytokine Production and T Cell Activation. *J. Leuk. Biol.* 57 (3), 450–454. doi: 10.1002/jlb.57.3.450

Larsson, S., and Linden, M. (1998). Effects of a Corticosteroid, Budesonide, on Production of Bioactive IL-12 by Human Monocytes. *Cytokine* 10 (10), 786–789. doi: 10.1006/cyto.1998.0362

Leahy, T.R., McManus, R., Doherty, D. G., Grealy, R., Coulter, T., Smyth, P., et al. (2016). Interleukin-15 Is Associated with Disease Severity in Viral Bronchiolitis. *Eur. Respir. J.* 47 (1), 212–222. doi: 10.1183/13993003.00642-2015

Li, C. K.-f., Wu, H., Yan, H., Ma, S., Wang, L., Zhang, M., et al. (2008). T Cell Responses to Whole SARS Coronavirus in Humans. *J. Immunol.* 181 (8), 5490–5500. doi: 10.4049/jimmunol.181.8.5490

Li, S., Jiang, L., Li, X., Lin, F., Wang, Y., Li, B., et al. (2020). Clinical and Pathological Investigation of Patients with Severe COVID-19. *JCI Insight* 5 (12), 1–13. doi: 10.1172/jci.insight.138070

Liao, Y.-C., Liang, W.-G., Chen, F.-W., Hsu, J.-H., Yang, J.-J., and Chang, M.-S. (2002). IL-19 Induces Production of IL-6 and TNF-α and Results in Cell Apoptosis Through TNF-α. *J. Immunol.* 169 (8), 4288–4297. doi: 10.4049/jimmunol.169.8.4288

Lucas, C., Wong, P., Klein, J., Tiago, B. R. C., Silva, J., Sundaram, M., et al. (2020). Longitudinal Analyses Reveal Immunological Misfiring in Severe COVID-19. *Nature* 584 (7821), 463. doi: 10.1038/s41586-020-2588-y

Mallett, G., Laurence, A., and Amarnath, S. (2019). Programmed Cell Death-1 Receptor (Pd-1)-Mediated Regulation of Innate Lymphoid Cells. *Int. J. Mol. Sci.* 20 (11), 1–13. doi: 10.3390/ijms20112836

Mescher, M. F., Curtsinger, J. M., Agarwal, P., Casey, K. A., Gerner, M., Hammerbeck, C. D., et al. (2006). Signals Required for Programming Effector and Memory Development by CD8+ T Cells. *Immunol. Rev.* 211 (June), 81–92. doi: 10.1111/j.0105-2896.2006.00382.x

Min, C. K., Cheon, S., Ha, N. Y., Sohn, K. M., Kim, Y., Aigerim, A., et al. (2016). Comparative and Kinetic Analysis of Viral Shedding and Immunological Responses in MERS Patients Representing a Broad Spectrum of Disease Severity. *Sci. Rep.* 6 (1), 1–12. doi: 10.1038/srep25359

Morris, O. (1998). Expression of T Lymphocyte Adhesion Molecules: Regulation during Antigen-Induced T Cell Activation and Differenciation. *Crit. Reves Immunol. Immunol.* 18, 153–184. doi: 10.1615/critrevimmunol.v18.i3.10

Mosmann, T. R., and Sad, S. (1996). The Expanding Universe of T-Cell Subsets: Th1, Th2 and More. *Immunol. Today* 17 (3), 138–146. doi: 10.1016/0167-5699(96)80606-2

Mousset, C. M., Hobo, W., Woestenenk, R., Preijers, F., Dolstra, H., and van der Waart, A. B. (2019). Comprehensive Phenotyping of T Cells Using Flow Cytometry. *Cytometry Part A* 95 (6), 647–654. doi: 10.1002/cyto.a.23724

Neidleman, J., Luo, X., Frouard, J., Xie, G., Gill, G., Stein, E. S., et al. (2020). SARS-CoV-2-Specific T Cells Exhibit Phenotypic Features of Robust Helper Function, Lack of Terminal Differentiation, and High Proliferative Potential. *Cell Rep. Med.* 1 (6):100081. doi: 10.1016/j.xcrm.2020.100081

Oppenheimer-marks, N., Brezinschek, R. I., Mohamadzadeh, M., Randi, V., and Peter, E.L. (1998). Interleukin 15 Is Produced by Endothelial Cells and Increases the Transendothelial Migration of T Cells In Vitro and in the SCID Mouse - Human Rheumatoid Arthritis Model In Vivo. *J. Clin.* 101 (6), 1261–1272. doi: 10.1172/JCI1986

Ozdemir, C., Kucuksezer, U. C., and Tamay, Z. U. (2020). Is BCG Vaccination Affecting the Spread and Severity of COVID-19?" *Allergy* 75 (7), 1824–1827. doi: 10.1111/all.14344

Peiris, J. S. M., Lai, S. T., Poon, L. L. M., Guan, Y., Yam, L. Y. C., Lim, W., et al. (2003). Coronavirus as a Possible Cause of Severe Acute Respiratory Syndrome. *Lancet* 361 (9366), 1319–1325. doi: 10.1016/S0140-6736(03)13077-2

Perera, P.-y., Lichy, J. H., Waldmann, T. A., and Perera, L. P. (2012). The Role of Interleukin-15 in Inflammation and Immune Responses to Infection : Implications for Its Therapeutic Use. *Microbes Infect.* 14 (3), 247–261. doi: 10.1016/j.micinf.2011.10.006

Qin, C., Zhou, L., Hu, Z., Zhang, S., Yang, S., Tao, Y., et al. (2020). Dysregulation of Immune Response in Patients with COVID-19 in Wuhan, China. *Clin. Infect. Dis.* 71 (15), 762–768. doi: 10.1093/cid/ciaa248/5803306

Ramírez, F. (1998). Glucocorticoids Induce a Th2 Response in Vitro. *Dev. Immunol.* 6 (3–4), 223–243. doi: 10.1155/1998/73401

Rocio, L.-G., Utrero-Rico, A., Talayero, P., Lasa-Lazaro, M., Ramirez-Fernandez, A., Naranjo, L., et al. (2020). Interleukin-6-Based Mortality Risk Model for Hospitalised COVID-19 Patients. *J. Allergy Clin. Immunol.* 146 (4): 799–807. doi: 10.1016/j.jaci.2020.07.009

Roncati, L., Nasillo, V., Lusenti, B., and Riva, G. (2020). Signals of Th2 Immune Response from COVID-19 Patients Requiring Intensive Care. *Ann. Hematol.* 99 (6), 1419–1420. doi: 10.1007/s00277-020-04066-7

Rothan, H. A., and Byrareddy, S. N. (2020). The Epidemiology and Pathogenesis of Coronavirus Disease (COVID-19) Outbreak. *J. Autoimmun.* 109, 102433 doi: 10.1016/j.jaut.2020.102433

Sähr, A., Förmer, S., Hildebrand, D., and Heeg, K. (2015). T-Cell Activation or Tolerization: The Yin and Yang of Bacterial Superantigens. *Front. Microbiol.* 6, 1153. doi: 10.3389/fmicb.2015.01153

Sakata-Kaneko, S., Wakatsuki, Y., Matsunaga, Y., Usui, T., and Kita, T. (2000). Altered Th1/Th2 Commitment in Human CD4+ T Cells with Ageing. *Clin. Exp. Immunol.* 120 (2), 267–273. doi: 10.1046/j.1365-2249.2000.01224.x

Schett, G., Sticherling, M., and Neurath, M. F. (2020). COVID-19: Risk for Cytokine Targeting in Chronic Inflammatory Diseases?" *Nat. Rev. Immunol.* 20 (5), 271–272. doi: 10.1038/s41577-020-0312-7

Song, C. Y., Xu, J., He, J. Q., and Lu, Y. Q. (2020). Immune Dysfunction Following COVID-19, Especially in Severe Patients. *Sci. Rep.* 10 (1), 1–11. doi: 10.1038/s41598-020-72718-9

Spellberg, B., and Edwards, J. E. (2001). Type 1/Type 2 Immunity in Infectious Diseases. *Clin. Infect. Dis.* 32 (1), 76–102. doi: 10.1086/317537

Tan, L., Wang, Q., Zhang, D., Ding, J., Huang, Q., Tang, Y. Q., et al. (2020). Lymphopenia Predicts Disease Severity of COVID-19: A Descriptive and Predictive Study. *Signal Transduct. Target. Ther.* 52 (1), 33. doi: 10.1038/s41392-020-0148-4

Vabret, N., Britton, G. J., Gruber, C., Hegde, S., Kim, J., Kuksin, M., et al. (2020). Immunology of COVID-19: Current State of the Science. *Immunity* 52 (6), 910–941. doi: 10.1016/j.immuni.2020.05.002

Vardhana, S. A., and Wolchok, J. D. (2020). The Many Faces of the Anti-COVID Immune Response. *J. Exp. Med.* 217 (6). doi: 10.1084/JEM.20200678

Vieira, P. L., Kaliński, P., Wierenga, E. A., Kapsenberg, M. L., and de Jong, E. C. (1998). Glucocorticoids Inhibit Bioactive IL-12p70 Production by In Vitro-Generated Human Dendritic Cells Without Affecting Their T Cell Stimulatory Potential. *J. Immunol.* 161, (10).

Wan, Y. Y. (2010). Multi-Tasking of Helper T Cells. *Immunology* 130 (2), 166–171. doi: 10.1111/j.1365-2567.2010.03289.x

Wang, W. K., Chen, S. Y., Jung Liu, I., Kao, C. L., Chen, H. L., Chiang, B. L., et al. (2004). Temporal Relationship of Viral Load, Ribavirin, Interleukin (IL)-6, IL-8, and Clinical Progression in Patients with Severe Acute Respiratory Syndrome. *Clin. Infect. Dis.* 39 (7), 1071–1075. doi: 10.1086/423808

Wang, F., Nie, J., Wang, H., Zhao, Q., Xiong, Y., Deng, L., et al. (2020). Characteristics of Peripheral Lymphocyte Subset Alteration in COVID-19 Pneumonia. *J. Infect. Dis.* 221 (11), 1762–1769. doi: 10.1093/infdis/jiaa150

Wang, F., Hou, H., Luo, Y., Tang, G., Wu, S., Huang, M., et al. (2020). The Laboratory Tests and Host Immunity of COVID-19 Patients with Different Severity of Illness. *JCI Insight* 5 (10), e137799. doi: 10.1172/jci.insight.137799

Ward, E. J., Fu, H., and Marelli-Berg, F. (2017). Monitoring Migration of Activated T Cells to Antigen-Rich Non-Lymphoid Tissue." In *Methods Mol. Biol.* 1591, 215–224. doi: 10.1007/978-1-4939-6931-9_15

Wei, L.-l., Wang, W.-j., Chen, D.-x., and Xu, B. (2020). Dysregulation of the Immune Response Affects the Outcome of Critical COVID-19 Patients. *J. Med. Virol.* 92 (11), 2768–2776 doi: 10.1002/jmv.26181

Weiskopf, D., Schmitz, K. S., Raadsen, M. P., Grifoni, A., Okba, N. M. A., Endeman, H., et al. (2020). Phenotype and Kinetics of SARS-CoV-2-Specific T Cells in COVID-19 Patients with Acute Respiratory Distress Syndrome. *Sci. Immunol.* 5 (48), eabd2071. doi: 10.1126/sciimmunol.abd2071

WHO (2020). *"Clinical Management of COVID-19 : interim guidance, 27 May 2020. World Health Organization. Document number: WHO/2019-nCoV/clinical/2020.5."* World Health Organization. Available from: https://apps.who.int/iris/handle/10665/332196. License: CC BY-NC-SA 3.0 IGO

Willheim, M., Ebner, C., Baier, K., Kern, W., Schrattbauer, K., Thien, R., et al. (1997). Cell Surface Characterization of T Lymphocytes and Allergen-Specific T Cell Clones: Correlation of CD26 Expression with TH1 Subsets. *J. Allergy Clin. Immunol.* 100 (3), 348–355. doi: 10.1016/S0091-6749(97)70248-3

Wolff, D., Nee, S., Hickey, N. S., and Marschollek, M. (2020). Risk Factors for Covid-19 Severity and Fatality: A Structured Literature Review. *Infection* 49 (1), 1 doi: 10.1007/s15010-020-01509-1

Wong, R. S. M., Wu, A., To, K. F., Lee, N., Lam, C. W. K., Wong, C. K., et al. (2003). Haematological Manifestations in Patients with Severe Acute Respiratory Syndrome: Retrospective Analysis. *Br. Med. J.* 326 (7403), 1358–1362. doi: 10.1136/bmj.326.7403.1358

Wong, C. K., Lam, C. W. K., Wu, A. K. L., Ip, W. K., Lee, N. L. S., Chan, I. H. S., et al. (2004). Plasma Inflammatory Cytokines and Chemokines in Severe Acute Respiratory Syndrome. *Clin. Exp. Immunol.* 136 (1), 95–103. doi: 10.1111/j.1365-2249.2004.02415.x

Wu, D., and Yang, X. O. (2020). TH17 Responses in Cytokine Storm of COVID-19: An Emerging Target of JAK2 Inhibitor Fedratinib. *J. Microbiol. Immunol. Infect.* 53 (3), 368–370. doi: 10.1016/j.jmii.2020.03.005

Xu, H., Zhong, L., Deng, J., Peng, J., Dan, H., Zeng, X., et al. (2020). High Expression of ACE2 Receptor of 2019-NCoV on the Epithelial Cells of Oral Mucosa. *Int. J. Oral. Sci.* 12 (1), 1–5. doi: 10.1038/s41368-020-0074-x

Xu, X., Han, M., Li, T., Sun, W., Wang, D., Fu, B., et al. (2020). Effective Treatment of Severe COVID-19 Patients with Tocilizumab. *Proc. Natl. Acad. Sci. United States America* 117 (20), 10970–10975. doi: 10.1073/pnas.2005615117

Yang, A. P., Liu, J. p., Tao, W. q., and ming Li, H. (2020). The Diagnostic and Predictive Role of NLR, d-NLR and PLR in COVID-19 Patients. *Int. Immunopharmacol.* 84 (July), 106504. doi: 10.1016/j.intimp.2020.106504

Yao, X. H., Li, T. Y., He, Z. C., Ping, Y. F., Liu, H. W., Yu, S. C., et al. (2020). [A Pathological Report of Three COVID-19 Cases by Minimally Invasive Autopsies]. *Zhonghua Bing Li Xue Za Zhi = Chin. J. Pathol.* 49 (0), E009. doi: 10.3760/cma.j.cn112151-20200312-00193

Yuki, K., Fujiogi, M., and Koutsogiannaki, S. (2020). COVID-19 Pathophysiology: A Review. *Clin. Immunol.* 215 (June), 108427. doi: 10.1016/j.clim.2020.108427

Zhang, Y., Li, J., Zhan, Y., Wu, L., Yu, X., Zhang, W., et al. (2004). Analysis of Serum Cytokines in Patients with Severe Acute Respiratory Syndrome. *Infect. Immun.* 72 (8), 4410–4415. doi: 10.1128/IAI.72.8.4410-4415.2004

Zheng, H. Y., Zhang, M., Yang, C. X., Zhang, N., Wang, X. C., Yang, X. P., et al (2020). Elevated Exhaustion Levels and Reduced Functional Diversity of T Cells in Peripheral Blood May Predict Severe Progression in COVID-19 Patients. *Cell. Mol. Immunol. Springer Nat.* 17 (5), 541–43. doi: 10.1038/s41423-020-0401-3

Zheng, M., Gao, Y., Wang, G., Song, G., Liu, S., Sun, D., et al. (2020). Functional Exhaustion of Antiviral Lymphocytes in COVID-19 Patients. *Cell. Mol. Immunol.* 17 (5), 533–535. doi: 10.1038/s41423-020-0402-2

Zheng, Z., Peng, F., Xu, B., Zhao, J., Liu, H., Peng, J., et al. (2020). Risk Factors of Critical & Mortal COVID-19 Cases: A Systematic Literature Review and Meta-Analysis. *J. Infect.* 81 (2), e16–e25. doi: 10.1016/j.jinf.2020.04.021

Zhou, Y., Fu, B., Zheng, X., Wang, D., Zhao, C., qi, Y., et al. Aberrant Pathogenic GM-CSF + T Cells and Inflammatory CD14 + CD16 + Monocytes 1 in Severe Pulmonary Syndrome Patients of a New Coronavirus 2 3. *BioRxiv* doi: 10.1101/2020.02.12.945576

Zhou, Y., Yang, Z., Guo, Y., Geng, S., Gao, S., Ye, S., et al. (2020). A New Predictor of Disease Severity in Patients with COVID-19 in Wuhan, China" *MedRxiv* doi: 10.1101/2020.03.24.20042119. March, 2020.03.24.20042119.

Zhu, J., Yamane, H., and Paul, W. E. (2010). Differentiation of Effector CD4 T Cell Populations" *Annu. Rev. Immunol.* 28 (1), 445–489. doi: 10.1146/annurev-immunol-030409-101212

8

Fluticasone Propionate Suppresses Poly(I:C)-Induced ACE2 in Primary Human Nasal Epithelial Cells

Akira Nakazono[1], Yuji Nakamaru[1], Mahnaz Ramezanpour[2], Takeshi Kondo[3], Masashi Watanabe[3], Shigetsugu Hatakeyama[3], Shogo Kimura[1], Aya Honma[1], P. J. Wormald[2], Sarah Vreugde[2], Masanobu Suzuki[1] and Akihiro Homma[1]*

[1] Department of Otolaryngology-Head and Neck Surgery, Faculty of Medicine and Graduate School of Medicine, Hokkaido University, Sapporo, Japan, [2] Department of Surgery–Otorhinolaryngology Head and Neck Surgery, Central Adelaide Local Health Network and the University of Adelaide, Adelaide, SA, Australia, [3] Department of Biochemistry, Faculty of Medicine and Graduate School of Medicine, Hokkaido University, Sapporo, Japan

***Correspondence:**
Masanobu Suzuki
masanobuwork@med.hokudai.ac.jp

Background: From the first detection in 2019, SARS-CoV-2 infections have spread rapidly worldwide and have been proven to cause an urgent and important health problem. SARS-CoV-2 cell entry depends on two proteins present on the surface of host cells, angiotensin-converting enzyme 2 (ACE2) and transmembrane protease serine 2 (TMPRSS2). The nasal cavity is thought to be one of the initial sites of infection and a possible reservoir for dissemination within and between individuals. However, it is not known how the expression of these genes is regulated in the nasal mucosa.

Objective: In this study, we examined whether the expression of ACE2 and TMPRSS2 is affected by innate immune signals in the nasal mucosa. We also investigated how fluticasone propionate (FP), a corticosteroid used as an intranasal steroid spray, affects the gene expression.

Methods: Primary human nasal epithelial cells (HNECs) were collected from the nasal mucosa and incubated with Toll-like receptor (TLR) agonists and/or fluticasone propionate (FP), followed by quantitative PCR, immunofluorescence, and immunoblot analyses.

Results: Among the TLR agonists, the TLR3 agonist Poly(I:C) significantly increased ACE2 and TMPRSS2 mRNA expression in HNECs (ACE2 36.212±11.600-fold change, $p<0.0001$; TMPRSS2 5.598±2.434-fold change, $p=0.031$). The ACE2 protein level was also increased with Poly(I:C) stimulation (2.884±0.505-fold change, $p=0.003$). The Poly(I:C)-induced ACE2 expression was suppressed by co-incubation with FP (0.405±0.312-fold change, $p=0.044$).

Conclusion: The activation of innate immune signals *via* TLR3 promotes the expression of genes related to SARS-CoV2 cell entry in the nasal mucosa, although this expression is suppressed in the presence of FP. Further studies are required to evaluate whether FP suppresses SARS-CoV-2 viral cell entry.

Keywords: SARS-CoV-2, TMPRSS2, virus infection, toll-like receptors, intranasal steroid spray, NFκB, interferon, COVID-19

INTRODUCTION

Corona virus disease 2019 (COVID-19) has rapidly spread to become the most urgent health issue around the world. Severe acute respiratory syndrome coronavirus 2 (SARS-CoV-2) has been identified as the responsible virus for COVID-19. SARS-CoV-2 can infect multiple organs, including the intestines, esophagus, liver, heart, kidneys, bladder, testes, brain, lung and nasal cavity (Chen et al., 2020; Huang et al., 2020; Zhang et al., 2020; Zou et al., 2020).

Among these organs, the nasal cavity is assumed to be one of the organs most susceptible to SARS-CoV-2 infection (Hou et al., 2020). It has been reported that more than half of COVID-19 patients had nasal symptoms including olfactory dysfunction and nasal obstruction (Paderno et al., 2020; Sakalli et al., 2020). A high SARS-CoV-2 viral load was indeed detected in nasal swabs from COVID-19 patients (Zou et al., 2020). The nasal cavity is also considered to be the initial site of the infection and is thought to act as a possible reservoir for dissemination within and between individuals (Hou et al., 2020; Sungnak et al., 2020). Therefore, it is important to elucidate the mechanism of SARS-CoV-2 infection in the nasal mucosa, not only to evaluate how it affects local inflammation in the nasal cavity but also to understand whether topical therapies might affect infection efficiency and potentially reduce the development of systemic infection and transmission to other individuals.

For its entry into host cells, SARS-CoV-2 depends on angiotensin-converting enzyme 2 (ACE2) and transmembrane protease serine 2 (TMPRSS2) expressed on the surface of the cells (Li et al., 2003; Hoffmann et al., 2020). SARS-CoV-2 attaches to the cell membrane using spike (S) proteins to bind to ACE2 on the host cells. The viral cell entry also requires S protein-priming by TMPRSS2 (Hoffmann et al., 2020). Therefore, the expression of ACE2 and TMPRSS2 is assumed to be associated with host susceptibility to and severity of COVID-19 (Bunyavanich et al., 2020; Devaux et al., 2020; Saheb Sharif-Askari et al., 2020; Sharif-Askari et al., 2020; Wu et al., 2020). Notably, differences in ACE2 and TMPRSS2 expression levels in the lower airway might contribute to COVID-19 severity (Matsumoto and Saito, 2020; Saheb Sharif-Askari et al., 2020). In the nasal epithelium, ACE2 and TMPRSS2 have been shown to be expressed at high levels (Sungnak et al., 2020; Ziegler et al., 2020), and their expression has been related to the susceptibility of the nasal cavity mucosa to SARS-CoV2 infection (Bunyavanich et al., 2020; Sharif-Askari et al., 2020). These proteins have also been targeted as a possible therapeutic strategy for COVID-19 (Hoffmann et al., 2020; Patel and Verma, 2020; Wu et al., 2020).

Recent research has shown that ACE2 expression is induced by interferons (IFNs), suggesting that ACE2 expression could be regulated by the activation of innate immune signals such as Toll-like receptor (TLR) signals (Ziegler et al., 2020). Also, corticosteroids, which are a regulator of innate immunity (Kato et al., 2007; Zhang et al., 2007), might affect ACE2 expression. However, it is not known whether the activation or suppression of innate immune signaling affects ACE2 expression in the nasal mucosa.

In this study, we examined whether TLR agonist activation alters ACE2 and TMPRSS2 expression levels in primary human nasal epithelial cells (HNECs). We also investigated whether fluticasone propionate (FP), a corticosteroid widely used as intranasal steroid spray, affects the expression of SARS-CoV-2 cell entry-related genes.

MATERIALS AND METHODS

Primary Human Nasal Epithelial Cell Cultures

This study was approved by the Institutional Review Board for Clinical Research of Hokkaido University Hospital, Sapporo, Japan (019–0242) and by The Queen Elizabeth Hospital Human Research Ethics Committee (reference HREC/15/TQEH/132), and was conducted in accordance with the Declaration of Helsinki. Written informed consent was obtained from study participants prior to tissue or cell collection. Primary human nasal epithelial cells (HNECs) were taken from the nasal mucosa of the inferior turbinates of seven patients treated for deviation of the nasal septum as previously described (Cooksley et al., 2015; Suzuki et al., 2018; Ramezanpour et al., 2019). The cells were suspended in Bronchial Epithelial Growth Medium (BEGM, CC-3170, Lonza, Walkersville, MD, USA) supplemented with Amphotericin B (Fujifilm, Osaka, Japan) and Penicillin/Streptomycin (Fujifilm, Osaka, Japan). Monocytes were depleted from the cell suspension using anti-CD68 antibody (Dako, Glostrup, Denmark) -coated cell culture dishes. HNECs were incubated at 37°C in humidified conditions under 5% CO_2 in collagen-coated flasks (Thermo Scientific, Waltham, MA, USA) until passage 2.

TLR Stimulation and Agents

HNECs were seeded onto 6-well dishes coated with collagen type I (Kurabo, Osaka, Japan) at 0.6×10^6 cells/well for 24 hours prior to subsequent analysis. The cells were washed with phosphate-buffered saline (PBS), followed by the addition of TLR agonists (Invivogen, San Diego, CA, USA) for 24 hours, unless otherwise described. The following dosages were used: TLR1/2 (Pam3CSK4) 1 μg/ml, TLR2 (HKLM) 10^8 cells/ml, TLR3 (Poly(I:C)) 10 μg/ml, TLR4 (LPS) 10 μg/ml, TLR5 (Flagellin) 10 μg/ml, TLR6/2 (FSL-1) 1 μg/ml, TLR7 (Imiquimod) 10 μg/ml, TLR8 (ssRNA40) 10 μg/ml, and TLR9 (ODN2006) 5 μM. In some experiments, fluticasone propionate (FP; Cayman Chemical Company, Ann Arbor, MI, USA) and JSH-23 (NFκB transcriptional activity inhibitor; Abcam, Cambridge, MA, USA), was added to the cells, 1 hour prior to TLR stimulation. The following dosages were used: FP 10 nM and JSH-23 30 μM, unless otherwise described. FP and JSH-23 were dissolved in dimethyl sulfoxide (DMSO). In experiments where FP or JSH-23 was used, corresponding DMSO control solutions were also used in parallel as controls.

RNA Extraction, Reverse Transcription, and qPCR

HNECs were incubated in 6-well dishes in BEGM media. After incubation with the TLR agonists, FP and/or JSH-23, HNECs were collected and washed with PBS, followed by RNA extraction using ISOGEN in accordance with the manufacturer's instructions

(Nippon Gene, Tokyo, Japan). Extracted RNA was quantified using a Nanodrop 1000 spectrophotometer (Thermo Fisher Scientific, Waltham, MA, USA). RNA was reverse transcribed into cDNA using a ReverTra Ace qPCR RT Kit (TOYOBO, Osaka, Japan) with a LifeECO Thermal Cycler (Hangzhou Bioer Technology, Hangzhou, China). The resulting cDNA was subjected to qPCR using a StepOne Realtime PCR System (Applied Biosytems, Foster City, CA, USA) with Power SYBR Green PCR Master Mix (Thermo Fisher Scientific, Waltham, MA, USA) and nuclease-free water (Thermo Fisher Scientific, Waltham, MA, USA). The average threshold cycle (Ct) was determined from three or more independent experiments and the level of gene expression relative to glyceraldehyde 3-phosphate dehydrogenase (GAPDH) was determined using the comparative CT method. The following primers were used for the qPCR: GAPDH forward (Fw) 5'-TGCACCACCAACTGCTTAGC-3', GAPDH reverse (Rev) 5'-GGCATGGACTGTGGTCATGAG-3', ACE2 (Fw) 5'-CTCTACAGAAGCTGGACAGAAAC-3', ACE2 (Rev) 5'-GAG CAGTGGCCTTACATTCA-3', TMPRSS2 (Fw) 5'-GGAG TGTACGGGAATGTGATG-3', TMPRSS2 (Rev) 5'-GGAC GAAGACCATGTGGATTAG-3', TNF-α (Fw) 5'-GAGGC CAAGCCCTGGTATG-3', TNF-α (Rev) 5'-CGGGCCGATTG ATCTCAGC-3', IL-6 (Fw) 5'-ATGTAGCCGCCCCACACAGA-3', IL-6 (Rev) 5'-ATTTGCCGAAGAGCCCTCAG-3', IFN-β (Fw) 5'-AGGACAGGATGAACTTTGAC-3', IFN-β (Rev) 5'-TGATAGACATTAGCCAGGAG-3', CXCL10 (Fw) 5'-GCTCTACTGAGGTGCTATGTTC-3', CXCL10 (Rev) 5'-GGA GGATGGCAGTGGAAGTC-3', IFN-γ (Fw) 5'-TCGGTAAC TGACTTGAATGTCCA-3', and IFN-γ (Rev) 5'-TCGCTTCC CTGTTTTAGCTGC-3'.

Immunoblotting

HNECs were incubated with 10 μg/ml of Poly(I:C), 10 nM of FP for 28 hours. The cells were lysed in glycoprotein denaturing buffer containing sodium dodecyl sulfate (0.5% (w/v)) and 40 mM dithiothreitol. The cell lysates were then boiled and sonicated in glycoprotein denaturing buffer. PNGase F (New England Biolabs, Ipswich, MA, USA) was used to remove oligosaccharides from the glycoproteins following the manufacturer's protocol. After removing oligosaccharides, SDS sample buffer containing 50 mM Tris-HCl (pH 6.8), 2-mercaptoethanol (6% (v/v)), sodium dodecyl sulfate (2% (w/v)), glycerol (10% (v/v)) and bromophenol blue (0.01% (w/v)) was added to the supernatant. Immunoblot analysis was performed with the antibodies indicated below. Immune complexes were detected with horseradish peroxidase-conjugated antibodies to rabbit (1:10000 dilution, Promega, Madison, WI, USA) and an enhanced chemiluminescence system (Thermo Fisher Scientific, Waltham, MA, USA). The acquired bands were quantified using ImageJ 1.50i (National Institutes of Health, Bethesda, MD, USA) and expressed as the ratio relative to GAPDH. The antibodies used in immunoblotting were as follows: rabbit monoclonal anti-ACE2 (1:1000; SN0754, Thermo Fisher Scientific, Waltham, MA, USA), rabbit monoclonal anti-TMPRSS2 (1:1000; ab92323, Abcam, Cambridge, United Kingdom), and monoclonal anti-GAPDH HRP-DirecT (1:5000; M171-7, MBL, Nagoya, Japan).

Immunofluorescence

HNECs were incubated for 48 hours with or without 10 μg/ml Poly(I:C) and 10 nM fluticasone propionate (FP). HNECs were fixed with 2.5% formalin in PBS for 10 minutes at room temperature (RT) followed by washing twice with PBS. Fixed samples were blocked for 1 hour with Protein Block (SFB; Dako, Glostrup, Denmark). Rabbit anti-ACE2 polyclonal antibody (1:100, Invitrogen, Carlsbad, CA, USA) and rabbit anti-TMPRSS2 antibody (1:100, Abcam, Cambridge, MA, USA) were added overnight at 4°C. Excess primary antibody was removed, and 2 μg/ml anti-mouse Alexa-Fluor 488 conjugated secondary antibody (Jackson ImmunoResearch Labs Inc., West Grove, PA, USA) was added and incubated for 1 hour at RT. The samples were rinsed in TBST, and after the third wash, 200 ng/ml of 4', 6-diamidino-2-phenylindole (DAPI; Sigma, Aldrich, USA) was added to resolve nuclei. Samples were visualized using a LSM700 confocal laser scanning microscope (Zeiss Microscopy, Oberkochen, Germany). Processing was performed using ZEN Imaging Software (Carl Zeiss AG, Oberkochen, Germany). The threshold of each image was adjusted for each channel to remove background fluorescence and evaluation was performed in a blinded fashion. ACE2 and TMPRSS2 fluorescence intensities were quantified and normalized to the DAPI intensity. Results are expressed as the relative value of mean arbitrary fluorescence units as provided by the ZEN imaging software.

Statistical Analysis

All data was expressed as mean ± standard deviation (SD). Shapiro-Wilk test and Kolmogrov test were applied to examine whether the data fitted normal and lognormal distributions, respectively. In cases where the data fitted the lognormal distribution, log transformation was performed before statistical analysis. Fold changes in relative gene expression were compared by a two-tailed t-test. When 3 or more groups were compared, one-way Analysis of Variance (ANOVA) followed by Dunnetts's test was used to analyze differences among the groups. P values of <0.05 were considered statistically significant. All analyses were performed using JMP® 11 software (SAS Institute Inc., Cary, NC, USA).

RESULTS

Poly(I:C) Increases ACE2 and TMPRSS2 mRNA Expression Levels

To determine whether TLR stimulation affects ACE2 and TMPRSS2 expression in HNECs, we examined mRNA expression in HNECs after stimulation with several TLR agonists for 24 hours. ACE2 mRNA expression was significantly increased upon TLR3-stimulation with Poly(I:C) (a 36.212±11.600-fold change, $p<0.0001$, **Figure 1A**). TMPRSS2 mRNA expression was also significantly increased upon TLR3-stimulation with Poly(I:C) (a 5.598±2.434-fold change, $p=0.003$, **Figure 1B**). These findings indicate that TLR3 stimulation with Poly(I:C) increases the expression levels of ACE2 and TMPRSS2.

Poly(I:C) Upregulates Expression of NFκB Target Genes and an IFN-Stimulated Gene

We also examined the mRNA expression of TNF-α and IL-6 (NFκB target genes), as well as IFN-β, IFN-γ, and CXCL10 (an IFN-stimulated gene) in HNECs (**Supplementary Figure 1**). Poly(I:C) significantly promoted TNF-α (a 101.65±26.85-fold change, p<.0001) and IL-6 (a 215.85±34.82-fold change, p<.0001, **Supplementary Figures 1A, B**). Other than Poly(I:C), Pam3CSK4 (TLR1/2 agonist) significantly upregulated TNF-α (a 5.97±0.70-fold change, p=0.0046) and IL-6 (a 4.43±0.83-fold change, p=0.0233). FSL-1 (TLR6/2 agonist) also significantly upregulated TNF-α (a 7.68±2.56-fold change, p=0.002) and IL-6 (a 5.35±1.80-fold change, p=0.0132). Flagellin (a TLR5 agonist) and ODN2006 (a TLR9 agonist) significantly increased TNF-α (Flagellin; a 7.048±3.18-fold change, p=0.0051, ODN2006; a 5.15±1.92-fold change, p=0.0180).

As for the genes related to the IFN signaling pathway, Poly(I:C) also significantly upregulated the expression of IFN-β (a 14.19±4.37-fold change, p=0.0065) and CXCL10 (a 7496.34±1862.24-fold change, p<.0001). On the contrary, neither Pam3CSK4 nor FSL1 increased IFN-β or CXCL10 (**Supplementary Figures 1C, D**). IFN-γ was not upregulated by any TLR agonist (**Supplementary Figure 1E**). These results suggested that TLR3 stimulation with Poly(I:C) activates both the NFκB and IFN signaling pathways in HNECs.

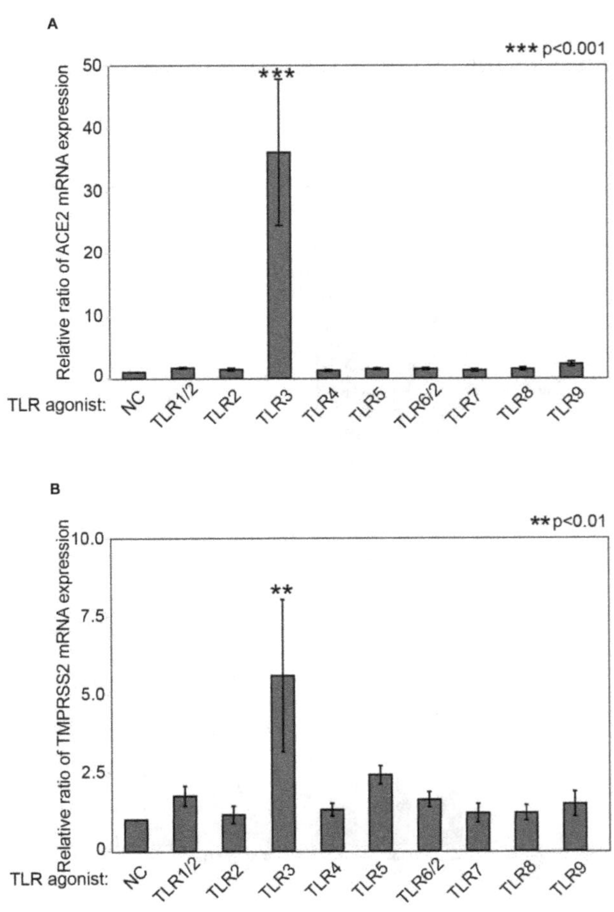

FIGURE 1 | Poly(I:C) increases ACE2 mRNA as well as TMPRSS2 expression. Relative mRNA expression of ACE2 **(A)** and TMPRSS2 **(B)** after stimulation with TLR agonists for 24 hours. The following TLR agonists were used: Pam3CSK4 for TLR1/2, HKLM for TLR2, Poly(I:C) for TLR3, LPS for TLR4, Flagellin for TLR5, FSL-1 for TLR6/2, Imiquimod for TLR7, ssRNA40 for TLR8, and ODN2006 for TLR9. Relative mRNA expression was determined by normalization against untreated control cells and GAPDH. Data are means ± standard deviation (s.d.) of values from three independent experiments. **p < 0.01 ***p < 0.001.

Poly(I:C) Induces ACE2 and TMPRSS2 mRNA Expression in a Time-Dependent Manner

We determined the time course of ACE2 mRNA expression after Poly(I:C) stimulation. A significant increase in ACE2 mRNA expression was found at 4, 8, 12, 16, 20 and 24 hours after stimulation with Poly(I:C) (**Figure 2A**). Similarly, a significant increase in TMPRSS2 mRNA expression was found at 4, 8, 12, 16, and 20 hours after stimulation with Poly(I:C) (**Figure 2B**).

We also examined ACE2 and TMPRSS2 mRNA expression in HNECs incubated with different concentrations of Poly(I:C). A significant increase in ACE2 mRNA expression was found after stimulation with 0.1, 1 and 10 μg/ml Poly(I:C) in a dose-dependency manner (**Supplementary Figure 2A**). On the other hand, a significant increase in TMPRSS2 mRNA expression was only observed after stimulation with 10 μg/ml Poly(I:C) (**Supplementary Figure 2B**).

The Poly(I:C)-Induced Increase in ACE2 mRNA Expression Is Significantly Suppressed by FP

We investigated how FP affects ACE2 and TMPRSS2 expression in HNECs. A tendency for ACE2 expression to be suppressed by FP was seen at the indicated time points, and significant suppression of Poly(I:C)-induced ACE2 expression was observed at 16, 20, and 24 hours (**Figure 2A**). To the contrary, no suppression of TMPRSS2 mRNA expression by FP was observed at the indicated time points (**Figure 2B**).

We also examined the inhibitive effect on the Poly(I:C)-induced increases in ACE2 and TMPRSS2 mRNA expression of different concentrations of FP. Significant suppression of the Poly(I:C)-induced increases in ACE2 expression was observed for 1 and 10 nM FP (**Supplementary Figure 3A**). To the contrary, no suppression of TMPRSS2 mRNA expression was observed for any concentration of FP (**Supplementary Figure 3B**).

We also examined how FP affects the mRNA expression of genes related to the NFκB and IFN signaling pathways in HNECs. FP significantly suppressed the Poly(I:C)-induced increases in TNF-α and IL-6 expression as well as that of ACE2, while FP did not alter the Poly(I:C)-induced increases in IFN-β or CXCL10 expression (**Supplementary Figure 4**). Further, JSH-23, a NFκB transcriptional activity inhibitor, significantly suppressed the Poly(I:C)-induced increases in ACE2 (**Supplementary Figure 5A**) as well as those of the other NFκB target genes, TNF-α and IL-6, in HNECs (**Supplementary Figures 5B, C**), while JSH-23 did not alter the

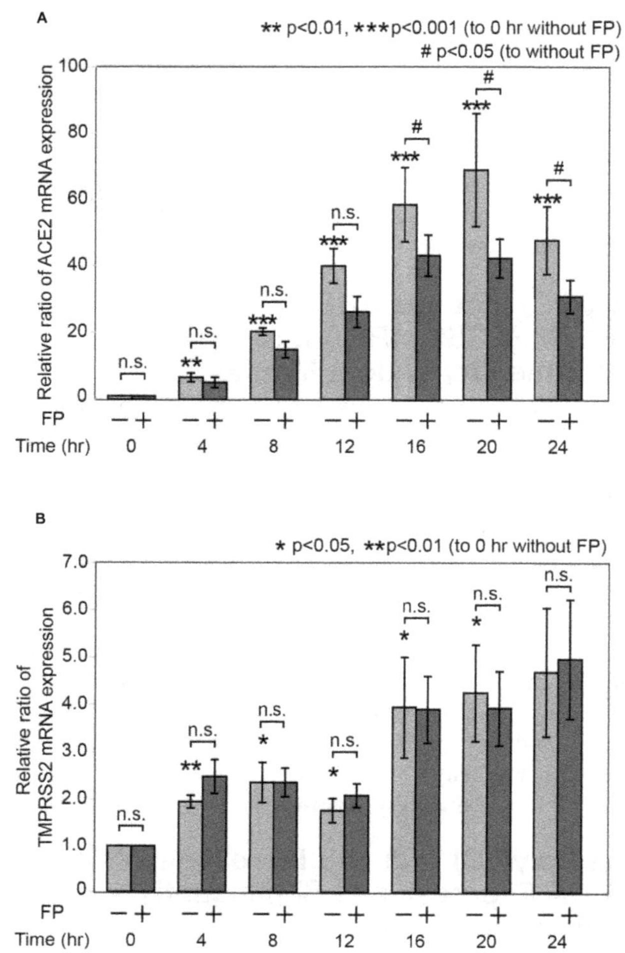

FIGURE 2 | Time course of ACE2 and TMPRSS2 mRNA expression after Poly (I:C) stimulation with and without fluticasone propionate. HNECs were incubated for the indicated times with or without 10 µg/ml Poly(I:C) and 10 nM fluticasone propionate (FP), followed by qPCR using primer sets for ACE2 **(A)** and TMPRSS2 **(B)**. Data are means ± standard deviation (s.d.) of values from five independent experiments. P values for the indicated comparisons were determined by t-test with (ACE2) and without log transformation (TMPRSS2). *p < 0.05, **p < 0.01, ***p < 0.001 (for comparison between untreated cells and cells treated with Poly(I:C)), and #p < 0.05 (for comparison between cells treated with and without FP at the indicated times, respectively).

Poly(I:C)-induced increases in the expression of TMPRSS2 or the IFN-stimulated genes, IFN-β or CXCL10 (**Supplementary Figures 5D–F**). These results suggested that the Poly(I:C)-induced increases in ACE2 mRNA expression is induced *via* the NFκB signaling pathway, but not the IFN signaling pathway.

Poly(I:C) and FP Significantly Affect ACE2, but Not TMPRSS2, Expression at the Protein Level

Last, we examined whether Poly(I:C) and FP alter ACE2 and TMPRSS2 protein expression. Immunoblot analysis showed that Poly(I:C) significantly increased ACE2 protein expression (a 1.377±0.069-fold change *vs.* untreated cells, p=0.002). The Poly(I:C)-induced increase in ACE2 protein expression was significantly suppressed by FP (a 0.770±0.017-fold change *vs.* Poly(I:C)-treated cells, p<0.001, **Figures 3A, B**). On the other hand, there was no significant induction of TMPRSS2 protein expression by Poly(I:C) (a 1.083±0.0394-fold change *vs.* untreated cells, p=0.213) or subsequent suppression by FP (a 0.946±0.0340-fold change *vs.* Poly(I:C)-treated cells, p=0.208, **Figures 3A, C**).

We further examined ACE2 and TMPRSS2 protein expression using immunofluorescent analysis (**Figure 4**). The ACE2 intensity in HNECs was significantly promoted by Poly(I:C) (a 2.884±0.505-fold change *vs.* untreated cells, p=0.003). This Poly(I:C)-induced change was significantly suppressed by FP (a 0.405±0.312-fold change *vs.* Poly(I:C)-treated cells, p=0.044, **Figures 4A, B**). The TMPRSS2 intensity was also altered by Poly (I:C) and FP, but the changes were not statistically significant (a 2.423±2.937-fold change *vs.* untreated cells p=0.449 and a 0.795±0.472-fold change *vs.* Poly(I:C)-treated cells, p=0.611, **Figures 4C, D**).

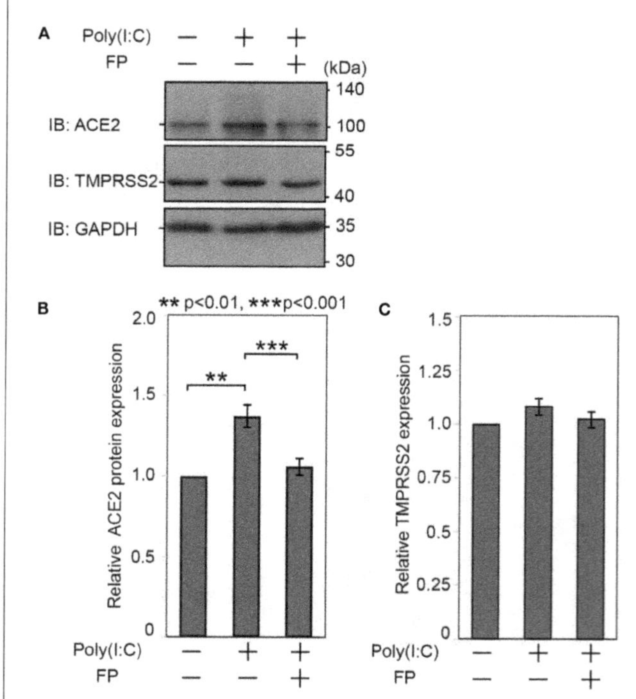

FIGURE 3 | Immunoblotting for ACE2 and TMPRSS2 proteins in HNECs treated with Poly(I:C) and/or fluticasone propionate. HNECs were incubated for 28 hours with or without 10 µg/ml Poly(I:C) and 10 nM fluticasone propionate (FP). After removing oligosaccharides by PNGase F, the cell lysates were subjected to immunoblotting for ACE2 **(A, B)**, TMPRSS2 **(A, C)** and GAPDH. The obtained bands were quantified and calculated as relative ratios to GAPDH, using ImageJ 1.50i (National Institutes of Health, Bethesda, MD, USA). Data are means ± standard deviation (s.d.) of values from four independent experiments. P values for indicated comparisons were determined by t-test. **p < 0.01, ***p < 0.001.

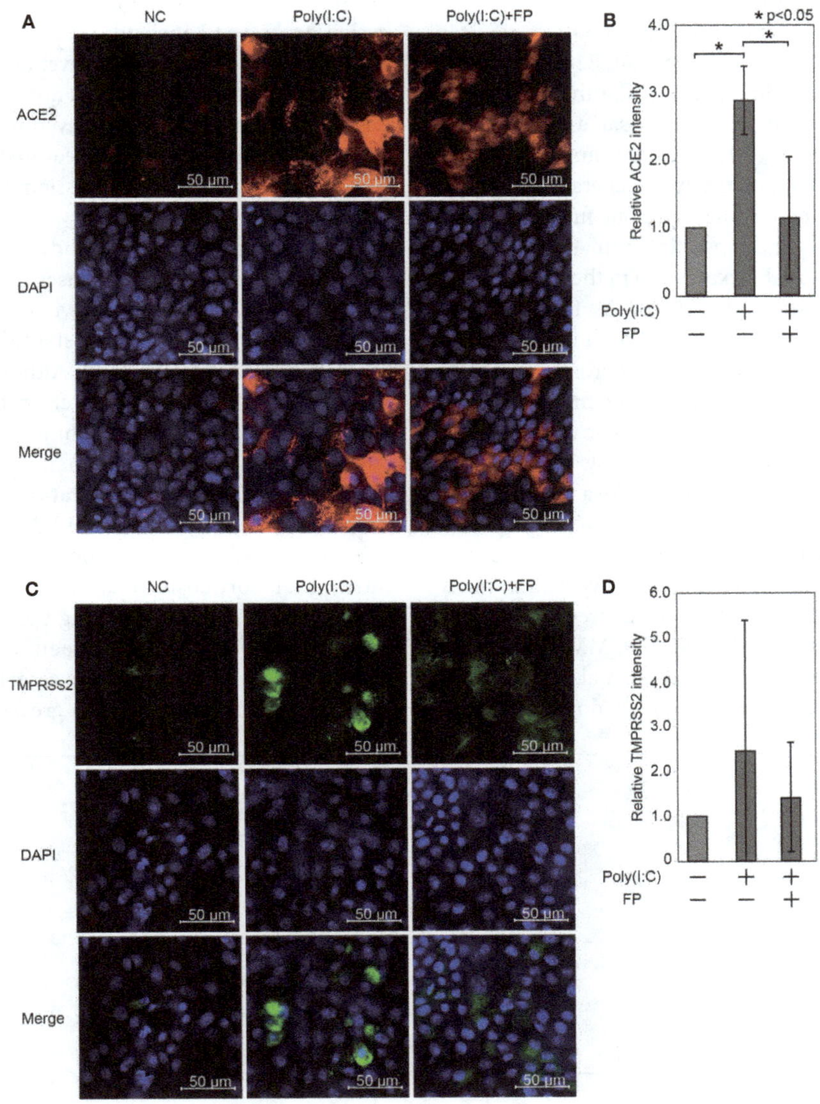

FIGURE 4 | Immunofluorescent analysis for ACE2 and TMPRSS2 in HNECs treated with Poly(I:C) with and without fluticasone propionate. HNECs were incubated for 48 hours with or without 10 μg/ml Poly(I:C) and 10 nM fluticasone propionate (FP), followed by immunofluorescent analysis for ACE2 **(A, B)** and TMPRSS2 **(C, D)**. The average fluorescence intensity was standardized compared to the DAPI intensity and represented as the relative value to those of untreated cells. Data are means ± standard deviation (s.d.) of values from three independent experiments. P values for indicated comparisons were determined by t-test. *$p < 0.05$. The white bar is 50 μm and 20× magnification.

DISCUSSION

In this study, we demonstrated that innate immune signaling activation, in particular TLR3 activation, significantly promotes ACE2 expression in nasal epithelial cells. FP, a routinely used intranasal corticosteroid, suppressed the Poly(I:C)-induced increase in ACE2 expression but did not affect TMPRSS2 expression.

Understanding the regulation of SARS-CoV2 cell entry-related gene expression is important as it can directly lead to the study and development of preventive and therapeutic strategies against COVID-19 (Wu et al., 2020). To date, the focus has been mainly on ACE2 expression in the lower airway, rather than in the upper airway. In the lower airway, Poly(I:C), IFN-α, β, and γ, TNF-α, IL-6, and IL-1α and β were reported to activate the promoter of ACE2 (Zhuang et al., 2020; Ziegler et al., 2020). Also, viral infection and smoking promote ACE2 expression (Kimura et al., 2020; Sharif-Askari et al., 2020; Zhuang et al., 2020). Conversely, type 2 inflammatory cytokines have been shown to suppress ACE2 expression

(Jackson et al., 2020; Kimura et al., 2020). Notably, this is thought to potentially contribute to a decreased risk of COVID-19 in patients with asthma (Matsumoto and Saito, 2020).

On the other hand, little is known about ACE2 expression in the upper airway. Significant differences in the innate immune response have been reported between nasal and bronchial epithelial cells (Cooksley et al., 2015). Hence, findings specific to the lower airway cannot automatically be generalized to apply to the upper airway immune response without further detailed studies. To date, only IFN-γ and type 2 inflammatory cytokines have been reported to affect ACE2 expression in the upper airway (Kimura et al., 2020; Ziegler et al., 2020). As for TMPRSS2 expression, current knowledge is limited for both the upper and lower airway, with only the androgen receptor reported to upregulate TMPRSS2 expression, although this finding has not been confirmed in the airway (Lin et al., 1999; Lucas et al., 2014). Whether TMPRSS2 expression is regulated by the activated innate immune signals in the nasal mucosa has not yet been elucidated.

In this study, we found that ACE2 expression in HNECs was significantly increased by stimulation with Poly(I:C), as many other genes in HNECs were found to do in previous reports, including IL-6 (Cooksley et al., 2015), MMP9, MMP1, MMP10, TIMP-1 (Suzuki et al., 2018), TSLP (Golebski et al., 2016), TNF-α and IL-8 (Ohkuni et al., 2011). Poly(I:C) is a double-stranded RNA (dsRNA) often used as a model for viral infection, as most viruses induce the synthesis of dsRNA during their replication cycle (Jacobs and Langland, 1996). This finding might afford an important insight into the prevention and treatment of acute rhinosinusitis by viral infection, not only in terms of relieving its nasal symptoms but also in preventing secondary SARS-CoV-2 infection. Further research is required to evaluate the potential role of increased ACE2 expression in enhancing SARS-CoV-2 infection.

Another highlight of this study was the suppressive effect of FP on Poly(I:C)-induced increases in ACE2 expression in nasal epithelial cells. From a clinical view point, controversy remains surrounding the use of corticosteroids for COVID-19 (Russell et al., 2020; Shang et al., 2020). Although clinical evidence does not support systemic corticosteroid treatment for COVID-19 (Russell et al., 2020), ciclesonide, a widely-used inhalant corticosteroid, could be beneficial against COVID-19 in preventing SARS-CoV-2 replication (Matsuyama et al., 2020). As for intra-nasal corticosteroids, The European Academy of Allergy and Clinical Immunology (EAACI) has stated that intra-nasal corticosteroids can be continued for cases of allergic rhinitis and that halting their use is not advised as no immunosuppression has been shown after intranasal corticosteroid use and the increase in sneezing after halting their application may lead to a greater spread of SARS-CoV-2

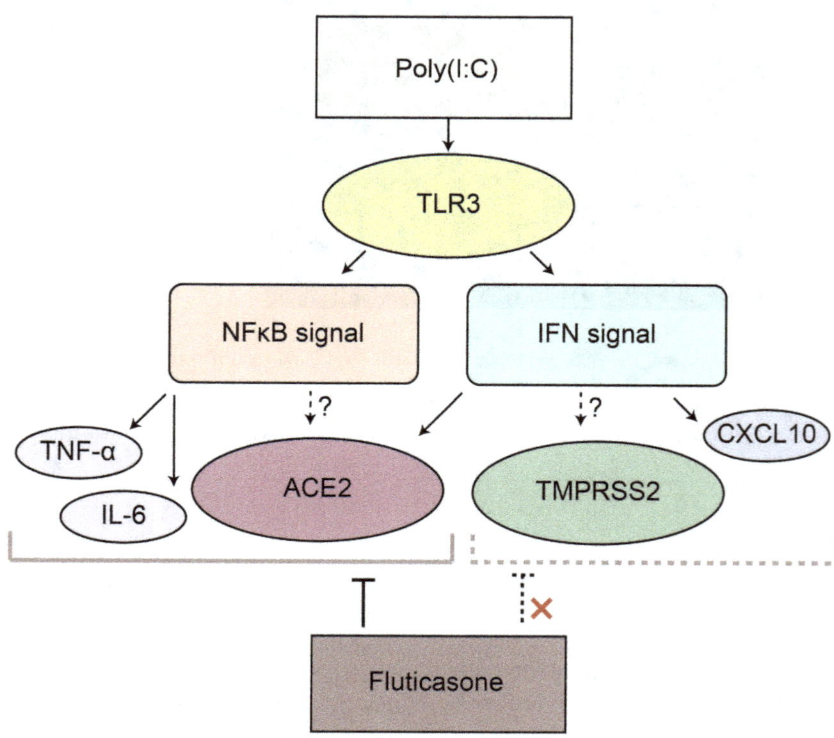

FIGURE 5 | Poly(I:C) significantly increased ACE2 and TMPRSS2 possibly via the IFN and NFκB signaling pathways in HNECs. Poly(I:C) activates both the IFN and NFκB signaling pathways by binding to TLR3, resulting in the induction of ACE2 and TMPRSS2. IFN-β upregulates ACE2 expression; however, ACE2 as well as the target genes of the NFκB signaling pathway such as TNF-α and IL-6 is suppressed by fluticasone propionate, while TMPRSS2 and an interferon-stimulated gene are not. This suggested that ACE2 in HNECs is regulated not only *via* the IFN signaling pathway but also *via* the NFκB signaling pathway.

(Bousquet et al., 2020). However, intranasal corticosteroids might impair anti-viral immune responses and increase viral titers, as they do for rhinovirus (Singanayagam et al., 2015). Further studies are needed to clarify the clinical significance of intranasal steroid spray for COVID-19.

Interestingly, we found different responses to FP in the NFκB and IFN signaling pathways. While FP suppressed the NFκB target genes, FP did not suppress IFN-β itself or IFN-stimulated genes in HNECs. Glucocorticoids including FP induced gene transcription and protein synthesis of the NFκB inhibitor, IκB. Activated glucocorticoid cytosolic receptors also antagonized NFκB activity through protein–protein interaction involving direct complexing with, and inhibition of, NFκB binding to DNA (Almawi and Melemedjian, 2002). On the other hand, it is reported that the response to the IFN signaling pathway by glucocorticoids varies depending on cell type (Flammer et al., 2010). In HNECs, the Poly(I:C)-induced increase in ACE2 was also suppressed by FP, suggesting that ACE2 is significantly regulated *via* the NFκB signaling pathway, as well (Hou et al., 2020). To the contrary, the Poly(I:C)-induced increase in TMPRSS2 was not suppressed by FP, implying that the NFκB signaling pathway plays a limited role in the regulation of TMPRSS2 expression (**Figure 5**). Furthermore, we found that a NFκB inhibitor significantly suppressed the Poly(I:C)-induced increase in ACE2 expression, suggesting this increase is regulated *via* the NFκB signaling pathway in nasal epithelial cells.

As a limitation, although we demonstrated that activated innate immune signals promoted the expression of SARS-CoV2 cell entry-related genes on which SARS-CoV-2 cell entry is dependent the association between the upregulated expression of the genes and host susceptibility to SARS-CoV-2 remains to be investigated. Also, it is unknown whether the suppression of ACE2 expression by FP can indeed prevent SARS-CoV-2 infection. Although further biological and epidemiological studies are necessary, it can be concluded that the regulation of inflammation in the nasal cavity is increasingly important and should be of greater focus in the COVID-19 era than ever before.

CONCLUSION

The activation of innate immune signals *via* TLR3 promotes the expression of SARS-CoV2 cell entry-related genes in the nasal mucosa, which is suppressed in the presence of the intranasal corticosteroid FP. Further studies are required to evaluate whether FP suppresses SARS-CoV-2 viral cell entry.

AUTHOR CONTRIBUTIONS

AN, YN, and MS designed the experiments. SH, PW, SV, and AkH supervised the project. AN, MR, MW, and TK performed most of the experiments. AN, SK, AyH, and MS compiled the data. AN, SV, SH and MS wrote the manuscript. All authors contributed to the article and approved the submitted version.

ACKNOWLEDGMENTS

We are grateful to Ayaka Kubota, Yuka Masuta, Shizuka Sugawara, Yumiko Kimura, Yumi Matsuzaki, and Shiho Sakata for their help in culturing the HNECs and preparing the manuscript.

SUPPLEMENTARY MATERIAL

Supplementary Figure 1 | Poly(I:C) significantly increases the expression of NFκB target genes and genes related to the IFN signaling pathway in HNECs. Relative mRNA expression of TNF-α **(A)**, IL-6 **(B)**, IFN-β **(C)**, CXCL10 **(D)**, and IFN-γ (E) after stimulation with TLR agonists for 24 hours. The following TLR agonists were used: Pam3CSK4 for TLR1/2, HKLM for TLR2, Poly(I:C) for TLR3, LPS for TLR4, Flagellin for TLR5, FSL-1 for TLR6/2, Imiquimod for TLR7, ssRNA40 for TLR8, and ODN2006 for TLR9. Relative mRNA expression was determined by normalization against untreated control cells and GAPDH. Data are means ± standard deviation (s.d.) of values from five independent experiments. *p<0.05 **p<0.01 ***p<0.001.

Supplementary Figure 2 | ACE2 and TMPRSS2 mRNA expression in HNECs incubated with different concentrations of Poly(I:C). Relative mRNA expression of ACE2 **(A)** and TMPRSS2 **(B)** after stimulation with 0.1, 1 and 10 µg/ml Poly(I:C) for 20 hours. Relative mRNA expression was determined by normalization against untreated control cells and GAPDH. Data are means ± standard deviation (s.d.) of values from five independent experiments. *p<0.05 ***p<0.001.

Supplementary Figure 3 | ACE2 and TMPRSS2 mRNA expression in HNECs incubated with different concentrations of fluticasone propionate. HNECs were incubated for 20 hours with 10 µg/ml Poly(I:C) and/or 0.1, 1 and 10 nM fluticasone propionate (FP), followed by qPCR using primer sets for ACE2 **(A)** and TMPRSS2 **(B)**. Relative mRNA expression was determined by normalization against untreated control cells and GAPDH. Data are means ± standard deviation (s.d.) of values from four independent experiments. *p<0.05.

Supplementary Figure 4 | Fluticasone propionate significantly suppressed the Poly(I:C)-induced increase in the expression of NFκB target genes but not genes related to the IFN signaling pathway. HNECs were incubated for 8 hours with 10 µg/ml Poly(I:C) and/or 10 nM fluticasone propionate (FP), followed by qPCR using primer sets for TNF-α **(A)**, IL-6 **(B)**, IFN-β **(C)** and CXCL10 **(D)**. Data are means ± standard deviation (s.d.) of values from three or four independent experiments. P values for indicated comparisons were determined by t-test with log transformation. *p<0.05, **p<0.01, ***p<0.001.

Supplementary Figure 5 | A NFκB inhibitor significantly suppressed ACE2 expression in HNECs. Relative mRNA expression of ACE2 **(A)**, TNF-α **(B)**, IL-6 **(C)**, TMPRSS2 **(D)**, IFN-β **(E)** and CXCL10 **(F)** in HNECs incubated with 10 µg/ml Poly(I:C) and 30 µM JSH-23 (NFκB transcriptional activity inhibitor) for 20 hours (for ACE2 and TMPRSS2) and for 8 hours (for TNF-α, IL-6, IFN-β, and CXCL10), respectively. Relative mRNA expression was determined by normalization against untreated control cells and GAPDH. Data are means ± standard deviation (s.d.) of values from four independent experiments. *p<0.05 **p<0.01 ***p<0.001.

REFERENCES

Almawi, W. Y., and Melemedjian, O. K. (2002). Negative Regulation of Nuclear Factor-Kappab Activation and Function by Glucocorticoids. *J. Mol. Endocrinol.* 28 (2), 69–78. doi: 10.1677/jme.0.0280069

Bousquet, J., Akdis, C., Jutel, M., Bachert, C., Klimek, L., Agache, I., et al. (2020). Intranasal Corticosteroids in Allergic Rhinitis in COVID-19 Infected Patients:

An ARIA-EAACI Statement. *Allergy* 75 (10), 2440–2444. doi: 10.1111/all.14302

Bunyavanich, S., Do, A., and Vicencio, A. (2020). Nasal Gene Expression of Angiotensin-Converting Enzyme 2 in Children and Adults. *JAMA* 323 (23), 2427–2429. doi: 10.1001/jama.2020.8707

Chen, N., Zhou, M., Dong, X., Qu, J., Gong, F., Han, Y., et al. (2020). Epidemiological and Clinical Characteristics of 99 Cases of 2019 Novel Coronavirus Pneumonia in Wuhan, China: A Descriptive Study. *Lancet* 395 (10223), 507–513. doi: 10.1016/S0140-6736(20)30211-7

Cooksley, C., Roscioli, E., Wormald, P. J., and Vreugde, S. (2015). TLR Response Pathways in Nuli-1 Cells and Primary Human Nasal Epithelial Cells. *Mol. Immunol.* 68 (2 Pt B), 476–483. doi: 10.1016/j.molimm.2015.09.024

Devaux, C. A., Rolain, J.-M., and Raoult, D. (2020). ACE2 Receptor Polymorphism: Susceptibility to SARS-Cov-2, Hypertension, Multi-Organ Failure, and COVID-19 Disease Outcome. *J. Microbiol. Immunol. Infect.* 53 (3), 425–435. doi: 10.1016/j.jmii.2020.04.015

Flammer, J. R., Dobrovolna, J., Kennedy, M. A., Chinenov, Y., Glass, C. K., Ivashkiv, L. B., et al. (2010). The Type I Interferon Signaling Pathway is a Target for Glucocorticoid Inhibition. *Mol. Cell. Biol.* 30 (19), 4564–4574. doi: 10.1128/MCB.00146-10

Golebski, K., van Tongeren, J., van Egmond, D., de Groot, E. J., Fokkens, W. J., and van Drunen, C. M. (2016). Specific Induction of TSLP by the Viral RNA Analogue Poly(I:C) in Primary Epithelial Cells Derived From Nasal Polyps. *PloS One* 11 (4), e0152808. doi: 10.1371/journal.pone.0152808

Hoffmann, M., Kleine-Weber, H., Schroeder, S., Krüger, N., Herrler, T., Erichsen, S., et al. (2020). SARS-Cov-2 Cell Entry Depends on ACE2 and TMPRSS2 and is Blocked by a Clinically Proven Protease Inhibitor. *Cell* 181 (2), 271–280.e8. doi: 10.1016/j.cell.2020.02.052

Hou, Y. J., Okuda, K., Edwards, C. E., Martinez, D. R., Asakura, T., Dinnon, K. H.,. 3., et al. (2020). SARS-Cov-2 Reverse Genetics Reveals a Variable Infection Gradient in the Respiratory Tract. *Cell* 182 (2), 429–446.e14. doi: 10.1016/j.cell.2020.05.042

Huang, C., Wang, Y., Li, X., Ren, L., Zhao, J., Hu, Y., et al. (2020). Clinical Features of Patients Infected With 2019 Novel Coronavirus in Wuhan, China. *Lancet* 395 (10223), 497–506. doi: 10.1016/S0140-6736(20)30183-5

Jackson, D. J., Busse, W. W., Bacharier, L. B., Kattan, M., O'Connor, G. T., Wood, R. A., et al. (2020). Association of Respiratory Allergy, Asthma, and Expression of the SARS-Cov-2 Receptor ACE2. *J. Allergy Clin. Immunol.* 146 (1), 203–206.e3. doi: 10.1016/j.jaci.2020.04.009

Jacobs, B. L., and Langland, J. O. (1996). When Two Strands are Better Than One: The Mediators and Modulators of the Cellular Responses to Double-Stranded RNA. *Virology* 219 (2), 339–349. doi: 10.1006/viro.1996.0259

Kato, A., Favoreto, S.Jr., Avila, P. C., and Schleimer, R. P. (2007). TLR3- and Th2 Cytokine-Dependent Production of Thymic Stromal Lymphopoietin in Human Airway Epithelial Cells. *J. Immunol. (Baltimore Md 1950)* 179 (2), 1080–1087. doi: 10.4049/jimmunol.179.2.1080

Kimura, H., Francisco, D., Conway, M., Martinez, F. D., Vercelli, D., Polverino, F., et al. (2020). Type 2 Inflammation Modulates ACE2 and TMPRSS2 in Airway Epithelial Cells. *J. Allergy Clin. Immunol.* 146 (1), 80–88. doi: 10.1016/j.jaci.2020.05.004

Li, W., Moore, M. J., Vasilieva, N., Sui, J., Wong, S. K., Berne, M. A., et al. (2003). Angiotensin-Converting Enzyme 2 is a Functional Receptor for the SARS Coronavirus. *Nature* 426 (6965), 450–454. doi: 10.1038/nature02145

Lin, B., Ferguson, C., White, J. T., Wang, S., Vessella, R., True, L. D., et al. (1999). Prostate-Localized and Androgen-Regulated Expression of the Membrane-Bound Serine Protease TMPRSS2. *Cancer Res.* 59 (17), 4180–4184.

Lucas, J. M., Heinlein, C., Kim, T., Hernandez, S. A., Malik, M. S., True, L. D., et al. (2014). The Androgen-Regulated Protease TMPRSS2 Activates a Proteolytic Cascade Involving Components of the Tumor Microenvironment and Promotes Prostate Cancer Metastasis. *Cancer Discovery* 4 (11), 1310–1325. doi: 10.1158/2159-8290.CD-13-1010

Matsumoto, K., and Saito, H. (2020). Does Asthma Affect Morbidity or Severity of COVID-19? *J. Allergy Clin. Immunol.* 146 (1), 55–57. doi: 10.1016/j.jaci.2020.05.017

Matsuyama, S., Kawase, M., Nao, N., Shirato, K., Ujike, M., Kamitani, W., et al. (2020). The Inhaled Corticosteroid Ciclesonide Blocks Coronavirus RNA Replication by Targeting Viral NSP15. *bioRxiv* 2020, 03.11.987016. doi: 10.1101/2020.03.11.987016

Ohkuni, T., Kojima, T., Ogasawara, N., Masaki, T., Fuchimoto, J., Kamekura, R., et al. (2011). Poly(I:C) Reduces Expression of JAM-a and Induces Secretion of IL-8 and TNF-Alpha Via Distinct NF-Kappab Pathways in Human Nasal Epithelial Cells. *Toxicol. Appl. Pharmacol.* 250 (1), 29–38. doi: 10.1016/j.taap.2010.09.023

Paderno, A., Schreiber, A., Grammatica, A., Raffetti, E., Tomasoni, M., Gualtieri, T., et al. (2020). Smell and Taste Alterations in COVID-19: A Cross-Sectional Analysis of Different Cohorts. *Int. Forum Allergy Rhinol.* 10 (8), 955–962. doi: 10.1002/alr.22610

Patel, A. B., and Verma, A. (2020). Nasal ACE2 Levels and COVID-19 in Children. *JAMA* 323 (23), 2386–2387. doi: 10.1001/jama.2020.8946

Ramezanpour, M., Bolt, H., Psaltis, A., Wormald, P. J., and Vreugde, S. (2019). Inducing a Mucosal Barrier-Sparing Inflammatory Response in Laboratory-Grown Primary Human Nasal Epithelial Cells. *Curr. Protoc. Toxicol.* 80 (1), e69. doi: 10.1002/cptx.69

Russell, C. D., Millar, J. E., and Baillie, J. K. (2020). Clinical Evidence Does Not Support Corticosteroid Treatment for 2019-Ncov Lung Injury. *Lancet* 395 (10223), 473–475. doi: 10.1016/S0140-6736(20)30317-2

Saheb Sharif-Askari, N., Saheb Sharif-Askari, F., Alabed, M., Temsah, M. H., Al Heialy, S., Hamid, Q., et al. (2020). Airways Expression of SARS-Cov-2 Receptor, ACE2, and TMPRSS2 is Lower in Children Than Adults and Increases With Smoking and COPD. *Mol. Ther. Methods Clin. Dev.* 18, 1–6. doi: 10.1016/j.omtm.2020.05.013

Sakalli, E., Temirbekov, D., Bayri, E., Alis, E. E., Erdurak, S. C., and Bayraktaroglu, M. (2020). Ear Nose Throat-Related Symptoms With a Focus on Loss of Smell and/or Taste in COVID-19 Patients. *Am. J. Otolaryngol.* 41 (6), 102622. doi: 10.1016/j.amjoto.2020.102622

Shang, L., Zhao, J., Hu, Y., Du, R., and Cao, B. (2020). On the Use of Corticosteroids for 2019-Ncov Pneumonia. *Lancet* 395 (10225), 683–684. doi: 10.1016/S0140-6736(20)30361-5

Sharif-Askari, F. S., Sharif-Askari, N. S., Goel, S., Fakhri, S., Al-Muhsen, S., Hamid, Q., et al. (2020). Are Patients With Chronic Rhinosinusitis With Nasal Polyps At a Decreased Risk of COVID-19 Infection? *Int. Forum Allergy Rhinol.* 10 (10), 1182–1185. doi: 10.1002/alr.22672

Singanayagam, A., Glanville, N., Bartlett, N., and Johnston, S. (2015). Effect of Fluticasone Propionate on Virus-Induced Airways Inflammation and Anti-Viral Immune Responses in Mice. *Lancet* 385 (Suppl 1), S88. doi: 10.1016/S0140-6736(15)60403-2

Sungnak, W., Huang, N., Bécavin, C., Berg, M., Queen, R., Litvinukova, M., et al. (2020). SARS-Cov-2 Entry Factors are Highly Expressed in Nasal Epithelial Cells Together With Innate Immune Genes. *Nat. Med.* 26 (5), 681–687. doi: 10.1038/s41591-020-0868-6

Suzuki, M., Ramezanpour, M., Cooksley, C., Li, J., Nakamaru, Y., Homma, A., et al. (2018). Sirtuin-1 Controls Poly (I:C)-Dependent Matrix Metalloproteinase 9 Activation in Primary Human Nasal Epithelial Cells. *Am. J. Respir. Cell Mol. Biol.* 59 (4), 500–510. doi: 10.1165/rcmb.2017-0415OC

Wu, J., Deng, W., Li, S., and Yang, X. (2020). Advances in Research on ACE2 as a Receptor for 2019-Ncov. *Cell. Mol. Life Sci. CMLS* 11, 1–14. doi: 10.1007/s00018-020-03611-x

Zhang, Y., Geng, X., Tan, Y., Li, Q., Xu, C., Xu, J., et al. (2020). New Understanding of the Damage of SARS-Cov-2 Infection Outside the Respiratory System. *Biomed. Pharmacother.* 127, 110195. doi: 10.1016/j.biopha.2020.110195

Zhang, N., Truong-Tran, Q. A., Tancowny, B., Harris, K. E., and Schleimer, R. P. (2007). Glucocorticoids Enhance or Spare Innate Immunity: Effects in Airway Epithelium are Mediated by CCAAT/Enhancer Binding Proteins. *J. Immunol. (Baltimore Md 1950)* 179 (1), 578–589. doi: 10.4049/jimmunol.179.1.578

Zhuang, M. W., Cheng, Y., Zhang, J., Jiang, X. M., Wang, L., Deng, J., et al. (2020). Increasing Host Cellular Receptor-Angiotensin-Converting Enzyme 2 (ACE2) Expression by Coronavirus May Facilitate 2019-Ncov (or SARS-Cov-2) Infection. *J. Med. Virol.* doi: 10.1101/2020.02.24.963348

Ziegler, C. G. K., Allon, S. J., Nyquist, S. K., Mbano, I. M., Miao, V. N., Tzouanas, C. N., et al. (2020). SARS-Cov-2 Receptor ACE2 is an Interferon-Stimulated Gene in Human Airway Epithelial Cells and is Detected in Specific Cell Subsets Across Tissues. *Cell* 181 (5), 1016–1035.e19. doi: 10.1016/j.cell.2020.04.035

Zou, L., Ruan, F., Huang, M., Liang, L., Huang, H., Hong, Z., et al. (2020). SARS-Cov-2 Viral Load in Upper Respiratory Specimens of Infected Patients. *New Engl. J. Med.* 382 (12), 1177–1179. doi: 10.1056/NEJMc2001737

9

SARS-CoV-2: Structure, Biology and Structure-Based Therapeutics Development

Mei-Yue Wang[†], *Rong Zhao*[†], *Li-Juan Gao*, *Xue-Fei Gao*, *De-Ping Wang*[*] *and Ji-Min Cao*[*]

Key Laboratory of Cellular Physiology at Shanxi Medical University, Ministry of Education, Key Laboratory of Cellular Physiology of Shanxi Province, and the Department of Physiology, Shanxi Medical University, Taiyuan, China

***Correspondence:**
De-Ping Wang
wangdeping@sxmu.edu.cn
Ji-Min Cao
caojimin@sxmu.edu.cn

[†]*These authors have contributed equally to this work*

The pandemic of the novel severe acute respiratory syndrome coronavirus 2 (SARS-CoV-2) has been posing great threats to the world in many aspects. Effective therapeutic and preventive approaches including drugs and vaccines are still unavailable although they are in development. Comprehensive understandings on the life logic of SARS-CoV-2 and the interaction of the virus with hosts are fundamentally important in the fight against SARS-CoV-2. In this review, we briefly summarized the current advances in SARS-CoV-2 research, including the epidemic situation and epidemiological characteristics of the caused disease COVID-19. We further discussed the biology of SARS-CoV-2, including the origin, evolution, and receptor recognition mechanism of SARS-CoV-2. And particularly, we introduced the protein structures of SARS-CoV-2 and structure-based therapeutics development including antibodies, antiviral compounds, and vaccines, and indicated the limitations and perspectives of SARS-CoV-2 research. We wish the information provided by this review may be helpful to the global battle against SARS-CoV-2 infection.

Keywords: severe acute respiratory syndrome coronavirus 2, protein structure, antibodies, antiviral compounds, vaccines

GENERAL INFORMATION OF SARS-COV-2

Current Situation of SARS-CoV-2 Epidemic

In December 2019, the World Health Organization (WHO) was informed about an outbreak of pneumonia in Wuhan, Hubei Province, China, and the etiology was not identified. On January 30, 2020, WHO declared that the severe acute respiratory syndrome coronavirus 2 (SARS-CoV-2) epidemic is a public health emergency of international concern (PHEIC). On February 11, 2020, the WHO officially named the current outbreak of coronavirus disease as Coronavirus Disease-2019 (COVID-19) (Sun P. et al., 2020) and the International Committee on Taxonomy of Viruses (ICTV) named the virus as SARS-CoV-2 (Hu B. et al., 2020). Data as received by WHO from national authorities by October 11, 2020, there were more than 37 million confirmed cases with COVID-19 and 1 million deaths. Globally, the United States, India, and Brazil are the three countries with the largest cumulative number of confirmed cases in the world (https://www.who.int/docs/default-source/coronaviruse/situation-reports/20201012-weekly-epi-update-9.pdf). The total cumulative number of confirmed cases have far exceeded the number during SARS period (Wang and Jin, 2020). After the emergence of SARS-CoV and MERS-CoV, SARS-CoV-2 is the third zoonotic human coronavirus of the century (Gralinski and Menachery, 2020).

The Origin and Evolution of SARS-CoV-2

Bioinformatic analyses showed that SARS-CoV-2 had characteristics typical of coronavirus family. It belongs to the betacoronavirus 2B lineage (Lai et al., 2020). Early in the pneumonia epidemic in Wuhan, scientists obtained the complete genome sequences from five patients infected with SARS-CoV-2. These genome sequences share 79.5% sequence identity to SARS-CoV. Obviously, SARS-CoV-2 is divergent from SARS-CoV. It is considered to be a new betacoronavirus that infects human (Zhou P. et al., 2020). Scientists aligned the full-length genome sequence of SARS-CoV-2 and other available genomes of betacoronaviruses. Results indicate the closest relationship of SARS-CoV-2 with the bat SARS-like coronavirus strain BatCov RaTG13, with an identity of 96%. These studies suggest that SARS-CoV-2 could be of bat origin, and SARS-CoV-2 might be naturally evolved from bat coronavirus RaTG13 (Zhang C. et al., 2020; Zhou P. et al., 2020).

One study analyzed the genomes of SARS-CoV-2 and similar isolates from the GISATD and NCBI (Xiong C. et al., 2020). Results indicate that an isolate numbered EPI_ISL_403928 shows different genetic distances of the whole length genome and different phylogenetic trees, the coding sequences of spike protein (S), nucleoprotein (N), and polyprotein (P) from other SARS-CoV-2, with 4, 2, and 22 variations in S, N, and P at the level of amino acid residues respectively. The results show that at least two SARS-CoV-2 strains are involved in the outbreak (Xiong C. et al., 2020).

After aligning the coding sequences (CDSs) based on the protein alignments, open reading frame 8 (ORF8) and open reading frame 10 (ORF10) of SARS-CoV-2 are different from other viruses. However, most ORFs annotated from SARS-CoV-2 are conserved. The overall genomic nucleotides identity between SARS-CoV-2 and SARS-like coronavirus strain BatCov RaTG13 is 96%. Compared with other viruses, the divergence of SARS-CoV-2 at neutral site is 17%, much larger than previously assessed. The spike gene exhibits larger dS (synonymous substitutions per synonymous site) values than other genes, which could be caused either by natural selection that accelerates synonymous substitutions or by a high mutation rate. Researchers obtained 103 SARS-CoV-2 genomes to recognize the genetic variants (Tang X. et al., 2020). Among the 103 strains, a total of 149 mutations are identified and population genetic analyses indicate that these strains are mainly divided into two types. Results suggest that 101 of the 103 SARS-CoV-2 strains show significant linkage between the two single nucleotide polypeptides (SNPs). The major types of SARS-CoV-2 (L type and S type) are distinguished by two SNPs which locate at the sites of 8,782 and 28,144. L type accounts for 70% of the 103 strains and S type accounts for 30%, suggesting L type is more prevalent than the S type. However, S type is the ancestral version of SARS-CoV-2 (Tang X. et al., 2020).

To date, 13 mutations in the spike protein have been identified. The mutation D614G should be paid special attention. In early February, the mutation Spike D614G began spreading in Europe. When introduced to new regions, it rapidly replaced the original strain to become the dominant strain (Korber B. et al., 2020). The D614G mutation in the spike protein would increase infectivity. S^{G614} is more stable than S^{D641} and less S1 shedding are observed, so the SARS-CoV-2 with S^{G614} could transmit more efficiently (Zhang et al., 2020b). One study shows that in multiple cell lines, the SARS-CoV-2 carrying the D614G mutation is eight times more effective at transducing cells than wild-type spike protein, providing evidence that the D614G mutation in SARS-CoV-2 spike protein could increase the transduction of multiple human cell types (Daniloski Z. et al., 2020). The D614G mutation could also decrease neutralization sensitivity to the sera of convalescent COVID-19 patients (Hu J. et al., 2020).

The Epidemiological Characteristics of COVID-19

Bats appear to be the natural reservoir of SARS-CoV-2 (Zhang C. et al., 2020; Zhou P. et al., 2020). In one study, betacoronavirus isolated from pangolins has a sequence similarity of up to 99% with the currently infected human strain (Liu et al., 2020). Another study indicates that SARS-CoV-2 and the coronavirus from a pangolin in Malaysia has high genetic similarity. The gene similarity between these two viruses in terms of E, M, N, and S genes is 100, 98.6, 97.8, and 90.7%, respectively, suggesting the potential for pangolins to be the intermediate host (Xiao et al., 2020). Among the animals in close contact with humans, dogs, chickens, ducks, and pigs are not permissive to infection. SARS-CoV-2 replicates efficiently in cats and ferrets (Shi J. et al., 2020). SARS-CoV-2 can also transmit in golden hamster (Sia et al., 2020).

SARS-CoV-2 is transmitted *via* fomites and droplets during close unprotected contact between the infected and uninfected. Symptomatic and asymptomatic patients are the main source of infection. The virus can also spread through indirect contact transmission. Virus-containing droplets contaminate hands, people then contact the mucous membranes of the mouth, nose, and eyes, causing infection. The transmission of SARS-CoV-2 is not limited to the respiratory tract (Du et al., 2020). Some studies have demonstrated the aerosol transmission of SARS-CoV-2. During the COVID-19 outbreak, one study investigated the aerodynamic nature of SARS-CoV-2 by measuring viral RNA in aerosols in two Wuhan hospitals, indicating that SARS-CoV-2 has the potential to spread through aerosols. There may be a possibility of airborne transmission in health care facilities due to aerosols generated by medical procedures. Of note, in the spread of COVID-19, airborne transmission is the dominant route. (Chan et al., 2020; Meselson, 2020; Morawska and Cao, 2020; Sommerstein et al., 2020; Tang S. et al., 2020; van Doremalen et al., 2020; Zhang R. et al., 2020). In some pediatric SARS-CoV-2 infection cases, although children's nasopharyngeal swabs are negative, rectal swabs are consistently positive, indicating the possibility of fecal-oral transmission (Xu et al., 2020). Recent studies demonstrate that SARS-CoV-2 could replicate effectively in human intestinal organoids and intestinal epithelium. As a result, SARS-CoV-2 has the potential to spread through intestinal tract. SARS-CoV-2 can also infect the intestinal cells of bats (Lamers et al., 2020; Zhou J. et al., 2020). A COVID-19 patient's urine also contains infectious SARS-CoV-2 (Sun J. et al., 2020). After studying COVID-19 infection in nine pregnant women, the result suggests that there is no evidence that pregnant women who were infected SARS-CoV-2 in late pregnancy can transmit the virus to infant through intrauterine vertical transmission (Chen N. et al., 2020). However, recently, some studies demonstrated the possibility of vertical transmission of SARS-CoV-2 (Chen H. et al., 2020; Deniz and Tezer, 2020; Egloff et al., 2020; Hu X. et al., 2020; Mahyuddin et al., 2020; Oliveira et al., 2020; Parazzini et al., 2020; Peyronnet et al., 2020; Vivanti et al., 2020; Yang and Liu, 2020). In one case, the newborn whose mother was diagnosed with SARS-CoV-2 in the last trimester was infected with SARS-CoV-2, with neurological compromise. In another case, the cytokine levels and anti-SARS-CoV-2 IgM antibodies of the neonate is higher than normal, with no physical contact, suggesting the possibility of transplacental transmission (Dong et al., 2020). The risk of perinatal transmission of SARS-CoV-2 is relatively low. Compared with SARS-CoV-2, pregnant women infected with SARS and MERS showed more severe symptoms, such as miscarriage and abortion (Fan et al., 2020; Parazzini et al., 2020). According to current reports, the perinatal transmission can occur but the rate is low and the information about exposition during the first or second trimester of pregnancy remains unknown (Egloff et al., 2020; Parazzini et al., 2020). The major spread route of SARS-CoV-2 is person-to-person, it could happen in family, hospital, community, and other gathering of people. Most cases of the person-to-person transmission of the early stage in China happened in family clusters (Chan et al., 2020; Ghinai et al., 2020a; Ghinai et al., 2020b). This kind of spreading has the possibility to occur during the incubation period (Yu P. et al., 2020). It is worth noting that SARS-CoV-2 has high transmissibility during asymptomatic period or mild disease (Hu B. et al., 2020; Li et al., 2020). SARS-CoV-2 can also transmit from human to animal. Some animals, such as tiger, dog, and cat, are found to be infected with the virus through close contact with the infected people (Singla et al., 2020). A 17-years-old dog in Hong Kong was affected and it was the first case of human-to-animal transmission (https://www.afcd.gov.hk/english/publications/publi cationspress/pr2342.html). One study shows that the viral genetic sequences of SARS-CoV-2 detected in two dogs are the same with the SARS-CoV-2 in the corresponding human cases, suggesting the human-to-animal transmission. However, it remains unknown whether infected dogs can transmit the virus back to humans (Sit et al., 2020). SARS-CoV-2 is believed to transmit from the animal kingdom to human. According to the sequence analysis, bats are natural hosts for SARS-CoV-2 (Cui et al., 2019; Salata et al., 2019). SARS-CoV-2 and the coronavirus from a pangolin in Malaysia have high genetic similarity (Xiao et al., 2020), and the CoVs isolated from pangolins have the highest closeness to SARS-CoV-2 (Zhang T. et al., 2020), suggesting the potential for pangolins to be the intermediate host. The intermediate hosts could transmit the virus to susceptible people, leading to the newly appear diseases in humans (Ye et al., 2020; Zhang T. et al., 2020). SARS-CoV-2 can also transmit between animals. SARS-CoV-2 infected cats could transmit the virus to naïve cats with close contact (Halfmann et al., 2020). SARS-CoV-2 could also transmit in naïve ferrets, through direct or indirect contact (Kim et al., 2020).

According to current observed epidemiologic characteristics, everyone is considered susceptible and the median age is about 50 years (Chen N. et al., 2020; Guan et al., 2020; Huang et al., 2020; Wang D. et al., 2020; Wu and McGoogan, 2020).

The clinical manifestations differ with age. One study indicates that the cases over 60 years old have higher levels of blood urea nitrogen, inflammatory indicators, and more lobes bilateral lesions. The patients older than 60 years old have a greater chance of respiratory failure and longer disease courses. However, in those under 60, the severity is milder (Liu et al., 2020). One study reports a total of 72,314 confirmed cases in China, the majority of the patients (87%) are between the ages of 30 and 79. In the group no older than nine, no deaths occurred. However, in the group aged 70–79 years, the case-fatality rate (CFR) is 8.0%, in the group aged 80 years and older, the CFR is 14.8%. As to the patients with different comorbid conditions, such as cardiovascular disease, diabetes, chronic respiratory disease, hypertension, and cancer, the CFR is 10.5, 7.3, 6.3, 6.0, and 5.6%, respectively. These results suggest that comorbid conditions are high risk factors for COVID-19 patients and higher fatality rates are observed than those without underlying diseases (Wu and McGoogan, 2020). Among the 1,099 cases confirmed with COVID-19, patients with severe disease were 7 years older than those with non-severe disease (Guan et al., 2020). Of the 1,391 infected children, the median age is 6.7 years and most children show milder symptoms (non-pneumonia or mild pneumonia) than adults (Lu X. et al., 2020). The patients who aged ≥65 years old have a higher risk of mortality from COVID-19, especially the patients with acute respiratory distress syndrome (ARDS) and comorbidities (Du et al., 2020; Wu C. et al., 2020; Yang X. et al., 2020; Zhou F. et al., 2020).

Clinical Characteristics of COVID-19

The most common manifestations of COVID-19 are fever and dry cough. The majority of the patients showed bilateral pneumonia. Old males with comorbidities are more likely to be affected by SARS-CoV-2 (Chen N. et al., 2020). The blood counts of patients showed leucopenia and lymphopenia. The content of IL2, IL7, IL10, GSCF, IP10, MCP1, MIP1A, and TNFα in the plasma of ICU patients is higher than non-ICU patients (Huang et al., 2020).

COVID-19 is divided into three levels according to the severity of the disease: mild, severe, and critical. The majority of patients only have mild symptoms and recover (Hu B. et al., 2020). Asymptomatic infection cases were also reported, but most of the asymptomatic patients went on to develop disease since the data of identification (Huang et al., 2020). **Table 1** shows the clinical

TABLE 1 | Clinical manifestations and three different levels of COVID-19.

Clinical manifestations	fever, dry cough, fatigue, shortness of breath, muscle ache, confusion, headache, sore throat, rhinorrhea, chest pain, diarrhea, nausea, vomiting, chills, sputum production, haemoptysis, dyspnea, bilateral pneumonia anorexia, chest pain, leucopenia, lymphopenia, olfactory and taste disorders, higher levels of plasma cytokines (IL2, IL7, IL10, GSCF, IP10, MCP1, MIP1A, and TNFα) (ICU patients)	
Three different levels of COVID-19	Mild	fever, cough, fatigue, ground-glass opacities, non-pneumonia, and mild pneumonia
	Severe	dyspnea, blood oxygen saturation ≤93%, respiratory frequency ≥30/min, partial pressure of arterial oxygen to fraction of inspired oxygen ratio <300, and/or lung infiltrates >50% within 24 to 48 h, ICU needed
	critical	acute respiratory distress syndrome (ARDS), respiratory failure, septic shock, and/or multiple organ dysfunction or failure, hard-to-correct metabolic acidosis, septic shock, coagulation dysfunction

manifestations of COVID-19 (Chen T. et al., 2020; Hu B. et al., 2020; Huang et al., 2020; Wang Y. et al., 2020; Wu and McGoogan, 2020) and three different levels of COVID-19 divided according to the severity (Chen T. et al., 2020; Hu B. et al., 2020; Huang et al., 2020; Wang Y. et al., 2020; Wu and McGoogan, 2020). Besides respiratory illness, COVID-19 disease could lead to myocardial injury and arrhythmic complications (Bansal, 2020; Kochi et al., 2020), neurological complications, such as myalgia, headache, dizziness, impaired consciousness, intracranial hemorrhage, hypogeusia, and hyposmia (Berger, 2020; Paybast et al., 2020), and even stroke (Hess et al., 2020; Trejo-Gabriel-Galán, 2020). Digestive symptoms and liver injury (Lee et al., 2020), hypercoagulability and thrombotic complications (Haimei, 2020) have also been reported. Critical patients could quickly progress to ARDS, hard-to-correct metabolic acidosis, septic shock, coagulation dysfunction, and multiple organ functional failure. Severe complications included ARDS, RNAaemia (detectable serum SARS-CoV-2 viral load), multiple organ failure, and acute cardiac injury. About 26.1% patients were admitted to the ICU because of complications caused by COVID-19 (Huang et al., 2020). With proper diagnosis and treatments for COVID-19, most patients had a good prognosis (Wang Y. et al., 2020). The elderly and the patients with underlying diseases have worse prognosis (Deng and Peng, 2020).

THE STRUCTURE OF SARS-COV-2

Coronaviruses belongs to the subfamily *Coronavirinae* in the family of Coronaviridae and the subfamily contains four genera: *Alphacoronavirus*, *Betacoronavirus*, *Gammacoronavirus*, and *Deltacoronavirus*. The genome of CoVs (27–32 kb) is a single-stranded positive-sense RNA (+ssRNA) which is larger than any other RNA viruses. The nucleocapsid protein (N) formed the capsid outside the genome and the genome is further packed by an envelope which is associated with three structural proteins: membrane protein (M), spike protein (S), and envelope protein (E) (Brian and Baric, 2005). As a member of coronavirus family, the genome size of SARS-CoV-2 which was sequenced recently is approximately 29.9 kb (Lu R. et al., 2020). SARS-CoV-2 contains four structural proteins (S, E, M, and N) and sixteen non-structural proteins (nsp1–16). Nsp1 mediates RNA processing and replication. Nsp2 modulates the survival signaling pathway of host cell. Nsp3 is believed to separate the translated protein. Nsp4 contains transmembrane domain 2 (TM2) and modifies ER membranes. Nsp5 participates in the process of polyprotein during replication. Nsp6 is a presumptive transmembrane domain. The presence of nsp7 and nsp8 significantly increased the combination of nsp12 and template-primer RNA. Nsp9 functions as an ssRNA-binding protein. Nsp10 is critical for the cap methylation of viral mRNAs. Nsp12 contains the RNA-dependent RNA polymerase (RdRp), which is a critical composition of coronavirus replication/transcription. Nsp13 binds with ATP and the zinc-binding domain in nsp13 participates in the process of replication and transcription. Nsp14 is a proofreading exoribonuclease domain. Nsp15 has Mn(2+)-dependent endoribonuclease activity. Nsp16 is a 2'-O-ribose methyltransferase (Naqvi et al., 2020). One study shows that there are some NSP-mediated effects on splicing, translation, and protein trafficking to inhibit host defenses. Upon SARS-CoV-2 infection, NSP16 binds mRNA recognition domains of the U1 and U2 snRNAs to suppress mRNA splicing. NSP1 binds to 18S ribosomal RNA in the mRNA entry channel of the ribosome to interfere with the translation of mRNA. NSP8 and NSP9 binds to the 7SL RNA which locates at the Signal Recognition Particle to disrupt protein trafficking to the cell membrane (Banerjee et al., 2020). Followings are some SARS-CoV-2 proteins which may potentially serve as antiviral drug targets based on their structures.

Spike Glycoprotein

The coronaviruses entry into host cells is mediated by spike glycoprotein (S protein) (Li et al., 2003; Li et al., 2005; Li, 2016). The transmembrane spike glycoproteins form homotrimers that protrude from the viral surface. The spike glycoprotein is critical for the entry of the coronaviruses so it is an attractive antiviral target. S protein is composed of two functional subunits, including the S1 and S2 subunits. The S1 subunit consists of N-terminal domain (NTD) and receptor binding domain (RBD). The function of S1 subunit is bind to the receptor on host cell. S2 subunit contains fusion peptide (FP), heptad repeat 1 (HR1), central helix (CH), connector domain (CD), heptad repeat 2 (HR2), transmembrane domain (TM), and cytoplasmic tail (CT) (**Figure 1A**). The function of S2 subunit is to fuse the membranes of viruses and host cells. The cleavage site at the border between the S1 and S2 subunits is called S1/S2 protease cleavage site. For all the coronaviruses, host proteases cleave the spike glycoprotein at the S2' cleavage site to activate the proteins which is critical to fuse the membranes of viruses and host cells through irreversible conformational changes. N-linked glycans are critical for proper folding, neutralizing antibodies, and decorating the spike protein trimers extensively (Walls et al., 2020; Wrapp et al., 2020).

Overall, the structure of SARS-CoV-2 S protein resembles the closely related SARS-CoV S protein. In the prefusion

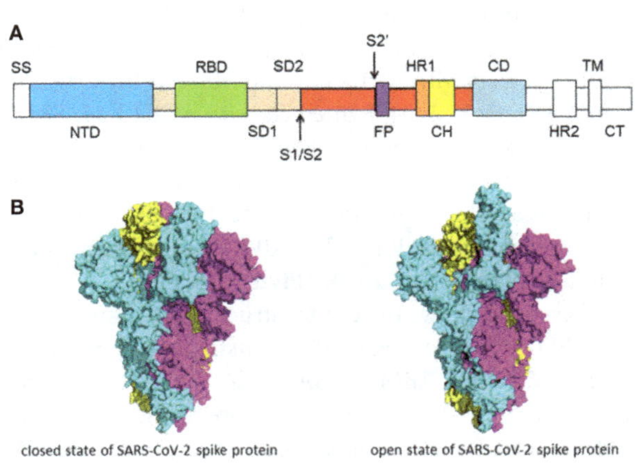

FIGURE 1 | **(A)** Schematic of SARS-CoV-2 spike protein primary structure. Different domains are shown by different colors. SS, single sequence; NTD, N-terminal domain; RBD, receptor-binding domain; SD1, subdomain 1; SD2, subdomain 2; S1/S2, S1/S2 protease cleavage site; S2', S2' protease cleavage site; FP, fusion peptide; HR1, heptad repeat 1; CH, central helix; CD, connector domain; HR2, heptad repeat 2; TM, transmembrane domain; CT, cytoplasmic tail. The protease cleavage site is indicated by arrows. **(B)** Cryo-EM structure of the SARS-CoV-2 spike protein. The closed state (PDB: 6VXX) of the SARS-CoV-2 S glycoprotein (left) the open state (PDB: 6VYB) of the SARS-CoV-2 S glycoprotein (right).

conformation, S1 and S2 subunits remain non-covalently bound. Different kinds of coronaviruses utilize special domains in the S1 subunit to recognize different entry receptors. In the case of SARS-CoV and SARS-CoV-2, to enter host cells, they recognize the receptor angiotensin-converting enzyme 2 (ACE2) on host cells *via* the receptor binding domain (RBD). The S protein has two forms of structure, including the closed state and the open state (**Figure 1B**). In the closed state, the three recognition motifs do not protrude from the interface formed by three spike protein protomers. In the open state, the RBD is in the "up" conformation. The open state is necessary for the fusion of the SARS-CoV-2 and the host cell membranes, thereby facilitating SARS-CoV-2 to enter the host cells (Walls et al., 2020).

HR1 and HR2

The six-helical bundle (6-HB) is formed by HR1 and HR2 and is critical for membrane fusion which is dominated by the spike protein of SARS-CoV or SARS-CoV-2, making HR1 and HR2 an attractive drug target (Liu et al., 2004; Xia et al., 2020b). The difference between the 6-HB of SARS-CoV-2 and SARS-CoV may stabilize 6-HB conformation of SARS-CoV-2 and enhance the interactions between HR1 and HR2, resulting in the increased infectivity of SARS-CoV-2. The HR1-L6-HR2 complex contains most parts of HR1 and HR2 domain and a linker (Xia et al., 2020a). This fusion protein exhibits a rod-like shape and it is the standard structure of 6-HB. Three HR1 domains come together to form a spiral coil trimer in a parallel manner. Three HR2 domains are entwined around the coiled-coil center in an antiparallel manner which is mainly mediated by hydrophobic force. Hydrophobic residues on theHR2 domian binds with the hydrophobic groove formed by every two two neighboring HR1 helices. The overall 6-HB structure of SARS-CoV and SARS-CoV-2 is very similar, especially the S2 subunit (Xia et al., 2020a). The identity of the HR1 of SARS-CoV and SARS-CoV-2 is 96% and HR2 is 100%. There are eight distinct residues in the fusion core region of HR1 domain. In the HR1 domain of SARS-CoV, lysine 911 binds to the glutamic acid 1176 in HR2 domain through a salt bridge. As to SARS-CoV-2, the salt bridge is replaced by a strong hydrogen bond between serine 929 in HR1 and serine 1,196 in HR2. In SARS-CoV HR1, glutamine 915 has no interaction with HR2. However, as to SARS-CoV-2, there is a salt bridge between lysine 933 in HR1 and asparagine 1,192 in HR2 (Xia et al., 2020a). In SARS-CoV, there is a weak salt bridge between glutamic acid 918 in HR1 and arginine 1,166. However, aspartic acid 936 in the HR1 of SARS-CoV-2 binds to the arginine 1,158 through a salt bridge. In the SARS-CoV, lysine 929 binds to the glutamic acid 1,163 in the HR2 domain through a salt bridge and threonine 925 does not bind to the glutamic acid 1,163. However, serine 943 and lysine 947 in the SARS-CoV-2 bind to the glutamic acid 1,182 in HR2 through a hydrogen bond and a salt bridge. These differences may result in increased infectivity of SARS-CoV-2 (Xia et al., 2020a).

The Receptor Binding Domain (RBD)

The spike protein of SARS-CoV-2 contains an RBD that recognizes the receptor ACE2 specifically. RBD is a critical target for antiviral compounds and antibodies (Letko et al., 2020). SARS-CoV-2 RBD includes two structural domains: the core and the external subdomains. The core subdomain is highly conserved. It is composed of five β strands arranged in antiparallel manner and a disulfide bond between two β strands. The external subdomain is mainly dominated by the loop which is stabilized by the disulfide bond (Wang Q. et al., 2020). The SARS-CoV-2 RBD core consists of five β sheets arranged in antiparallel manner and connected by loops and short helices. Between the antiparallel β4 and β7 strands is the receptor-binding motif (RBM) which consists of loops and α helices, as well as short β5 and β6 strands. RBM contains most binding sites for SARS-CoV-2 and ACE2. Eight of the nine Cys residues in the RBD form four pairs of disulfide bonds. Three disulfide bonds are in the core of RBD, enhancing the stabilization of the β sheet (C336-C361, C379-C432, and C391-C525). With respect to the remaining disulfide bond (C480-C488), it promotes the connections between the loops in RBM. The peptidase domain in the N-terminal of ACE2 contains the binding site, which is formed by two lobes of RBM and ACE2. RBM binds to the small lobe of the ACE2 on the bottom side. The surface of RBM is slightly concave inward to make room for ACE2 (Lan et al., 2020).

One study obtained a 3.5 Å-resolution structure of spike protein trimer with one RBD in the in the "up" conformation (receptor-accessible state). Receptor binding destabilizes the prefusion structure, triggered by this process, the S1 subunit dissociates and the S2 subunit refolds into a stable postfusion conformation, which has been captured in SARS-CoV. RBD goes through conformational transitions like a hinge, leading to the hide or exposure of the determinants of the spike protein to engage a host cell receptor. This process will form the following two states: "down" conformation and "up" conformation. In the "down" conformation, SARS-CoV-2 could not recognize the ACE2 on the host cells. The structure of SARS-CoV-2 is highly similar with SARS-CoV. One of the larger differences is in the down conformation, SARS-CoV RBD packs tightly against the NTD of the neighboring protomer, while the angle of SARS-CoV-2 RBD is near to the central cavity of the spike protein trimer. When aligned the individual structural domains corresponding to SARS-CoV-2 and SARS-CoV, highly similar structures were observed (Wrapp et al., 2020). The overall structure of SARS-CoV-2 RBM is also nearly identical to that identified in previous studies, with only one observed difference on the distal end (Lan et al., 2020).

RBD-ACE2 Complex

It is important to understand the receptor recognition mechanism of the SARS-CoV-2, which determines the infectivity, host range, and pathogenesis of the virus. Both SARS-CoV-2 and SARS-CoV recognize the ACE2 in humans (Li et al., 2003; Li et al., 2005; Sia et al., 2020). The crystal structure of SARS-CoV-2 RBD bound with ACE2 has been determined (**Figure 2A**). The overall combination mode of SARS-CoV-2 RBD-ACE2 complex is highly similar with that of the identified SARS-CoV RBD-ACE2 complex in previous study. Seventeen of the 20 residues of the ACE2 interacting with the RBD of SARS-CoV and SARS-CoV-2 are the same.

However, there are subtle distinct ACE2 interactions which lead to the variation in binding affinity between SARS-CoV-2 and SARS-CoV RBD to ACE2. The affinity between ACE2 and SARS-CoV-2 is higher than the affinity between ACE2 and SARS-CoV. At the F486/L472 position, SARS-CoV-2 F486 interacts with ACE2 Q24, L79, M82, and Y83, and SARS-CoV L472 only interacts with ACE2 L79 and M82. At the Q493/N479 position, SARS-CoV-2 Q493 interacts with ACE2 K31, E35, and H34. There is a hydrogen bond between Q493 and E35. SARS-CoV N479 only interacts with ACE2 H34. Outside SARS-CoV-2 RBM, there is a salt bridge between ACE2 D30 and SARS-CoV-2 K417. However, the SARS-CoV V404 failed to participate in ACE2 binding (Lan et al., 2020) (**Figure 2B**).

Another study shows the crystal structure of chimeric SARS-CoV-2 RBD-ACE2 complex. The constructed chimeric RBD which contains the RBM of SARS-CoV-2 as the function-related unit and the SARS-CoV RBD core as the crystallization scaffold could facilitate crystallization. The side loop from SARS-CoV-2 (away from the main binding interface) maintains a salt bridge between RBD R426 and ACE2 E329. This side loop could further facilitate crystallization. The structure of chimeric RBD-ACE2 complex is highly similar with the wild-type RBD-ACE2 complex as introduced above, especially in the RBM region. SARS-CoV-2 RBM forms a surface which is gently concave, binding to the claw-like structure on the exposed outer surface of ACE2. There is a N-O bridge between R439 of the chimeric RBD and E329 of ACE2. The N-O bridge is non-natural, resulting from the SARS-CoV-based chimaera. The binding affinity between chimeric RBD and ACE2 is higher than the binding affinity between wild-type SARS-CoV-2 RBD and ACE2. It is obvious that the ACE2-binding affinity of SARS-CoV RBD is lower than SARS-CoV-2 and chimeric RBDs (Shang et al., 2020).

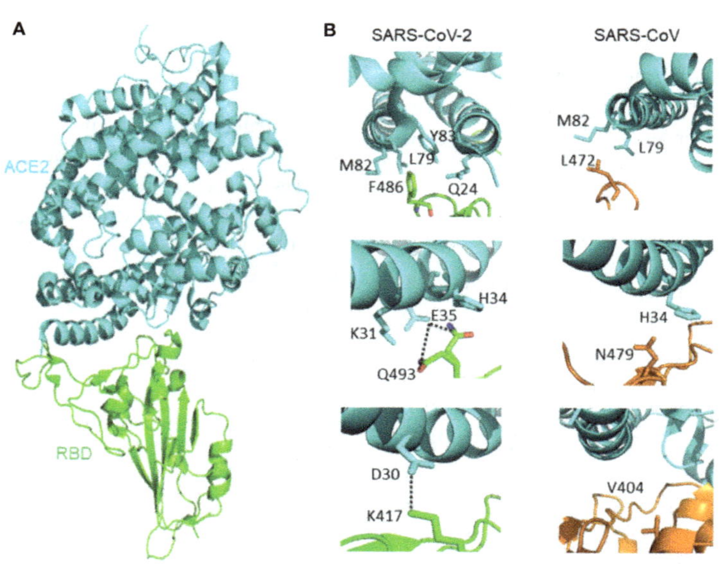

FIGURE 2 | **(A)** The overall structure of SARS-CoV-2 RBD bound with ACE2. ACE2 is colored cyan, SARS-CoV-2 RBD core is colored green (PDB: 6M0J). **(B)** Different interactions between SARS-CoV-2 RBD/ACE2 (PDB: 6M0J) and SARS-CoV RBD/ACE2 (PDB: 2AJF) that contribute to binding affinity difference. ACE2 is colored cyan. The RBD of SARS-CoV-2 is green, and the RBD of SARS-CoV is orange. Hydrogen bond between Q493 and E35 is represented by dash lines. Salt-bridge between ACE2 D30 and SARS-CoV-2 K417 is represented by dash lines.

Furin Cleavage Site of the Spike Protein

The S1/S2 boundary of SARS-CoV-2 spike protein constitutes the cleavage site for the subtilisin-like host cell protease furin, which sets SARS-CoV-2 S apart from SARS-CoV S. The furin cleavage site includes four residues (P681, R682, R683, and A684) and is located at the boundary between the S1 and S2 subunit. Functionally, R682, R683, A684, and R685 constitute the minimal polybasic furin cleavage site, RXYR, where X or Y is a positively charged arginine or lysine (Li, 2020). Such polybasic cleavage sites are not present in SARS-CoV and SARS-CoV-related group 2b betacoronaviruses found in humans, which may contribute to the high virulence of SARS-CoV-2 as a result of furin proteases required for proteolytic activation of S are ubiquitously expressed in humans, providing expanded tissue tropism and pathogenesis (Sternberg and Naujokat, 2020).

Additionally, a study has generated a SARS-CoV-2 mutant virus lacking the furin cleavage site (δPRRA) in the spike protein. The mutant virus had reduced spike protein processing in Vero E6 cells as compared to wild type SARS-CoV-2 virus. The mutant virus also had reduced replication in Calu3 human respiratory cells and had attenuated disease in a hamster pathogenesis model. These results showed an important role of the furin cleavage site in SARS-CoV-2 replication and pathogenesis (Johnson et al., 2020).

The RNA-Dependent RNA Polymerase (RdRp)

The replication of SARS-CoV-2 is dominated by a replication/transcription complex which contains several subunits. The complex is composed of viral non-structural proteins (nsp) and the core of the complex is the RdRp in nsp12. The functions of the nsp12 require accessory factors, including nsp7 and nsp8. Nsp12 alone has little activity. The presence of nsp7 and nsp8 significantly increased the combination of nsp12 and template-primer RNA. The crystal structure of nsp12-nsp7-nsp8 complex has been identified (**Figure 3A**). RNA-dependent RNA polymerase, which catalyzes the synthesis of viral RNA, is a critical composition of coronavirus replication/transcription. RdRp is an important antiviral drug target. The structures on the SARS-CoV-2 nsp12 contain a nidovirus-unique N-terminal extension domain which adopts a nidovirus RdRp-associated nucleotidyltransferase (NiRAN) structure and a "right hand" RNA-dependent RNA polymerase domain in the C-terminal. These two domains are connected by an interface domain. A unique β-hairpin is observed in the N-terminal extension domain. The β-hairpin forms close contacts to stabilize the overall structure. The RNA-dependent RNA polymerase domain contains three subdomains: a fingers subdomain, a palm subdomain, and a thumb subdomain. The β-hairpin structure inserts into the clamping groove formed by the palm subdomain and the NiRAN domain. In the plam domain, polymerase motifs A–G which is highly conserved form the active site chamber of SARS-CoV-2 RdRp domain. The RdRp motifs mediate template-directed RNA synthesis in a central cavity through four positively charged solvent-accessible paths, including template entry path, primer entry path, the NTP entry channel, and the nascent strand exit path (Gao Y. et al., 2020). A recent study shows the cryo-electron microscopic structure of the nsp12-nsp7-nsp8 complex in active form (Yin et al., 2020) (**Figure 3B**).

When added a minimal RNA hairpin substrate, the complex nsp12-nsp7-nsp8 exhibited RNA-dependent RNA extension activity. The structure of RdRp-RNA complex shows nsp12-nsp7-nsp8 complex engaged with more than two turns of duplex RNA. The RdRp-RNA structure is similar to that of the free enzyme with some unique characteristics. Compared with free enzyme, the RdRp-RNA complex contains an extended protein region in nsp8 and a protruding RNA. The subunit nsp12 binds with the first turn of RNA between its thumb subdomains and fingers subdomains. The palm subdomain contains the active site

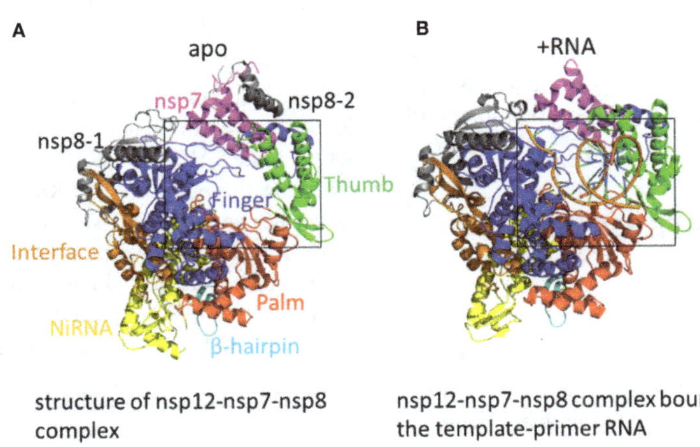

FIGURE 3 | **(A)** The structure of nsp12-nsp7-nsp8 complex. Color marks: nsp7, magenta; nsp8-1 and nsp8-2, grey; β-hairpin, cyan; NiRAN, yellow; the interface, orange; the fingers domain, blue; the palm domain, red; the thumb domain, green. (PDB: 6M71) **(B)** The structure of the SARS-CoV-2 RNA-dependent RNA polymerase (RdRp) in active form. The nsp12-nsp7-nsp8 complex bound to the template-primer RNA. (PDB: 7BV2).

which is formed by five nsp12 motifs A–E. Motif C interacts with the 3' end of RNA and includes the aspartic acid 760 and 761. The nsp12 motifs F and G lies in the fingers subdomain and have the function of positioning the RNA template. As the RNA duplex leaves the cleft of the RdRp, it forms a second helical turn, protruding from the surface of nsp12. No structural factors in the RdRp will limit RNA duplex extension. Between the α-helical extensions is the RNA duplex. The N-terminal regions, which are located in the two nsp8 subunits and are highly conserved, form the α-helical extensions. These nsp8 extensions use the positively charged residues to interact with the RNA backbones. The nsp8 could function as the "sliding poles", sliding along the protruding RNA to prevent RdRp from dissociating prematurely during replication. The triphosphate-binding site is conserved. Residues D623, S682, and N691 are likely to interacts with the 2'-OH group of the triphosphate (NTP), making the RdRp special for the synthesis of RNA instead of DNA (Hillen et al., 2020).

The Main Protease

The main protease (M^{pro}) of SARS-CoV-2 plays a pivotal role in mediating the replication and transcription of viral gene. M^{pro} hydrolyzes the polyprotein at least eleven conserved sites and begins with cleaving the pp1a and pp1b of M^{pro}. Considering the absence of closely related homologues in humans, together with the functional importance of the main protease in the life cycle of the virus, the main protease is an attractive antiviral target. The crystallographic symmetry shows that M^{pro} forms a homodimer (protomer A and protomer B). Each protomer contains three subdomains, namely domain I, domain II, and domain III. A long loop connects domain II and domain III. The cleft between domain I and domain II lies the substrate-binding pocket, which features the catalytic dyad residues His41 and Cys145 (Jin et al., 2020a). As to all the coronaviruses, the active sites of M^{pro} are highly conserved and consists of four sites: S1', S1, S2, and S4. In the S1' site, the thiol of a cysteine anchors inhibitors by a covalent linkage. For inhibitors, the covalent linkage is critical to maintain its antiviral activity (Yang et al., 2005).

The spike protein is critical in the process of SARS-CoV-2 invading host cells. The main protease and RdRp have important functions in the replication of SARS-CoV-2. As a result, the spike protein, main protease, and RdRp are important anti-SARS-CoV-2 drug targets, providing ideas for the development of antibodies, drugs, and vaccines.

STRUCTURE-BASED ANTIBODIES AGAINST SARS-COV-2

Meplazumab

Recently, the study indicates that SARS-CoV-2 invades host cells through a new route: CD147-spike protein, through which spike protein bound to CD147, a transmembrane glycoprotein belongs to the immunoglobulin superfamily, thereby mediating the invasion of SARS-CoV-2. Meplazumab is an anti-CD147 humanized antibody. It could block CD147 and significantly prevent the SARS-CoV-2 from entering host cells. BIOcore experiment shows that the affinity constant between CD147 and RBD is 1.85×10^{-7} M. Unlike ACE2, CD147 is highly expressed in inflamed tissues, pathogen infected cells, and tumor tissues. It has low cross-reaction with normal cells. As a result, CD147 targeted drugs are safe and reliable (Wang K. et al., 2020).

Monoclonal Antibody 4A8

One study isolated monoclonal antibodies (MAbs) from ten SARS-CoV-2 infected patients in recovery period. Among these antibodies, MAb 4A8, exhibits high neutralization activities against SARS-CoV-2. The crystal structure of spike protein-4A8 complex at 3.1 Å resolution shows that three 4A8 monoclonal antibodies binds the N-terminal domain (NTD) of the spike protein trimer. Each of the 4A8 monoclonal antibody interacts with one N-terminal domain (NTD) of the spike protein.

The crystal structure of spike protein-4A8 complex at 3.1 Å resolution shows that each one of the three 4A8 monoclonal antibodies binds to one N-terminal domain (NTD) of the spike protein trimer. The asymmertric conformation of the trimeric spike protein exhibits one of three RBD in "up" conformation and two RBDs in "down" conformation. The interface between 4A8 and the corresponding NTD is identical. Among the five new constructed loops for NTD which are designed as N1 which are designated as N1–N5, N3 and N5 loops dominate the interactions with 4A8. Three complementarity-determining regions (CDRs) which are designated as CDR1, CDR2, and CDR3 on the heavy chain of 4A8 binds with NTD. R246 on the N5 loop interacts with the Y27 and E31 of 4A8 on the CDR1. K150 and K147 on the N3 loop form salt bridges with E54 and E72 of 4A8 respectively. There are hydrogen bonds between K150 and 4A8-Y111, H146 and 4A8-T30 (Chi et al., 2020).

Monoclonal Antibody 47D11

A human monoclonal antibody (mAb) 47D11 is found to potently block SARS-CoV-2 infection. The target of 47D11 is the RBD and spike ectodomain (S_{ecto}) of the SARS-CoV-2 spike protein. The 47D11 binds to the RBD of SARS-CoV and SARS-CoV-2 with similar affinity constant. However, the binding affinity between 47D11 and SARS-CoV-2 S_{ecto} was lower than that of SARS-CoV. The binding of 47D11 to SARS-CoV-RBD and SARS-CoV-2-RBD did not compete with the binding of 47D11 to the ACE2 receptor on the cell surface (Wang C. et al., 2020). Despite the relatively high degree of structural similarity between the SARS-CoV RBD and the SARS-CoV-2 RBD, when using the three reported SARS-CoV RBD-directed monoclonal antibodies which have a strong binding to the SARS-CoV RBD, there is no detectable binding for any of the three mABs (S230, m396, 80R) at the tested concentration. Because of the different antigenicity, SARS-directed mAbs have no absolute cross reactions with SARS-CoV-2-directed mAbs (Wrapp et al., 2020).

Monoclonal Antibody CR3022

The SARS-CoV-specific antibody, which was discovered in the plasma of a SARS-infected patient in recovery period, CR3022, could also bind with the RBD of SARS-CoV-2 potently. After saturating the streptavidin biosensors which labelled with biotinylated SARS-CoV-2 RBD, followed by the mixture of

CR3022 and ACE2, the results indicated that the binding sites of CR3022 on RBD is different from ACE2. The mixture of CR3022 and CR3014 (a potent SARS-CoV-specific neutralizing antibody) neutralized SARS-CoV-2 in a collaborative way, with different epitopes on RBD. In conclusion, CR3022 has the potential to function as one kind of therapeutics, alone or with other neutralizing antibodies (Tian et al., 2020). The crystal structure of CR3022-RBD complex has been determined (**Figure 4A**). The light chain, heavy chain, and six CDR loops (H1, H2, H3, L1, L2, and L3) of CR3022 are used to interact with the RBD of SARS-CoV-2.

CR3022's recognition of SARS-CoV-2 is mainly mediated by hydrophobic interactions. As to SARS-CoV and SARS-CoV-2, 24 of 28 residues buried by antibody CR3022 are the same, which is the cause of the cross-reactivity of CR3022. Although the high similarities of sequence, the affinity between CR3022 and SARS-CoV RBD is much higher than the affinity between CR3022 and SARS-CoV-2 RBD, likely resulting from the non-conserved residues in the epitope. Only when the RBD is in the "up" conformation, the epitope of CR3022 is exposed. If only one RBD on the trimeric S protein is in the "up" conformation, there would exist some clashes between CR3022 and RBD to hinder the bind. First, the variable region of CR3022 collides with S2 subunit of RBD, as well as the adjacent RBD in "down" conformation. Second, the constant region of CR3022 collides with NTD. When the targeted-RBD are in the double-"up" conformation (at least two) with a slight rotation, the binding epitope of the RBD can be accessed by CR3022 and all the clashes can be resolved (Yuan et al., 2020).

Monoclonal Antibodies B38 and H4

The monoclonal antibodies B38 and H4 isolated from a convalescent patient display neutralization ability. The crystal structure of B38-RBD complex has been identified (**Figure 4B**). B38 and H4 are able to hinder the binding between SARS-CoV-2 RBD and cellular receptor ACE2. The epitopes of B38 and H4 on the RBD are different. As a result, B38 and H4 has the potential to function as the noncompeting monoclonal antibody pair to treat COVID-19. In infected lungs, B38 and H4 can reduce virus titers. The crystal structures of RBD-B38 indicates that two CDRs on the light chain and all the three CDRs on the heavy chain of CR3022 interacts with RBD. A total of 21 amino acids in the RBD binds with the heavy chain and 15 residues with the light chain. Among the 36 residues, only 15 residues are conserved between SARS-CoV and SARS-CoV-2. Hydrophilic interactions mediate most of the contacts between B38 and RBD. Water molecules play a significant role in the binding between SARS-CoV-2 RBD and B38. The comparison of RBD/B38-Fab complex and RBD/hACE2 complex shows no obvious conformational changes and 18 of 21 amino acids on the RBD are conserved between B38 and ACE2. This explains why antibody B38 blocks SARS-CoV-2 from binding to receptor ACE2 (Wu et al., 2020b).

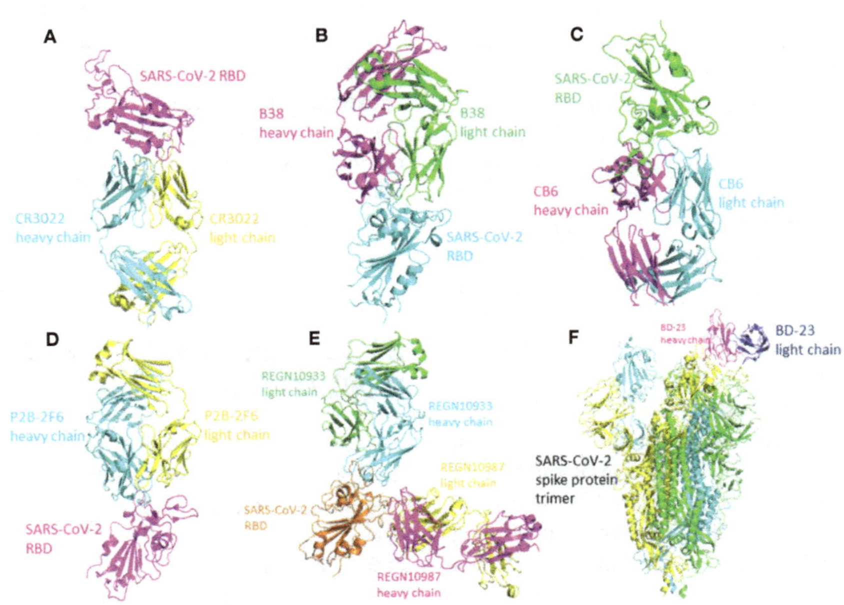

FIGURE 4 | The crystal structure of the antibody-RBD/spike protein complex. **(A)** Crystal structure of CR3022 in complex with SARS-CoV-2 RBD. CR3022 heavy chain is colored in cyan and light chain in yellow. The SARS-CoV-2 RBD in colored in magenta (PDB: 6W41). **(B)** The crystal structure of B38/SARS-CoV-2 RBD. The heavy chain of B38 is colored magenta and the light chain is colored green. The RBD is colored cyan (PDB: 7BZ5). **(C)** The crystal structure of CB6-Fab/SARS-CoV-2-RBD. The heavy chain of CB6 is colored magenta and the light chain of CB6 is colored cyan. The SARS-CoV-2-RBD is colored green (PDB: 7C01). **(D)** The crystal structure of P2B-2F6 Fab/SARS-CoV-2 RBD complex. The light chain of P2B-2F6 Fab is colored yellow and the heavy chain is colored cyan. The SARS-CoV-2 RBD is colored magenta (PDB: 7BWJ). **(E)** The crystal structure of the complex of SARS-CoV-2 spike RBD bound to Fab fragments of REGN10933 and REGN10987. REGN10933 heavy and light chains are cyan and green, and REGN10987 heavy and light chains are magenta and yellow, respectively (PDB: 6XDG). **(F)** The crystal structure of BD-23 Fab/spike protein trimer complex. The light chain of BD-23 Fab is colored blue and the heavy chain is colored magenta. The three protomers in the spike protein trimer are colored cyan **(A)**, green **(B)**, and yellow **(C)** (PDB: 7BYR).

Monoclonal Antibodies CA1 and CB6

Two human monoclonal antibodies CA1 and CB6 could potently neutralize the SARS-CoV-2 *in vitro*. Particularly, CB6 could reduce lung damage and inhibit the titer of SARS-CoV-2 in rhesus monkeys, thereby having the potential to treat and prevent SARS-CoV-2 infection. The crystal structure of CB6-Fab/SARS-CoV-2-RBD complex indicates that CB6 binds to the RBD of SARS-CoV-2 (**Figure 4C**). CDR1, CDR2, and CDR3 loops in the CB6 V_H dominate the interaction between the CB6 and SARS-CoV-2-RBD, forming concentrated hydrophobic interactions and polar contacts. CB6 light chain has limited interactions with SARS-CoV-2-RBD, with only one hydrogen bond between Y505 and Y92. The superimposition of CB6/SARS-CoV-2-RBD complex and hACE2/SARS-CoV2-RBD complex indicated the steric competition between hACE2 and CB6 for RBD binding. The steric hindrance caused by CB6 is dominated by both the light chain and heavy chain of CB6, thus resulting in structure clashes with the SARS-CoV-2-RBD. CB6 and hACE2 have many overlapping binding sites on the RBD. In conclusion, steric hindrance caused by the V_H and V_L of CB6 and the overlapped binding areas inhibit the binding of SARS-CoV-RBD and hACE2 (Shi R. et al., 2020).

Monoclonal Antibody P2B-2F6

Total 206 kinds of RBD-specific monoclonal antibodies have been isolated from the B cells of 8 COVID-19 patients. The most potent neutralizing antibodies are P2C-1F11, P2B-2F6, and P2C-1A3. The crystal structure of P2B-2F6/SARS-CoV-2 RBD complex has been determined at 2.85 Å resolution (**Figure 4D**). The interactions between P28-2F6 and the SARS-CoV-2 RBD is dominated by the heavy chain of P28-2F6. The paratope contains 3 light chain residues and 14 heavy chain residues. All the 12 epitopes residues are in the RBM, including lysine 444, glycine 446 and 447, asparagine 448, tyrosine 449, asparagine 450, leucine 452, valine 483, glutamic acid 484, glycine 485, phenylalanine 490, and serine 494. At the binding interface, there are hydrophobic interactions between P2B-2F6 and SARS-CoV-2 RBD residues Y449, L452, and F490, facilitating P2B-2F6 attachment. Hydrophilic interactions also exit at the binding interface. Structural superimposition of SARS-CoV-2 RBD/ACE2 complex and SARS-CoV-2 RBD/P2B-2F6 complex shows that the light chain of P2B-2F6 clashes with ACE2 residues aspartic acid 67, lysine 68, alanine 71, lysine 74, glutamic acid 110, and lysine 114, inhibiting the binding of ACE2 and RBD. The residues in RBD recognized by both P2B-2F6 and ACE2 are Y449 and G446. Compared with the binding affinity between ACE2 and RDB, the binding affinity between P2B-2F6 and RBD is higher. P2B-2F6 Fab could connect with both the "up" and "down" conformations of the RBDs of the trimer spike protein, while ACE2 only binds the "up" conformation of RBD (Ju et al., 2020).

Antibody Cocktail: REGN10987 and REGN10933

One study used both genetically modified mice and B cells from SARS-CoV-2 convalescent patients to collect monoclonal antibodies. It has been identified that REGN10987 and REGN10933 are a pair of highly potent individual antibodies. The epitope of REGN10933 is located at the top of the RBD while the epitope of REGN10987 is located at the side of the RBD. They can bind to the RBD of SARS-CoV-2 simultaneously without competition. As a result, REGN10987 and REGN10933 can be paired in a therapeutic antibody cocktail. The bind of REGN10933 to RBD overlap the binding site for ACE2 extensively. However, the binding of REGN10987 has no or little overlap with the binding site of ACE2. The crystal structure has been identified (Hansen et al., 2020) (**Figure 4E**).

Monoclonal Antibody BD-23

High-throughput single-cell RNA and VDJ sequencing were used to identify SARS-CoV-2 neutralizing antibodies from the B cells of 60 convalescent patients and 14 antibodies with strong neutralization ability were discovered, including the neutralizing antibody BD-23. The crystal structure of BD-23-Fab/spike protein at 3.8 Å resolution has been solved (**Figure 4F**). The spike adopts an asymmetric conformation. Two RBDs of the spike protein trimer adopt "down" conformation and the other adopts "up" conformation. Structural superimposition of SARS-CoV-2 RBD/ACE2 complex and SARS-CoV-2 RBD/BD-23 complex shows that BD-23 could clash with ACE2 to inhibit the RBD-ACE2 binding, endowing BD-23 with the SARS-CoV-2 neutralizing ability (Cao et al., 2020).

A variety of other antibodies are found targeting the spike protein of the SARS-CoV-2. Antibody n3130 and n3088 target the S_{RBD} and S1 subunit with the affinity of 55.4 nM (Wu et al., 2020a). Antibody S309 comes from B cells of SARS rehabilitation patients. It has cross-reaction with SARS-CoV and the affinity with its target S^B is 0.1 nM. The crystal structure of S309 has been identified (Pinto et al., 2020). Antibodies n3103, n3088, and S309 do not block the binding of SARS-CoV-2 with its receptor ACE2. Horse F(ab')2 comes from horse serum immunized with RBD and the affinity between F(ab')2 and RBD is 0.76 nM (Pan et al., 2020).

STRUCTURE-BASED SARS-COV-2 INHIBITORS

Currently, some small-molecule compounds have been developed which showed inhibitory effects on the SARS-CoV-2 infection, as described below.

Remdesivir

Remdesivir is an adenosine analogue and is a potent inhibitor of RdRp. Remdesivir could potently inhibit the replication of SARS-CoV-2 *in vitro*. Remdesivir shows broad-spectrum antiviral effects against RNA virus infection in cultured cells, nonhuman primate models, and mice. As an adenosine analogue, remdesivir functions after virus entry, *via* incorporating into nascent viral RNA to terminate the replication before the RNA become mature (Gurwitz, 2020). Remdesivir is a kind of prodrug. In target cells, it would transform into the triphosphate form (RTP) and become active (Siegel et al., 2017). Like other nucleotide analog prodrugs, remdesivir inhibits the RdRp activity through covalently binds the primer strand to terminate RNA chain. Upon adding ATP, the nsp12-nsp7-nsp8 complex exhibits the function of RNA polymerase. However, with the addition of the active triphosphate form of remdesivir (RTP), the RNA polymerization activity would be significantly inhibited. The structure of the apo RdRp is composed of nsp12, nsp7, and nsp8. Besides, the template-RTP RdRp complex is composed of a 14-base RNA in the template strand as well as 11-base RNA in the primer strand. Of note, the remdesivir is in the monophosphate form (RMP) in the complex. The RMP is covalently linked to the primer strand, three magnesium ions, and a pyrophosphate. The three magnesium ions locate near the active site and promote catalysis. The RMP locates in the catalytic active site center. The catalytic active site is composed of seven motifs. There are base-stacking interactions between RMP and the base of the primer strand in the upstream. Hydrogen bonds also exists between RMP and the uridine base of the template strand. There are also interactions between RMP and side chains (K545 and R555). Twenty-nine residues from nsp12 participate the binding of the RNA directly. No residue from nsp7 or nsp8 mediates the RNA interactions (Yin et al., 2020).

Similar to remdesivir, favipiravir is also an inhibitor of the RdRp. The structure of favipiravir resembles the endogenous guanine. Clinical trial demonstrated that favipiravir had little side effect as the first anti-SARS-CoV-2 compound conducted in China (Furuta et al., 2017; Tu et al., 2020).

N3

A mechanism-based inhibitor, N3, which was identified by the drug design aided by computer, could fit inside the substrate-binding pocket of the main protein and is a potent irreversible inhibitor of the main protein. Two of the Mpro-N3 complex associate to form a dimer (the two complexes are named protomer A and protomer B, respectively). Each protomer contains three domains which are designated as domain I–III. Both domain I and domain II have a β-barrel structure arranged in antiparallel manner. Domain III has five α-helices which associate to form a globular cluster structure in antiparallel manner. Domain III connects to domain II with a long loop. The cleft between domain I and domain II contains the substrate binding site. The backbone atoms of the compound N3 form an antiparallel sheet with residues 189–191 of the loop that connects domain II and domain III on one side, and with residues 164–168 of the long strand (residues 155–168) on the other (Jin et al., 2020a) (**Figure 5A**).

11a and 11b

Two compounds, namely 11a and 11b which target the M^{pro}, exhibit excellent inhibitory effects on SARS-CoV-2 infection *in vitro*. The inhibitory activity of 11a and 11b at 1 μM is 100 and 96%. In vivo, the 11a and 11b exhibit good pharmacokinetics (PK) properties. Of note, 11a showed low toxicity as well. The -CHO group of 11a and 11b bond to the cysteine 145 of M^{pro} covalently. Different parts of 11a (designated as P1', P1, P2, and P3) fits into different parts of the substrate-binding site. The (S)-γ-lactam ring of 11a at P1 inserts into the S1 site. The cyclohexyl moiety of 11a at P2 fits into the S2 site. At the part P3 of 11a, the indole group is exposed to the S4 site (in the solvent). The oxygen atom of -CHO forms a hydrogen bond with the cysteine 145 in the S1' site. In addition, many water molecules (designated as W1–W6) are critical for binding 11a. The SARS-CoV-2 M^{pro}-11b complex is similar to the SARS-CoV-2 M^{pro}-11a complex and the 11a and 11b exhibit similar inhibitor binding mode (Dai W. et al., 2020) (**Figures 5B, C**).

Camostat Mesylate

TMPRSS2 and TMPRSS4 are two mucosa-specific serine proteases which facilitate the fusogenic activity of SARS-CoV-2 spike protein and facilitate the virus to enter host cells (Zang et al., 2020). SARS-CoV-2 employs the TMPRSS2 in cells to prime the spike protein. TMPRSS2 activity is critical for the

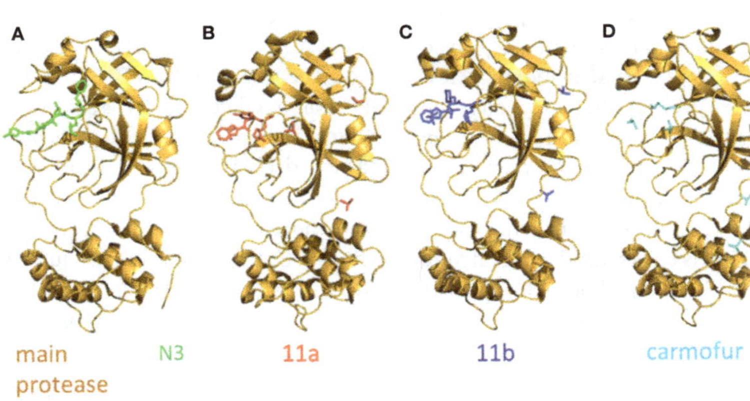

FIGURE 5 | The crystal structure of N3 and its inhibitors. **(A)** The crystal structure of N3-main protease complex. The main protease is colored brightorange. N3 is colored green (PDB: 6LU7). **(B)** The crystal structure of 11a-main protease complex. The main protease is colored brightorange, 11a is blue (PDB: 6LZE). **(C)** The crystal structure of 11b-main protease complex. The main protease is brightorange, 11b is red (PDB: 6M0K). **(D)** The crystal structure of Carmofur-main protease complex. The main protease is brightorange, carmofur is cyan (PDB: 7BUY).

spread of SARS-CoV-2 as well as the pathogenesis in the infected host. Therefore, TMPRSS2 is a potential antiviral target. The spectrum of cell lines mediated entry by the S protein of SARS-CoV-2 and SARS-CoV are similar. Camostat mesylate, a clinical TMPRSS2 inhibitor, can partially block SARS-CoV-2 spike-driven entry into lung cells. In addition, camostat mesylate exhibits potent inhibit activity on SARS-CoV, SARS-CoV-2, and MERS-CoV, inhibiting them from entering lung cell line Calu-3, without cytotoxicity. In conclusion, camostat mesylate has the potential to treat and prevent COVID-19 (Hoffmann et al., 2020).

Carmofur

The antineoplastic drug carmofur can inhibit the main protease (M^{pro}) of SARS-CoV-2. The crystal structure of carmofur-main protease complex has been solved. Carmofur inhibits the activity of SARS-CoV-2 main protein *in vitro* and the half-maximum inhibitory concentration (IC50) is 1.82 μM. Carmofur is an approved antineoplastic agent used for colorectal cancer. It is a derivative of 5-fluoroyracil (5-FU). The molecular details of how carmofur inhibits the activity of SARS-CoV-2 main protein have not been resolved. One study showed the crystal structure of SARS-CoV-2 M^{pro}-carmofur complex. The electron density figure indicates that the fatty acid moiety ($C_7H_{14}NO$) of carmofur links with the Sγ atom of SARS-CoV-2 main protein catalytic residue Cys145 covalently. The electrophilic carbonyl group of carmofur is attacked by the sulfhydryl group of Cys145. This process modifies the Cys145 covalently and releases the 5-FU motif. Notably, numerous hydrogen bonds and hydrophobic interactions stabilize the inhibitor carmofur. The fatty acid tail of carmofur (an extended conformation) inserts into the S2 subunit of SARS-CoV-2. Most of the hydrophobic interactions are contributed by His41, Met165, and Met49 in the side chain (Jin et al., 2020b) (**Figure 5D**).

Lipopeptide EK1C4

The complex (6-HB) formed by the HR1 and HR2 of the SARS-CoV-2 S protein could facilitate the infection of the viruses (Xia et al., 2020b). EK1 is one kind of coronavirus fusion inhibitor and has an inhibitory effect on various coronaviruses. It targets the HR1 of the S protein of human coronavirus and has been proved to effectively inhibit the infection of five HCoVs, including SARS-CoV and MERS-CoV. Peptide EK1 could intervene the formation of viral 6-HB (Xia et al., 2020a). A recent study shows that the peptide EK1 could also inhibit the membrane fusion mediated by SARS-CoV-2 spike protein as well as SARS-CoV-2 pseudovirus infection in a dose-dependent manner (Xia et al., 2020a; Xia et al., 2020b). EK1C is constructed by covalently attaching the cholesterol acid to the C-terminal of EK1 sequence. It is noteworthy that the lipopeptide EK1C4 has the strongest inhibitory effect on the membrane fusion which is mediated by the spike protein, with IC50 of 4.3 nM. However, the IC50 of EK1 is 409.3 nM. EK1C4 could also potently inhibit the infection caused by live coronavirus *in vitro* with little, or even no, toxic effect. In conclusion, EK1C4 has the potential to be used for the treatment and prevention of COVID-19 (Xia et al., 2020a).

VACCINES OF SARS-COV-2

It is urgent to develop effective and safe vaccines to control the new occurrence of COVID-19 and to reduce SARS-CoV-2-infection-related morbidity and mortality (Amanat and Krammer, 2020). Chinese Health Commission announced that more than five kinds of vaccines are currently developed for COVID-19 in China, including subunit protein vaccine, nucleic acid vaccine, inactivated vaccine, adenoviral vector vaccine, and influenza viral vector vaccine (Lu, 2020; Sun J. et al., 2020). As of October 17, 2020, there are 177 vaccine candidates for COVID-19 and 54 are in human trials in the world (https://biorender.com/covid-vaccine-tracker). For example, the non-replicating Ad5 vectored COVID-19 vaccine produced by CanSino Biologics lnc, the mRNA-1273 COVID-19 vaccine developed by Moderna, the DNA vaccine of Inovio Pharmaceuticals, the BioNTech's mRNA COVID-19 vaccine, the vaccine ChAdOx1 nCoV-19 of University of Oxford (Zhu et al., 2020), the adenovirus serotype 26 vector-based vaccine Ad26.COV2.S, the Novavax's protein subunit vaccine NVX-CoV2373, the Sinovac's inactive vaccine CoronaVac, the Chulalongkorn University's mRNA vaccine ChulaCov19, etc. (https://biorender.com/covid-vaccine-tracker). Currently, clinically approved vaccines are not widely available (Hu B. et al., 2020). The safety and efficacy of the vaccines should be kept in mind in the efforts of vaccine development. Following are some notable SARS-CoV-2 vaccines in development.

mRNA-1273

Moderna's mRNA-based vaccine stimulates the expression of target antigen after injection of mRNA encapsulated in nanoparticles (Amanat and Krammer, 2020). The vaccine is called mRNA-1273, it is a synthetic mRNA strand, which can encode the viral spike protein that is stable before fusion. After being injected into the body intramuscularly, the vaccine mRNA-1273 could stimulate antiviral response that targets the spike protein of SARS-CoV-2 specifically. Different from conventional route of vaccine development, the lipid mRNA nanoparticle-encapsulated mRNA vaccine can be synthesized and made without the virus (Tu et al., 2020). At present, mRNA-1273 has completed phase I clinical trial (ClinicalTrials.gov Identifier: NCT04283461) and phase II clinical trial. The results of the mRNA-1273 vaccine phase I clinical trial in 45 healthy adults (18–55 years old) show a strong antibody and cellular immune response in participants and no safety concerns are identified (Jackson et al., 2020). Phase II clinical trial is a dose-conformation study used to evaluate the safety, reactogenicity, and immunogenicity of mRNA-1273 in healthy adults. The phase III clinical trial has started on July 27, 2020 (ClinicalTrials.gov Identifier: NCT04470427). This is a randomized, stratified study to evaluate the efficacy, immunogenicity, and safety of the vaccine in healthy adults.

Recombinant Adenovirus Type-5 (Ad5) Vectored Vaccine

The phase I clinical trial of an Ad5 vectored COVID-19 vaccine has been done in Wuhan, China. The Ad5 vectored COVID-19 vaccine targets the spike protein of SARS-CoV-2. This trial is a dose-escalation, non-randomized, open-label, and first-in-human trial. The vaccine trial had three dose groups, including 5×10^{10}, 1×10^{11}, and 1.5×10^{11} viral particles. A total of 108 participants who were healthy and aged between 18–60 years old were allocated to one of the three dose group and each group contains 36 participants. The vaccine is injected intramuscularly into the human body. Results indicated that participants in all the dose groups exhibited at least one adverse reaction within 7 days post-vaccination. The most reported adverse reaction at the injection site was pain. Fever and fatigue were the most common systematic symptoms, 46 and 44% of the recipients exhibited such symptoms, respectively. However, most reported adverse reactions were mild or moderate in severity. Within 28 days after vaccination, no serious adverse reactions were reported. Humoral responses against SARS-CoV-2 peaked 28 days after vaccination in participants. From 14 days after vaccination, the specific T-cell responses were notable and rapid. Results demonstrate that this vaccine is immunogenic and tolerable in healthy adults and has the potential to control the outbreak of COVID-19. However, further investigations are needed to identify the immunogenicity and safety of this vaccine (Zhu et al., 2020). The phase II trial in China (NCT04341389) has started. This is a randomized, double-blinded and placebo-controlled clinical trial in healthy adults. The purpose of the study is to evaluate the safety and immunogenicity of Ad5 vectored vaccine.

PiCoVacc

In a recent study, a purified inactivated SARS-CoV-2 virus vaccine candidate (PiCoVacc) is developed in a pilot-scale production. The target of PiCoVacc is the entire virus. The study indicated that PiCoVacc could induce neutralizing antibodies which neutralized 10 representative SARS-CoV-2 strains in mice, rats, and non-human primates, suggesting its strong potential to neutralizing the other SARS-CoV-2 strains that are circulating. Six μg per dose of the PiCoVacc could protect the macaques from SARS-CoV-2 infection completely and systematic evaluation suggests its safety (Gao Q. et al., 2020).

DNA Vaccines

A recent study (Yu J. et al., 2020) has produced a series of DNA vaccine candidates which express six variants of the spike protein of the SARS-CoV-2. DNA vaccines targets the spike protein of SARS-CoV-2. The candidates were evaluated in 35 rhesus macaques. At week 0 and week 3, rhesus macaques were injected 5 mg DNA vaccines intramuscularly. S-specific binding antibodies and neutralizing antibodies (NAbs) were detected after the boost immunization at week 5. Neutralizing antibody (NAb) titers in the vaccinated macaques were comparable to the Nab titers in 9 convalescent rhesus macaques and 27 convalescent patients who were infected with SARS-CoV-2. Cellular immune responses targeting the S peptides were observed in most of the vaccinated rhesus macaques at week 5. At week 6, all rhesus macaques were challenged with 1.2×10^{8} VP SARS-CoV-2 intranasally and intratracheally. Compared to the control groups, lower levels of SARS-CoV-2 RNA were observed in the vaccine groups. Reduced levels of subgenomic mRNA (sgmRNA) in bronchoalveolar lavage (BAL) and nasal swabs (NS) were observed in vaccine groups. In conclusion, these DNA vaccines prevent rhesus macaques from being infected by SARS-CoV-2 and may accelerate the development of SARS-CoV-2 vaccine which are urgently needed to protect humans from SARS-CoV-2 infections.

A Universal Betacoronavirus Vaccine Against COVID-19, MERS, and SARS

The RBD of coronaviruses is an attractive vaccine target. However, RBD-based vaccines have relatively low immunogenicity. One study describes the dimeric form of MERS-CoV RBD. Compared to monomeric form, the RBD-dimer could expose double receptor-binding motifs and increase neutralizing antibody (NAb) titers significantly, so as to overcome the limitation of low immunogenicity. RBD-sc-dimer is a stable version of RBD-dimer with high vaccine efficacy. When using this strategy to design vaccines against SARS and COVID-19, 10–100-fold enhancement of Nab titers were achieved. Notably, the Nab titers caused by two-dose of RBD-sc-dimer is much higher than the RBD-sc-dimer, reaching ~4,096 (Dai L. et al., 2020).

On June 23, 2020, the clinical phase III trial of the inactivated SARS-CoV-2 vaccine developed by the SINOPHARM CNBG launched officially. This is the first international clinical phase III trial of inactivated SARS-CoV-2 vaccine. The clinical phase III trial takes about half a year to evaluate the safety and effectiveness of the vaccine in a larger population.

DISCUSSION

The rapid global pandemic of SARS-CoV-2 has already posed a great threat to human health, social health system, global economy, and even the global governance, and these influences may likely continue for a longer time. We need to learn the epidemic logic of SARS-CoV-2 and study the unknown viruses carried by wild animals in nature in advance to make early warning. There may be an outbreak caused by other kinds of viruses next time except for SARS-CoV-2. Study experiences and lessons on different viruses may be referenced each other.

Sufficient understanding on the differences of structural and non-structural proteins among SARS-CoVs and other coronaviruses may help to the development of therapeutics for SARS-CoV-2 infection. The non-structural proteins of the coronaviruses which can infect humans are relatively similar with SARS-CoV-2 in structure. Except S protein, most of the structural proteins, such as E protein and M protein, showed no significant difference in protein architecture between SARS-CoV-2 and other known human CoVs. The S protein of CoVs is responsible for binding the host cell-surface receptor during host cell entry. Different CoVs recognize different cell surface receptor. For instance, MERS-CoVs recognize the dipeptidyl peptidase 4 receptor. Nevertheless, SARS-CoV and SARS-CoV-2 recognize the ACE2 receptor. This may be the reason why different CoVs have various host entry mechanism. In addition, the SARS-CoV-2 RBD has higher hACE2 binding affinity than SARS-CoV RBD, supporting efficient cell entry. Unlike SARS-CoV, the entry of SARS-CoV-2 is preactivated by proprotein convertase furin, reducing its dependence on target cell proteases for entry. The high hACE2 binding affinity of the RBD and the furin preactivation of the spike allow SARS-CoV-2 to maintain efficient cell entry while evading immune surveillance. These features may contribute to the wide spread of the virus.

Due to the limited knowledge about SARS-CoV-2 at present, there is no approved therapeutic drugs or vaccines available for the treatment of COVID-19. As the global epidemic worsens, effective and safe vaccines, antibodies, and specific anti-SARS-CoV-2 drugs are in urgent need. Neutralizing antibodies are expected effective for SARS-CoV-2 infection, but their costs, production scales, and covering rates are still questions. Vaccine development also faces difficulties such as timeliness and ineffectiveness due to inconsiderate vaccine design and/or virus mutation.

Unlike the vaccine which has a relatively clear mechanism and route in development, antiviral drugs with high potency and high safety may be more difficult to develop at present because of our incomplete understanding on the virus world and the host responsiveness. This may be the reason why there is no one satisfactory antiviral drug available till now. The potential *in vivo* toxic effect of an antiviral drug which is claimed effective *in vitro* may disappointingly overwhelm its pharmacological applause. New and unconventional ideas and routes of antiviral drug design and development are needed to overcome the shortcomings of the present reductionism-based drug research. In this aspect, the holism-based traditional Chinese medicine especially the Chinese medical herb formulae could be considered which are proved effective in the fight against COVID-19 in China (Ang et al., 2020; Luo et al., 2020; Ren et al., 2020; Zhang et al., 2020a; Zhong et al., 2020), although further mechanistic studies and large-scale clinical trials are warranted.

Recently, many countries in the world have increased their investment in the research and development of antiviral drugs, antibodies, and vaccines. Accelerating the development of vaccines is likely the current keyway to solve this global disaster. Through joint efforts around the world, people can develop effective anti-SARS-CoV-2 technologies hopefully in the near future.

AUTHOR CONTRIBUTIONS

M-YW and RZ wrote the manuscript. L-JG and X-FG helped drew the figures. D-PW and J-MC revised the manuscript. All authors contributed to the article and approved the submitted version.

REFERENCES

Amanat, F., and Krammer, F. (2020). SARS-CoV-2 Vaccines: Status Report. *Immunity* 52, 583–589. doi: 10.1016/j.immuni.2020.03.007

Ang, L., Lee, H. W., Kim, A., Lee, J. A., Zhang, J., and Lee, M. S. (2020). Herbal medicine for treatment of children diagnosed with COVID-19: A review of guidelines. *Complement. Therapies Clin. Pract.* 39, 101174. doi: 10.1016/j.ctcp.2020.101174

Banerjee, A. K., Blanco, M. R., Bruce, E. A., Honson, D. D., Chen, L. M., Chow, A., et al. (2020). SARS-CoV-2 disrupts splicing, translation, and protein trafficking to suppress host defenses. *Cell.* S0092-8674, 31310-6. doi: 10.1016/j.cell.2020.10.004

Bansal, M. (2020). Cardiovascular disease and COVID-19. *Diabetes Metab. Syndrome* 14, 247–250. doi: 10.1016/j.dsx.2020.03.013

Berger, J. R. (2020). COVID-19 and the nervous system. *J. Neurovirol.* 26, 143–148. doi: 10.1007/s13365-020-00840-5

Brian, D. A., and Baric, R. S. (2005). Coronavirus genome structure and replication. *Curr. Topics Microbiol. Immunol.* 287, 1–30. doi: 10.1007/3-540-26765-4_1

Cao, Y., Su, B., Guo, X., Sun, W., Deng, Y., Bao, L., et al. (2020). Potent Neutralizing Antibodies against SARS-CoV-2 Identified by High-Throughput Single-Cell Sequencing of Convalescent Patients' B Cells. *Cell* 182, 73–84.e16. doi: 10.1016/j.cell.2020.05.025

Chan, J. F., Yuan, S., Kok, K. H., To, K. K., Chu, H., Yang, J., et al. (2020). A familial cluster of pneumonia associated with the 2019 novel coronavirus indicating person-to-person transmission: a study of a family cluster. *Lancet (London England)* 395, 514–523. doi: 10.1016/s0140-6736(20)30154-9

Chen, H., Guo, J., Wang, C., Luo, F., Yu, X., Zhang, W., et al. (2020). Clinical characteristics and intrauterine vertical transmission potential of COVID-19 infection in nine pregnant women: a retrospective review of medical records. *Lancet (London England)* 395, 809–815. doi: 10.1016/s0140-6736(20)30360-3

Chen, N., Zhou, M., Dong, X., Qu, J., Gong, F., Han, Y., et al. (2020). Epidemiological and clinical characteristics of 99 cases of 2019 novel coronavirus pneumonia in Wuhan, China: a descriptive study. *Lancet (London England)* 395, 507–513. doi: 10.1016/s0140-6736(20)30211-7

Chen, T., Wu, D., Chen, H., Yan, W., Yang, D., Chen, G., et al. (2020). Clinical characteristics of 113 deceased patients with coronavirus disease 2019: retrospective study. *BMJ (Clin. Res. Ed.)* 368, m1091. doi: 10.1136/bmj.m1091

Chi, X., Yan, R., Zhang, J., Zhang, G., Zhang, Y., Hao, M., et al. (2020). A neutralizing human antibody binds to the N-terminal domain of the Spike protein of SARS-CoV-2. *Sci. (N. Y. N.Y.)* 369, 650–655. doi: 10.1126/science.abc6952

Cui, J., Li, F., and Shi, Z. L. (2019). Origin and evolution of pathogenic coronaviruses. *Nat. Rev. Microbiol.* 17, 181–192. doi: 10.1038/s41579-018-0118-9

Dai, L., Zheng, T., Xu, K., Han, Y., Xu, L., Huang, E., et al. (2020). A Universal Design of Betacoronavirus Vaccines against COVID-19, MERS, and SARS. *Cell* 182, 722–733.e711. doi: 10.1016/j.cell.2020.06.035

Dai, W., Zhang, B., Jiang, X. M., Su, H., Li, J., Zhao, Y., et al. (2020). Structure-based design of antiviral drug candidates targeting the SARS-CoV-2 main protease. *Sci. (N. Y. N.Y.)* 368, 1331–1335. doi: 10.1126/science.abb4489

Daniloski, Z., Guo, X., and Sanjana, N. E.. (2020). The D614G mutation in SARS-CoV-2 spike increases transduction of multiple human cell types. *Preprint Server Biol.* doi: 10.1101/2020.06.14.151357

Deng, S. Q., and Peng, H. J. (2020). Characteristics of and Public Health Responses to the Coronavirus Disease 2019 Outbreak in China. *J. Clin. Med.* 9, 575. doi: 10.3390/jcm9020575

Deniz, M., and Tezer, H. (2020). Vertical transmission of SARS CoV-2: a systematic review. *J. Maternal-fetal Neonatal Med. Off. J. Eur. Assoc. Perinatal Med. Fed. Asia Oceania Perinatal Soc. Int. Soc. Perinatal Obstet.* doi: 10.1080/14767058.2020.1793322

Dong, L., Tian, J., He, S., Zhu, C., Wang, J., Liu, C., et al. (2020). Possible Vertical Transmission of SARS-CoV-2 From an Infected Mother to Her Newborn. *Jama* 323, 1846–1848. doi: 10.1001/jama.2020.4621

Du, R. H., Liang, L. R., Yang, C. Q., Wang, W., Cao, T. Z., Li, M., et al. (2020). Predictors of mortality for patients with COVID-19 pneumonia caused by SARS-CoV-2: a prospective cohort study. *Eur. Respirat. J.* 55, 2000524. doi: 10.1183/13993003.00524-2020

Egloff, C., Vauloup-Fellous, C., Picone, O., Mandelbrot, L., and Roques, P. (2020). Evidence and possible mechanisms of rare maternal-fetal transmission of SARS-CoV-2. *J. Clin. Virol. Off. Publ. Pan Am. Soc. Clin. Virol.* 128, 104447. doi: 10.1016/j.jcv.2020.104447

Fan, C., Lei, D., Fang, C., Li, C., Wang, M., Liu, Y., et al. (2020). Perinatal Transmission of COVID-19 Associated SARS-CoV-2: Should We Worry? *Clin. Infect. Dis. Off. Publ. Infect. Dis. Soc. America.* doi: 10.1093/cid/ciaa226

Furuta, Y., Komeno, T., and Nakamura, T. (2017). Favipiravir (T-705), a broad spectrum inhibitor of viral RNA polymerase. *Proc. Japan Acad. Ser. B. Phys. Biol. Sci.* 93, 449–463. doi: 10.2183/pjab.93.027

Gao, Q., Bao, L., Mao, H., Wang, L., Xu, K., Yang, M., et al. (2020). Rapid development of an inactivated vaccine candidate for SARS-CoV-2. *Science.* 369, 77–81. doi: 10.1126/science.abc1932

Gao, Y., Yan, L., Huang, Y., Liu, F., Zhao, Y., Cao, L., et al. (2020). Structure of the RNA-dependent RNA polymerase from COVID-19 virus. *Sci. (N. Y. N.Y.)* 368, 779–782. doi: 10.1126/science.abb7498

Ghinai, I., Woods, S., Ritger, K. A., McPherson, T. D., Black, S. R., Sparrow, L., et al. (2020a). Community Transmission of SARS-CoV-2 at Two Family Gatherings - Chicago, Illinois, February-March 2020. *MMWR. Morbidity Mortality Weekly Rep.* 69, 446–450. doi: 10.15585/mmwr.mm6915e1

Ghinai, I., McPherson, T. D., Hunter, J. C., Kirking, H. L., Christiansen, D., Joshi, K., et al. (2020b). First known person-to-person transmission of severe acute respiratory syndrome coronavirus 2 (SARS-CoV-2) in the USA. *Lancet (London England)* 395, 1137–1144. doi: 10.1016/s0140-6736(20)30607-3

Gralinski, L. E., and Menachery, V. D. (2020). Return of the Coronavirus: 2019-nCoV. *Viruses* 12, 135. doi: 10.3390/v12020135

Guan, W. J., Ni, Z. Y., Hu, Y., Liang, W. H., Ou, C. Q., He, J. X., et al. (2020). Clinical Characteristics of Coronavirus Disease 2019 in China. *New Engl. J. Med.* 382, 1708–1720. doi: 10.1056/NEJMoa2002032

Gurwitz, D. (2020). Angiotensin receptor blockers as tentative SARS-CoV-2 therapeutics. *Drug Dev. Res.* 81, 537–540. doi: 10.1002/ddr.21656

Haimei, M. A. (2020). Pathogenesis and Treatment Strategies of COVID-19-Related Hypercoagulant and Thrombotic Complications. *Clin. Appl. Thrombosis/Hemostasis Off. J. Int. Acad. Clin. Appl. Thrombosis/Hemostasis* 26:1076029620944497. doi: 10.1177/1076029620944497

Halfmann, P. J., Hatta, M., Chiba, S., Maemura, T., Fan, S., Takeda, M., et al. (2020). Transmission of SARS-CoV-2 in Domestic Cats. *New Engl. J. Med.* 383, 592–594. doi: 10.1056/NEJMc2013400

Hansen, J., Baum, A., Pascal, K. E., Russo, V., Giordano, S., Wloga, E., et al. (2020). Studies in humanized mice and convalescent humans yield a SARS-CoV-2 antibody cocktail. *Sci. (N. Y. N.Y.)* 369, 1010–1014. doi: 10.1126/science.abd0827

Hess, D. C., Eldahshan, W., and Rutkowski, E. (2020). COVID-19-Related Stroke. *Trans. Stroke Res.* 11, 322–325. doi: 10.1007/s12975-020-00818-9

Hillen, H. S., Kokic, G., Farnung, L., Dienemann, C., Tegunov, D., and Cramer, P. (2020). Structure of replicating SARS-CoV-2 polymerase. *Nature* 584, 154–156. doi: 10.1038/s41586-020-2368-8

Hoffmann, M., Kleine-Weber, H., Schroeder, S., Krüger, N., Herrler, T., Erichsen, S., et al. (2020). SARS-CoV-2 Cell Entry Depends on ACE2 and TMPRSS2 and Is Blocked by a Clinically Proven Protease Inhibitor. *Cell* 181, 271–280.e278. doi: 10.1016/j.cell.2020.02.052

Hu, B., Guo, H., Zhou, P., and Shi, Z.-L. (2020). Characteristics of SARS-CoV-2 and COVID-19. *Nat. Rev. Microbiol.* doi: 10.1038/s41579-020-00459-7

Hu, J., He, C., Gao, Q., Zhang, G., Cao, X., Long, Q., et al. (2020). The D614G mutation of SARS-CoV-2 spike protein enhances viral infectivity and decreases neutralization sensitivity to individual convalescent sera. *Preprint Server Biol.* doi: 10.1101/2020.06.20.161323

Hu, X., Gao, J., Luo, X., Feng, L., Liu, W., Chen, J., et al. (2020). Severe Acute Respiratory Syndrome Coronavirus 2 (SARS-CoV-2) Vertical Transmission in Neonates Born to Mothers With Coronavirus Disease 2019 (COVID-19) Pneumonia. *Obstetr. Gynecol.* 136, 65–67. doi: 10.1097/aog.0000000000003926

Huang, C., Wang, Y., Li, X., Ren, L., Zhao, J., Hu, Y., et al. (2020). Clinical features of patients infected with 2019 novel coronavirus in Wuhan, China. *Lancet (London England)* 395, 497–506. doi: 10.1016/s0140-6736(20)30183-5

Jackson, L. A., Anderson, E. J., Rouphael, N. G., Roberts, P. C., Makhene, M., Coler, R. N., et al. (2020). An mRNA Vaccine against SARS-CoV-2 - Preliminary Report. *New Engl. J. Med.* doi: 10.1056/NEJMoa2022483

Jin, Z., Du, X., Xu, Y., Deng, Y., Liu, M., Zhao, Y., et al. (2020a). Structure of M (pro) from SARS-CoV-2 and discovery of its inhibitors. *Nature* 582, 289–293. doi: 10.1038/s41586-020-2223-y

Jin, Z., Zhao, Y., Sun, Y., Zhang, B., Wang, H., Wu, Y., et al. (2020b). Structural basis for the inhibition of SARS-CoV-2 main protease by antineoplastic drug carmofur. *Nat. Struct. Mol. Biol.* 27, 529–532. doi: 10.1038/s41594-020-0440-6

Johnson, B. A., Xie, X., Kalveram, B., Lokugamage, K. G., Muruato, A., Zou, J., et al. (2020). Furin Cleavage Site Is Key to SARS-CoV-2 Pathogenesis. *Preprint Server Biol.* doi: 10.1101/2020.08.26.268854

Ju, B., Zhang, Q., Ge, J., Wang, R., Sun, J., Ge, X., et al. (2020). Human neutralizing antibodies elicited by SARS-CoV-2 infection. *Nature* 584, 115–119. doi: 10.1038/s41586-020-2380-z

Kim, Y.II, Kim, S. G., Kim, S. M., Kim, E. H., Park, S. J., Yu, K. M., et al. (2020). Infection and Rapid Transmission of SARS-CoV-2 in Ferrets. *Cell Host Microbe* 27, 704–709.e702. doi: 10.1016/j.chom.2020.03.023

Korber, B., Fischer, W. M., Gnanakaran, S., Yoon, H., Theiler, J., Abfalterer, W., et al. (2020). Spike mutation pipeline reveals the emergence of a more transmissible form of SARS-CoV-2. *Preprint Server Biol.* doi: 10.1101/2020.04.29.069054

Kochi, A. N., Tagliari, A. P., Forleo, G. B., Fassini, G. M., and Tondo, C. (2020). Cardiac and arrhythmic complications in patients with COVID-19. *J. Cardiovasc. Electrophysiol.* 31, 1003–1008. doi: 10.1111/jce.14479

Lai, C. C., Shih, T. P., Ko, W. C., Tang, H. J., and Hsueh, P. R. (2020). Severe acute respiratory syndrome coronavirus 2 (SARS-CoV-2) and coronavirus disease-2019 (COVID-19): The epidemic and the challenges. *Int. J. Antimicrobial Agents* 55, 105924. doi: 10.1016/j.ijantimicag.2020.105924

Lamers, M. M., Beumer, J., van der Vaart, J., Knoops, K., Puschhof, J., Breugem, T.II, et al. (2020). SARS-CoV-2 productively infects human gut enterocytes. *Sci. (N. Y. N.Y.)* 369, 50–54. doi: 10.1126/science.abc1669

Lan, J., Ge, J., Yu, J., Shan, S., Zhou, H., Fan, S., et al. (2020). Structure of the SARS-CoV-2 spike receptor-binding domain bound to the ACE2 receptor. *Nature* 581, 215–220. doi: 10.1038/s41586-020-2180-5

Lee, I. C., Huo, T.II, and Huang, Y. H. (2020). Gastrointestinal and liver manifestations in patients with COVID-19. *J. Chin. Med. Assoc. JCMA* 83, 521–523. doi: 10.1097/jcma.0000000000000319

Letko, M., Marzi, A., and Munster, V. (2020). Functional assessment of cell entry and receptor usage for SARS-CoV-2 and other lineage B betacoronaviruses. *Nat. Microbiol.* 5, 562–569. doi: 10.1038/s41564-020-0688-y

Li, W., Moore, M. J., Vasilieva, N., Sui, J., Wong, S. K., Berne, M. A., et al. (2003). Angiotensin-converting enzyme 2 is a functional receptor for the SARS coronavirus. *Nature* 426, 450–454. doi: 10.1038/nature02145

Li, F., Li, W., Farzan, M., and Harrison, S. C. (2005). Structure of SARS coronavirus spike receptor-binding domain complexed with receptor. *Sci. (N. Y. N.Y.)* 309, 1864–1868. doi: 10.1126/science.1116480

Li, R., Pei, S., Chen, B., Song, Y., Zhang, T., Yang, W., et al. (2020). Substantial undocumented infection facilitates the rapid dissemination of novel coronavirus (SARS-CoV-2). *Sci. (N. Y. N.Y.)* 368, 489–493. doi: 10.1126/science.abb3221

Li, F. (2016). Structure, Function, and Evolution of Coronavirus Spike Proteins. *Annu. Rev. Virol.* 3, 237–261. doi: 10.1146/annurev-virology-110615-042301

Li, W. (2020). Delving deep into the structural aspects of a furin cleavage site inserted into the spike protein of SARS-CoV-2: A structural biophysical perspective. *Biophys. Chem.* 264, 106420. doi: 10.1016/j.bpc.2020.106420

Liu, S., Xiao, G., Chen, Y., He, Y., Niu, J., Escalante, C. R., et al. (2004). Interaction between heptad repeat 1 and 2 regions in spike protein of SARS-associated coronavirus: implications for virus fusogenic mechanism and identification of fusion inhibitors. *Lancet (London England)* 363, 938–947. doi: 10.1016/s0140-6736(04)15788-7

Liu, Y., Mao, B., Liang, S., Yang, J. W., Lu, H. W., Chai, Y. H., et al. (2020). Association between age and clinical characteristics and outcomes of COVID-19. *Eur. Respirat. J.* 55, 2001112. doi: 10.1183/13993003.01112-2020

Lu, R., Zhao, X., Li, J., Niu, P., Yang, B., Wu, H., et al. (2020). Genomic characterisation and epidemiology of 2019 novel coronavirus: implications for virus origins and receptor binding. *Lancet (London England)* 395, 565–574. doi: 10.1016/s0140-6736(20)30251-8

Lu, X., Zhang, L., Du, H., Zhang, J., Li, Y. Y., Qu, J., et al. (2020). SARS-CoV-2 Infection in Children. *New Engl. J. Med.* 382, 1663–1665. doi: 10.1056/NEJMc2005073

Lu, S. (2020). Timely development of vaccines against SARS-CoV-2. *Emerg. Microbes Infect.* 9, 542–544. doi: 10.1080/22221751.2020.1737580

Luo, H., Tang, Q. L., Shang, Y. X., Liang, S. B., Yang, M., Robinson, N., et al. (2020). Can Chinese Medicine Be Used for Prevention of Corona Virus Disease 2019 (COVID-19)? A Review of Historical Classics, Research Evidence and Current Prevention Programs. *Chin. J. Integr. Med.* 26, 243–250. doi: 10.1007/s11655-020-3192-6

Mahyuddin, A. P., Kanneganti, A., Wong, J. J. L., Dimri, P. S., Su, L. L., Biswas, A., et al. (2020). Mechanisms and evidence of vertical transmission of infections in pregnancy including SARS-CoV-2s. *Prenatal Diagn.* doi: 10.1002/pd.5765

Meselson, M. (2020). Droplets and Aerosols in the Transmission of SARS-CoV-2. *New Engl. J. Med.* 382, 2063. doi: 10.1056/NEJMc2009324

Morawska, L., and Cao, J. (2020). Airborne transmission of SARS-CoV-2: The world should face the reality. *Environ. Int.* 139, 105730. doi: 10.1016/j.envint.2020.105730

Naqvi, A. A. T., Fatima, K., Mohammad, T., Fatima, U., Singh, I. K., Singh, A., et al. (2020). Insights into SARS-CoV-2 genome, structure, evolution, pathogenesis and therapies: Structural genomics approach. *Biochim. Biophys. Acta Mol. Basis Dis.* 1866, 165878. doi: 10.1016/j.bbadis.2020.165878

Oliveira, L. V., Silva, C., Lopes, L. P., and Agra, I. K. R. (2020). Current evidence of SARS-CoV-2 vertical transmission: an integrative review. *Rev. Da Associacao Med. Bras.* 1992) 66Suppl 2, 130–135. doi: 10.1590/1806-9282.66.S2.130

Pan, X., Zhou, P., Fan, T., Wu, Y., Zhang, J., Shi, X., et al. (2020). Immunoglobulin fragment F(ab')(2) against RBD potently neutralizes SARS-CoV-2 in vitro. *Antiviral Res.* 182, 104868. doi: 10.1016/j.antiviral.2020.104868

Parazzini, F., Bortolus, R., Mauri, P. A., Favilli, A., Gerli, S., and Ferrazzi, E. (2020). Delivery in pregnant women infected with SARS-CoV-2: A fast review. *Int. J. Gynaecol. Obstetr.: Off. Organ Int. Fed. Gynaecol. Obstetr.* 150, 41–46. doi: 10.1002/ijgo.13166

Paybast, S., Emami, A., Koosha, M., and Baghalha, F. (2020). Novel Coronavirus Disease (COVID-19) and Central Nervous System Complications: What Neurologist Need to Know. *Acta Neurol. Taiwanica* 29 (1), 24–31.

Peyronnet, V., Sibiude, J., Deruelle, P., Huissoud, C., Lescure, X., Lucet, J. C., et al. (2020). SARS-CoV-2 infection during pregnancy. Information and proposal of management care. CNGOF. *Gynecol. Obstetr. Fertilite Senol.* 48, 436–443. doi: 10.1016/j.gofs.2020.03.014

Pinto, D., Park, Y. J., Beltramello, M., Walls, A. C., Tortorici, M. A., Bianchi, S., et al. (2020). Structural and functional analysis of a potent sarbecovirus neutralizing antibody. *Preprint Server Biol.* doi: 10.1101/2020.04.07.023903

Ren, X., Shao, X. X., Li, X. X., Jia, X. H., Song, T., Zhou, W. Y., et al. (2020). Identifying potential treatments of COVID-19 from Traditional Chinese Medicine (TCM) by using a data-driven approach. *J. Ethnopharmacol.* 258, 112932. doi: 10.1016/j.jep.2020.112932

Salata, C., Calistri, A., Parolin, C., and Palù, G. (2019). Coronaviruses: a paradigm of new emerging zoonotic diseases. *Pathog. Dis.* 77, ftaa006. doi: 10.1093/femspd/ftaa006

Shang, J., Ye, G., Shi, K., Wan, Y., Luo, C., Aihara, H., et al. (2020). Structural basis of receptor recognition by SARS-CoV-2. *Nature* 581, 221–224. doi: 10.1038/s41586-020-2179-y

Shi, J., Wen, Z., Zhong, G., Yang, H., Wang, C., Huang, B., et al. (2020). Susceptibility of ferrets, cats, dogs, and other domesticated animals to SARS-coronavirus 2. *Sci. (N. Y. N.Y.)* 368, 1016–1020. doi: 10.1126/science.abb7015

Shi, R., Shan, C., Duan, X., Chen, Z., Liu, P., Song, J., et al. (2020). A human neutralizing antibody targets the receptor-binding site of SARS-CoV-2. *Nature* 584, 120–124. doi: 10.1038/s41586-020-2381-y

Sia, S. F., Yan, L. M., Chin, A. W. H., Fung, K., Choy, K. T., Wong, A. Y. L., et al. (2020). Pathogenesis and transmission of SARS-CoV-2 in golden hamsters. *Nature* 583, 834–838. doi: 10.1038/s41586-020-2342-5

Siegel, D., Hui, H. C., Doerffler, E., Clarke, M. O., Chun, K., Zhang, L., et al. (2017). Discovery and Synthesis of a Phosphoramidate Prodrug of a Pyrrolo[2,1-f][triazin-4-amino] Adenine C-Nucleoside (GS-5734) for the Treatment of Ebola and Emerging Viruses. *J. Med. Chem.* 60, 1648–1661. doi: 10.1021/acs.jmedchem.6b01594

Singla, R., Mishra, A., Joshi, R., Jha, S., Sharma, A. R., Upadhyay, S., et al. (2020). Human animal interface of SARS-CoV-2 (COVID-19) transmission: a critical appraisal of scientific evidence. *Veterinary Res. Commun.* 44, 119–130. doi: 10.1007/s11259-020-09781-01-12

Sit, T. H. C., Brackman, C. J., Ip, S. M., Tam, K. W. S., Law, P. Y. T., To, E. M. W., et al. (2020). Infection of dogs with SARS-CoV-2. *Nature* 586, 776–778. doi: 10.1038/s41586-020-2334-5

Sommerstein, R., Fux, C. A., Vuichard-Gysin, D., Abbas, M., Marschall, J., Balmelli, C., et al. (2020). Risk of SARS-CoV-2 transmission by aerosols, the rational use of masks, and protection of healthcare workers from COVID-19. *Antimicrobial Resist. Infect. Control* 9, 100. doi: 10.1186/s13756-020-00763-0

Sternberg, A., and Naujokat, C. (2020). Structural features of coronavirus SARS-CoV-2 spike protein: Targets for vaccination. *Life Sci.* 257, 118056. doi: 10.1016/j.lfs.2020.118056

Sun, J., Zhu, A., Li, H., Zheng, K., Zhuang, Z., Chen, Z., et al. (2020). Isolation of infectious SARS-CoV-2 from urine of a COVID-19 patient. *Emerg. Microbes Infect.* 9, 991–993. doi: 10.1080/22221751.2020.1760144

Sun, P., Lu, X., Xu, C., Sun, W., and Pan, B. (2020). Understanding of COVID-19 based on current evidence. *J. Med. Virol.* 92, 548–551. doi: 10.1002/jmv.25722

Tang, S., Mao, Y., Jones, R. M., Tan, Q., Ji, J. S., Li, N., et al. (2020). Aerosol transmission of SARS-CoV-2? Evidence, prevention and control. *Environ. Int.* 144, 106039. doi: 10.1016/j.envint.2020.106039

Tang, X., Wu, C., Li, X., Song, Y., Yao, X., Wu, X., et al. (2020). On the origin and continuing evolution of SARS-CoV-2. *Natl. Sci. Rev.* 7, 10121023. doi: 10.1093/nsr/nwaa036

Tian, X., Li, C., Huang, A., Xia, S., Lu, S., Shi, Z., et al. (2020). Potent binding of 2019 novel coronavirus spike protein by a SARS coronavirus-specific human monoclonal antibody. *Emerg. Microbes Infect.* 9, 382–385. doi: 10.1080/22221751.2020.1729069

Trejo-Gabriel-Galán, J. M. (2020). Stroke as a complication and prognostic factor of COVID-19. *Neurol. (Barcelona Spain)* 35, 318–322. doi: 10.1016/j.nrl.2020.04.015

Tu, Y. F., Chien, C. S., Yarmishyn, A. A., Lin, Y. Y., Luo, Y. H., Lin, Y. T., et al. (2020). A Review of SARS-CoV-2 and the Ongoing Clinical Trials. *Int. J. Mol. Sci.* 21, 2657. doi: 10.3390/ijms21072657

van Doremalen, N., Bushmaker, T., Morris, D. H., Holbrook, M. G., Gamble, A., Williamson, B. N., et al. (2020). Aerosol and Surface Stability of SARS-CoV-2 as Compared with SARS-CoV-1. *New Engl. J. Med.* 382, 1564–1567. doi: 10.1056/NEJMc2004973

Vivanti, A. J., Vauloup-Fellous, C., Prevot, S., Zupan, V., Suffee, C., Do Cao, J., et al. (2020). Transplacental transmission of SARS-CoV-2 infection. *Nat. Commun.* 11, 3572. doi: 10.1038/s41467-020-17436-6

Walls, A. C., Park, Y. J., Tortorici, M. A., Wall, A., McGuire, A. T., and Veesler, D. (2020). Structure, Function, and Antigenicity of the SARS-CoV-2 Spike Glycoprotein. *Cell* 181, 281–292.e286. doi: 10.1016/j.cell.2020.02.058

Wang, G., and Jin, X. (2020). The progress of 2019 novel coronavirus event in China. *J. Med. Virol.* 92, 468–472. doi: 10.1002/jmv.25705

Wang, C., Li, W., Drabek, D., Okba, N. M. A., van Haperen, R., Osterhaus, A., et al. (2020). A human monoclonal antibody blocking SARS-CoV-2 infection. *Nat. Commun.* 11, 2251. doi: 10.1038/s41467-020-16256-y

Wang, D., Hu, B., Hu, C., Zhu, F., Liu, X., Zhang, J., et al. (2020). Clinical Characteristics of 138 Hospitalized Patients With 2019 Novel Coronavirus-Infected Pneumonia in Wuhan, China. *Jama* 323, 1061–1069. doi: 10.1001/jama.2020.1585

Wang, K., Chen, W., Zhou, Y., Lian, J., Zhang, Z., Du, P., et al. (2020). SARS-CoV-2 invades host cells via a novel route: CD147-spike protein. *Preprint Server Biol.* doi: 10.1101/2020.03.14.988345

Wang, Q., Zhang, Y., Wu, L., Niu, S., Song, C., Zhang, Z., et al. (2020). Structural and Functional Basis of SARS-CoV-2 Entry by Using Human ACE2. *Cell* 181, 894–904.e899. doi: 10.1016/j.cell.2020.03.045

Wang, Y., Wang, Y., Chen, Y., and Qin, Q. (2020). Unique epidemiological and clinical features of the emerging 2019 novel coronavirus pneumonia (COVID-19) implicate special control measures. *J. Med. Virol.* 92, 568–576. doi: 10.1002/jmv.25748

Wrapp, D., Wang, N., Corbett, K. S., Goldsmith, J. A., Hsieh, C. L., Abiona, O., et al. (2020). Cryo-EM structure of the 2019-nCoV spike in the prefusion conformation. *Sci. (N. Y. N.Y.)* 367, 1260–1263. doi: 10.1126/science.abb2507

Wu, Z., and McGoogan, J. M. (2020). Characteristics of and Important Lessons From the Coronavirus Disease 2019 (COVID-19) Outbreak in China: Summary of a Report of 72 314 Cases From the Chinese Center for Disease Control and Prevention. *Jama* 323, 1239–1242. doi: 10.1001/jama.2020.2648

Wu, C., Chen, X., Cai, Y., Xia, J., Zhou, X., Xu, S., et al. (2020). Risk Factors Associated With Acute Respiratory Distress Syndrome and Death in Patients With Coronavirus Disease 2019 Pneumonia in Wuhan, China. *JAMA Internal Med.* 180, 934–943. doi: 10.1001/jamainternmed.2020.0994

Wu, Y., Li, C., Xia, S., Tian, X., Kong, Y., Wang, Z., et al. (2020a). Identification of Human Single-Domain Antibodies against SARS-CoV-2. *Cell Host Microbe* 27, 891–898.e895. doi: 10.1016/j.chom.2020.04.023

Wu, Y., Wang, F., Shen, C., Peng, W., Li, D., Zhao, C., et al. (2020b). A noncompeting pair of human neutralizing antibodies block COVID-19 virus binding to its receptor ACE2. *Science* 368, 1274–1278. doi: 10.1126/science.abc2241

Xia, S., Liu, M., Wang, C., Xu, W., Lan, Q., Feng, S., et al. (2020a). Inhibition of SARS-CoV-2 (previously 2019-nCoV) infection by a highly potent pan-coronavirus fusion inhibitor targeting its spike protein that harbors a high capacity to mediate membrane fusion. *Cell Res.* 30, 343–355. doi: 10.1038/s41422-020-0305-x

Xia, S., Zhu, Y., Liu, M., Lan, Q., Xu, W., Wu, Y., et al. (2020b). Fusion mechanism of 2019-nCoV and fusion inhibitors targeting HR1 domain in spike protein. *Cell. Mol. Immunol.* 17, 765–767. doi: 10.1038/s41423-020-0374-2

Xiao, K., Zhai, J., Feng, Y., Zhou, N., Zhang, X., Zou, J. J., et al. (2020). Isolation of SARS-CoV-2-related coronavirus from Malayan pangolins. *Nature* 583, 286–289. doi: 10.1038/s41586-020-2313-x

Xiong, C., Jiang, L., Chen, Y., and Jiang, Q. (2020). Evolution and variation of 2019-novel coronavirus. *Preprint Server Biol.* doi: 10.1101/2020.01.30.926477

Xu, Y., Li, X., Zhu, B., Liang, H., Fang, C., Gong, Y., et al. (2020). Characteristics of pediatric SARS-CoV-2 infection and potential evidence for persistent fecal viral shedding. *Nat. Med.* 26, 502–505. doi: 10.1038/s41591-020-0817-4

Yang, Z., and Liu, Y. (2020). Vertical Transmission of Severe Acute Respiratory Syndrome Coronavirus 2: A Systematic Review. *Am. J. Perinatol.* 37, 1055–1060. doi: 10.1055/s-0040-1712161

Yang, H., Xie, W., Xue, X., Yang, K., Ma, J., Liang, W., et al. (2005). Design of wide-spectrum inhibitors targeting coronavirus main proteases. *PLoS Biol.* 3, e324. doi: 10.1371/journal.pbio.0030324

Yang, X., Yu, Y., Xu, J., Shu, H., Xia, J., Liu, H., et al. (2020). Clinical course and outcomes of critically ill patients with SARS-CoV-2 pneumonia in Wuhan, China: a single-centered, retrospective, observational study. *Lancet Respiratory Med.* 8, 475–481. doi: 10.1016/s2213-2600(20)30079-5

Ye, Z. W., Yuan, S., Yuen, K. S., Fung, S. Y., Chan, C. P., and Jin, D. Y. (2020). Zoonotic origins of human coronaviruses. *Int. J. Biol. Sci.* 16, 1686–1697. doi: 10.7150/ijbs.45472

Yin, W., Mao, C., Luan, X., Shen, D. D., Shen, Q., Su, H., et al. (2020). Structural basis for inhibition of the RNA-dependent RNA polymerase from SARS-CoV-2 by remdesivir. *Sci. (N. Y. N.Y.)* 368, 1499–1504. doi: 10.1126/science.abc1560

Yu, J., Tostanoski, L. H., Peter, L., Mercado, N. B., McMahan, K., Mahrokhian, S. H., et al. (2020). DNA vaccine protection against SARS-CoV-2 in rhesus macaques. *Sci. (N. Y. N.Y.)* 369, 806–811. doi: 10.1126/science.abc6284

Yu, P., Zhu, J., Zhang, Z., and Han, Y. (2020). A Familial Cluster of Infection Associated With the 2019 Novel Coronavirus Indicating Possible Person-to-Person Transmission During the Incubation Period. *J. Infect. Dis.* 221, 1757–1761. doi: 10.1093/infdis/jiaa077

Yuan, M., Wu, N. C., Zhu, X., Lee, C. D., So, R. T. Y., Lv, H., et al. (2020). A highly conserved cryptic epitope in the receptor binding domains of SARS-CoV-2 and SARS-CoV. *Sci. (N. Y. N.Y.)* 368, 630–633. doi: 10.1126/science.abb7269

Zang, R., Gomez Castro, M. F., McCune, B. T., Zeng, Q., Rothlauf, P. W., Sonnek, N. M., et al. (2020). TMPRSS2 and TMPRSS4 promote SARS-CoV-2 infection of human small intestinal enterocytes. *Sci. Immunol.* 5, eabc358. doi: 10.1126/sciimmunol.abc3582

Zhang, C., Zheng, W., Huang, X., Bell, E. W., Zhou, X., and Zhang, Y. (2020). Protein Structure and Sequence Reanalysis of 2019-nCoV Genome Refutes Snakes as Its Intermediate Host and the Unique Similarity between Its Spike Protein Insertions and HIV-1. *J. Proteome Res.* 19, 1351–1360. doi: 10.1021/acs.jproteome.0c00129

Zhang, L., Yu, J., Zhou, Y., Shen, M., and Sun, L. (2020a). Becoming a Faithful Defender: Traditional Chinese Medicine against Coronavirus Disease 2019 (COVID-19). *Am. J. Chin. Med.* 48, 763–777. doi: 10.1142/s0192415x2050038x

Zhang, L., Jackson, C. B., Mou, H., Ojha, A., Rangarajan, E. S., Izard, T., et al. (2020b). The D614G mutation in the SARS-CoV-2 spike protein reduces S1 shedding and increases infectivity. *Preprint Server Biol.* doi: 10.1101/2020.06.12.148726

Zhang, R., Li, Y., Zhang, A. L., Wang, Y., and Molina, M. J. (2020). Identifying airborne transmission as the dominant route for the spread of COVID-19. *Proc. Natl. Acad. Sci. U. S. A.* 117, 14857–14863. doi: 10.1073/pnas.2009637117

Zhang, T., Wu, Q., and Zhang, Z. (2020). Probable Pangolin Origin of SARS-CoV-2 Associated with the COVID-19 Outbreak. *Curr. Biol. CB* 30, 1346–1351.e1342. doi: 10.1016/j.cub.2020.03.022

Zhong, L. L. D., Lam, W. C., Yang, W., Chan, K. W., Sze, S. C. W., Miao, J., et al. (2020). Potential Targets for Treatment of Coronavirus Disease 2019 (COVID-19): A Review of Qing-Fei-Pai-Du-Tang and Its Major Herbs. *Am. J. Chin. Med.* 48, 1051–1071. doi: 10.1142/s0192415x20500512

Zhou, F., Yu, T., Du, R., Fan, G., Liu, Y., Liu, Z., et al. (2020). Clinical course and risk factors for mortality of adult inpatients with COVID-19 in Wuhan, China: a retrospective cohort study. *Lancet (London England)* 395, 1054–1062. doi: 10.1016/s0140-6736(20)30566-3

Zhou, J., Li, C., Liu, X., Chiu, M. C., Zhao, X., Wang, D., et al. (2020). Infection of bat and human intestinal organoids by SARS-CoV-2. *Nat. Med.* 26, 1077–1083. doi: 10.1038/s41591-020-0912-6

Zhou, P., Yang, X. L., Wang, X. G., Hu, B., Zhang, L., Zhang, W., et al. (2020). A pneumonia outbreak associated with a new coronavirus of probable bat origin. *Nature* 579, 270–273. doi: 10.1038/s41586-020-2012-7

Zhu, F. C., Li, Y. H., Guan, X. H., Hou, L. H., Wang, W. J., Li, J. X., et al. (2020). Safety, tolerability, and immunogenicity of a recombinant adenovirus type-5 vectored COVID-19 vaccine: a dose-escalation, open-label, non-randomised, first-in-human trial. *Lancet (London England)* 395, 1845–1854. doi: 10.1016/s0140-6736(20)31208-3

10

Deleterious Effects of SARS-CoV-2 Infection on Human Pancreatic Cells

Syairah Hanan Shaharuddin[1,2†], Victoria Wang[1,2†], Roberta S. Santos[1,2†], Andrew Gross[1,2], Yizhou Wang[3,4], Harneet Jawanda[5], Yi Zhang[5], Wohaib Hasan[3,5,6], Gustavo Garcia Jr.[7], Vaithilingaraja Arumugaswami[7,8] and Dhruv Sareen[1,2,3,9*]*

[1] Board of Governors Regenerative Medicine Institute, Cedars-Sinai Medical Center, Los Angeles, CA, United States, [2] Cedars-Sinai Biomanufacturing Center, Cedars-Sinai Medical Center, Los Angeles, CA, United States, [3] Department of Biomedical Sciences, Cedars-Sinai Medical Center, Los Angeles, CA, United States, [4] Genomics Core, Cedars-Sinai Medical Center, Los Angeles, CA, United States, [5] Biobank and Translational Research Core, Samuel Oschin Comprehensive Cancer Institute (SOCCI), Cedars-Sinai Medical Center, Los Angeles, CA, United States, [6] Department of Pathology and Laboratory Medicine, Cedars-Sinai Medical Center, Los Angeles, CA, United States, [7] Department of Molecular and Medical Pharmacology, David Geffen School of Medicine, University of California, Los Angeles, Los Angeles, CA, United States, [8] Eli and Edythe Broad Center of Regenerative Medicine and Stem Cell Research, University of California, Los Angeles, Los Angeles, CA, United States, [9] iPSC Core, David and Janet Polak Foundation Stem Cell Core Laboratory, Cedars-Sinai Medical Center, Los Angeles, CA, United States

***Correspondence:**
Dhruv Sareen
dhruv.sareen@cshs.org
Vaithilingaraja Arumugaswami
varumugaswami@mednet.ucla.edu

[†]These authors have contributed equally to this work

COVID-19 pandemic has infected more than 154 million people worldwide and caused more than 3.2 million deaths. It is transmitted by the Severe Acute Respiratory Syndrome Coronavirus 2 (SARS-CoV-2) and affects the respiratory tract as well as extra-pulmonary systems, including the pancreas, that express the virus entry receptor, Angiotensin-Converting Enzyme 2 (ACE2) receptor. Importantly, the endocrine and exocrine pancreas, the latter composed of ductal and acinar cells, express high levels of ACE2, which correlates to impaired functionality characterized as acute pancreatitis observed in some cases presenting with COVID-19. Since acute pancreatitis is already one of the most frequent gastrointestinal causes of hospitalization in the U.S. and the majority of studies investigating the effects of SARS-CoV-2 on the pancreas are clinical and observational, we utilized human iPSC technology to investigate the potential deleterious effects of SARS-CoV-2 infection on iPSC-derived pancreatic cultures containing endocrine and exocrine cells. Interestingly, iPSC-derived pancreatic cultures allow SARS-CoV-2 entry and establish infection, thus perturbing their normal molecular and cellular phenotypes. The infection increased a key cytokine, CXCL12, known to be involved in inflammatory responses in the pancreas. Transcriptome analysis of infected pancreatic cultures confirmed that SARS-CoV-2 hijacks the ribosomal machinery in these cells. Notably, the SARS-CoV-2 infectivity of the pancreas was confirmed in post-mortem tissues from COVID-19 patients, which showed co-localization of SARS-CoV-2 in pancreatic endocrine and exocrine cells and increased the expression of some pancreatic ductal stress response genes. Thus, we demonstrate that SARS-CoV-2 can directly infect human iPSC-derived pancreatic cells with strong supporting evidence of presence of the virus in post-mortem pancreatic tissue of confirmed COVID-19 human cases. This novel model of iPSC-derived pancreatic cultures will open new avenues for the comprehension of the SARS-CoV-2 infection and potentially establish a platform for endocrine and exocrine pancreas-specific antiviral drug screening.

Keywords: COVID-19, SARS-CoV-2, iPSCs, pancreas, acinar cells, ductal cells, islets, pancreatitis

INTRODUCTION

The novel coronavirus disease 2019 (COVID-19), caused by SARS-CoV-2 (Severe Acute Respiratory Syndrome Coronavirus-2), initiated in China at the end of 2019 and rapidly escalated to global outbreak, infecting more than 154 million people and resulting in related fatalities in more than 3.2 million by beginning of May 2021 (JHU Dataset 2021). Although predominantly considered a respiratory disease, nearly one quarter of COVID-19 patients present other symptoms not related to the respiratory tract but to the gastrointestinal (GI) system (Cevik et al., 2020; Liu et al., 2020). SARS-CoV-2 enters host cells through binding of virus Spike protein (S) to ACE2 (Angiotensin-Converting Enzyme 2) receptor and activation of the virus by TMPRSS2 (Transmembrane Protease, serine 2). Interestingly, many other cells besides lung alveolar epithelial cells express ACE2 receptors, including heart, pancreas, GI tract, kidney, testis and other organs (Liu et al., 2020), thus making them a target for the virus. This is supported by studies demonstrating that virus can affect other tissues, including the heart (Sharma et al., 2020), vascular endothelial cells (Varga et al., 2020), kidney (Pelayo et al., 2020), liver (Amin, 2020) and the pancreas (Mukherjee et al., 2020; Pinte and Baicus, 2020; Tuttolomondo et al., 2020; Müller et al., 2021).

The pancreas, specifically the exocrine compartment (acinar and ductal cells), has high expression of ACE2 as analyzed by bulk RNA-seq data (GTEx database) and single-cell RNA-seq of the pancreas (NCBI-GEO database) (Liu et al., 2020). GTEx and TCGA (Genomic Data Commons Data Portal) datasets from human pancreas indicate no differences in ACE2 expression between males or females, as well as between younger (age ≤ 49 years) and older (age ≥ 49 years) populations (Li et al., 2020). In addition, recent findings have shown protein expression of ACE2 and TMPRSS2 in pancreatic cells from healthy humans, both in the endocrine and exocrine pancreas (Coate et al., 2020; Kusmartseva et al., 2020; Müller et al., 2021). Furthermore, few clinical reports provide evidence that some patients infected with SARS-CoV-2 who never presented pancreatic injuries show signs of acute pancreatitis-like symptoms, including elevated levels of serum amylase and lipase, and enlargement of the pancreas as seen in imaging evaluation (Kumaran et al., 2020; Liu et al., 2020). SARS-CoV-2 infection of the pancreas is certainly plausible as pancreatic ductal, acinar and islet cells express ACE2, so the virus could spread from the duodenal epithelium to the pancreas duct and then to acinar and islet cells. In fact, the virus was isolated easily from stool and from a pseudocyst of a COVID-19 patient with acute pancreatitis (de-Madaria and Capurso, 2021).

Acute pancreatitis is the major GI cause of hospitalization in the U.S.A., and despite the most common etiologies of this disease being related to gallstones and alcohol abuse, 10% of the cases are caused by infectious microorganisms including viruses (Rawla et al., 2017). Pertinent to the endocrine pancreas, it is now well-established that patients with type I (T1D) and II (T2D) diabetes have a higher risk for COVID-19 associated mortality, especially patients with associated comorbidities such as cardiovascular diseases and renal impairment, as indicated by a study with a large cohort of diabetic patients infected with SARS-CoV-2 (Holman et al., 2020). Diabetic patients (mostly T2D) infected with SARS-CoV-2 presented worse outcomes compared to non-diabetic patients, such as admission to the ICU, mechanical ventilation requirement and higher mortality rates (Apicella et al., 2020). These results were sustained by the *in vitro* evidence where replication of SARS-CoV-2 was demonstrated within pancreatic islet cultures, which led to impaired glucose-stimulated insulin secretion (Müller et al., 2021). Nevertheless, there is a paucity of knowledge whether and how SARS-CoV-2 can infect and impact the pancreas. This highlights the need for additional investigations to dissect and understand the potential influence of SARS-CoV-2 on human endocrine and exocrine pancreas.

Since primary human pancreatic cells are largely inaccessible and established cell lines do not fully represent human pancreas pathophysiology, we have developed novel methods to generate pancreatic progenitors from human induced pluripotent stem cells (iPSCs), which can be differentiated into endocrine (islet β-cells) and exocrine (acinar and ductal) cells. These cultures contain cells that are representative of human endocrine pancreas expressing endocrine NKX6.1 and C-peptide, exocrine acinar Amylase and Chymotrypsin (CTRC) and exocrine ductal Cytokeratin19 (CK19) and SOX9 cells. We show that iPSC-derived pancreatic cells including endocrine and exocrine cell types allow SARS-CoV-2 entry and establish infection, resulting in morphological perturbations as well as impaired expression of key markers. Importantly, these cellular phenotypes corresponded with inflammatory signatures. Infection of pancreatic tissue was also confirmed in post-mortem pancreatic tissues from COVID-19 patients. Thus, these results suggest the pancreatic cells can be directly infected by SARS-CoV-2. The iPSC-based model described here provides a valuable novel platform for understanding the pancreas-specific cellular responses to SARS-CoV-2 as well as for antiviral drug development against SARS-CoV-2.

METHODS

Human iPSC Culture

The induced pluripotent stem cell (iPSC) line, CS0007iCTR-n7, utilized in this study was generated from a healthy volunteer at the iPSC Core at Cedars-Sinai Medical Center from the peripheral blood mononuclear cells (PMBCs) utilizing non-integrating oriP/EBNA1-based episomal plasmid vectors, as described in (Rajamani et al., 2018). This approach results in highly cytogenetically stable iPSCs as tested by G-band karyotyping. All undifferentiated iPSCs were maintained in mTeSR$^+$ media (StemCell Technologies, Cat 05825) onto BD Matrigel™ matrix-coated plates.

Generation of iPSC-differentiated Pancreatic Progenitors.

iPSCs were single-cell dissociated using Accutase and plated onto Matrigel-coated plates at a density of 300,000 cells/cm^2 using mTeSR$^+$ and 10 μM Rho kinase Inhibitor (Stem Cell Tech). The following day, cells were directed into Definitive Endoderm (DE) using Phase I medium, which was composed of base medium MCDB 131 (Fisher Sci) supplemented with 100 ng/ml Activin A (R&D), 2 μM CHIR99021 (Stemgent), and 10 μM Rho kinase Inhibitor (Stem Cell Tech.) for 1 day. For the next two days, the same base medium was used, but supplemented instead with 100 ng/mL Activin A and 5 ng/mL FGF2 (Peprotech). Following this phase, cells were directed to form Posterior Foregut (PFG) using Phase II medium, which was composed of the same base medium as Phase I but supplemented with 50 ng/mL FGF10 (Peprotech), 0.25 μM CHIR99021 and 50 ng/ml Noggin (Peprotech), for 2 days. To reach a Pancreatic Progenitor (PP) stage, cells were fed with Phase III medium, which was composed of DMEM supplemented with 50 ng/mL Noggin, 50 ng/mL FGF10, 2 μM Retinoic Acid (Sigma), and 0.25 μM SANT1 (Sigma), for four days. More details about base medium formulation are described at **Supplementary Table 1**. This protocol was based on a published protocol to differentiate iPSCs into Pancreatic Progenitors (Memon et al., 2018).

Generation of iPSC-Differentiated Pancreatic Endocrine (iPan^{ENDO}), Acinar (iPan^{EXO} Acinar), and Ductal (iPan^{EXO} Ductal) Cells

To generate iPan^{EXO} Ductal cells, on Day 7 of differentiation, cells were single cell dissociated and seeded at 103.1k cells/cm^2 in Phase III medium supplemented with 10 μM Rho kinase Inhibitor on a Matrigel-coated plate. From Day 8 to Day 26, cells were grown in iPan^{EXO} Ductal phase media, which consisted of Phase III base medium supplemented with 25 ng/ml FGF10, 50 ng/ml EGF (Peprotech), and 25 ng/ml sDLL-1 (Peprotech). To generate iPan^{ENDO} and iPan^{EXO} Acinar cells, based on Hohwieler et al. (2017) protocol, after 4 days of Phase III media, PPs were fed with Phase III base medium supplemented with 20 ng/mL FGF10, 1μM XXI (Sigma Aldrich), 50 ng/mL Noggin, 10 mM Nicotinamide (Sigma-Aldrich), and 25 ng/mL Wnt3a (Peprotech) for seven days, daily feeding (Hohwieler et al., 2017). More details about base medium formulation are described at **Supplementary Table 1**.

Generation and Maintenance of iPan^{EXO} Organoid Cultures

On the last day of Phase III, PPs were roughly dissociated *via* scraping and trituration. They were centrifuged at 170 x G for 3 minutes, and then resuspended with a solution composed of Phase III medium and Matrigel at a 1:4 ratio (1 of medium and 4 of Matrigel). 30 μL of this solution with cells was plated into each well of a 96 round bottom plate and then incubated at 37°C for 20 minutes, before the plate was flipped upside down for 10 minutes. 100 μL of Phase III base medium supplemented with 20 ng/mL FGF10, 50 ng/mL Noggin, 10 mM Nicotinamide, and 25 ng/mL Wnt3a was then added to the cells. Cells were fed every other day with the same media until Day 57 or when organoids contained lumen and were at least 150 μm large.

SARS-CoV-2 Stock

SARS-CoV-2, isolate USA-WA1/2020, was obtained from the Biodefense and Emerging Infections (BEI) Resources of the National Institute of Allergy and Infectious Diseases (NIAID). Importantly, all studies involving SARS-CoV-2 infection of iPSC-derived pancreatic cells were conducted within a Biosafety Level 3 high containment facility at UCLA. SARS-CoV-2 was passed once in Vero-E6 cells and viral stocks were aliquoted and stored at – 80°C. Virus titer was measured in Vero-E6 cells by TCID50 assay. Vero-E6 cells were cultured in DMEM growth media containing 10% FBS, 2 mM glutamine, pen/step, and 10 mM HEPES. Cells were incubated at 37°C with 5% CO_2.

SARS-CoV-2 Infection of iPSC-Derived Pancreatic (iPan) Cultures

SARS-CoV-2 viral inoculum (MOI of 0.05 and 0.1) was prepared using acinar or ductal cell specific media. Human iPSCs were differentiated into iPSC-derived pancreatic (iPan) cultures containing iPan^{ENDO}, iPan^{EXO} Acinar and iPan^{EXO} Ductal cells in 96-well or 24-well plates before infection as detailed above, and the culture media at Day 26 of differentiation for iPan^{EXO} Ductal and Day 16 for iPan^{EXO} Acinar were replaced with 100 μl of prepared inoculum. For mock infection, cell type specific media (100 μl/well) alone was added. The inoculated plates were incubated for 1 hour at 37°C with 5% CO_2. At the end of incubation, the inoculum was replaced with fresh iPan^{EXO} Acinar or iPan^{EXO} Ductal culture medium. Cells remained at 37°C with 5% CO_2 for 24 hours (Day 1) or 72 hours (Day 3) before analysis. All studies involving active SARS-CoV-2 infection of iPSC-derived pancreatic cell cultures were conducted within a Biosafety Level 3 facility at University of California in Los Angeles (UCLA), CA, USA.

Immunofluorescence and Imaging of Cells

Cells subjected to immunofluorescence were fixed with 4% paraformaldehyde (PFA) in phosphate-buffered saline (PBS) for 20 minutes and subsequently washed with PBS. Fixed cells were then permeabilized and blocked for 1 hour in a blocking buffer containing PBS with 10% donkey serum (Millipore) and 0.1% Triton-X (Bio-Rad). Primary antibodies were diluted in the blocking buffer and added to the cells overnight at 4°C. The following primary antibodies and dilutions were used: SARS Coronavirus (1:400, NR-10361, BEI Resources), SARS-CoV-2 Spike S1 (1:100, 40150-R007, SinoBiological), eCAD (1:100, AF68, R&D Systems), MIST1 (1:100, MA1517, Invitrogen), CK19 (1:100, PIMA512663, Thermofisher), SOX9 (1:250,

AB5535, Millipore), ACE2 (1:100, AB15348, abcam), Chymotrypsin (1:100, MAB1476, Millipore), TMPRSS2 (1:250, AB92323, Abcam) and Amylase (1:100, A8273, Sigma). After washing using PBS with 0.1% Tween-20 (ThermoFisher), cells were incubated with appropriate species-specific Alexa Fluor-conjugated secondary antibodies (ThermoFisher) diluted in a blocking buffer (1:1,000) for 1 hour at room temperature. After washing in PBS with 0.1% Tween-20, cells were incubated in Hoechst 33342 diluted in PBS (1:2,500) for 15 min. Immunofluorescence images were visualized using appropriate fluorescent filters using ImageXpress Micro XLS (Molecular Devices) and analyzed using ImageJ Software. Image quantification was performed using CellProfiler Software (v3.1.9).

Real-Time qPCR

Relative gene expression was quantified using RT-qPCR. For this, cells were washed with PBS to remove any possible remaining viral inoculum and the total RNA was isolated with RLT (Qiagen). RNA was then extracted with RNeasy Micro Kit (Qiagen) according to the manufacturer's instructions. The concentration of RNA was determined by spectrophotometric analysis (Qubit 4 Fluorometer, ThermoFisher) and the purity with NanoDrop (ThermoFisher); all samples had a $A_{260/280}$ ratio around 2.0 (Desjardins and Conklin, 2010). After, RNA (1 µg) was reverse transcribed to cDNA with oligo(dT) using the High Capacity cDNA Reverse Transcription kit (ThermoFisher). Real-time qPCR was performed in triplicates using SsoAdvanced Universal SYBR Green Supermix (Biorad) and specific primer sequences to each gene (**Supplementary Table 2**), on a CFX384 Real Time system (Bio-Rad). Human *RPL13* was used as the reference gene and relative expression was determined using $2^{-\Delta\Delta}$ Ct method.

Post-Mortem Human Pancreatic Tissues

a) Real-Time qPCR From Snap-Frozen Tissues

Post-mortem pancreatic samples were isolated from the head of the pancreas (preferably) from patients that were infected with SARS-CoV-2 and passed from complications related to the disease (*COVID-19 patients*), or patients that were not infected with SARS-CoV-2 and passed from complications not related to it (*Control patients*). These samples were isolated 1-3 days after the patient's death and were snap-frozen in liquid nitrogen. Samples were stored for longer in -80 °C before used for RNA extraction. For RNA isolation, Trizol (Thermo) was used and for RNA extraction, RNeasy Mini Kit (Qiagen) was used according to the manufacturer's instructions. The concentration of RNA was determined by spectrophotometric analysis (Qubit 4 Fluorometer) and the purity with NanoDrop, as described above; all samples had a $A_{260/280}$ ratio around 2.0. After, RNA (2 µg) was reverse transcribed to cDNA with oligo(dT) using the High Capacity cDNA Reverse Transcription kit. Real-time qPCR was performed in triplicates using SsoAdvanced Universal SYBR Green Supermix (Bio-Rad) and specific primer sequences to each gene can be found in **Supplementary Table 3**. qPCR was performed on a CFX384 Real Time system. Human *β-ACTIN* was used as the reference gene and relative expression was determined using $2^{-\Delta\Delta}$ Ct method.

b) Immunohistochemistry From Paraffin Embedded Tissues

Pancreatic tissues were fixed in 10% formalin and then paraffin embedded. Blocks were sectioned at 4 µm thickness and mounted at microscope slides (Superfrost Plus microscope slides, Fisher). Slides were washed 2x in Xylene for 10 minutes each. This was followed by 2x 5-minute washes with 100% ethyl alcohol, 1x 3-minute wash with 95% ethyl alcohol, and 1x 3-minute wash with 75% alcohol for rehydration. They were then washed 3x with PBS for 5 minutes before beginning antigen retrieval. Samples were submerged in 10mM pH 6.0 sodium citrate Buffer, and then microwaved for 10 minutes at 80% power. Once cooled at room temperature for one hour, they were washed 3x for 5 minutes each with PBS. Samples were blocked for 2 hours in the same blocking buffer as mentioned above (PBS with 10% donkey serum and 0.1% Triton-X). Samples were incubated 4°C overnight with primary antibodies in the same concentrations as mentioned above. The following day, they were washed 3x for 10 minutes each in PBS, incubated one hour at room temperature with the secondary antibodies at concentrations of 1:1000, and then finally washed 3x for 10 minutes each before mounted with ProLong™ Gold Antifade Mountant with DAPI (Invitrogen).

RNA Sequencing (RNASeq)

a) RNA Extraction and Sequencing

RNA was extracted from pelleted cells using RNeasy Micro Kit (Qiagen) and was prepared for sequencing with the Illumina TruSeq Stranded mRNA library preparation kit (Illumina, San Diego, CA) by the Cedars-Sinai Applied Genomics, Computation, and Translational Core. Concentration and quality of RNA was assessed on a Qubit fluorometer (ThermoFisher Scientific, Waltham, MA) and 2100 Bioanalyzer (Agilent Technologies, Santa Clara, CA) respectively. Complementary DNA was reverse transcribed using Invitrogen's Reverse Transcriptase kit (Carlsbad, CA) and converted into double-stranded DNA (dsDNA). The dsDNA was then enriched using PCR before purification with Agencourt AMPure XP beads (Beckman Coulter, Brea, CA). The enriched purified DNA was then quantified and resolved *via* Qubit and Bioanalyzer. Sample libraries were then multiplexed and sequenced on Illumina's NextSeq 500 platform (San Diego, CA) using 75 bp single-end sequencing.

b) Analysis

Raw reads were quantified by mapping them with the STAR aligner (version 2.5.0) (Dobin et al., 2013)/RSEM (version 1.2.25) (Li and Dewey, 2011) to the GRCh38 human reference transcriptome based on human GENCODE version 33 (www.gencodegenes.org) as well as the GenBank: MT246667.1 SARS-CoV-2 reference viral genome. Expression tables were post-processed with a custom R script that filtered out non-coding RNA based on the transcript biotype assigned by biomaRt. Initial analyses were performed on the BioJupies platform. Principal

Component Analysis was then performed in R using the prcomp package. Differential expression tables were calculated in R using the DESeq2 package. Differential expression tables were used to plot heatmaps and volcano plots in ggplot. Enrichment analysis was performed by uploading the top 500 upregulated and downregulated transcripts to the Enrichr gene enrichment analysis portal (Chen et al., 2013; Kuleshov et al., 2016). Enrichment results of interest (including Gene Ontology enrichment and COVID-related gene enrichment) were exported from Enrichr as text files and imported into R for plotting using ggplot. All analysis and plotting scripts in R are available on github.com at github.com/Sareen-Lab/COVID. Gene transcript tables as well as the original FASTQ files are available through NCBI's GEO database at accession number GSE165890.

Statistical Analyses

Data are presented as mean ± standard error of the mean (SEM). Statistical significance between groups was determined by One-way ANOVA followed by Dunnet post-test. Two-tailed paired Student's test was used as appropriate. *P* values <.05 were considered statistically significant. Statistical analyses and graphs were generated using GraphPad Prism 7 for Windows Software (GraphPad Software).

RESULTS

iPSC-Derived Pancreatic Cells Exhibit ACE2 and TMPRSS2 Expression

Human iPSCs were differentiated into pancreatic adherent (2D) and organoid (3D) cultures. Protocols for differentiation after the pancreatic progenitor stage were directed to bias the cell fate of the cultures containing either exocrine acinar cells (iPan^{EXO} Acinar) or exocrine ductal cells (iPan^{EXO} Ductal). iPan^{EXO} Acinar cultures express some markers that are characteristic of mature acinar cultures such as cytoplasmic staining of digestive enzymes Amylase (AMY) and Chymotrypsin C (CTRC), and greater staining of nuclear transcription factor MIST1, which is characteristic of acinar cells that are not fully mature. In these cultures, cells that are AMY$^-$ are MIST1$^+$, which indicates we have mixed cultures of acinar progenitor and mature cells. Acinar cultures also contain some C-peptide expressing endocrine islet β-cells (iPan^{ENDO}). iPan^{EXO} Ductal cultures express cytoskeletal staining of Cytokeratin 19 (CK19). Interestingly, both AMY$^+$ iPan^{EXO} Acinar and CK19$^+$ iPan^{EXO} Ductal cultures exhibit ACE2 and TMPRSS2 protein expression (**Figures 1A, B**), which play a critical part in allowing SARS-CoV-2 cell entry (Hoffmann et al., 2020). Notably, while co-expression is seen, not all C-peptide$^+$ cells express ACE2 (**Figure 1C**), and this seems to be consistent with current literature, which shows lower ACE2 expression in endocrine cells (Coate et al., 2020; Kusmartseva et al., 2020). *ACE2* and *TMPRSS2* gene expression was also measured in iPSC-derived pancreatic cultures. As a negative control, pluripotent iPS cells were used, while cadaveric pancreatic acinar tissues, human pancreatic duct epithelium cell line H6C7, and lung tissues from healthy donors were used as positive controls. Human iPSC-derived neurons were also included as the brain-derived neural tissue lacks ACE2 expression (Lonsdale et al., 2013; Carithers et al., 2015). The results show that cadaveric pancreatic acinar tissues and immortalized human pancreatic duct epithelium cell line H6C7 have high *ACE2* expression. Relative to iPSCs, iPan^{EXO} Acinar and iPan^{EXO} Ductal cultures also contain significantly higher levels of *ACE2*. There is also a significantly higher expression of *TMPRSS2* in iPan^{EXO} Acinar and human acinar tissues, with low levels in iPan^{EXO} Ductal cells (**Figure 1D**). It is known that occasionally different normal and diseased tissues can be differently correlated in their protein and gene expression and there can be some discordance between protein and gene expression for a subset of genes within pancreas (Kosti et al., 2016). Differentiated iPan^{EXO} 3D organoids also show co-localization of ACE2 protein along with acinar and ductal markers (**Supplementary Figure 1**).

SARS-CoV-2 Can Directly Infect iPan^{EXO} Ductal Cultures and Elicit Abnormal Cellular Phenotypes

After 26 days of pancreatic ductal differentiation starting from iPSCs, cultures were infected with SARS-CoV-2 at a multiplicity of infection (MOI) 0.05 and 0.1, and cells were collected for analysis after one day (Day 1) or after three days (Day 3) (**Figure 2A**). These MOIs allowed for establishing *de novo* infection and active viral replication for the viral kinetics studies. The mock condition was treated with ductal media with no virus. MOI 0.05 infection shows 4% and 19% of cells infected with SARS-CoV-2 on Day 1 and Day 3 respectively, while MOI 0.1 infection shows 10% and 19% of infected cells, respectively (**Figure 2B**), showing viral infectivity increased from Day 1 to Day 3 in both MOIs. Although more cells got infected from Day 1 to Day 3, less cells were observed in culture comparing infected cultures with uninfected cultures, which suggests that the virus possibly decreased cell viability (data not shown). As expected, the mock condition has negative SARS-CoV-2-Spike S1 staining (**Figure 2B**). RT-qPCR for SARS-CoV-2 nucleocapsid gene *N1* shows SARS-CoV-2 mRNA production increased in the infected conditions compared to mock condition as seen in **Figure 2C**. Thus, iPSC-derived pancreatic cultures allow SARS-CoV-2 entry and establish infection.

SOX9 is a well-established nuclear transcription factor involved in determining ductal specification from pancreatic progenitors. Interestingly, SARS-CoV-2 positive cells in the infected iPan^{EXO} Ductal cultures at both MOIs show a more enlarged cellular morphology as observed by CK19 and SOX9 staining pattern (**Figure 3A**) and abnormal cytoplasmic SOX9 localization instead of the typical nuclear localization observed in normal ductal cells as evident in the mock condition and uninfected cells (**Figure 3B**). In fact, we observe a higher number of ductal cells with mislocalization of SOX9 in the cytoplasm of infected cells at both Day 1 and Day 3 compared with mock cells, and both MOIs seem to have a similar pattern of mislocalization (no statistical difference between MOIs in both

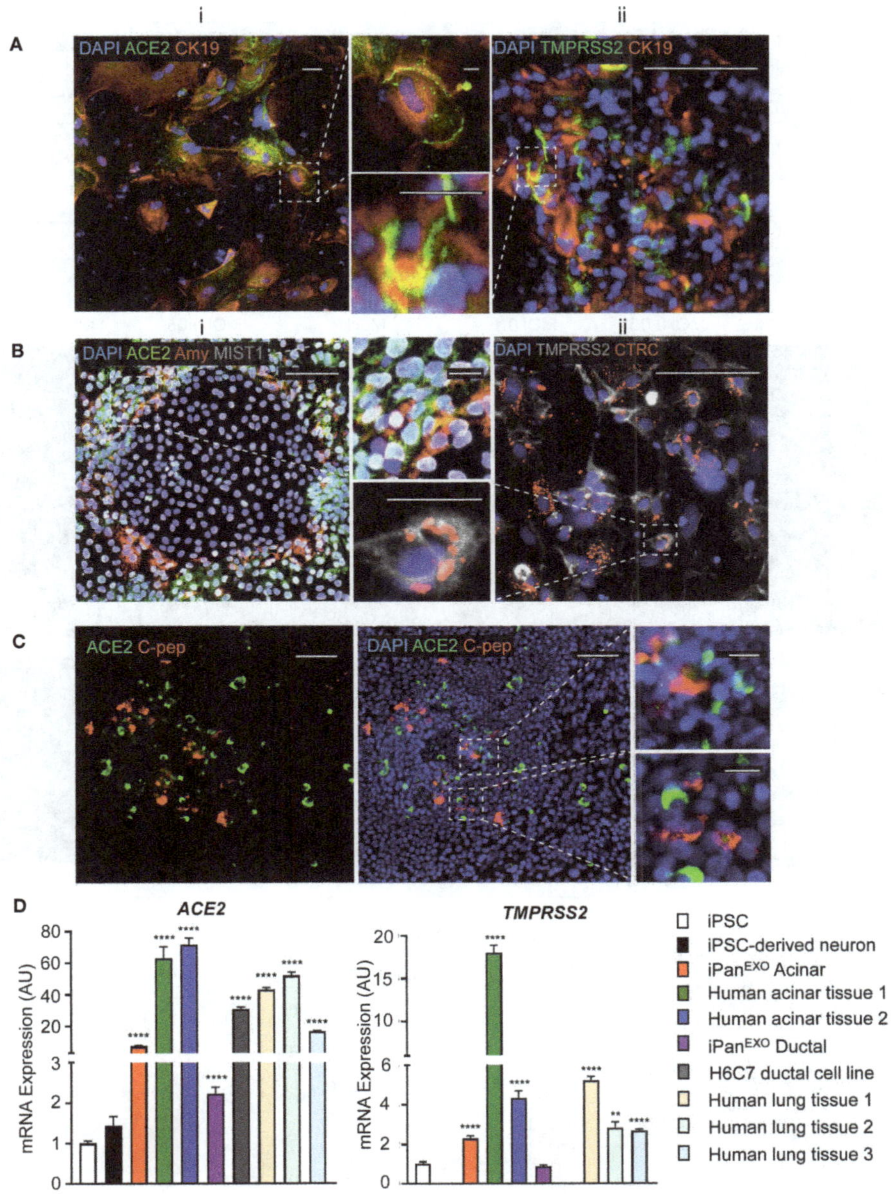

FIGURE 1 | Expression of ACE2 and TMPRSS2 in exocrine pancreatic cells. **(A)** iPan^{EXO} Ductal cells CK19 (red) exhibiting **i.** ACE2 (green) and **ii.** TMPRSS2 (green) expression. **(B)** iPan^{EXO} Acinar cells Amylase (red), MIST1 (gray) exhibit **i.** ACE2 (green) expression and **ii.** iPan^{EXO} Acinar CTRC (red) exhibit TMPRSS2 (green). **(C)** iPan^{EXO} Acinar and iPan^{ENDO} cultures contain some endocrine C-peptide expressing cells, which also co-stain with ACE2. **(D)** iPSC-derived pancreatic exocrine cells as well as human acinar tissues and human ductal cell line H6C7 express *ACE2* and *TMPRSS2*. Data is shown as mean ± SEM with statistical significance determined by unpaired two-tailed t-test. $^{**}p < 0.01$ and $^{****}p < 0.0001$. Scale bar represents 100 μm, and 20 μm for zoomed panels adjacent to main images. ICC images shown here are representative results from 27 independent sites acquired. RNA was extracted from aggregates of 2-3 biological replicates (using 12 well-plates), and qPCR was run with 3 technical replicates per sample. These results were pooled from 2 independent rounds of infection experiments.

Day 1 and Day 3) (**Figure 3C**). Meanwhile, CK19 is present across all treatments and timepoints, with no obvious differences in staining localization of the infected population. ACE2 expression is observed in Day 3 cells with no distinct differences between mock and MOI 0.05 and 0.1 conditions (**Supplementary Figure 2**). CK19^{+} ductal cells become multinucleated when infected with SARS-CoV-2 (MOI 0.1), while uninfected ductal cells remain mononucleated (Mock) (**Figure 3D**). This phenomenon has been described as syncytia formation, the fusion of multiple mononucleated cells, and known to amplify apoptotic signals in response to viral infection (Scheller and Jassoy, 2001; Salsman et al., 2005; Nardacci et al., 2015). In MOI 0.1 treatment of Day 3 culture, the percentage of multinucleated infected ductal cells is 81.6%,

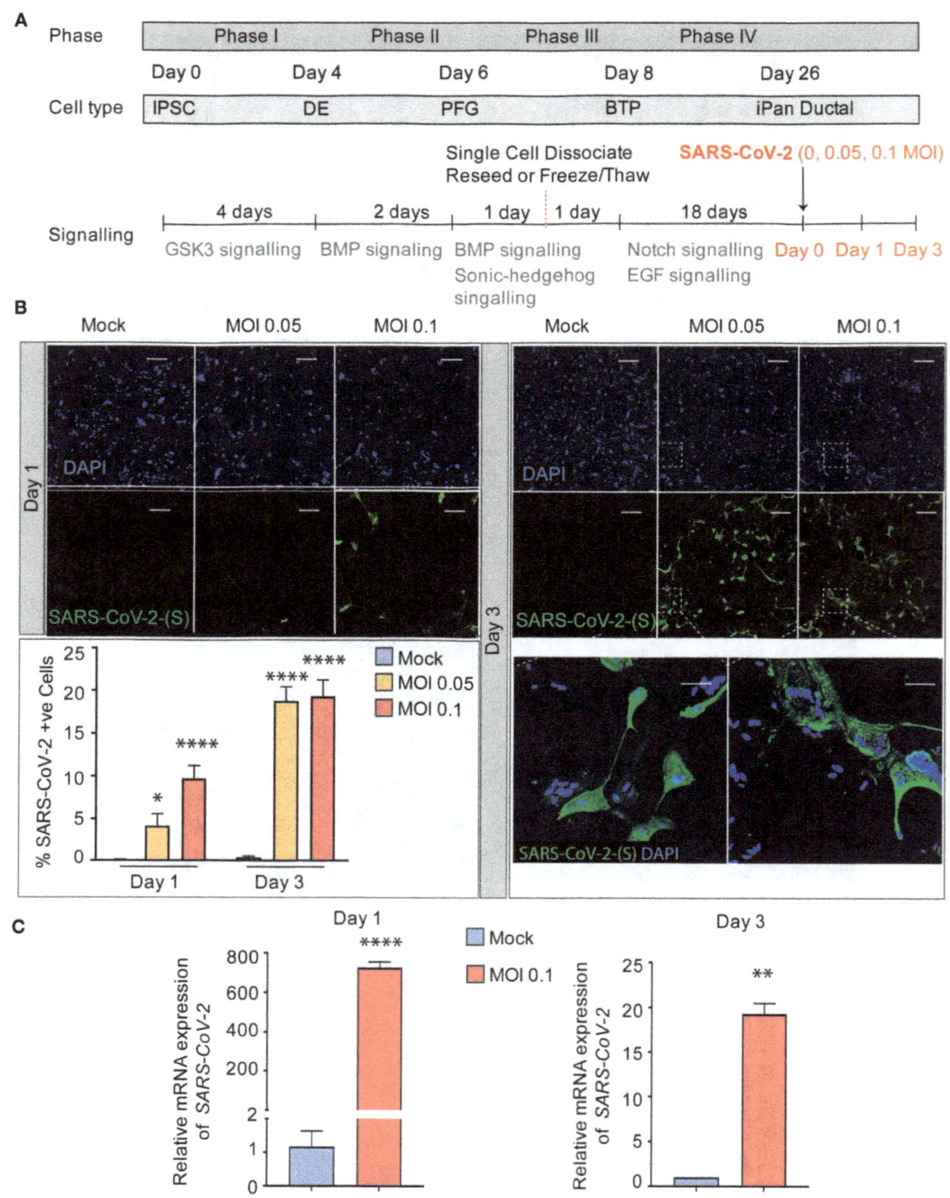

FIGURE 2 | SARS-CoV-2 can infect iPan^{EXO} Ductal Cells. **(A)** Differentiation scheme of pancreatic ductal cells and infection of SARS-CoV-2 on Day 26. **(B)** Immunocytochemistry staining of SARS-(S) at Day 1 and Day 3 (Scale bar is 200 μm). **(C)** RT-qPCR showing upregulation of *SARS-CoV-2 N1* from mock to infected cells at different days. Data is shown as mean ± SEM with statistical significance determined by unpaired two-tailed t-test. *p < 0.05, **p < 0.01, ****p < 0.0001. Scale bar represents 200 μm. ICC images shown here are representative results from 36 independent sites acquired. RNA was extracted from aggregates of 6-15 biological replicates (using 96 well-plates), and qPCR was run in 3 technical replicates per sample. These results were pooled from 2 independent rounds of infection experiments.

which is significantly higher than the percentage of multinucleated non-infected ductal cells, 12.2% (**Figure 3E**).

SARS-CoV-2 Can Infect iPan^{EXO} Acinar and iPan^{ENDO} Cells Resulting in Activation of Proinflammatory Genes

iPan^{EXO} Acinar cultures containing predominantly Chymotrypsin C (CTRC) and Amylase (AMY) positive cells and few iPan^{ENDO} C-peptide positive islet β-cells were differentiated for 16 days before being infected with SARS-CoV-2 at a MOI of 0.1. A separate mock condition was cultured in parallel and not infected. Like the iPan^{EXO} Ductal cultures, infected and uninfected cultures were fixed or lysed after one day or three days of infection (**Figure 4A**). CTRC-positive cells, which have a granular morphology that likely reflects zymogen granule formation, showed direct infection by SARS-CoV-2 (**Figure 4B**). Interestingly, a subpopulation of SARS-CoV-2 positive cells in these cultures were also C-peptide positive

(**Supplementary Figure 3**). On Day 1 post-infection, 0.63% of total cells were infected, which increased to 1.12% by Day 3. For both days, the difference in percentage of infected cells was statistically significant compared to mock condition (**Figure 4C**), which was similarly seen on mRNA level by RT-qPCR for SARS-CoV-2 nucleocapsid gene *N1*, showing high mRNA production of SARS-CoV-2 in the infected conditions (**Figure 4D**).

To investigate whether SARS-CoV-2 infection perturbed the inflammatory pathway, multiple genes known to be associated with pancreatitis-related inflammation were assessed using RT-qPCR. Among those, the genes *CXCL12*, *NFKB1*, and *STAT3*

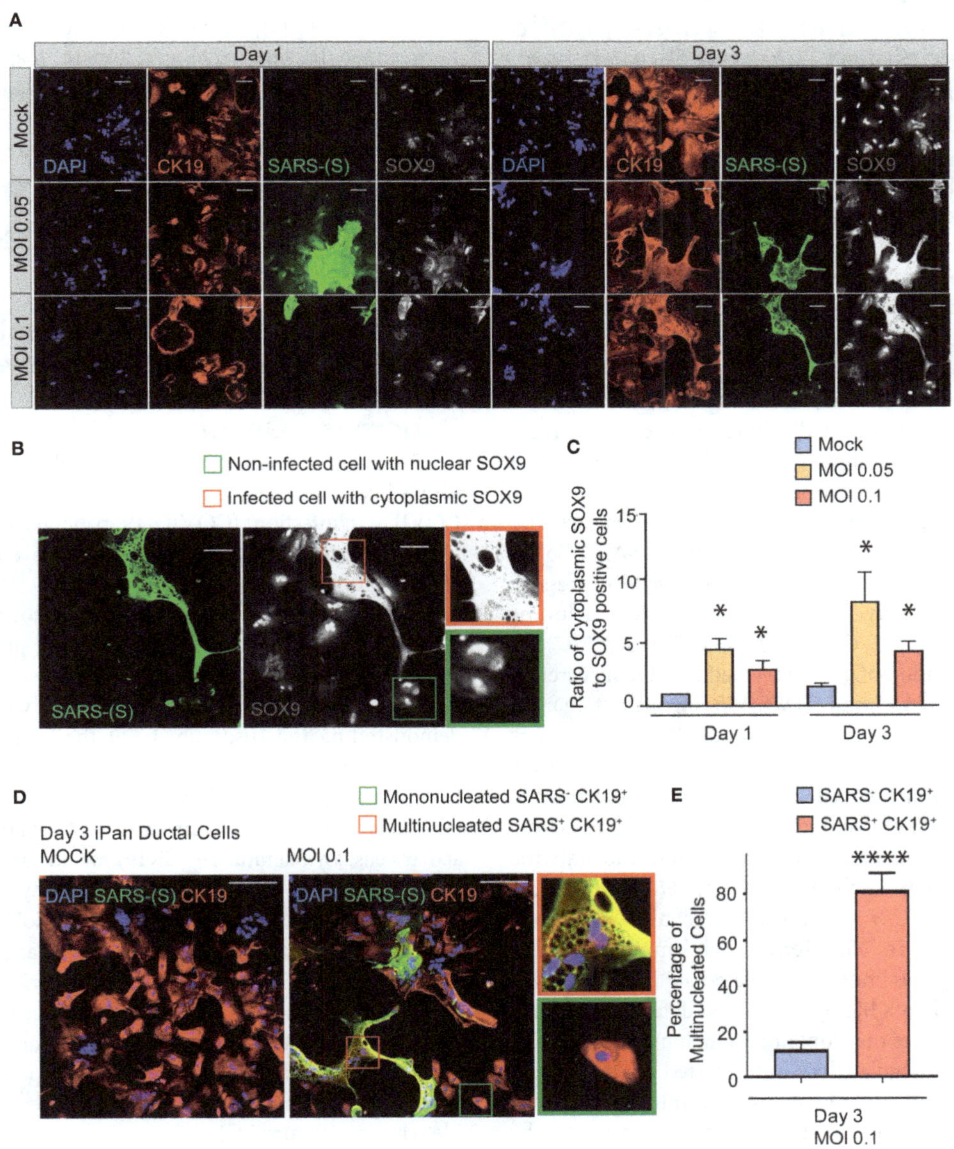

FIGURE 3 | SARS-CoV-2 elicits abnormal cellular phenotypes in iPan^{EXO} Ductal cultures. **(A)** Day 1 and Day 3 of post infected iPan^{EXO} Ductal cells. Immunocytochemistry staining of ductal cell markers CK19 (red), SOX9 (gray), and SARS-CoV-2 infected cells (green) on Day 1 and Day 3 with varying titers of virus (Mock, MOI 0.05, and 0.1). **(B)** SOX9 translocation in infected cells. (Scale bar is 200 µm). **(C)** Histogram is showing the ratio of cells with mis localized cytoplasmic SOX9 over total nuclear SOX9 positive cells in the culture, comparing mock vs SARS-CoV-2 infected ductal cultures at MOI 0.05 and 0.1. Data is shown as mean ± SEM with statistical significance determined by unpaired two-tailed t-test. *$p < 0.05$. Scale bar represents 200 µm. Zoomed panels adjacent to main images are 2.3x larger. ICC images shown here are representative results from 36 independent sites acquired. These results were pooled from 2 independent rounds of infection experiments. **(D)** Immunocytochemistry staining of SARS-(S) at Day 3 Mock and MOI 0.1. Zoom in panels indicate mononucleated SARS$^-$ CK19$^+$ cell (green box) and multinucleated SARS$^+$ CK19$^+$ cell (red box). Scale bar represents 200 µm. ICC images shown here are representative results from 9 independent sites acquired. **(E)** Histogram is showing the percentage of multinucleated cells in non-infected SARS$^-$ CK19$^+$ population and infected SARS$^+$ CK19$^+$ population. Data is shown as mean ± SEM with statistical significance determined by unpaired two-tailed t-test. ****$p < 0.0001$.

showed significant upregulation at Day 3 in infected cells compared to mock condition (**Figure 4E**), while no significant change was observed on infected cells by Day 1 compared to the mock condition (**Supplementary Figure 4**). No significant change in expression was seen on other inflammatory markers, such as *IL1B* and *TNFA*, on both days (**Supplementary Figure 4**).

Transcriptional Analysis of SARS-CoV-2 Infected iPSC-Derived Pancreatic Cultures Demonstrates Viral and Pancreas-Specific COVID-19 Associated Disease Signatures

The iPan cultures containing $iPan^{EXO}$ Acinar and $iPan^{ENDO}$ cells infected with 0.1 MOI SARS-CoV-2 were harvested on Day 1 and Day 3 post-infection for transcriptomic analysis after mRNA sequencing, as well as cells that were not infected (mock conditions). After mapping genomic reads in infected cultures, mapped reads were detected from the SARS-CoV-2 genome that confirm active SARS-CoV-2 viral replication within infected cultures (**Supplementary Table 3**). Principal component analysis (PCA) of Day 1 and Day 3 infected cultures demonstrated that 37.9% and 41.1% of the variance in the gene expression differences could be attributed to principal component 1 (PC1) in Day 1 and Day 3 infected cultures, respectively (**Figure 5A**). Both PCA and the heatmaps of differentially expressed genes clearly demonstrated transcriptomic clustering of samples in either the mock or infected condition in both days (**Figure 5B**). Upon further interrogation of the Day 3 data, SARS-CoV-2 infection induced significant pancreas-specific gene expression changes within iPSC-derived pancreatic cultures including upregulation of *PDX1, INS, GCG, CHGA, CFTR, IGFBP7* and *GHRL* and downregulation of genes involved in cellular secretory pathway such as *GOLGA8A* and *GOLGA8B*. Significant changes in expression of chemokine and immunomodulatory genes were detected. Most were upregulated such as *PTGES, MIF, CCR7, CXCL6* and *CXCL12*, which encodes immune cytokines known to be transcriptionally upregulated during SARS-CoV infection. Similarly, genes reflecting pathogenic interaction and antiviral responses in host cells such as *THOC1, TRIM28, CD37, TRAF3IP1, DDX17, NCBP3, HYAL2*, were also perturbed (**Supplementary Table 4**). Gene enrichment analysis comparing the 500 genes most upregulated in infected day 3 samples to Gene Ontology's Biological Process database identified several biological processes that contained a high number of genes found among those upregulated in our infected sample. These included the "[Signal Recognition Particle]-dependent cotranslational protein targeting to membranes" process, the "protein targeting to ER" process, and several processes associated with viral infection (**Figure 6A**) consisting of mainly ribosomal complex large and small subunit genes. This is consistent with the idea that SARS-CoV-2 like many other viruses requires recruitment of a variety of host cell factors including ribosomal proteins to participate in viral protein biosynthesis, in order to survive, accumulate and propagate in the pancreatic cells. A gene enrichment analysis comparing the 500 most downregulated genes in our samples to Gene Ontology's cellular components data set found that the most significant cellular components that appear to be downregulated include nuclear body, nuclear specks and nucleoplasm (**Figure 6B**), which is also consistent with the downregulation of the specific nuclear pore complex (NPC) genes such as *NPIPB3, 4, 5* (**Figure 5C**). Numerous viral pathogens have evolved different mechanisms to hijack the NPC in order to regulate trafficking of viral proteins, genomes and even capsids into and out of the nucleus thus promoting virus replication (Le Sage and Mouland, 2013). As expected, the cytosolic ribosomal units are the most significantly upregulated cellular component (**Figure 6B**). Performing the same gene enrichment analysis against NCBI's COVID-19 associated transcripts dataset available on the Enrichr database (Kuleshov et al., 2020) identified several dozen downregulated genes classified as downregulated by SARS-CoV-2 in pancreatic organoids (**Figure 6C**). Taken together, these results indicate that SARS-CoV- 2 infection induces significant transcriptional changes within iPSC-derived pancreatic cultures.

Post-Mortem Human Pancreatic Tissues From *COVID-19 Patients* Show Infectivity and Perturbed Expression of Pancreatic Genes

Post-mortem human pancreatic samples were obtained from individuals who succumbed from complications related to COVID-19 infection (COVID-19 patients) or from those who were not infected by SARS-CoV-2 and were deceased due to complications unrelated to COVID-19 (Control patients). Samples were processed for immunohistochemistry of SARS-CoV-2-Spike S1 and pancreatic markers or processed for analysis of changes in gene expression. As shown in **Figures 7A-C**, SARS-CoV-2-S was detected in pancreas of COVID-19 patients, demonstrating the susceptibility of the human pancreas to the virus. To better understand which cell types were infected by SARS-CoV-2 in the pancreas, cells were stained for specific endocrine and exocrine markers, such as Amylase and Chymotrypsin (CTRC) for acinar cells, Cytokeratin 19 (CK19) for ductal cells, and C-peptide for endocrine islet β-cells. Interestingly, many of the pancreatic cell types tested here co-localized with SARS-CoV-2-S. The virus was present in the majority of the $CTRC^+$ and some clusters of $Amylase^+$ cells (**Figures 7A, B**). However, SARS-CoV-2-S was not detected in ductal $CK19^+$ cells (**Supplementary Figure 5**) in the limited set of histology specimens from COVD19 patients examined. In the pancreatic endocrine compartment, interestingly, SARS-CoV-2 staining was frequently concentrated in $C\text{-}Peptide^+$ islet clusters (**Figure 7C**).

To examine whether the infected pancreatic tissues from COVID-19 patients may have differential expression of specific genes, snap-frozen post-mortem tissues from COVID-19 patients and Control subjects were assessed changes in expression of pancreas-specific genes. Interestingly, mRNA expression of ductal markers was increased in the COVID-19 samples, such as *KRT19, CFTR, CA2*, and *HNF1B* as seen in **Figure 7D**. Other pancreatic and inflammatory markers were also tested and although showed trends of perturbations, they were not statistically different between the groups likely due to

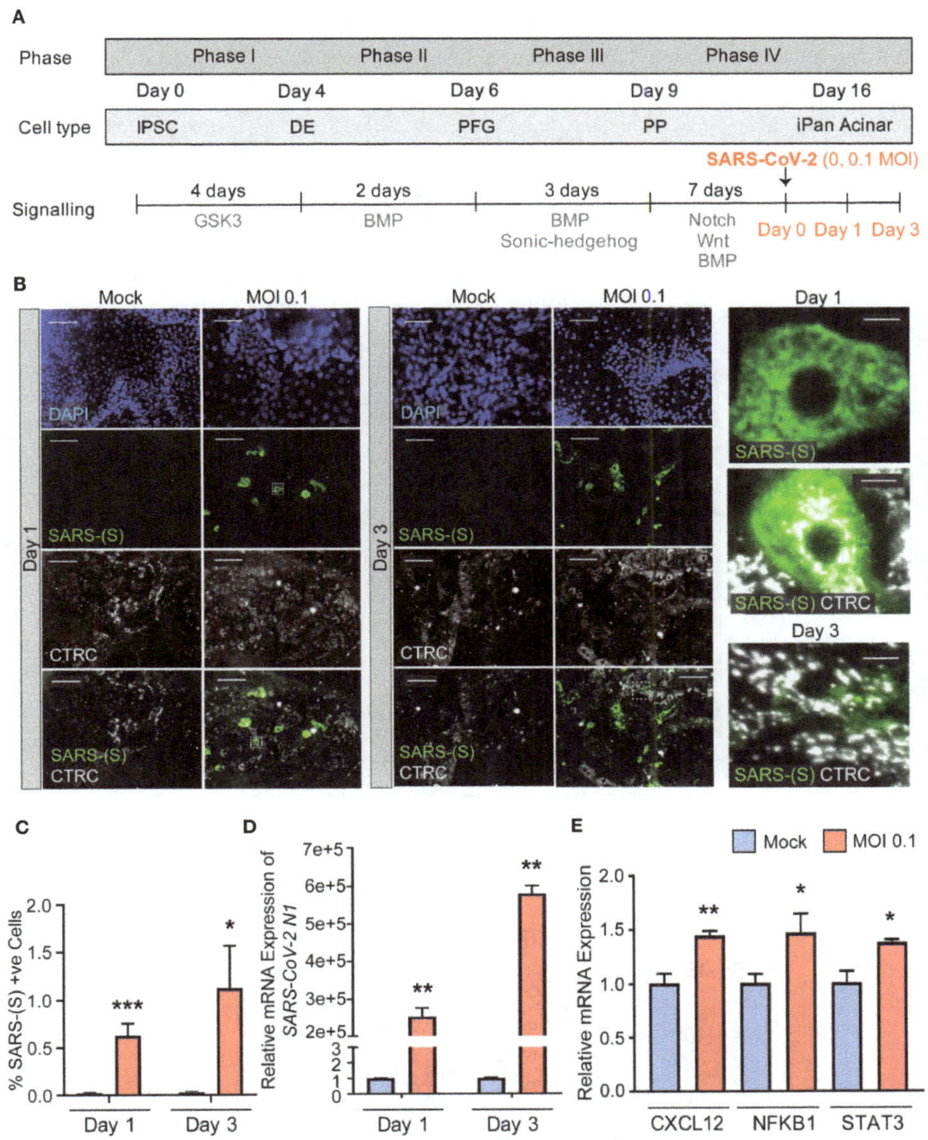

FIGURE 4 | iPan^{EXO} Acinar cultures can be infected with SARS-CoV-2 and result in upregulation of some proinflammatory genes. **(A)** Differentiation and infection timeline for the iPan^{EXO} Acinar cells. Cells were grown 16 days before being infected. Cells were fixed or lysed on the first and third days of infection. **(B)** Immunocytochemistry staining of SARS-(S) on Day 1 and 3 of mock and infected cells. **(C)** Quantification of immunocytochemistry images shows significant increase in SARS-(S) positive cells in the population treated with the virus at MOI 0.1. **(D)** qPCR shows upregulation of *SARS-CoV-2 N1* in infected cells. **(E)** qPCR of inflammation markers *CXCL12, NFKB1*, and *STAT3* show significant upregulation between mock and infected cells on day 3 of infection. Data is shown as mean ± SEM with statistical significance determined by unpaired two-tailed t-test. *$p < 0.05$, **$p < 0.01$, ***$p < 0.001$. Scale bar represents 130 μm, and 10 μm for zoomed panels adjacent to main images. ICC images shown here are representative results from 27 independent sites acquired. RNA was extracted from an aggregate of 6-16 biological replicates (using 96-well plates), and qPCR was run in 3 technical replicates per sample. These results were pooled from 2 independent rounds of infection experiments.

the higher variability in this subset of COVID-19 patients (**Supplementary Figure 6**). These results from COVID-19 and Control human tissues corroborate our novel results in iPan cell cultures, where we show that both pancreatic endocrine and exocrine cells can be infected by SARS-CoV-2, and the infection causes perturbations in pancreas-specific genes and the pancreatic cellular machinery.

DISCUSSION

In this novel study, by observing gene and protein expression in live human iPSC-derived pancreatic cultures and post-mortem pancreatic tissue from COVID-19 patients, we have described the ability of SARS-CoV-2 to infect pancreatic cells. Both approaches indicated that endocrine islets and exocrine

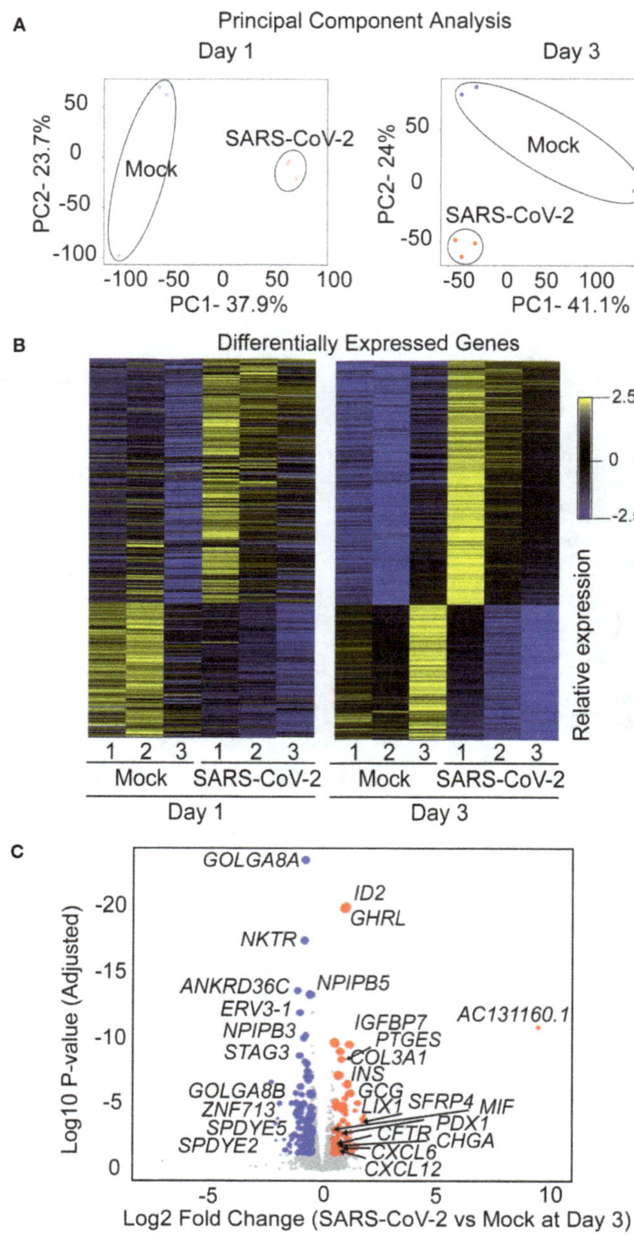

FIGURE 5 | RNAseq analysis of infected iPan^{EXO} cells on days 1 and 3 post infection. **(A)** Principal Component Analysis of infected and mock samples collected on day 1 and day 3, respectively. **(B)** Differentially Expressed Genes Heat map showing the relative expression levels of transcripts differentially expressed with adjusted p-values less than 0.01. **(C)** Volcano plot of the log10 adjusted p-value of each expressed transcript on day 3 versus the log2 fold change. Transcripts that did not demonstrate differential expression with an adjusted p-value of less than 0.05 and a log2 fold-change in either direction greater than 0.5 are plotted in grey. Those that did were sized proportionally to their mean expression level, and genes of interest have been labeled.

acinar and ductal cells within the pancreas allow SARS-CoV-2 entry and establish infection. These cell types are known to express the ACE2 and TMPRSS2 transmembrane proteins recognized as the entry points for SARS-CoV-2 (Coate et al., 2020; Shang et al., 2020; Verdecchia et al., 2020; Müller et al., 2021). In our iPSC-derived pancreatic models, ACE2 and TMPRSS2 expression was observed in both acinar and ductal cells. These cultures also presented C-peptide^{+} cells, and some of these endocrine cells expressed ACE2. Interestingly, recent clinical findings suggested pancreatic dysfunction following SARS-CoV-2 infection in COVID-19 patients (Apicella et al., 2020; Kusmartseva et al., 2020; Li et al., 2020; Liu et al., 2020). The iPSC-derived pancreatic cultures tested here were actively infected by SARS-CoV-2, as demonstrated by viral antigen expression and genomic replication. The cell culture observations were supported by similar results in

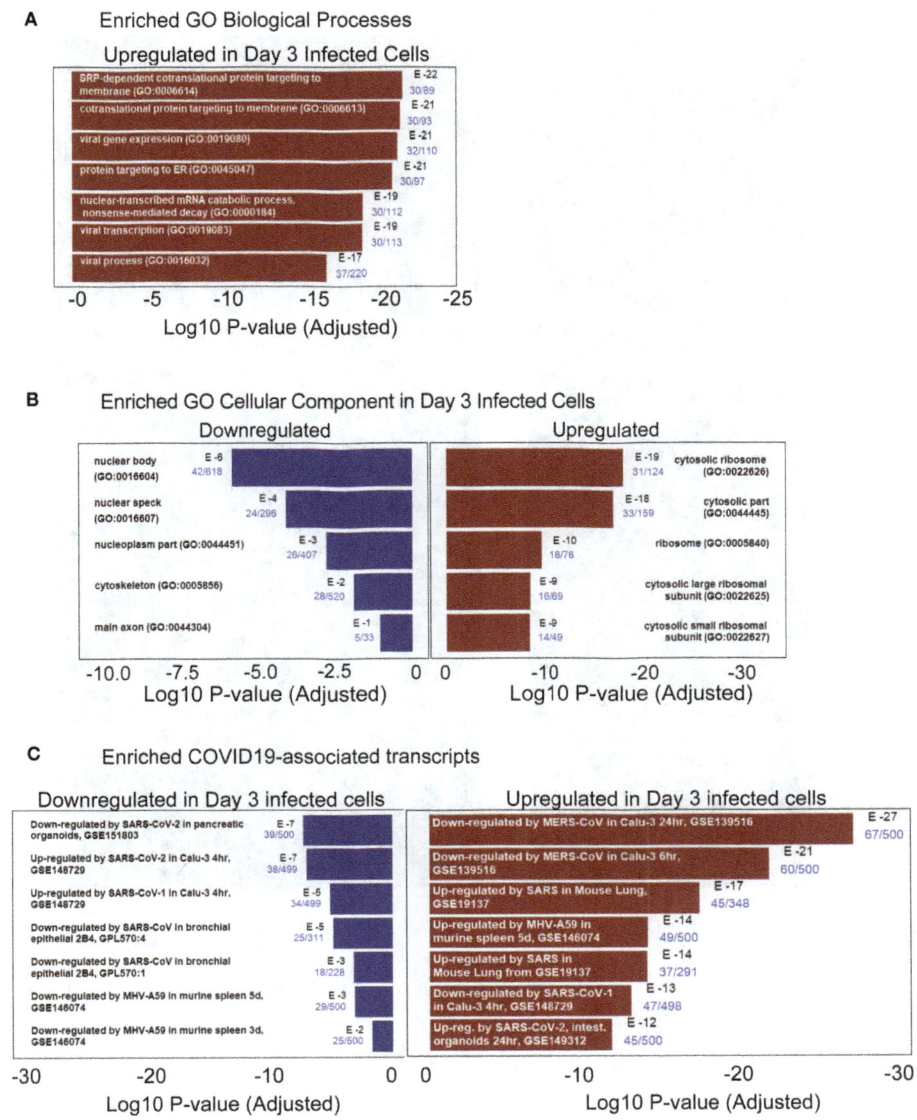

FIGURE 6 | RNAseq pathway and cellular component analysis of infected iPan^{EXO} cells on day 3 post infection. **(A)** Enriched GO Biological Processes: Upregulated biological processes were predicted based on the statistical overrepresentation of upregulated transcripts. The 500 most upregulated genes were submitted to Enrichr, and the Biological Processes in the Gene Ontology database which contained a statistically unlikely fraction of upregulated transcripts were plotted based on the probability of the observed enrichment. The fraction of genes in the gene set which were present in the 500 transcripts under analysis are listed in blue text. **(B)** Enriched GO Cellular Component: Upregulated and downregulated cellular components were predicted based on the statistical over representation of transcripts associated with these components. Nuclear bodies were predicted to be downregulated based on the presence of 42 out of 618 genes associated with this component in the list of 500 most downregulated transcripts in day 3 infected samples. Cytosolic ribosomes were predicted to be upregulated based on the presence of 31 out of 124 genes associated with this component among the 500 most upregulated transcripts on day 3 when compared to the Gene Expression Omnibus' cellular component gene sets (Barrett et al., 2013) **(C)** Enriched COVID19-associated transcripts: Gene sets identified as potentially similar to day 3 infected samples were plotted based on the statistical overrepresentation of the top 500 upregulated and downregulated transcripts.

post-mortem pancreatic tissues from COVID-19 patients. SARS-CoV-2-S protein was expressed in the pancreas of infected patients, specifically co-localizing in exocrine acinar cells and endocrine β-cells. Although we observed SARS-CoV-2-S protein expression in CK19$^+$ ductal cells in culture and not in CK19$^+$ cells from the limited set of post-mortem human pancreatic tissues of COVID-19 patients, a recent study did observe SARS-CoV-2-N protein expression in CK19$^+$ ductal cells in human tissues, suggesting some extent SARS-CoV-2 infection is possible in human pancreatic ductal compartment (Müller et al., 2021). It is likely that there is some level of variability in susceptibility pancreatic ductal infection between patients that could be related to timing of virus infection their mortality. Interestingly, we also observed

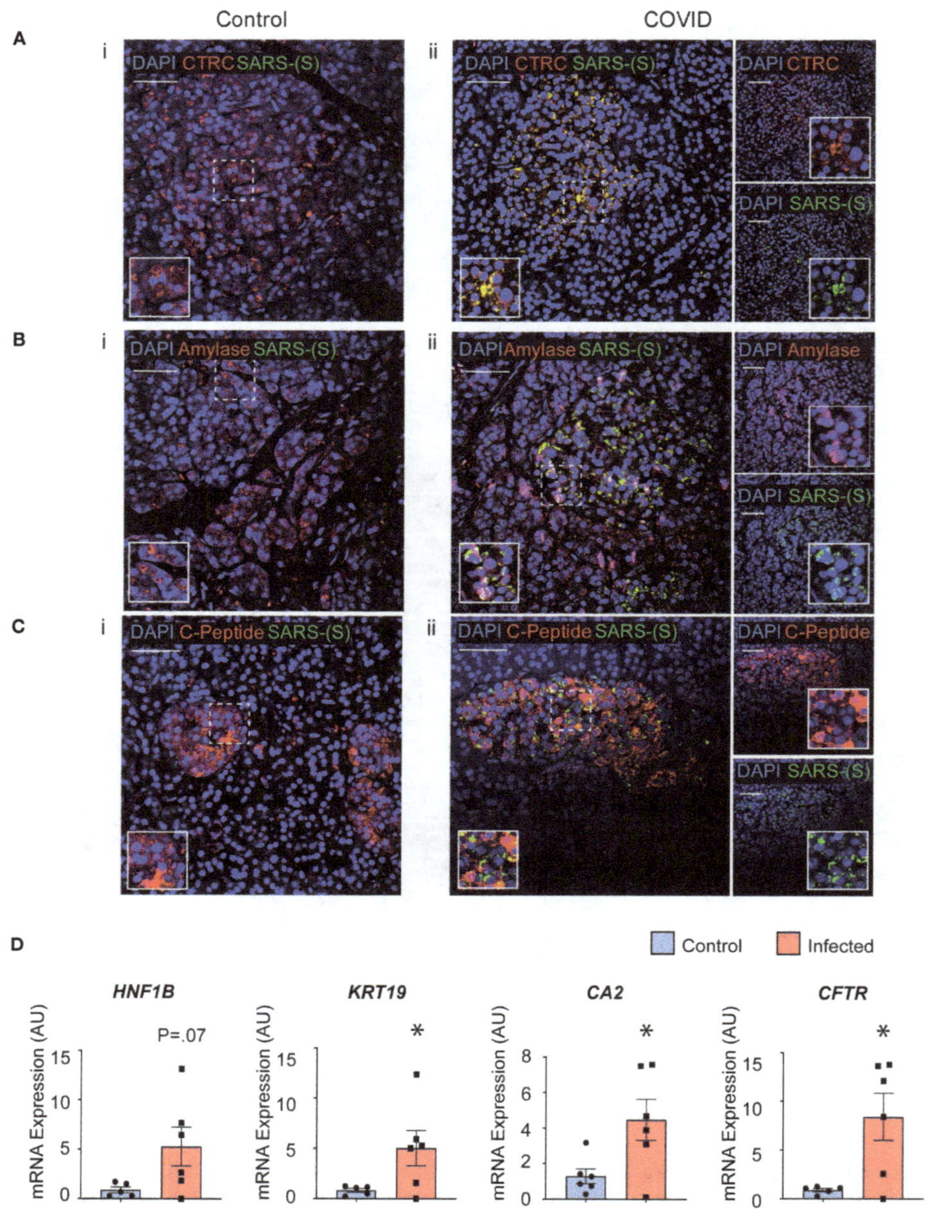

FIGURE 7 | Post-mortem human pancreas shows SARS-CoV-2 infectivity and co-localization with multiple pancreatic cell types. Immunohistochemistry results from pancreatic tissues of patients with COVID-19 show SARS-CoV-2-Spike S1 staining in green and pancreatic acinar markers in red, such as **(A) ii.** Chymotrypsin, **(B) ii.** Amylase; and pancreatic endocrine marker **(C) ii.** C-peptide. **(A–C) i.** Corresponding sets of staining on non-COVID patients indicate no SARS-CoV-2-Spike S1 staining. **(D)** Pancreatic tissues from COVID-19 patients (n=5) and Control subjects (n=6) were utilized for RNA extraction. Real-time qPCR results show increased mRNA expression of ductal markers CA2, CFTR, KRT19 and CFTR. Data is shown as mean ± SEM with statistical significance determined by unpaired two-tailed t-test. *$p < 0.05$. Scale bar represents 50 μM. IHC was performed in 3 non-COVID controls and 3 COVID patients. The results shown here are representative results from 3-10 independent sites acquired per patient. RNA was extracted from 6 non-COVID controls and 5 COVID patients, and qPCR was run in 3 technical replicates per sample.

SARS-CoV-2 infection in endocrine cells both *in vitro* and in post-mortem human tissues, and this was also observed by (Müller et al., 2021), where the infection of endocrine cells *in vitro* led to malfunction of cells and decreased glucose-stimulated insulin secretion. This is notable given that diabetes and related complications are considered independent risk factors associated with higher mortality rates in COVID-19 (Holman et al., 2020).

Upon assessing cellular and molecular perturbations in iPSC-derived pancreatic cultures, it was observed that SARS-CoV-2 infected ductal cells in culture were enlarged and the nuclear compartmentalization of the ductal-specific transcription factor

SOX9, which is typically observed in normal ductal cells, was absent. Instead, a cytoplasmic staining pattern, suggesting a mislocalization of SOX9 as a potential indicator of cellular stress imposed by the virus in infected cells (Chakravarty et al., 2011). The elongated morphology of the infected ductal cells is also a feature that is common in cancerous or inflamed epithelial cells converting to fibrotic cells undergoing a dynamic process known as epithelial-mesenchymal transition (EMT) (Kalluri and Weinberg, 2009; Krantz et al., 2012). Furthermore, SARS-CoV-2 infected pancreatic cultures exhibit a large percentage of multinucleated fused CK19$^+$ cells, a phenomenon described as syncytia formation; the fusion of multiple ACE2$^+$ cells upon SARS-CoV-2 infection (Buchrieser et al., 2020). The histology of 41 lung samples from COVID-19 patients show that 87% of them display dysmorphic pneumocytes with syncytia (Bussani et al., 2020). In vitro studies have also shown syncytia formation in hiPSC-derived neurons, hiPSC-derived astrocytes, U2OS-ACE2, Vero-ACE2, and 293T-ACE2 after viral infection (Buchrieser et al., 2020; Wang et al., 2021; Zhang et al., 2021). Recent papers propose that a unique bi-arginine motif within the S1/S2 cleavage site of SARS-CoV-2 spike glycoprotein mediates the fusion of neighboring ACE2$^+$ cells and formation of syncytia (Braga et al., 2021; Zhang et al., 2021). Furthermore, previous studies have found that syncytia mediated by SARS-CoV-2 as well as other viruses such as human immunodeficiency virus-1 (HIV-1) and reovirus-associated FAST proteins can lead to apoptosis (Scheller and Jassoy, 2001; Salsman et al., 2005; Nardacci et al., 2015; Buchrieser et al., 2020), This suggests that apoptosis in virus infected cultures becomes exacerbated *via* syncytia formation and cytopathy affects can be alleviated by targeting the relevant downstream processes specific to that cell type and virus. Pancreatic tissues from COVID-19 patients showed perturbation with upregulation of key ductal genes such as *KRT19*, *CA2* and *CFTR*. Increased *KRT19* expression is associated with pancreas-specific intracellular stress in patients with poor prognosis of pancreatic ductal adenocarcinoma (PDAC) (Yao et al., 2017). Cytoskeletal protein responses are known to be dysregulated under conditions of intracellular stress imposed by a viral infection and similar disturbances have also been reported to be an important in both immune and adaptive immunity (Kopecki et al., 2016; Ong et al., 2020) Yet, further elucidation of the mechanisms of pancreatic injury involved in response to the SARS-CoV-2 infection in pancreatic ductal cells is necessary. Granular morphology was noted in all SARS-CoV-2 positive cells and could be representative of viral replication and transportation occurring in membrane vesicles. This would be consistent with previous findings that SARS-CoV-2 associates with the host endo membrane system, with 40% of SARS-CoV-2-interacting proteins having functions in the endomembrane system (Gordon et al., 2020).

In infected acinar cell cultures, the gene *CXCL12* was upregulated. This gene, in particular, was found expressed ten-fold in blood plasma by (Xu et al., 2020), and is consistent with the overexpression of similar cytokines and chemokines widely seen during the cytokine storm frequently observed in COVID-19 patients (Coperchini et al., 2020; Song et al., 2020). Although CXCL12 seems to promote tumor invasion, proliferation, angiogenesis, epithelial to mesenchymal transition and metastasis in pancreatic cancer (Righetti et al., 2019), its roles seem to be pleiotropic, and this could be due to the presence of at least six CXCL12 splicing isoforms, each with different roles (Righetti et al., 2019). To date, CXCL12 was reported to function as an anti-inflammatory chemokine during autoimmune inflammatory responses (Karin, 2010). In our SARS-CoV-2 infected iPSC-derived acinar cells, we believe CXCL12 could be playing either pro-inflammatory roles since other known pro-inflammatory transcription factors were also upregulated, such as *NKFB1* and *STAT3* (Ji et al., 2019), or a defensive anti-inflammatory defensive to viral infection. The mechanistic role of CXCL12 upon SARS-CoV-2 infection of pancreatic cultures needs to be further investigated.

Upon probing the pathways disrupted by SARS-CoV-2 upon infection of pancreatic cells, the most dramatic transcriptional change was the over-expression of transcriptional machinery and SRP-dependent protein-targeting processes. The transcripts contributing to these pathways were identified as hallmarks of viral replication by gene enrichment analysis. It has been previously reported that a common feature of coronaviruses is the use of virus-engineered double membrane vesicles from host cell components as a central site for viral RNA synthesis (Snijder et al., 2020; Wolff et al., 2020). The upregulation of SRP-protein targeting processes could be a reflection of host cell machinery being repurposed for viral replication. Conversely, the top three downregulated cellular components were nuclear. Other coronaviruses, including avian infectious bronchitis virus (IBV) and murine hepatitis virus (MHV), and SARS-CoV have been found to arrest cell cycle in the nucleus, leading to increased viral replication (Chen and Makino, 2004; Dove et al., 2006; Yuan et al., 2006). Our results for the most upregulated and downregulated transcripts within the COVID-19-related Drug and Gene Set Library aligned with that of other coronaviruses, particularly SARS-CoV and MHV, with the top two downregulated transcripts being SARS-CoV-2 related. Taken all together, our results suggest that SARS-CoV-2, like other coronaviruses, elicits similar transcript-level signatures to promote viral replication in pancreatic cells. Future studies are necessary to confirm these mechanistic implications of these findings.

With this study, we provide novel patient-specific models for future mechanistic studies of SARS-CoV-2 impact on the pancreas. This study supports the utility of iPSC-derived pancreatic cells as an excellent platform to explore the detrimental impacts of SARS-CoV-2 on pancreatic cells. Further, detailed studies are required to better understand and perhaps the 3D organoids and Organ-Chip systems can be utilized to explore the short-term and long-term detrimental effects SARS-CoV-2 has on the pancreas.

ETHICS STATEMENT

Human cell lines, tissues and histology specimens were obtained or created at Cedars-Sinai under the auspices of the Cedars-Sinai

Medical Center Institutional Review Board (IRB) approved protocols. Specifically, the iPSC cell lines and differentiation protocols in the present study were carried out in accordance with the guidelines approved by Stem Cell Research Oversight committee (SCRO) and IRB, under the auspices of IRB-SCRO Protocols Pro00032834 (iPSC Core Repository and Stem Cell Program) and Pro00036896 (Sareen Stem Cell Program). Infections of iPSC-derived cells were performed under the auspices of UCLA's Stem Cell Oversight Committee under protocol #2020-004-01 and UCLA Biosafety Committee protocol BUA-2020-015-004-A. Post-mortem pancreatic tissues were collected by Cedars-Sinai's Biobank and Translational Research core in accordance with protocol Pro00036514, and lung tissues in accordance with the protocol Pro00035396. In vitro studies using human cell lines were conducted from participants that provided written informed consent for research studies. Remaining studies were conducted with post-mortem human specimens with appropriate IRB approvals.

AUTHOR CONTRIBUTIONS

SS: conception and design of the study, data collection, analysis, and interpretation, and manuscript writing. VW: conception and design of the study, data collection, analysis, and interpretation, and manuscript writing. RS: conception and design of the study, data collection, analysis, and interpretation, and manuscript writing. AG: data analysis and interpretation, and viral count analysis. YW: Next generation sequencing for mRNA-sequencing experiments and data analysis. HJ, YZ, and WH: provision of study material (human pancreatic post-mortem tissues and slides). GG: SARS-CoV-2 infection of *in vitro* samples. VA: conception and design of the study, SARS-CoV-2 infection of *in vitro* samples. DS: conception and design of study, financial and administrative support, data analysis and interpretation, manuscript writing, and final approval of manuscript. All authors contributed to the article and approved the submitted version.

ACKNOWLEDGMENTS

We would like to acknowledge the support of the Cedars-Sinai Biomanufacturing Center facility and Cedars-Sinai Research Institute in supporting this project. We would like to thank The David and Janet Polak Foundation. The following reagents were obtained through BEI Resources, NIAID, NIH: Polyclonal Anti-SARS Coronavirus (antiserum, Guinea Pig), NR-10361; The following reagent was deposited by the Centers for Disease Control and Prevention and obtained through BEI Resources, NIAID, NIH: SARS-Related Coronavirus 2, Isolate USA-WA1/2020, NR-52281. We are grateful to Barbara Dillon, UCLA High Containment Program Director for BSL3 work. We would like to acknowledge Stephen Beil and Dr. Barry Stripp for kindly providing us human lung tissues (Lung Institute, Cedars-Sinai Medical Center, and to Aaron Frank (iPSC Core, Cedars-Sinai Medical Center) for kindly providing us human iPSC-derived neuron samples.

REFERENCES

Amin M.. (2021). COVID-19 and the Liver: Overview. *Eur. J. Gastroenterol. Hepatol.* 68, 309–311. doi: 10.1097/MEG.0000000000001808

Apicella M., Campopiano M. C., Mantuano M., Mazoni L., Coppelli A., and Del Prato S. (2020) Covid-19 in People With Diabetes: Understanding the Reasons for Worse Outcomes. *Lancet Diabetes Endocrinol.* 8, 782–792. doi: 10.1016/S2213-8587(20)

Barrett T., Wilhite S. E., Ledoux P., Evangelista C., Kim I. F., Tomashevsky M., et al. (2013). Ncbi GEO: Archive for Functional Genomics Data Sets - Update.. *Nucleic Acids Res.* 41, 991–995 doi: 10.1093/nar/gks1193

Braga L., Ali H., Secco I., Chiavacci E., Neves G., Goldhill D., et al. (2021). Drugs That Inhibit TMEM16 Proteins Block SARS-CoV-2 Spike-Induced Syncytia. *Nature.* doi: 10.1038/s41586-021-03491-6

Buchrieser J., Dufloo J., Hubert M., Monel B., Planas D., Rajah M. M., et al. (2020). Syncytia Formation by SARS-CoV-2-Infected Cells. *EMBO J.* 39, e106267. doi: 10.15252/embj.2020106267

Bussani R., Schneider E., Zentilin L., Collesi C., Ali H., Braga L., et al. (2020). Persistence of Viral RNA, Pneumocyte Syncytia and Thrombosis are Hallmarks of Advanced COVID-19 Pathology. *EBioMedicine* 61, 103104. doi: 10.1016/j.ebiom.2020.103104

Carithers L. J., Ardlie K., Barcus M., Branton P. A., Britton A., Buia S. A., et al. (2015). A Novel Approach to High-Quality Postmortem Tissue Procurement: The Gtex Project. *Biopreserv. Biobank.* 13, 311–317. doi: 10.1089/bio.2015.0032

Cevik M., Bamford C. G. G., and Ho A. (2020). Covid-19 Pandemic—A Focused Review for Clinicians. *Clin. Microbiol. Infect.* 26, 842–847. doi: 10.1016/j.cmi.2020.04.023

Chakravarty G., Moroz K., Makridakis N. M., Lloyd S. A., Galvez S. E., Canavello P. R., et al. (2011). Prognostic Significance of Cytoplasmic SOX9 in Invasive Ductal Carcinoma and Metastatic Breast Cancer. *Exp. Biol. Med.* 236, 145–155. doi: 10.1258/ebm.2010.010086

Chen C.-J., and Makino S. (2004). Murine Coronavirus Replication Induces Cell Cycle Arrest in G0/G1 Phase. *J. Virol.* 78, 128. doi: 10.1128/JVI.78.11.5658-5669.2004

Chen E. Y., Tan C. M., Kou Y., Duan Q., Wang Z., Meirelles G. V., et al. (2013). Enrichr: Interactive and Collaborative HTML5 Gene List Enrichment Analysis Tool. *BMC Bioinf.* 14. doi: 10.1186/1471-2105-14-128

Coate K. C., Cha J., Shrestha S., Wang W., Gonçalves L. M., Almaça J., et al. (2020). SARS-Cov-2 Cell Entry Factors ACE2 and TMPRSS2 are Expressed in the Pancreas But are Not Enriched in Islet Endocrine Cells. *BioRxiv Prepr. Serv. Biol.* doi: 10.1101/2020.08.31.275719

Coperchini F., Chiovato L., Croce L., Magri F., and Rotondi M. (2020). The Cytokine Storm in COVID-19: An Overview of the Involvement of the Chemokine/Chemokine-Receptor System. *Cytokine Growth Factor Rev.* 53, 25–32. doi: 10.1016/j.cytogfr.2020.05.003

Dataset (2020). GitHub - CSSEGISandData/COVID-19: Novel Coronavirus (COVID-19) Cases, provided by JHU CSSE.

de-Madaria E., and Capurso G. (2021). Covid-19 and Acute Pancreatitis: Examining the Causality. *Nat. Rev. Gastroenterol. Hepatol.* 18, 3–4. doi: 10.1038/s41575-020-00389-y

Desjardins P, and Conklin D. (2010) NanoDrop Microvolume Quantitation of Nucleic Acids. *J. Vis. Exp.* (45), 2565. doi: 10.3791/2565

Dobin A., Davis C. A., Schlesinger F., Drenkow J., Zaleski C., Jha S., et al. (2013). Star: Ultrafast Universal RNA-seq Aligner. *Bioinformatics* 29, 15–21. doi: 10.1093/bioinformatics/bts635

Dove B., Brooks G., Bicknell K., Wurm T., and Hiscox J. A. (2006). Cell Cycle Perturbations Induced by Infection With the Coronavirus Infectious Bronchitis Virus and Their Effect on Virus Replication. *J. Virol.* 80, 4147–4156. doi: 10.1128/JVI.80.8.4147-4156.2006

Gordon D. E., Jang G. M., Bouhaddou M., Xu J., Obernier K., White K. M., et al. (2020). A SARS-CoV-2 Protein Interaction Map Reveals Targets for Drug Repurposing. *Nature* 583, 459–468. doi: 10.1038/s41586-020-2286-9

Hoffmann M., Kleine-Weber H., Schroeder S., Krüger N., Herrler T., Erichsen S., et al. (2020). SARS-Cov-2 Cell Entry Depends on ACE2 and TMPRSS2 and Is Blocked by a Clinically Proven Protease Inhibitor. *Cell* 181, 271–280. e8. doi: 10.1016/j.cell.2020.02.052

Hohwieler M., Illing A., Hermann P. C., Mayer T., Stockmann M., Perkhofer L., et al. (2017). Human Pluripotent Stem Cell-Derived Acinar/Ductal Organoids Generate Human Pancreas Upon Orthotopic Transplantation and Allow Disease Modelling. *Gut* 66, 473–486. doi: 10.1136/gutjnl-2016-312423

Holman N., Knighton P., Kar P., O'Keefe J., Curley M., Weaver A., et al. (2020). Risk Factors for COVID-19-related Mortality in People With Type 1 and Type 2 Diabetes in England: A Population-Based Cohort Study. *Lancet Diabetes Endocrinol.* 8, 823–833. doi: 10.1016/S2213-8587(20)30271-0

Ji Z., He L., Regev A., and Struhl K. (2019). Inflammatory Regulatory Network Mediated by the Joint Action of NF-kB, STAT3, and AP-1 Factors is Involved in Many Human Cancers. *Proc. Natl. Acad. Sci. USA* 116, 9453–9462. doi: 10.1073/pnas.1821068116

Kalluri R., and Weinberg R. A. (2009). The Basics of Epithelial-Mesenchymal Transition. *J. Clin. Invest.* 119, 1420–1428. doi: 10.1172/JCI39104

Karin N. (2010). The Multiple Faces of CXCL12 (Sdf-1α) in the Regulation of Immunity During Health and Disease. *J. Leukoc. Biol.* 88, 463–473. doi: 10.1189/jlb.0909602

Kopecki Z., Ludwig R. J., and Cowin A. J. (2016). Cytoskeletal Regulation of Inflammation and its Impact on Skin Blistering Disease Epidermolysis Bullosa Acquisita. *Int. J. Mol. Sci.* 17, 1116. doi: 10.3390/ijms17071116

Kosti I., Jain N., Aran D., Butte A. J., and Sirota M. (2016). Cross-Tissue Analysis of Gene and Protein Expression in Normal and Cancer Tissues OPEN. *Nat. Publ. Gr.* 6, 24799. doi: 10.1038/srep24799

Krantz S. B., Shields M. A., Dangi-Garimella S., Munshi H. G., and Bentrem D. J. (2012). Contribution of Epithelial-to-Mesenchymal Transition and Cancer Stem Cells to Pancreatic Cancer Progression. *J. Surg. Res.* 173, 105–112. doi: 10.1016/j.jss.2011.09.020

Kuleshov M. V., Jones M. R., Rouillard A. D., Fernandez N. F., Duan Q., Wang Z., et al. (2016). Enrichr: A Comprehensive Gene Set Enrichment Analysis Web Server 2016 Update. Nucleic Acids Res. 44, W90–W97. doi: 10.1093/nar/gkw377

Kuleshov M. V., Stein D. J., Clarke D. J. B., Kropiwnicki E., Jagodnik K. M., Bartal A., et al. (2020). The COVID-19 Drug and Gene Set Library. *Patterns* 1. doi: 10.1016/j.patter.2020.100090

Kumaran N. K., Karmakar B. K., and Taylor O. M. (2020). Coronavirus disease-19 (Covid-19) Associated With Acute Necrotising Pancreatitis (ANP). *BMJ Case Rep.* 13, e237903. doi: 10.1136/bcr-2020-237903

Kusmartseva I., Wu W., Syed F., van der Heide V., Jorgensen M., Joseph P., et al. (2020). Expression of SARS-CoV-2 Entry Factors in the Pancreas of Normal Organ Donors and Individuals With COVID-19. *Cell Metab.* 32, 1041-1051.e6. doi: 10.1016/j.cmet.2020.11.005

Le Sage V., and Mouland A. J. (2013). Viral Subversion of the Nuclear Pore Complex. *Viruses* 5, 2019–2042. doi: 10.3390/v5082019

Li B., and Dewey C. N. (2011). Rsem: Accurate Transcript Quantification From RNA-Seq Data With or Without a Reference Genome. *BMC Bioinf.* 12, 323. doi: 10.1186/1471-2105-12-323

Li M. Y., Li L., Zhang Y., and Wang X. S. (2020). Expression of the SARS-CoV-2 Cell Receptor Gene ACE2 in a Wide Variety of Human Tissues. *Infect. Dis. Poverty* 9, 45. doi: 10.1186/s40249-020-00662-x

Liu F., Long X., Zhang B., Zhang W., Chen X., and Zhang Z. (2020). Ace2 Expression in Pancreas may Cause Pancreatic Damage After SARS-CoV-2 Infection. *Clin. Gastroenterol. Hepatol.* 18, 2128–2130.e2. doi: 10.1016/j.cgh.2020.04.040

Lonsdale J., Thomas J., Salvatore M., Phillips R., Lo E., Shad S., et al. (2013). The Genotype-Tissue Expression (Gtex) Project. *Nature Genet* doi: 10.1038/ng.2653

Memon B., Karam M., Al-Khawaga S., and Abdelalim E. M. (2018). Enhanced Differentiation of Human Pluripotent Stem Cells Into Pancreatic Progenitors Co-Expressing PDX1 and NKX6.1. *Stem Cell Res. Ther.* 9, 15. doi: 10.1186/s13287-017-0759-z

Mukherjee R., Smith A., and Sutton R. (2020). Covid-19-related Pancreatic Injury. *Br. J. Surg.* 107, e1900. doi: 10.1002/bjs.11645

Müller J. A., Groß R., Conzelmann C., Krüger J., Merle U., Steinhart J., et al. (2021). Sars-CoV-2 Infects and Replicates in Cells of the Human Endocrine and Exocrine Pancreas. *Nat. Metab.* 3, 149–165. doi: 10.1038/s42255-021-00347-1

Nardacci R., Perfettini J., Grieco L., Thieffry D., Kroemer G., and Piacentini M. (2015). Syncytial Apoptosis Signaling Network Induced by the HIV-1 Envelope Glycoprotein Complex: An Overview. *Cell Death and Dis* 6, e1846. doi: 10.1038/cddis.2015.204

Ong M. S., Deng S., Halim C. E., Cai W., Tan T. Z., Huang R. Y. J., et al. (2020). Cytoskeletal Proteins in Cancer and Intracellular Stress: A Therapeutic Perspective. *Cancers (Basel)* 12, 238. doi: 10.3390/cancers12010238

Pelayo J., Lo K. B., Bhargav R., Gul F., Peterson E., Dejoy R., et al. (2020). Clinical Characteristics and Outcomes of Community- and Hospital-Acquired Acute Kidney Injury With COVID-19 in a US Inner City Hospital System. *Cardio Renal Med.* 10, 223–231. doi: 10.1159/000509182

Pinte L., and Baicus C. (2020). Pancreatic Involvement in SARS-CoV-2: Case Report and Living Review. *J. Gastrointestin. Liver Dis.* 29, 277–276. doi: 10.15403/jgld-2618

Rajamani U., Gross A. R., Hjelm B. E., Sequeira A., Vawter M. P., Tang J., et al. (2018). Super-Obese Patient-Derived Ipsc Hypothalamic Neurons Exhibit Obesogenic Signatures and Hormone Responses. *Cell Stem Cell* 22, 698–712.e9. doi: 10.1016/j.stem.2018.03.009

Rawla P., Bandaru S. S., and Vellipuram A. R. (2017). Review of Infectious Etiology of Acute Pancreatitis. *Gastroenterol. Res.* 10, 153–158. doi: 10.14740/gr858w

Righetti A., Giulietti M., Šabanović B., Occhipinti G., Principato G., and Piva F. (2019). CXCL12 and Its Isoforms: Different Roles in Pancreatic Cancer? *J. Oncol.* 2019. doi: 10.1155/2019/9681698

Salsman J., Top D., Boutilier J., and Duncan R. (2005). Extensive Syncytium Formation Mediated by the Reovirus Fast Proteins Triggers Apoptosis-Induced Membrane Instability. *J. Virol.* 79, 8090–8100. doi: 10.1128/JVI.79.13.8090-8100.2005

Scheller C., and Jassoy C. (2001). Syncytium Formation Amplifies Apoptotic Signals: A New View on Apoptosis in HIV Infection *In Vitro*. *Virology* 282, 48–55. doi: 10.1006/viro.2000.0811

Shang J., Wan Y., Luo C., Ye G., Geng Q., Auerbach A., et al. (2020). Cell Entry Mechanisms of SARS-CoV-2. *Proc. Natl. Acad. Sci. USA* 117, 11727–11734. doi: 10.1073/pnas.2003138117

Sharma A., Garcia G., Wang Y., Plummer J. T., Morizono K., Arumugaswami V., et al. (2020). Human Ipsc-Derived Cardiomyocytes are Susceptible to SARS-CoV-2 Infection. *Cell Rep. Med.* 1, 100052. doi: 10.1016/j.xcrm.2020.100052

Snijder E. J., Limpens R. W. A. L., de Wilde A. H., de Jong A. W. M., Zevenhoven-Dobbe J. C., Maier H. J., et al. (2020). A Unifying Structural and Functional Model of the Coronavirus Replication Organelle: Tracking Down RNA Synthesis. *PloS Biol.* 18, e3000715. doi: 10.1371/journal.pbio.3000715

Song P., Li W., Xie J., Hou Y., and You C. (2020). Cytokine Storm Induced by SARS-CoV-2. *Clin. Chim. Acta* 509, 280–287. doi: 1016/j.cca.2020.06.017

Tuttolomondo D., Frizzelli A., Aiello M., Bertorelli G., Majori M., and Chetta A. (2020). Beyond the Lung Involvement in COVID-19 Patients. A Review. *Minerva Med.* doi: 10.23736/S0026-4806.20.06719-1

Varga Z., Flammer A. J., Steiger P., Haberecker M., Andermatt R., Zinkernagel A. S., et al. (2020). Endothelial Cell Infection and Endotheliitis in COVID-19. *Lancet* 395, 1417–1418. doi: 10.1016/S0140-6736(20)30937-5

Verdecchia P., Cavallini C., Spanevello A., and Angeli F. (2020). The Pivotal Link Between ACE2 Deficiency and SARS-CoV-2 Infection. *Eur. J. Intern. Med.* 76, 14–20. doi: 10.1016/j.ejim.2020.04.037

Wang C., Zhang M., Garcia G., Tian E., Cui Q., Chen X., et al. (2021). Apoe-Isoform-Dependent SARS-CoV-2 Neurotropism and Cellular Response. *Cell Stem Cell* 28, 331–342.e5. doi: 10.1016/j.stem.2020.12.018

Wolff G., Melia C. E., Snijder E. J., and Bárcena M. (2020). Double-Membrane Vesicles as Platforms for Viral Replication. *Trends Microbiol.* 28, 1022–1033. doi: 10.1016/j.tim.2020.05.009

Xu Z. S., Shu T., Kang L., Wu D., Zhou X., Liao B. W., et al. (2020). Temporal Profiling of Plasma Cytokines, Chemokines and Growth Factors From Mild, Severe and Fatal COVID-19 Patients. *Signal Transduction Targeting Ther.* 5, 100. doi: 10.1038/s41392-020-0211-1

Yao H., Yang Z., Liu Z., Miao X., Yang L., Li D., et al. (2017). Glypican-3 and KRT19 are Markers Associating With Metastasis and Poor Prognosis of Pancreatic Ductal Adenocarcinoma. *Cancer Biomarkers* 17, 397–404. doi: 10.3233/CBM-160655

Yuan X., Wu J., Shan Y., Yao Z., Dong B., Chen B., et al. (2006). SARS Coronavirus 7a Protein Blocks Cell Cycle Progression at G0/G1 Phase *Via* the Cyclin D3/pRb Pathway. *Virology* 346, 74–85. doi: 10.1016/j.virol.2005.10.015

11

Next-Generation Sequencing Reveals the Progression of COVID-19

Xiaomin Chen[1], Yutong Kang[2,3,4], Jing Luo[5], Kun Pang[1], Xin Xu[1], Jinyu Wu[1], Xiaokun Li[6] and Shengwei Jin[7]**

[1] Institute of Genomic Medicine, Wenzhou Medical University, Wenzhou, China, [2] Wenzhou Key Laboratory of Sanitary Microbiology, Ministry of Education, Wenzhou, China, [3] Key Laboratory of Laboratory Medicine, Ministry of Education, Wenzhou, China, [4] School of Laboratory Medicine and Life Sciences, Wenzhou Medical University, Wenzhou, China, [5] Rheumatology Department, The First Affiliated Hospital of Wenzhou Medical University, Wenzhou, China, [6] Chemical Biology Research Center, School of Pharmaceutical Sciences, Wenzhou Medical University, Wenzhou, China, [7] Department of Anesthesia and Critical Care, Second Affiliated Hospital of Wenzhou Medical University, Wenzhou, China

***Correspondence:**
Shengwei Jin
18796242588@163.com
Xiaokun Li
xiaokunli@163.net

The novel coronavirus SARS-CoV-2 (causing the disease COVID-19) has caused a highly transmissible and ongoing pandemic worldwide. Due to its rapid development, next-generation sequencing plays vital roles in many aspects. Here, we summarize the current knowledge on the origin and human transmission of SARS-CoV-2 based on NGS analysis. The ACE2 expression levels in various human tissues and relevant cells were compared to provide insights into the mechanism of SAS-CoV-2 infection. Gut microbiota dysbiosis observed by metagenome sequencing and the immunogenetics of COVID-19 patients according to single-cell sequencing analysis were also highlighted. Overall, the application of these sequencing techniques could be meaningful for finding novel intermediate SARS-CoV-2 hosts to block interspecies transmission. This information will further benefit SARS-CoV-2 diagnostic development and new therapeutic target discovery. The extensive application of NGS will provide powerful support for our fight against future public health emergencies.

Keywords: next-generation sequencing, SARS coronavirus 2 (SARS-CoV-2), origin, gut microbiota, angiotensin-converting enzyme 2 (ACE2)

INTRODUCTION

In the end of 2019, the Chinese population was infected with a novel coronavirus, SARS coronavirus 2 (SARS-CoV-2, causing the disease COVID-19), which was identified from sequence-based analysis of isolates from the patients (Cui et al., 2019a). SARS-CoV-2 is the seventh known coronavirus that infects humans (Dallavilla et al., 2020). Phylogenetic analysis showed that SARS-CoV-2 belongs to the Sarbecovirus subtype of Betacoronavirus (Zhou et al., 2020b). SARS-CoV-2 uses angiotension-converting enzyme 2 (ACE2) as a receptor and primarily infects ciliated bronchial epithelial cells and type II pneumocytes (Kuhn et al., 2004). It has infected 78,939,299 individuals, with a mortality rate of 2.2%, across 109 countries as of the date 2020/12/24 (**Supplementary Figure 1**). The outbreaks of novel pneumonia add to evidence of the COVID-19 epidemic steadily growing by human-to-human transmission (Fang et al., 2020a). COVID-19 has very important clinical manifestations, such as high rates of transmission and mild to moderate clinical features, especially with more serious abnormalities found in the elderly (Yuen et al., 2020).

Infected patients present with respiratory symptoms, such as fever, dry cough, and even dyspnea, as well as sometimes with digestive and other systemic manifestations, and some progress with severe acute respiratory syndrome or even death (Liu et al., 2020b).

The COVID-19 epidemic was declared a public health emergency of international concern. Since the outbreak of COVID-19, there has been considerable discussion on the origin and human-to-human transmission of the causative virus. Interestingly, ACE2 receptors are also reported to be expressed in the kidney and gastrointestinal tract, tissues known to harbor SARS-CoV (Harmer et al., 2002; Leung et al., 2003). Reports also suggest that SARS-CoV-2 RNA can be detected in the stool of some patients with COVID-19 (Wu et al., 2020b). Thus, there is the distinct possibility of involvement of the lung-gut axis caused by the gut microbiota, which is supported by the fact that some COVID-19 patients have diarrhea. A total of 273,606 new coronavirus-related genome sequences has been uploaded to the EpiFlu™ database (belong to GISAID) worldwide as of 22nd December, 2020. Notably, next-generation sequencing (NGS) has been applied to the study of COVID-19 and has greatly promoted SARS-CoV-2 origin tracing. It is critical to explore the potential origins and mechanism of SARS-CoV-2 to control the spread of COVID-19 and further improve the therapeutic regimen.

NEXT-GENERATION SEQUENCING PROMOTES SARS-COV-2 ORIGIN TRACING

NGS plays an important role in finding the origin and intermediate host of SARS-CoV-2. Hundreds of coronaviruses and SARS-CoV-2 genomes which were determined with NGS are publicly available for researchers to study the origin of SARS-CoV-2 (Woo et al., 2010; Zhou et al., 2020e). A small number of people speculate that SARS-CoV-2 may be man-made, but there is probably no basis for speculation about artificial SARS-CoV-2 (Dallavilla et al., 2020). Kristian G Andersen et al. clearly showed that SARS-CoV-2 is not a laboratory structure or a deliberately manipulated virus (Andersen et al., 2020). In addition, two notable genomic features of SARS-CoV-2 were identified by NGS (**Figure 1B**): Spike protein contains two subunits, S1 and S2, whose boundary position is at 685/686 of the amino acid sequence. S1 mainly contains receptor binding domain (RBD), which is responsible for the recognition of cell receptors. S2 contains the basic elements required for membrane fusion. The RBD in the spike protein is the most variable part of the coronavirus genome. Six RBD amino acids have been shown to be critical for binding to ACE2 receptors and for defining the host range of SARS-CoV-like viruses (Wan et al., 2020); additionally, the spike protein of SARS-CoV-2 inserts 12 nucleotides with a functional multibase (furin) cleavage site (RRAR) at the S1-S2 boundary, which also leads to the expected three O-linked glycans around the site (Andersen et al., 2020).

During 2020.01.29-2020.02.03, Lu et al. performed NGS of bronchoalveolar lavage fluid samples (n=9) (Lu et al., 2020a). Zhou et al. used NGS to obtain the viruses from seven patients with severe pneumonia and carried out full-length sequencing on an RNA sample of *Rhinolophus affinis* (Global Initiative on Sharing All Influenza Data, GISAID). The metagenomic analysis of the bat sample (*Rhinolophus affinis*) showed that the most closely related virus to SARS-CoV-2 is RaTG13, with an identity of 96.2% (**Figure 1**) (Zhou et al., 2020e). Similarly, Zhang et al's phylogenomic analysis of the released genomic data of 27 isolates of SARS-CoV-2 showed that bat coronavirus and SARS-CoV-2 probably have a common ancestor (Hu et al., 2018). SARS-CoV-2 was first isolated from street vendors selling wild animals and mammals (Zhang et al., 2020b). On 2020.06.08, Zhou et al. reported a coronavirus named RmYN02 (identified from a metagenomic analysis of 227 bats) have 93.3% nucleotide identity with SARS-CoV-2 in the complete genome. However, RmYN02 has a low sequence identity with SARS-CoV-2 in the RBD (61.3%) (Zhou et al., 2020b). All these studies indicated that SARS-CoV-2 may have originated from bats.

During 2020.03–2020.05, Zhang et al. used reference genome of the *Manis javanica* (SRA), SARS-CoV-2, Bat-CoV-RaTG13 (NGDC), and 2,845 coronavirus from ViPR for genome analysis. In terms of sequence identity, in addition to Bat-CoV-RaTG13, Pangolin-CoV-2020 is the coronavirus most closely related to SARS-CoV-2 (**Figure 1C**). Because the six RBD amino acids residues (L, F, Q, S, N, and Y, **Figure 1B**) on the S1 protein of Pangolin-CoV-2020 are exactly the same as those of SARS-CoV-2 ((Wan et al., 2020), Receptor Recognition by the Novel Coronavirus from Wuhan: an Analysis Based on Decade-Long Structural Studies of SARS Coronavirus), while Bat-CoV-RaTG13 has only one amino acid residue that is the same as on the six RBD residues in SARS-CoV-2. Thus, they proposed that the pangolin is more likely than the bat to be the origin of SARS-CoV-2. However, Pangolin-CoV-2020 and Bat-CoV-RaTG13 have lost the key polybasic cleavage site (RRAR) at the junction of S1 and S2 (**Figure 1B**), the two subunits of the spike of SARS-CoV-2 (Zhang et al., 2020c). Furthermore, a similar debatable conclusion was also obtained (Liu et al., 2020b). In addition, NGS of frozen tissues (lungs, intestine, and blood) collected from 18 Malayan pangolins (*Manis javanica*) identified pangolin-associated coronaviruses as belonging to two SARS-CoV-2-associated coronavirus sublines, one of which has a strong similarity to SARS-CoV-2 in the RBD (Lam et al., 2020). These discoveries only suggest that pangolins may be the origin of SARS-CoV-2-like viruses.

During 2020.05–2020.07, Xiao et al. identified 34 highly related contigs in a set of pangolin viral metagenomes based on BLAST results. Subsequently, metagenomic sequencing of the lung tissue of four Chinese pangolins (*Manis pentadactyla*) and 25 Malayan pangolins (*Manis javanica*) showed surprising results. The sequence identity of the Pangolin-CoV genome, comparing with SARS-CoV-2 and Bat SARS-related (SARSr-CoV) RaTG13 is 80%–98% excluding the S gene, while the identity is 80%–91% including the S gene. Further comparison and analysis of the S gene revealed that these genomes may have

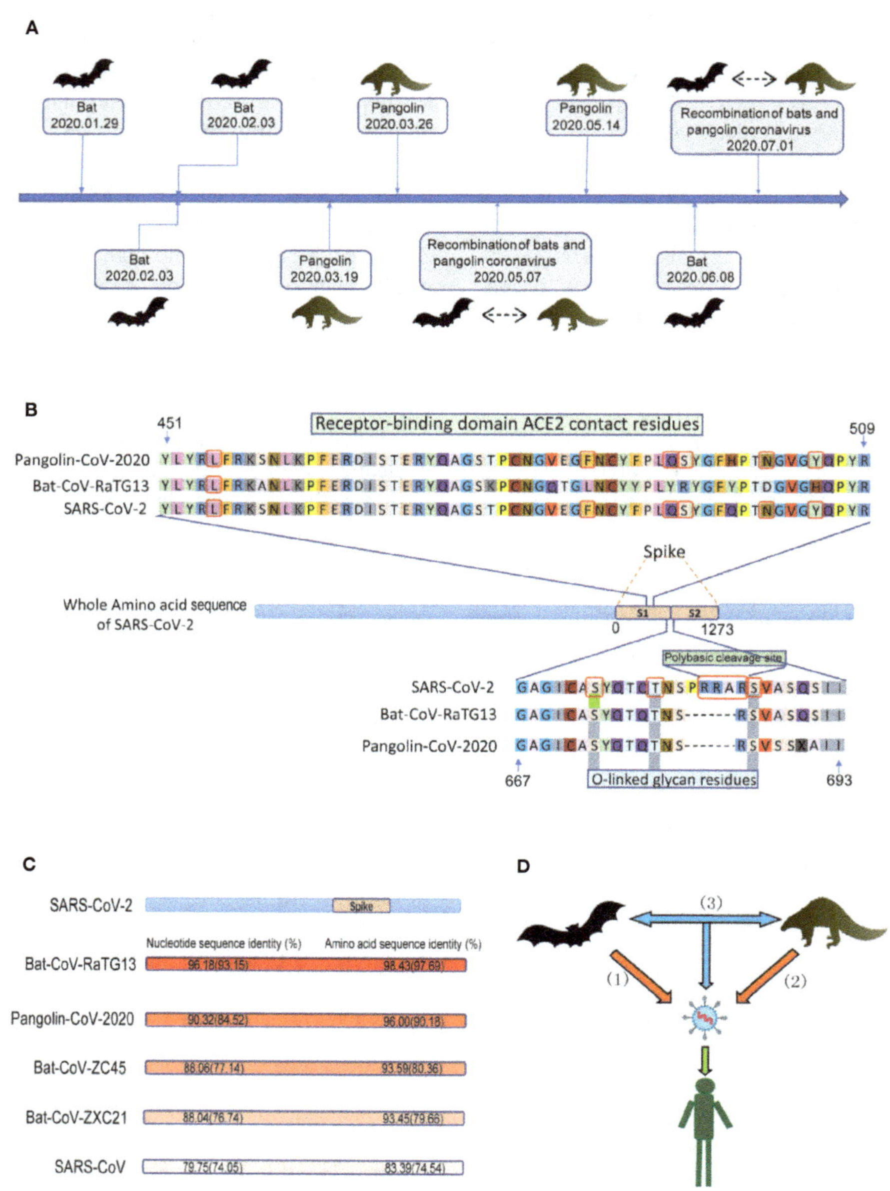

FIGURE 1 | Conjectures on the origin of SARS-CoV-2. **(A)** The discovery of the potential animal origin of SARS-CoV-2 at different times, such as Bat-2020.01.29 (Lu et al., 2020a), Bat-2020.02.03 (Zhou et al., 2020e), Bat-2020.02.03 (Zhang et al., 2020b), Pangolin-2020.03.19 (Zhang et al., 2020c), Pangolin-2020.03.26 (Lam et al., 2020), Recombination of bats and pangolin coronavirus-2020.05.07 (Xiao et al., 2020), Pangolin-2020.05.14 (Liu et al., 2020b), Bat-2020.06.08 (Zhou et al., 2020b), Recombination of bats and pangolin coronavirus-2020.07.01 (Li et al., 2020c). **(B)** Features of the spike protein in human SARS-CoV-2 and related coronaviruses. Key residues in the spike protein that make contact with the ACE2 receptor are marked with blue boxes. Both the polybasic cleavage site and the three adjacent predicted O-linked glycans are unique to SARS-CoV-2. The six key RBD amino acids are indicated by red. **(C)** Nucleotide sequence identity and protein sequence identity among the whole genome including S gene (indicated by brackets) of some representative coronaviruses with SARS-CoV-2 **(D)** Three conjectures about the origin of SARS-CoV-2. i) SARS-CoV-2 originated in bats, ii) pangolins, and iii) *via* recombination events during the evolution of different animal coronaviruses.

undergone recombination events. For example, Pangolin-CoV is more similar to Bat SARSr-CoV ZXC21 and Bat SARSr-CoV ZC45 in the region of nucleotides 1-914, while in the remaining part, it is more similar to SARS-CoV-2-like and Bat-CoV-RaTG13. According to the existing genome comparison, SARS-CoV-2 may have originated from the recombination of Pangolin-CoV-like viruses and Bat-CoV-RaTG13-like viruses (Xiao et al., 2020). Liu et al. also obtained similar results showing that a recombination event could have occurred during the evolution of these coronaviruses (Liu et al., 2020c). Li et al. analyzed 43 complete coronavirus genome sequences (Li et al., 2020c), including coronaviruses from bats, pangolins and humans. Their study showed that the currently sampled pangolin coronaviruses are unlikely to be precursors of SARS-

CoV-2, but these sequences contain the receptor-binding motif most likely to bind to human ACE2. Excluding S genes, SARS-CoV-2 has the greatest genetic similarity with RaTG13. In addition, researchers found recombination fracture sites before and after the ACE2 RBD in SARS-CoV-2. Therefore, they think that SARS-CoV-2 was produced by the selection and recombination of bat and pangolin coronaviruses.

Recently, the SARS-CoV-2 epidemic broke out in a newly developed market in Beijing. Relevant agencies have detected SARS-CoV-2 in the cutting board of imported salmon. Researchers discovered 3 new viruses in wild and farmed salmon in September 2019 by metatranscriptomic sequencing of dead and moribund cultured Chinook salmon (Mordecai et al., 2019). We analyzed the nucleotide sequences of SARS-CoV-2 (NCBI, GenBank: MN908947.3) and Pacific salmon nidovirus (PsNV, GenBank: MK611985.1), one from the three new viruses, and found only 22%–35% identity in partial protein sequence (**Supplementary Table 1**), and PsNV does not have key amino acid residues similar to the SARS-CoV-2 spike protein, which can bind to human ACE2. Therefore, the possibility that salmon is the origin or intermediate host of SARS-CoV-2 is low based on the genome data obtained by NGS. This result further supports the evidence that SARS-CoV-2 infects only mammals since it belongs to the Coronaviridae family, Betacoronavirus (Cui et al., 2019a).

Using NGS technology, the genome sequence information of unknown viruses can be obtained for the first time. This information provides the possibility to quickly trace the potential origin of novel SARS-CoV-2, which is vital to blocking interspecies transmission. However, this method is limited by the number of known sequences. At present, scientists and researchers upload whole genomic sequences of SARS-CoV-2 at GISAID EpiFlu™, and the number of genomes is still increasing. It may take time due to the massive diversity and evolution of the virus. We still believe that NGS technology will greatly promote the process of tracing the origin of SARS-CoV-2.

NEXT-GENERATION SEQUENCING PROMOTES TRACING INTERPERSONAL TRANSMISSION OF SARS-COV-2

SARS-CoV-2 is a positive-sense RNA virus belonging to the genus Betacoronavirus. Recent genotyping analysis of the SARS-CoV-2 population revealed a high frequency of mutations in various essential genes encoding S protein, N protein, and RNA polymerase (Yin, 2020). SARS-Cov-2 may first indirectly control mitochondria through ACE2 regulation of mitochondrial function. Once the virus enters the host cell, open reading frame (ORF) (e.g., ORF-9B) can directly manipulate mitochondrial function to evade the immune function of host cells and promote viral replication, causing COVID-19 disease (Singh et al., 2020). The evolutionary pattern of SARS-CoV-2 with highly frequent mutations can be observed in a short time using NGS. The monitoring of SARS-CoV-2's evolutionary patterns and spread dynamics by genome sequencing is essential for controlling and preventing COVID-19. High-resolution genomic epidemiology has become an effective tool for public health surveillance and disease control, and the large number of the real-time genome sequencing efforts for SARS-CoV-2 were triggered by the current COVID-19 pandemic (Sintchenko et al., 2009; Gardy and Loman, 2018; Grubaugh et al., 2019b). Analysis of the genetic sequence data of the pandemic SARS-CoV-2 can provide insights into the origin of the epidemic, global transmission, and epidemiological history.

The outbreak of COVID-19 started in mid-December 2019 in Wuhan, China, and rapidly spread throughout China. The haplotype evolution network can be utilized for recovering the direction of human-to-human transmission in a local area and spread in a larger area. A study conducted metagenomic NGS on 10 samples from COVID-19 patients in Hubei. Ten newly sequenced SARS-CoV-2 genomes and 136 genomes from the GISAID database were classified as 58 haplotypes. The network indicated that virus samples corresponding to the original haplotype found in patients living near the Huanan Seafood Wholesale Market. Although the patients had a high probability of subconscious contact with the market, it is impossible to draw a conclusion based on this clue regarding whether the market is the origin center of SARS-CoV-2. Among them, 16 genomes from the Huanan Seafood Wholesale Market were assigned to 10 haplotypes, indicating that the market experienced a circulating infection in the short term, which caused the outbreak of SARS-CoV-2 in Wuhan and other regions (Fang et al., 2020a).

Using both metagenomic sequencing and tiling amplicon approaches, viral genome sequences were generated from 53 patients in Guangdong. Combined genomic data and epidemiological data showed that the SARS-CoV-2 sequences in Guangdong Province are interspersed with virus clades from other provinces in China and other countries, indicating that most of the detected cases are related to travel, not local communities. Following the discovery of the first COVID-19 case in early January, most infections were attributed to viruses imported from elsewhere. The size and duration of the local transmission chain is limited (Lu et al., 2020a).

Since the emergence of COVID-19 in Asia at the end of last year, the disease has spread to all continents except Antarctica (Rodriguez-Morales et al., 2020). To reveal the source of SARS-CoV-2 introduction and the patterns of transmission in the United States, Fauver et al. sequenced the nine viral genomes of patients with COVID-19 reported early in Connecticut using the amplicon sequencing approach "PrimalSeq" (Grubaugh et al., 2019a), using "genomic epidemiology" to identify the likely sources of SARS-CoV-2 in Connecticut. The combined results of genomic epidemiology and travel pattern analysis indicated that family transmission has become an important source of new SARS-CoV-2 infection. The outbreak on the east coast (Connecticut) is related to the outbreak on the west coast (Washington), which indicates that transcontinental transmission has already occurred.

To investigate the genomic epidemiology and genetic diversity of SARS-CoV-2 in Northern California, 29 samples from patients diagnosed with COVID-19 infection were collected for whole-genome sequencing. Phylogenetic analysis showed that there are at least eight different SARS-CoV-2 lineages, indicating that the virus has been independently introduced into the state many times. To date, the cryptic transmission of SARS-CoV-2 in Northern California has been characterized by multiple transmission chains, whose origin is a unique introduction from international and interstate travel, rather than the widespread community transmission of a single main lineage (Deng et al., 2020).

To prospectively monitor the spread of incidents in New South Wales, Australia, SARS-CoV-2 was extracted from 209 patients diagnosed with COVID-19 infection for whole-genome sequencing from January 2020 to March 2020. Computational agent-based modeling and high-resolution SARS-CoV-2 genome surveillance were used to understand the evolution of this novel virus strain and the local transmission chain in the community. The 209 New South Wales SARS-CoV-2 genomes are scattered throughout the global SARS-CoV-2 phylogeny. Most genomes from imported New South Wales cases grouped with viral sequences from the origin country. The major genomic lineage is dominated by genomes from Australia, which are considered to be imported from Iran (Rockett et al., 2020).

A study collected genome data of 93 SARS-CoV-2 isolates covering 12 countries on 4 continents from the GISAID EpiFlu™ database (access date 12 February 2020). All the genomes were classified as 58 haplotypes (H1~H58). The results showed that H13 and H38 are the ancestral haplotypes of SARS-CoV-2. The virus samples corresponding to these two haplotypes were from patients from Shenzhen (the first case in Guangdong) and patients from Washington state (the first case in the United States). The potentially specific directions of human-to-human transmission were recovered by this approach, such as in the England family (H28 → H29), Shenzhen family (H13 → H14), Queensland tour group (H25 → H26), and Japanese group (H53 → H52). Phylogenetic network analysis showed that the source of SARS-CoV-2 in the Huanan Seafood Wholesale Market was imported from elsewhere (Yu et al., 2020).

Phylogenetics is very important to solve various biological problems, such as the relationship between species or genes, the origin and spread of viral infections, and the demographic changes and migration patterns of species (Avise and Wollenberg, 1997; Grenfell et al., 2004; Li and Durbin, 2011). The NGS technology and the rapid accumulation of genome sequence data have made phylogeny an indispensable tool for all branches of biology (Yang and Rannala, 2012). Phylogenetic network analysis of 160 complete SARS-CoV-2 genome sequences collected from around the world from December 24, 2019 to March 4, 2020 revealed that there are three distinct but closely related variants of SARS-CoV-2 called A, B, and C (**Figure 2**). Based on the bat outgroup coronavirus, A is an ancestral type. Data analysis found that the first type A virus was from an American individual living in Wuhan. At the same time, the type A virus itself was also detected in a large number of infected people in the United States and Australia, but surprisingly, type A is not the main type of virus in Wuhan city. The main virus type of patients in Wuhan is type B, and it has infected patients throughout East Asia. Type B virus is immunologically or environmentally suitable for most populations in East Asia, and if there is no further mutation, it will not spread much outside the region. People in Wuhan also exhibited type A infection, and the earliest cases were in American individuals. Type C virus is the main European type and was found in early patients from France, Italy, Sweden, and the United Kingdom. Type C virus did not appear in the Chinese patient samples in the study, but it was found in Singapore, Hong Kong, and South Korea (Forster et al., 2020).

The use of NGS technology has become a widely accepted method for outbreak tracking and genomic epidemiology in molecular typing in microbiology laboratories. Detecting new mutations in SARS-CoV-2 allows researchers to reconstruct unknown routes of infection and provide a molecular basis for SARS-CoV-2 vaccine design, drug discovery, and diagnostic development, which is a key technology in genomic epidemiology (Lourenco et al., 2020). Monitoring the SARS-

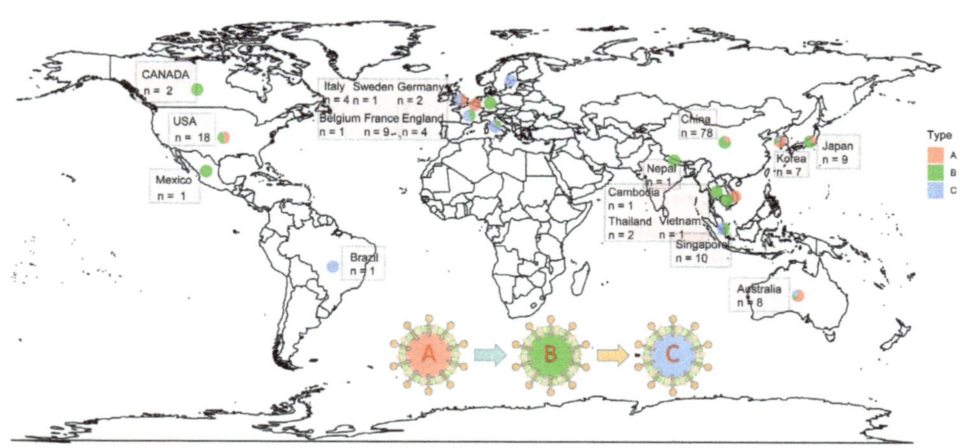

FIGURE 2 | The distribution of SARS-CoV-2 A\B\C types in some countries worldwide. The data were collected from 2019.12.24 to 2020.03.04. The type A was indicated by red; type B was indicated by green; and type C was indicated by green.

CoV-2 genome helps to achieve a more effective COVID-19 control strategy and to investigate cases with unclear sources of infection within a short turnaround time (Sintchenko and Holmes, 2015; Deng et al., 2020; Lu et al., 2020a; Lu et al., 2020b). The international sharing of SARS-CoV-2 genomic data collected by researchers and public health microbiology service providers enhances the power of such surveillance (Dos et al., 2018; Hadfield et al., 2018).

SARS-COV-2-SUSCEPTIBLE ORGANS WITH HIGH EXPRESSION OF ACE2 DETERMINED BY NEXT-GENERATION SEQUENCING

Over the past years, RNA sequencing technology has achieved dynamic improvement of genomes, including DNA and RNA quantitative and qualitative changes, which were widely applied into various genomic measurements especially transcriptomics studies (Consortium et al., 2007). However, ordinary RNA-seq was also confronted with several challenges including limited sequencing depth for low-abundance transcripts and ineffaceable influence of interferential cells' gene expression in tissues (Levin et al., 2009). Similar to the process of RNA-seq, scRNA-seq also have to undergo some required steps including RNA extraction, transcription into first-strand cDNA, second-strand synthesis, and cDNA amplification (Islam et al., 2014). Moreover, through preliminary single-cell extraction, scRNA-seq could overcome the influence of heterogeneous cells expression in tissues and accomplish various analysis including cell type identification, cell trajectory inference, cell hierarchy reconstruction, and other potential applications (Hwang et al., 2018). Hence, NGS technology could be applied to identify relative gene expression and detect special cell type in various diseases.

NGS technology was applied at either the molecular or protein level to further investigate the mechanism of SAS-CoV-2 infection. Only when bound to cell surface receptors can the virus enter the target cells for further replication, which is the prerequisite of coronavirus infection (Li, 2016). ACE2 is a cell surface protein that is expressed in the heart, blood vessels, kidney, and especially lung type II alveolar (AT2) epithelial cells (Richardson et al., 2020a). Two teams independently reported the discovery that ACE2 could serve as the receptor for SAS-CoV-2 (Xu et al., 2020b; Zhou et al., 2020d). Furthermore, SARS-CoV-2 could enhance infection by exploiting species-specific interferon-driven upregulation of ACE2 (Ziegler et al., 2020). Therefore, the different organs, tissues and cells with high ACE2 expression are considered targets with potential high infection risk for SARS-CoV-2. In **Figure 3A**, the mechanism for the binding of ACE2 and SARS-CoV-2 through spike protein, assisted by TMPRSS2, was clearly studied by massive researches (Hoffmann et al., 2020).

Specific comorbidities were found to increase the risk of infection with worse lung injury and death in COVID-19 and hypertension, obesity, and diabetes were identified as the most common comorbidities in COVID-19 according to a clinical research of 5,700 patients in the New York City Area (Richardson et al., 2020b). Moreover, the expression imbalance of ACE2 was found significantly associated with multiple comorbidities in COVID-19. A Mendelian randomization analysis revealed the high-expression level of ACE2 was causally associated with diabetes, which might interpret the high risk to COVID-19 in diabetic patients (Rao et al., 2020). In addition, Sammy et al. identified higher expression of ACE2 in visceral and subcutaneous adipose tissue than that in lung tissues, providing with a possible interpretation for susceptibility of infection in obese patients (Al-Benna, 2020). In China, about 23% of hypertensive COVID-19 patients were reported with 6% case fatality rate (Ma et al., 2020) and hypotensors, especially ACE2 inhibitors, and angiotensin receptor blockers (ARBs), were frequently used to control the levels of blood pressure, which also upregulated the expression of ACE2 receptor and leaded to increasing susceptibility to SARS-CoV-2 infection (Fang et al., 2020b). Further, other common comorbidities including chronic obstructive pulmonary disease (COPD), asthma, and cardiovascular disease (CVD) were also found more severe symptom and prognosis in COVID-19 with high expression of ACE2 (Contoli et al., 2006; Shi et al., 2020; Wan et al., 2020). Here, we summarize the expression features of ACE2 in the respiratory, cardiovascular, digestive, urinary, and reproductive systems through RNA sequencing (RNA-seq) and single-cell RNA sequencing (scRNA-seq) to investigate susceptibility to COVID-19.

Respiratory symptoms are usually the initial clinical presentation of COVID-19, including fever, chest pain, shortness of breath, dry cough, and fatigue, suggesting that the respiratory system is the most common target organ of SARS-CoV-2 infection (Ge et al., 2020; Zhou et al., 2020c). A previous study investigated the mRNA and protein expression of ACE2 from different human tissues by RT-qPCR and immunohistochemistry and found that ACE2 was concentrated in lung alveolar epithelial cells and enterocytes of the small intestine (Harmer et al., 2002; Hamming et al., 2004). Moreover, Xin Zou et al. analyzed scRNA-seq datasets of the human respiratory system, including the nasal mucosa, respiratory track, and bronchus, using lung tissues and airway epithelial cells. Lung ACE2 was further identified to be highly expressed in AT2 and respiratory epithelial cells, while nasal and bronchial cells showed low ACE2 expression (Zou et al., 2020). Zhao's study also found that ACE2 expression in AT2 cells significantly upregulated other genes relevant to viral reproduction and transmission through scRNA-seq (Zhao et al., 2020). Furthermore, lung type II pneumocytes and nasal goblet secretory cells were identified as ACE2 and TMPRSS2-coexpressing cells in both humans and nonhuman primates *via* scRNA-seq analysis. Based on the above studies, AT2, respiratory epithelial, and nasal goblet secretory cells with high expression of ACE2 based on NGS technology probably have a high SARS-CoV-2 infection risk.

Xin Zou et al. investigated scRNA-seq datasets from the esophagus, stomach, ileum, and liver and found extremely high ACE2 expression in epithelial cells of the ileal esophagus, which is

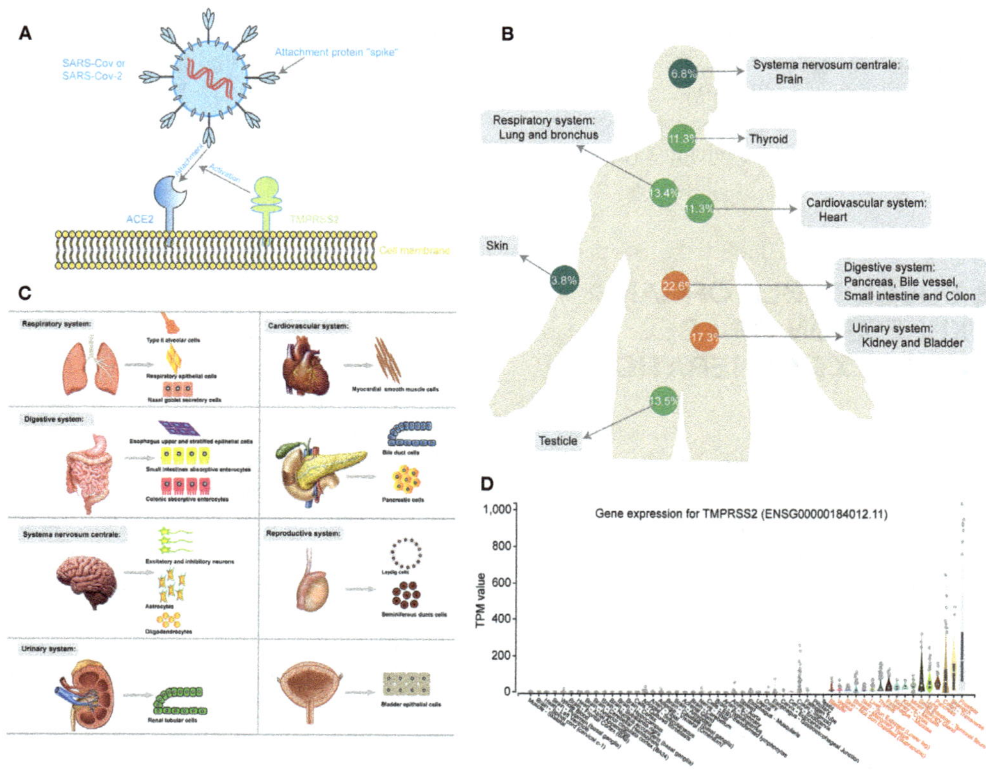

FIGURE 3 | **(A)** Schematic chart showing the mechanism of SARS-CoV-2 binding to the ACE2 receptor, assisted by TMPRSS2. **(B)** The human figure displays different expression levels of ACE2 in different organs. **(C)** The cell maps show different susceptible cells of different susceptible organs during SARS-CoV-2 infection. **(D)** The box diagram showing the different expression of TMPRSS2 in different human tissues.

consistent with the results of histopathology and immunohistochemical staining by (Hamming et al., 2004; Zou et al., 2020). Moreover, the distribution of ACE in the digestive system was systematically analyzed *via* scRNA-seq from surgically resected digestive organs tissues in Xu's study (Zhang et al., 2020a). High-level expression of ACE2 was identified not only in upper and stratified epithelial cells of the esophagus but also in absorptive enterocytes from the ileum and colon, consistent with previous studies (Hamming et al., 2004). Regarding other organs of the digestive system, it was reported by Liu et al. that the mRNA level of ACE2 was higher in the pancreas than in the lung and that ACE2 was expressed in both the exocrine glands and islets *via* scRNA-seq (Liu et al., 2020a). In addition, scRNA-seq analysis was also applied to identify specific ACE2 expression in cholangiocytes rather than hepatocytes, suggesting that liver abnormalities might be caused by cholangiocyte dysfunction (Chai et al., 2020). All these studies identified the specific cellular susceptibility to SARS-CoV-2 infection in the digestive system according to NGS and scRNA-seq technology, especially in esophageal upper and stratified epithelial cells, absorptive enterocytes from the ileum and colon, exocrine glands, islets, and cholangiocytes.

It has been reported that patients with SARS-CoV-2 infection have a high proportion of acute and chronic cardiac injury, based on clinical studies (Wu et al., 2020a; Zheng et al., 2020). Moreover, Li et al. analyzed the mRNA expression of ACE2 in 13 different human organs from the GTEx database with NGS and found that ACE2 expression levels were high in the small intestine, testes, kidneys, heart, thyroid, and adipose tissues but relatively low in the blood, spleen, bone marrow, brain, blood vessels, and muscle (Li et al., 2020b). Regarding specific cells, ACE2 was identified to be overexpressed in massive myocardial cells through scRNA-seq using cardiac cells from human embryos (Zou et al., 2020). Additionally, scRNA-seq also demonstrated high expression of ACE2 in specific cells of human fetal hearts, including cardiomyocytes (CM), macrophages, smooth muscle cells, and pericytes (SMC/Peri) (Cui et al., 2019b).

Using scRNA-seq from tissues of kidney transplant and bladder tissues homogenate, high expression of ACE2 was confirmed in kidney proximal tubule (PT) cells and bladder urothelial cells in Xin Zou's study, indicating that the kidney and bladder might also be the target organs for SARS-CoV-2 infection (Zou et al., 2020). Moreover, quite similar results showing that overexpressed ACE2 was identified in renal tubular cells of patients with COVID-19 were also validated in another study (Li et al., 2020d). In addition, both Fan's and Wang's studies (Fan et al., 2020; Wang and Xu, 2020) also found that ACE2 was highly expressed in Leydig cells and cells in seminiferous ducts in the testis, indicating that the urinary and reproductive systems are susceptible to SARS-CoV-2 infection due to high levels of ACE2.

In addition to atypical pneumonia, the central nervous system (CNS) symptoms of COVID-19 patients have been observed in the clinic, including dizziness, headache, impaired consciousness, acute cerebrovascular disease, ataxia, and epilepsy (Li et al., 2020d; Mao et al., 2020). Massive microarray, RNA-seq and scRNA-seq analyses have indicated that nuclear expression of ACE2 was identified in many neurons and some non-neuron cells in the human middle temporal gyrus and posterior cingulate cortex. These expression features of ACE2 were also validated in a mouse model using brain tissues (Chen et al., 2020).

Aside the CNS, several specific organs, such as the skin, thyroid, and adrenal gland, also exhibited high expression of ACE2, as detected by scRNA-seq analysis (Li et al., 2020b). In particular, Li et al. demonstrated that ACE2 is highly expressed in maternal-fetal interface cells, including stromal cells and perivascular cells of the decidua and cytotrophoblasts and syncytiotrophoblasts in the placenta. Moreover, high expression of ACE2 was also validated in human fetal organs, including the heart, liver, and lung but not the kidney (Li et al., 2020a).

Furthermore, Bian et al. directly detected SARS-CoV-2 RNA in the stomach, breast, testes, spleen, heart, hilar lymph nodes, liver, gallbladder, kidney, nasopharyngeal mucosa, oral mucosa and skin through virus nucleic acid RT-qPCR detection, immunohistochemical staining, and electron microscopy from 37 systematic autopsy and 54 percutaneous multiple organ biopsy cases, consistent with the results of RNA-seq (Wu and Team, 2020). On a cautionary note, the NGS data from Genotype-Tissue Expression (GTEx) project also clear exhibited the mRNA expression of TMPRSS2 in different human tissues (**Figure 3D**) (Consortium, 2013). Similar to the expression of ACE2, TMPRSS2 was not only high-expressed in respiratory (lungs) and digestive system (stomach, transverse-colon, pancreas, small intestine, esophagus -mucosa, and liver), but also up-regulated in urinary system (kidney-medulla and cortex, and bladder) and other glandular tissues (prostate, thyroid and mammary tissue), perhaps contributing to one explanation for non-respiratory symptoms in COVID-19 patients.

In conclusion, NGS and scRNA-seq were applied to reveal the expression features of ACE2 in different organ systems and specific cells after SARS-CoV-2 infection. The ratio of ACE2 expression in different organ systems was clearly exhibited, and the respiratory, digestive, cardiovascular, urinary, and reproductive systems were identified as high-risk organs with relatively high expression of ACE2, while relatively low expression of ACE2 was found in the CNS and skin (**Figure 3B**). Moreover, a susceptibility cell map of SARS-CoV-2 infection with high ACE2 expression is displayed in a systemic multiorgan depiction (**Figure 3C**). These findings will further benefit SARS-CoV-2 diagnostics and new therapeutic target identification.

THE CHANGES IN THE INTESTINAL FLORA REVEALED BY METAGENOMICS SEQUENCING

In addition to common clinical symptoms in the lungs, some COVID-19 patients have also developed gastrointestinal symptoms, such as diarrhea, nausea, and vomiting (Chen et al., 2020; Gu et al., 2020a; Wang et al., 2020a). It was recently reported that COVID-19 RNA was found in the fecal samples and anal swabs of infected patients (Wu et al., 2020b; Zhou et al., 2020a). Interestingly, intestinal epithelial cells, particularly the crypt surface of small intestine epithelial cells, also express ACE2 receptors. Researchers also found that ACE2 mutations may reduce the expression of antimicrobial peptides and change the composition of intestinal microbes (Hashimoto et al., 2012). In addition, the intestinal flora has been shown to affect lung health through important cross-talk between the intestinal flora and lungs, which is known as the gut-lung axis (Keely et al., 2012). The gut-lung axis is considered to be bidirectional, which means that endotoxins and microbial metabolites can affect the lungs through blood circulation, and inflammation of the lungs may change the gut microecology (Dumas et al., 2018). It is also known that respiratory viral infections can disturb the intestinal flora, such as influenza and respiratory syncytial virus (RSV) (Groves et al., 2018). This fact raises the interesting possibility that COVID-19 may also affect the intestinal flora.

The intestinal microbiota is a dynamic ecological community and can regulate promote or suppress response by invading viruses (Li et al., 2019). Prior studies have suggested that respiratory viral infections are associated with alterations of the gut microbiota, which made patients more susceptible to secondary bacterial infections (Hanada et al., 2018; Yildiz et al., 2018). A preliminary study using shotgun metagenomic sequencing of 15 patients with COVID-19 found that the fecal microbiome of COVID-19 patients had continuous changes during hospitalization compared with that of the control group. Many pathogens and opportunistic pathogens were enriched in the intestinal microbiome of patients with COVID-19, including Clostridium, *Bacteroides nordii*, and *Actinomyces viscosus*. Research on the oral and upper respiratory microbiome of patients with the COVID-19 also found an increase in the abundance of the opportunistic pathogen *Actinomyces viscosus* (Habib et al., 2018). Even after the clearance of SARS-CoV-2 (as determined by a throat swab) and relief of respiratory symptoms, depleted symbionts, and intestinal dysbiosis persisted. Correlation analysis between fecal microbe baseline abundance and COVID-19 severity showed that *Coprobacillus*, *Clostridium ramosum*, and *Clostridium hathewayi* were significantly positively correlated with COVID-19 severity, whereas *Faecalibacterium prausnitzii* (an anti-inflammatory bacteria) was inversely related to the severity (mild, moderate, severe, or critical) of disease (Zuo et al., 2020).

A recent study compared the fecal microbiome of COVID-19 patients with that of healthy controls (HCs) and H1N1 patients and obtained results similar to those of Tao et al. (Gu et al., 2020b) (**Table 1**). Compared with that in the gut microbiome of HCs, the relative abundance of opportunistic pathogens (such as Streptococcus, Rothia, Veillonella, and Actinomycetes) in the gut microbiome of COVID-19 patients was significantly higher, and the relative abundance of beneficial symbiotic bacteria was lower. Compared with COVID-19 patients, H1N1 patients showed lower diversity and different overall microbial compositions.

TABLE 1 | The change of gut microbiome in COVID-19 patients (Gu et al., 2020b).

Title	Subject	Sample	Sequencing method	Conclusion
Alterations in Gut Microbiota of Patients With COVID-19 During Time of Hospitalization	15 COVID-19 patients Six community-acquired pneumonia patients 15 healthy controls	fecal samples	shotgun metagenomic sequencing	enrichment of opportunistic pathogens and depletion of beneficial symbionts
Alterations of the Gut Microbiota in Patients with COVID-19 or H1N1 Influenza	30 COVID-19 patients 24 influenza A patients 30 healthy controls	fecal samples	16sRNA	

Intestinal flora regulation is very important for improving the immune system, preventing viral infections and reducing clinical signs. Some patients with COVID-19 show dysbiosis of the intestinal flora, and the abundance of probiotics, such as Lactobacillus and Bifidobacterium, is reduced. The use of prebiotics or probiotics may help to regulate intestinal flora balance and reduce the risk of secondary infections caused by bacterial translocation after coronavirus infection (Xu et al., 2020a). In addition, a fiber-rich diet not only changes the intestinal flora but also affects lung immunity (Trompette et al., 2014). Circulating short-chain fatty acids (SCFAs) produced during microbial metabolism of fermentable fibers in the diet may have a mitigating effect on lung allergic inflammation (Trompette et al., 2014). Intestinal flora diversity decreases in old age, and COVID-19 is fatal mainly in elderly patients, which again shows that the intestinal flora may play a role in the disease (Nagpal et al., 2018).

IMMUNOGENETICS OF COVID-19 REVEALED THROUGH SINGLE-CELL RNA SEQUENCING

Acute respiratory distress syndrome (ARDS) and multiple organ failure have been reported as the major causes of death due to SARS-CoV-2 infection, associated with high levels of circulating cytokines and substantial mononuclear cell infiltration in the heart, lungs, kidneys, and spleen through autopsy analysis (Diao et al., 2020b; Mehta et al., 2020; Xu et al., 2020c). The mechanism of the immune response is complex during SARS-CoV-2 infection, and Ronny et al. identified two distinct immunopathological profiles. One is high expression of interferon-stimulated genes (ISGs) and cytokines and high viral loads with limited pulmonary damage, and the other is severely damaged lungs with downregulated ISGs, low viral loads, and abundant immune infiltrates (Nienhold et al., 2020). A better understanding of the immune cells associated with differential responses in SARS-CoV-2-infected patients will be immensely helpful to better identifying therapeutic targets. However, the concrete mechanisms of the key immune cell subset changes remain unclear. Here, we summarized the major distinct immune cell compositions and states of different degrees of SARS-CoV-2 infection by scRNA-seq technology. Hyperinflammation similar to macrophage activation syndrome has been detected in patients with severe COVID-19, including massively increased production of cytokines, such as IL-6, IL-7, and tumor necrosis factor (TNF), and of inflammatory chemokines, such as CC-chemokine ligand 2 (CCL2), CCL3, and CXCL10 (Schulert and Grom, 2015; Mehta et al., 2020). Through scRNA-seq analysis based on bronchoalveolar fluid (BALF) from patients with COVID-19, Liao et al. found increased proportions of mononuclear macrophages accounting for 80% of total BALF cells and further identified a depletion of tissue-resident alveolar macrophages and an abundance of inflammatory monocyte-derived macrophages (Liao et al., 2020a). Moreover, a significant increase in the populations of CD14+ and CD16+ monocytes producing IL-6 was also validated in the peripheral blood samples of patients with COVID-19 through scRNA-seq analysis of peripheral blood mononuclear cells (Wen et al., 2020b). In addition, a special subset of macrophages of COVID-19 patients has been described, which is enriched in genes associated with tissue repair and promotes fibrosis generation, and scRNA-seq analysis also identified alternative M2-like macrophages that were functionally defined as a profibrotic subset (Ramachandran et al., 2019; Liao et al., 2020b). Dandan et al. (Wu and Yang, 2020) have detected high levels of IL-17-induced helper T cells (Th17 cells) in the periphery blood of patients infected with SARS-Cov-2 and those cells were considered as the main sources for IL17A which would lead to worse alveolar damage and multiple organ failures (Xu et al., 2020c). Moreover, Sodhi et al. demonstrated that ACE2 could regulate pneumonic neutrophilic infiltration through an IL17A-dependent manner in the bacterial pneumonia murine model and further found recombinant ACE2 could reduce neutrophilic infiltration by inhibiting IL17A-induced activation of STAT3 (Sodhi et al., 2019). High levels of IL18 and the reduction of mucosal-associated invariant T (MAIT) cells have also been identified in COVID-19 and significantly associated with the mortality and poor outcome in SARS-Cov-2 infection (Satis et al., 2021). Flament et al. validated the correlation between increasing cytotoxicity of circulating MAIT cells and severe inflammation response, particularly high levels of IL-18 through analysis data from 102 COVID-19 patients and 80 uninfected controls. Furthermore, these researchers proposed a two-step process of MAIT cell activation induced by type I IFN and later IL-18 through co-culture experiments of SARS-CoV-2-infected macrophages with MAIT cells *in vitro* (Gea-Mallorqui, 2020).

The T cell immune response, especially memory T cell activation, has been reported to be necessary for resolving

SARS-CoV infection in patients and mice (Channappanavar et al., 2014; Liu et al., 2017). However, previous studies have certified that coronavirus could cause an irregular T cell response by stimulating T cell apoptosis (Zhou et al., 2014), and substantial clinical studies have also demonstrated a reduction in and functional exhaustion of T cells (especially CD4+ and CD8+ T cells) based on data from 522 patients with laboratory-confirmed COVID-19 (Diao et al., 2020a). In addition, during the severe and mild stages of SARS-CoV-2 infection, a lower proportion of CD8+ T cells and a higher proportion of CD4+ T cells with high levels of effector molecules were detected in severe patients than in mild patients, according to scRNA-seq analysis based on BALF from three severe and three mild COVID-19 patients (Liao et al., 2020a). Furthermore, it was also confirmed that the ratio of naïve CD4+ T cells to CD8+ T cells decreased in early recovery-stage (ERS) COVID-19 patients, while the central memory CD4+ T cells were significantly higher than in HCs by scRNA-seq analysis of peripheral blood mononuclear cells during the recovery stage of COVID-19 (Wen et al., 2020a).

Similarly, B lymphocytes, especially plasma cells, are also immune effectors that protect against viral infection through producing immunoglobulin antibodies, and for respiratory viruses, these antibodies, which reside in upper respiratory tract tissues, are particularly effective in that they provide a first line of defense against the virus at its point of entry (Sealy et al., 2013). However, the number of B cells significantly decreased in COVID-19 patients, and severe cases had a lower level than mild cases, according to clinical studies (Wang et al., 2020b). Moreover, Liu et al. also further verified that the significant decrease in B cell levels was consistent with the degree of disease severity and was detected earlier in pleural effusion than in peripheral blood *via* scRNA-seq analysis (Liu et al., 2020d). Notably, compared with that in the severe stage of COVID-19, the percentage of plasma cells increased significantly, whereas naïve B cell levels decreased significantly in the recovery stage of COVID-19 in Wen's scRNA-seq analysis (Wen et al., 2020a).

It is well known that natural killer (NK) cells play a vital role in the control of pathogen infection by mediating cellular immunity and cytotoxic function as primary cytotoxic lymphocytes (Vivier et al., 2008). In one study, the absolute number of NK cells was found to be significantly decreased in severe and mild COVID-19 patients, and it tended to increase after remission in 32 COVID-19 patients with different severities (Jiang et al., 2020). However, Liao and her colleagues identified higher proportions of NK cells in COVID-19 patients than in controls, and severe patients contained a lower proportion of NK cells than mild patients, according to scRNA-seq analysis (Liao et al., 2020a). Regarding the recovery stage of COVID-19, the proportion of NK cells was found to be higher than that in the HCs, and these cells express higher levels of inflammatory genes. In contrast, during the later recovery stage, these patients have an increase in NK cell levels with lower expression of inflammatory genes (Wen et al., 2020b).

During the progression of SARS-CoV-2 infection, innate and adaptive immune responses are activated, with massive inflammatory factor release, which causes exhaustion of various types of immune cells, especially lymphocytes (Xiong et al., 2020). The recent research provides data of adaptive immunity in COVID-19 patients (Schultheiss et al., 2020). The application of NGS technology, including scRNA-seq analysis, clearly revealed the landscape of immune cells during the different stages of COVID-19, which could be a valuable resource for clinical guidance on anti-inflammatory medication and understanding the molecular mechanisms.

CONCLUSION

COVID-19 has pushed the world to the brink. Its outbreak has seriously threatened public health and caused general panic. This is perhaps one among the first reviews that focuses on the application of NGS to COVID-19. NGS, the ultra-rapid and cost-effective technology, has contributed to progress in determining novel SARS-CoV-2 hosts, evolution, and spread patterns, which are critical to designing effective disease control and prevention strategies. The rate of data acquisition and analysis has been inconceivably rapid which made the NGS methods applicable to monitor and counter the spread of SARS-CoV-2. Coordinated efforts are required to promote the principles of data sharing in order to facilitate more efficient data analysis of SARS-CoV-2.

In just very short time, NGS was applied to reveal the expression features of ACE2 in different organ systems and specific cells after infection with SARS-CoV-2 and to characterize the intestinal flora. This map might provide potential clues for interpreting different organ damage due to SARS-CoV-2 infection and help doctors better prevent target organ damage in the clinic, indicating the essential role of sequencing technology in filling the gap between molecular research and clinical application. Moreover, these findings are expected to provide further insight into the role of ACE2 and the pathogenesis of SARS-CoV-2 infection.

The importance of the intestinal flora in COVID-19 infection has been recognized and accepted by the Chinese government and the majority of frontline medical staff. Although there are currently no specific antiviral treatments, we speculate that probiotics can regulate the intestinal flora, thereby beneficially changing gastrointestinal symptoms and providing respiratory protection. Further study should focus on investigating whether the benefits of ACE2 for lung diseases may be mediated by regulating the intestinal and/or lung microbiota. The profiled immune cells also provide insight into adaptive immunity to SARS-CoV-2 for therapeutic guidance and vaccine development.

In conclusion, the application of NGS is crucial to understand the pathophysiologic mechanisms underlying the systemic manifestations of COVID-19 and its clinical significance. The insights from this review will add new dimensions to the understanding of infectious diseases and will benefit future decisive actions.

AUTHOR CONTRIBUTIONS

SJ, XL, and JW conceived this review. XC organized and critically revised the manuscript. YK and JL did major work of writing the manuscript. KP and XX made contributions to writing the manuscript. All authors contributed to the article and approved the submitted version.

SUPPLEMENTARY MATERIAL

Supplementary Figure 1 | (A) The cumulative number of confirmed cases, as well as the cumulative number of cured and deaths around the world. **(B)** Number of patients in the top 25 countries and China with the largest number of confirmed cases. **(C)** Cure and deaths rates in the top 25 countries and China with the largest number of confirmed cases. The data comes from the website which is daily updated. (https://voice.baidu.com/act/newpneumonia/newpneumonia/?from=osari_aladin_banner#tab4)

REFERENCES

Al-Benna, S. (2020). Association of high level gene expression of ACE2 in adipose tissue with mortality of COVID-19 infection in obese patients. *Obes. Med.* 19. 1–4. doi: 10.1016/j.obmed.2020.100283

Andersen, K. G., Rambaut, A., Lipkin, W. I., Holmes, E. C., and Garry, R. F. (2020). The proximal origin of SARS-CoV-2. *Nat. Med.* 26, 450–452. doi: 10.1038/s41591-020-0820-9

Avise, J. C., and Wollenberg, K. (1997). Phylogenetics and the origin of species. *Proc. Natl. Acad. Sci. U. S. A.* 94, 7748–7755. doi: 10.1073/pnas.94.15.7748

Chai, X., Hu, L., Zhang, Y., Han, W., Lu, Z., Ke, A., et al. (2020). Specific ACE2 Expression in Cholangiocytes May Cause Liver Damage After 2019-nCoV Infection. *BioRxiv*. doi: 10.1101/2020.02.03.931766

Channappanavar, R., Fett, C., Zhao, J., Meyerholz, D. K., and Perlman, S. (2014). Virus-specific memory CD8 T cells provide substantial protection from lethal severe acute respiratory syndrome coronavirus infection. *J. Virol.* 88, 11034–11044. doi: 10.1128/JVI.01505-14

Chen, N., Zhou, M., Dong, X., Qu, J., Gong, F., Han, Y., et al. (2020). Epidemiological and clinical characteristics of 99 cases of 2019 novel coronavirus pneumonia in Wuhan, China: a descriptive study. *Lancet* 395, 507–513. doi: 10.1016/S0140-6736(20)30211-7

Consortium, E. P., Birney, E., Stamatoyannopoulos, J. A., Dutta, A., Guigo, R., Gingeras, T. R., et al. (2007). Identification and analysis of functional elements in 1% of the human genome by the ENCODE pilot project. *Nature* 447, 799–816. doi: 10.1038/nature05874

Consortium, G. T. (2013). The Genotype-Tissue Expression (GTEx) project. *Nat. Genet.* 45, 580–585. doi: 10.1038/ng.2653

Contoli, M., Message, S. D., Laza-Stanca, V., Edwards, M. R., Wark, P. A., Bartlett, N. W., et al. (2006). Role of deficient type III interferon-lambda production in asthma exacerbations. *Nat. Med.* 12, 1023–1026. doi: 10.1038/nm1462

Cui, J., Li, F., and Shi, Z. L. (2019a). Origin and evolution of pathogenic coronaviruses. *Nat. Rev. Microbiol.* 17, 181–192. doi: 10.1038/s41579-018-0118-9

Cui, Y., Zheng, Y., Liu, X., Yan, L., Fan, X., Yong, J., et al. (2019b). Single-cell transcriptome analysis maps the developmental track of the human heart. *Cell Rep.* 26, 1934–1950.e5. doi: 10.1016/j.celrep.2019.01.079

Dallavilla, T., Bertelli, M., Morresi, A., Bushati, V., Stuppia, L., Beccari, T., et al. (2020). Bioinformatic analysis indicates that SARS-CoV-2 is unrelated to known artificial coronaviruses. *Eur. Rev. Med. Pharmacol. Sci.* 24, 4558–4564. doi: 10.26355/eurrev_202004_21041

Deng, X., Gu, W., Federman, S., Du Plessis, L., Pybus, O., Faria, N., et al. (2020). A genomic survey of SARS-CoV-2 reveals multiple introductions into Northern California without a predominant lineage. *medRxiv* 2020.03.27.20044925. doi: 10.1101/2020.03.27.20044925

Diao, B., Wang, C., Tan, Y., Chen, X., Liu, Y., Ning, L., et al. (2020a). Reduction and Functional Exhaustion of T Cells in Patients With Coronavirus Disease 2019 (COVID-19). *Front. Immunol.* 11, 827, 1–7. doi: 10.3389/fimmu.2020.00827

Diao, B., Wang, C., Wang, R., Feng, Z., Tan, Y., Wang, H., et al. (2020b). Human Kidney is a Target for Novel Severe Acute Respiratory Syndrome Coronavirus 2 (SARS-CoV-2) Infection. *medRxiv* 1–17. doi: 10.1101/2020.03.04.20031120

Dos, S. R. C., Koopmans, M. P., and Haringhuizen, G. B. (2018). Threats to timely sharing of pathogen sequence data. *Science* 362, 404–406. doi: 10.1126/science.aau5229

Dumas, A., Bernard, L., Poquet, Y., Lugo-Villarino, G., and Neyrolles, O. (2018). The role of the lung microbiota and the gut-lung axis in respiratory infectious diseases. *Cell Microbiol.* 20, e12966. doi: 10.1111/cmi.12966

Fan, C., Li, K., Ding, Y., Lu, W. L., and Wang, J. (2020). ACE2 Expression in Kidney and Testis May Cause Kidney and Testis Damage After 2019-nCoV Infection. *medRxiv*. doi: 10.1101/2020.02.12.20022418

Fang, B., Liu, L., Yu, X., Li, X., Ye, G., Xu, J., et al. (2020a). Genome-wide data inferring the evolution and population demography of the novel pneumonia coronavirus (SARS-CoV-2). *bioRxiv* 2020.03.04.976662. doi: 10.1101/2020.03.04.976662

Fang, L., Karakiulakis, G., and Roth, M. (2020b). Are patients with hypertension and diabetes mellitus at increased risk for COVID-19 infection? *Lancet Respir. Med.* 8, e21.10. doi: 10.1016/S2213-2600(20)30116-8

Forster, P., Forster, L., Renfrew, C., and Forster, M. (2020). Phylogenetic network analysis of SARS-CoV-2 genomes. *Proc. Natl. Acad. Sci. U. S. A.* 117, 9241–9243. doi: 10.1073/pnas.2004999117

Gardy, J. L., and Loman, N. J. (2018). Towards a genomics-informed, real-time, global pathogen surveillance system. *Nat. Rev. Genet.* 19, 9–20. doi: 10.1038/nrg.2017.88

Ge, H., Wang, X., Yuan, X., Xiao, G., Wang, C., Deng, T., et al. (2020). The epidemiology and clinical information about COVID-19. *Eur. J. Clin. Microbiol. Infect. Dis.* 39, 1011–1019. doi: 10.1007/s10096-020-03874-z

Gea-Mallorqui, E. (2020). IL-18-dependent MAIT cell activation in COVID-19. *Nat. Rev. Immunol.* 20, 719. doi: 10.1038/s41577-020-00467-x

Grenfell, B. T., Pybus, O. G., Gog, J. R., Wood, J. L., Daly, J. M., Mumford, J. A., et al. (2004). Unifying the epidemiological and evolutionary dynamics of pathogens. *Science* 303, 327–332. doi: 10.1126/science.1090727

Groves, H. T., Cuthbertson, L., James, P., Moffatt, M. F., Cox, M. J., and Tregoning, J. S. (2018). Respiratory disease following viral lung infection alters the murine gut microbiota. *Front. Immunol.* 9, 182. doi: 10.3389/fimmu.2018.00182

Grubaugh, N. D., Gangavarapu, K., Quick, J., Matteson, N. L., De Jesus, J. G., Main, B. J., et al. (2019a). An amplicon-based sequencing framework for accurately measuring intrahost virus diversity using PrimalSeq and iVar. *Genome Biol.* 20, 8. doi: 10.1186/s13059-018-1618-7

Grubaugh, N. D., Ladner, J. T., Lemey, P., Pybus, O. G., Rambaut, A., Holmes, E. C., et al. (2019b). Tracking virus outbreaks in the twenty-first century. *Nat. Microbiol.* 4, 10–19. doi: 10.1038/s41564-018-0296-2

Gu, J., Han, B., and Wang, J. (2020a). COVID-19: gastrointestinal manifestations and potential fecal-oral transmission. *Gastroenterology* 158, 1518–1519. doi: 10.1053/j.gastro.2020.02.054

Gu, S., Chen, Y., Wu, Z., Chen, Y., Gao, H., Lv, L., et al. (2020b). Alterations of the gut microbiota in patients with COVID-19 or H1N1 influenza. *Clin. Infect. Dis.* doi: 10.1093/cid/ciaa709

Habib, S., Siddiqui, A. H., Azam, M., Siddiqui, F., and Chalhoub, M. (2018). Actinomyces viscosus causing disseminated disease in a patient on methotrexate. *Respir. Med. Case Rep.* 25, 158–160. doi: 10.1016/j.rmcr.2018.08.009

Hadfield, J., Megill, C., Bell, S. M., Huddleston, J., Potter, B., Callender, C., et al. (2018). Nextstrain: real-time tracking of pathogen evolution. *Bioinformatics* 34, 4121–4123. doi: 10.1093/bioinformatics/bty407

Hamming, I., Timens, W., Bulthuis, M. L., Lely, A. T., Navis, G., and van Goor, H. (2004). Tissue distribution of ACE2 protein, the functional receptor for SARS coronavirus. A first step in understanding SARS pathogenesis. *J. Pathol.* 203, 631–637. doi: 10.1002/path.1570

Hanada, S., Pirzadeh, M., Carver, K. Y., and Deng, J. C. (2018). Respiratory Viral Infection-Induced Microbiome Alterations and Secondary Bacterial Pneumonia. *Front. Immunol.* 9, 2640. doi: 10.3389/fimmu.2018.02640

Harmer, D., Gilbert, M., Borman, R., and Clark, K. L. (2002). Quantitative mRNA expression profiling of ACE 2, a novel homologue of angiotensin converting enzyme. *FEBS Lett.* 532, 107–110. doi: 10.1016/s0014-5793(02)03640-2

Hashimoto, T., Perlot, T., Rehman, A., Trichereau, J., Ishiguro, H., Paolino, M., et al. (2012). ACE2 links amino acid malnutrition to microbial ecology and intestinal inflammation. *Nature* 487, 477–481. doi: 10.1038/nature11228

Hoffmann, M., Kleine-Weber, H., Schroeder, S., Kruger, N., Herrler, T., Erichsen, S., et al. (2020). SARS-CoV-2 Cell Entry Depends on ACE2 and TMPRSS2 and Is Blocked by a Clinically Proven Protease Inhibitor. *Cell* 181, 271–280.e8. doi: 10.1016/j.cell.2020.02.052

Hu, D., Zhu, C., Ai, L., He, T., Wang, Y., Ye, F., et al. (2018). Genomic characterization and infectivity of a novel SARS-like coronavirus in Chinese bats. *Emerg. Microbes Infect.* 7, 154. doi: 10.1038/s41426-018-0155-5

Hwang, B., Lee, J. H., and Bang, D. (2018). Single-cell RNA sequencing technologies and bioinformatics pipelines. *Exp. Mol. Med.* 50, 96. doi: 10.1038/s12276-018-0071-8

Islam, S., Zeisel, A., Joost, S., La Manno, G., Zajac, P., Kasper, M., et al. (2014). Quantitative single-cell RNA-seq with unique molecular identifiers. *Nat. Methods* 11, 163–166. doi: 10.1038/nmeth.2772

Jiang, Y., Wei, X., Guan, J., Qin, S., Wang, Z., Lu, H., et al. (2020). COVID-19 pneumonia: CD8(+) T and NK cells are decreased in number but compensatory increased in cytotoxic potential. *Clin. Immunol.* 218, 108516. doi: 10.1016/j.clim.2020.108516

Keely, S., Talley, N. J., and Hansbro, P. M. (2012). Pulmonary-intestinal cross-talk in mucosal inflammatory disease. *Mucosal Immunol.* 5, 7–18. doi: 10.1038/mi.2011.55

Kuhn, J. H., Li, W., Choe, H., and Farzan, M. (2004). Angiotensin-converting enzyme 2: a functional receptor for SARS coronavirus. *Cell. Mol. Life Sci.* 61, 2738–2743. doi: 10.1007/s00018-004-4242-5

Lam, T. T., Jia, N., Zhang, Y. W., Shum, M. H., Jiang, J. F., Zhu, H. C., et al. (2020). Identifying SARS-CoV-2-related coronaviruses in Malayan pangolins. *Nature* 583, 282–285. doi: 10.1038/s41586-020-2169-0

Leung, W. K., To, K. F., Chan, P. K., Chan, H. L., Wu, A. K., Lee, N., et al. (2003). Enteric involvement of severe acute respiratory syndrome-associated coronavirus infection. *Gastroenterology* 125, 1011–1017. doi: 10.1016/s0016-5085(03)01215-0

Levin, J. Z., Berger, M. F., Adiconis, X., Rogov, P., Melnikov, A., Fennell, T., et al. (2009). Targeted next-generation sequencing of a cancer transcriptome enhances detection of sequence variants and novel fusion transcripts. *Genome Biol.* 10, R115. doi: 10.1186/gb-2009-10-10-r115

Li, H., and Durbin, R. (2011). Inference of human population history from individual whole-genome sequences. *Nature* 475, 493–496. doi: 10.1038/nature10231

Li, N., Ma, W. T., Pang, M., Fan, Q. L., and Hua, J. L. (2019). The Commensal Microbiota and Viral Infection: A Comprehensive Review. *Front. Immunol.* 10, 1551. doi: 10.3389/fimmu.2019.01551

Li, M., Chen, L., Zhang, J., Xiong, C., and Li, X. (2020a). The SARS-CoV-2 receptor ACE2 expression of maternal-fetal interface and fetal organs by single-cell transcriptome study. *PLoS One* 15, e0230295. doi: 10.1371/journal.pone.0230295

Li, M. Y., Li, L., Zhang, Y., and Wang, X. S. (2020b). Expression of the SARS-CoV-2 cell receptor gene ACE2 in a wide variety of human tissues. *Infect. Dis. Poverty* 9, 45. doi: 10.1186/s40249-020-00662-x

Li, X., Giorgi, E. E., Marichann, M. H., Foley, B., Xiao, C., Kong, X. P., et al. (2020c). Emergence of SARS-CoV-2 through recombination and strong purifying selection. *Sci. Adv.* doi: 10.1101/2020.03.20.000885

Li, Y. C., Bai, W. Z., and Hashikawa, T. (2020d). The neuroinvasive potential of SARS-CoV2 may play a role in the respiratory failure of COVID-19 patients. *J. Med. Virol.* 92, 552–555. doi: 10.1002/jmv.25728

Li, F. (2016). Structure, function, and evolution of coronavirus spike proteins. *Annu. Rev. Virol.* 3, 237–261. doi: 10.1146/annurev-virology-110615-042301

Liao, M., Liu, Y., Yuan, J., Wen, Y., Xu, G., Zhao, J., et al. (2020a). The landscape of lung bronchoalveolar immune cells in COVID-19 revealed by single-cell RNA sequencing. *MedRxiv.* doi: 10.1101/2020.02.23.20026690

Liao, M., Liu, Y., Yuan, J., Wen, Y., Xu, G., Zhao, J., et al. (2020b). Single-cell landscape of bronchoalveolar immune cells in patients with COVID-19. *Nat. Med.* 26, 842–844. doi: 10.1038/s41591-020-0901-9

Liu, W. J., Zhao, M., Liu, K., Xu, K., Wong, G., Tan, W., et al. (2017). T-cell immunity of SARS-CoV: Implications for vaccine development against MERS-CoV. *Antiviral Res.* 137, 82–92. doi: 10.1016/j.antiviral.2016.11.006

Liu, F., Long, X., Zhang, B., Zhang, W., Chen, X., and Zhang, Z. (2020a). ACE2 expression in pancreas may cause pancreatic damage after SARS-CoV-2 infection. *Clin. Gastroenterol. Hepatol.* doi: 10.1016/j.cgh.2020.04.040

Liu, K., Fang, Y. Y., Deng, Y., Liu, W., Wang, M. F., Ma, J. P., et al. (2020b). Clinical characteristics of novel coronavirus cases in tertiary hospitals in Hubei Province. *Chin. Med. J. (Engl).* 133, 1025–1031. doi: 10.1097/CM9.0000000000000744

Liu, P., Jiang, J. Z., Wan, X. F., Hua, Y., Li, L., Zhou, J., et al. (2020c). Are pangolins the intermediate host of the 2019 novel coronavirus (SARS-CoV-2)? *PLoS Pathog.* 16, e1008421. doi: 10.1371/journal.ppat.1008421

Liu, X., Zhu, A., He, J., Chen, Z., Liu, L., Xu, Y., et al. (2020d). Single-cell analysis reveals macrophage-driven T cell dysfunction in severe COVID-19 patients. *medRxiv.* doi: 10.1101/2020.05.23.20100024

Lourenco, J., Paton, R., Ghafari, M., Kraemer, M., Thompson, C., Simmonds, P., et al. (2020). Fundamental principles of epidemic spread highlight the immediate need for large-scale serological surveys to assess the stage of the SARS-CoV-2 epidemic. *medRxiv* 2020.03.24.20042291. doi: 10.1101/2020.03.24.20042291

Lu, J., du Plessis, L., Liu, Z., Hill, V., Kang, M., Lin, H., et al. (2020a). Genomic epidemiology of SARS-CoV-2 in Guangdong Province, China. *Cell* 181, 997–1003 e9. doi: 10.1016/j.cell.2020.04.023

Lu, R., Zhao, X., Li, J., Niu, P., Yang, B., Wu, H., et al. (2020b). Genomic characterisation and epidemiology of 2019 novel coronavirus: implications for virus origins and receptor binding. *Lancet* 395, 565–574. doi: 10.1016/s0140-6736(20)30251-8

Ma, L. Y., Chen, W. W., Gao, R. L., Liu, L. S., Zhu, M. L., Wang, Y. J., et al. (2020). China cardiovascular diseases report 2018: an updated summary. *J. Geriatr. Cardiol.* 17, 1–8. doi: 10.11909/j.issn.1671-5411.2020.01.001

Mao, L., Jin, H., Wang, M., Hu, Y., Chen, S., He, Q., et al. (2020). Neurologic manifestations of hospitalized patients with coronavirus disease 2019 in Wuhan, China. *JAMA Neurol.* 77, 683–690. doi: 10.1001/jamaneurol.2020.1127

Mehta, P., McAuley, D. F., Brown, M., Sanchez, E., Tattersall, R. S., Manson, J. J., et al. (2020). COVID-19: consider cytokine storm syndromes and immunosuppression. *Lancet* 395, 1033–1034. doi: 10.1016/S0140-6736(20)30628-0

Mordecai, G. J., Miller, K. M., Di Cicco, E., Schulze, A. D., Kaukinen, K. H., Ming, T. J., et al. (2019). Endangered wild salmon infected by newly discovered viruses. *Elife* 8, 1–18. doi: 10.7554/eLife.47615

Nagpal, R., Mainali, R., Ahmadi, S., Wang, S., Singh, R., Kavanagh, K., et al. (2018). Gut microbiome and aging: Physiological and mechanistic insights. *Nutr. Healthy Aging* 4, 267–285. doi: 10.3233/NHA-170030

Nienhold, R., Ciani, Y., Koelzer, V. H., Tzankov, A., Haslbauer, J. D., Menter, T., et al. (2020). Two distinct immunopathological profiles in lungs of lethal COVID-19. *medRxiv Nat Commun.* 11, 5086. doi: 10.1101/2020.06.17.20133637

Ramachandran, P., Dobie, R., Wilson-Kanamori, J. R., Dora, E. F., Henderson, B. E. P., Luu, N. T., et al. (2019). Resolving the fibrotic niche of human liver cirrhosis at single-cell level. *Nature* 575, 512–518. doi: 10.1038/s41586-019-1631-3

Rao, S., Lau, A., and So, H. C. (2020). Exploring Diseases/Traits and Blood Proteins Causally Related to Expression of ACE2, the Putative Receptor of SARS-CoV-2: A Mendelian Randomization Analysis Highlights Tentative Relevance of Diabetes-Related Traits. *Diabetes Care* 43, 1416–1426. doi: 10.2337/dc20-0643

Richardson, P., Griffin, I., Tucker, C., Smith, D., Oechsle, O., Phelan, A., et al. (2020a). Baricitinib as potential treatment for 2019-nCoV acute respiratory disease. *Lancet* 395, e30–e31. doi: 10.1016/s0140-6736(20)30304-4

Richardson, S., Hirsch, J. S., Narasimhan, M., Crawford, J. M., McGinn, T., Davidson, K. W., et al. (2020b). Presenting Characteristics, Comorbidities, and Outcomes Among 5700 Patients Hospitalized With COVID-19 in the New York City Area. *JAMA* 323, 2052–2059. doi: 10.1001/jama.2020.6775

Rockett, R. J., Arnott, A., Lam, C., Sadsad, R., Timms, V., Gray, K.-A., et al. (2020). Revealing COVID-19 transmission by SARS-CoV-2 genome sequencing and agent based modelling. *bioRxiv* 2020.04.19.048751. doi: 10.1101/2020.04.19.048751

Rodriguez-Morales, A. J., MacGregor, K., Kanagarajah, S., Patel, D., and Schlagenhauf, P. (2020). Going global - Travel and the 2019 novel coronavirus. *Travel Med. Infect. Dis.* 33, 101578. doi: 10.1016/j.tmaid.2020.101578

Satis, H., Ozger, H. S., Aysert Yildiz, P., Hizel, K., Gulbahar, O., Erbas, G., et al. (2021). Prognostic value of interleukin-18 and its association with other inflammatory markers and disease severity in COVID-19. *Cytokine* 137, 155302. doi: 10.1016/j.cyto.2020.155302

Schulert, G. S., and Grom, A. A. (2015). Pathogenesis of macrophage activation syndrome and potential for cytokine- directed therapies. *Annu. Rev. Med.* 66, 145–159. doi: 10.1146/annurev-med-061813-012806

Schultheiss, C., Paschold, L., Simnica, D., Mohme, M., Willscher, E., von Wenserski, L., et al. (2020). Next-Generation Sequencing of T and B Cell Receptor Repertoires from COVID-19 Patients Showed Signatures Associated with Severity of Disease. *Immunity* 53, 442–455.e4. doi: 10.1016/j.immuni.2020.06.024

Sealy, R., Webby, R. J., Crumpton, J. C., and Hurwitz, J. L. (2013). Differential localization and function of antibody-forming cells responsive to inactivated or live-attenuated influenza virus vaccines. *Int. Immunol.* 25, 183–195. doi: 10.1093/intimm/dxs107

Shi, S., Qin, M., Shen, B., Cai, Y., Liu, T., Yang, F., et al. (2020). Association of Cardiac Injury With Mortality in Hospitalized Patients With COVID-19 in Wuhan, China. *JAMA Cardiol.* 5, 802–810. doi: 10.1001/jamacardio.2020.0950

Singh, K. K., Chaubey, G., Chen, J. Y., and Suravajhala, P. (2020). Decoding SARS-CoV-2 hijacking of host mitochondria in COVID-19 pathogenesis. *Am. J. Physiol. Cell Physiol.* 319, C258–C267. doi: 10.1152/ajpcell.00224.2020

Sintchenko, V., and Holmes, E. C. (2015). The role of pathogen genomics in assessing disease transmission. *BMJ* 350, h1314. doi: 10.1136/bmj.h1314

Sintchenko, V., Gallego, B., Chung, G., and Coiera, E. (2009). Towards bioinformatics assisted infectious disease control. *BMC Bioinformatics* 10 Suppl;2, S10. doi: 10.1186/1471-2105-10-S2-S10

Sodhi, C. P., Nguyen, J., Yamaguchi, Y., Werts, A. D., Lu, P., Ladd, M. R., et al. (2019). A Dynamic Variation of Pulmonary ACE2 Is Required to Modulate Neutrophilic Inflammation in Response to Pseudomonas aeruginosa Lung Infection in Mice. *J. Immunol.* 203, 3000–3012. doi: 10.4049/jimmunol.1900579

Trompette, A., Gollwitzer, E. S., Yadava, K., Sichelstiel, A. K., Sprenger, N., Ngom-Bru, C., et al. (2014). Gut microbiota metabolism of dietary fiber influences allergic airway disease and hematopoiesis. *Nat. Med.* 20, 159–166. doi: 10.1038/nm.3444

Vivier, E., Tomasello, E., Baratin, M., Walzer, T., and Ugolini, S. (2008). Functions of natural killer cells. *Nat. Immunol.* 9, 503–510. doi: 10.1038/ni1582

Wan, Y., Shang, J., Graham, R., Baric, R. S., and Li, F. (2020). Receptor Recognition by the Novel Coronavirus from Wuhan: an Analysis Based on Decade-Long Structural Studies of SARS Coronavirus. *J. Virol.* 94, 1–9. doi: 10.1128/JVI.00127-20

Wang, Z., and Xu, X. (2020). scRNA-seq profiling of human testes reveals the presence of the ACE2 receptor, a target for SARS-CoV-2 infection in spermatogonia, leydig and sertoli cells. *Cells* 9, 1–9. doi: 10.3390/cells9040920

Wang, D., Hu, B., Hu, C., Zhu, F., Liu, X., Zhang, J., et al. (2020a). Clinical characteristics of 138 hospitalized patients with 2019 novel coronavirus-infected pneumonia in Wuhan, China. *JAMA* 323, 1061–1069. doi: 10.1001/jama.2020.1585

Wang, F., Nie, J., Wang, H., Zhao, Q., Xiong, Y., Deng, L., et al. (2020b). Characteristics of peripheral lymphocyte subset alteration in COVID-19 pneumonia. *J. Infect. Dis.* 221, 1762–1769. doi: 10.1093/infdis/jiaa150

Wen, W., Su, W., Tang, H., Le, W., Zhang, X., Zheng, Y., et al. (2020a). Immune cell profiling of COVID-19 patients in the recovery stage by single-cell sequencing. *Cell Discov.* 6, 31. doi: 10.1038/s41421-020-0168-9

Wen, W., Wenru, S., and Hao, T. (2020b). Immune Cell Profiling of COVID-19 Patients in the Recovery Stage by Single-Cell Sequencing. *Cell Discov.* 6, 41. doi: 10.1101/2020.03.23.20039362

Woo, P. C., Huang, Y., Lau, S. K., and Yuen, K. Y. (2010). Coronavirus genomics and bioinformatics analysis. *Viruses* 2, 1804–1820. doi: 10.3390/v2081803

Wu, B. X., and Team, T. C.-P. (2020). Autopsy of COVID-19 victims in China. *Natl. Sci. Rev.* doi: 10.1093/nsr/nwaa123/5854209

Wu, D., and Yang, X. O. (2020). TH17 responses in cytokine storm of COVID-19: An emerging target of JAK2 inhibitor Fedratinib. *J. Microbiol. Immunol. Infect.* 53, 368–370. doi: 10.1016/j.jmii.2020.03.005

Wu, J., Li, J., Zhu, G., Zhang, Y., Bi, Z., Yu, Y., et al. (2020a). Clinical features of maintenance hemodialysis patients with 2019 novel coronavirus-infected pneumonia in Wuhan, China. *Clin. J. Am. Soc. Nephrol.* 15, 1139–1145 doi: 10.2215/CJN.04160320

Wu, Y., Guo, C., Tang, L., Hong, Z., Zhou, J., Dong, X., et al. (2020b). Prolonged presence of SARS-CoV-2 viral RNA in faecal samples. *Lancet Gastroenterol. Hepatol.* 5, 434–435. doi: 10.1016/S2468-1253(20)30083-2

Xiao, K., Zhai, J., Feng, Y., Zhou, N., Zhang, X., Zou, J., et al. (2020). Isolation of SARS-CoV-2-related coronavirus from Malayan pangolins. *Nature* 583, 286–289. doi: 10.1038/s41586-020-2313-x

Xiong, Y., Liu, Y., Cao, L., Wang, D., Guo, M., Jiang, A., et al. (2020). Transcriptomic characteristics of bronchoalveolar lavage fluid and peripheral blood mononuclear cells in COVID-19 patients. *Emerg. Microbes Infect.* 9, 761–770. doi: 10.1080/22221751.2020.1747363

Xu, K., Cai, H., Shen, Y., Ni, Q., Chen, Y., Hu, S., et al. (2020a). Management of corona virus disease-19 (COVID-19): the Zhejiang experience. *Zhejiang Da Xue Xue Bao Yi Xue Ban* 49, 147–157. doi: 10.3785/j.issn.1008-9292.2020.02.02

Xu, X., Chen, P., Wang, J., Feng, J., Zhou, H., Li, X., et al. (2020b). Evolution of the novel coronavirus from the ongoing Wuhan outbreak and modeling of its spike protein for risk of human transmission. *Sci. China Life Sci.* 63, 457–460. doi: 10.1007/s11427-020-1637-5

Xu, Z., Shi, L., Wang, Y., Zhang, J., Huang, L., Zhang, C., et al. (2020c). Pathological findings of COVID-19 associated with acute respiratory distress syndrome. *Lancet Respir. Med.* 8, 420–422. doi: 10.1016/S2213-2600(20)30076-X

Yang, Z., and Rannala, B. (2012). Molecular phylogenetics: principles and practice. *Nat. Rev. Genet.* 13, 303–314. doi: 10.1038/nrg3186

Yildiz, S., Mazel-Sanchez, B., Kandasamy, M., Manicassamy, B., and Schmolke, M. (2018). Influenza A virus infection impacts systemic microbiota dynamics and causes quantitative enteric dysbiosis. *Microbiome* 6, 9. doi: 10.1186/s40168-017-0386-z

Yin, C. (2020). Genotyping coronavirus SARS-CoV-2: methods and implications. *Genomics* 112, 3588–3596. doi: 10.1016/j.ygeno.2020.04.016

Yu, W. B., Tang, G. D., Zhang, L., and Corlett, R. T. (2020). Decoding the evolution and transmissions of the novel pneumonia coronavirus (SARS-CoV-2 / HCoV-19) using whole genomic data. *Zool. Res.* 41, 247–257. doi: 10.24272/j.issn.2095-8137.2020.022

Yuen, K., Ye, Z., Fung, S., Chan, C., and Jin, D. (2020). SARS-CoV-2 and COVID-19: The most important research questions. *Cell Biosci.* 10, 40. doi: 10.1186/s13578-020-00404-4

Zhang, H., Kang, Z., Gong, H., and Xu, H. (2020a). Digestive system is a potential route of COVID-19: an analysis of single-cell coexpression pattern of key proteins in viral entry process. *Gut Immun* 69, 1010–1018. doi: 10.1136/gutjnl-2020-320953

Zhang, L., Shen, F. M., Chen, F., and Lin, Z. (2020b). Origin and evolution of the 2019 novel coronavirus. *Clin. Infect. Dis* 71, 882–883. doi: 10.1093/cid/ciaa112

Zhang, T., Wu, Q., and Zhang, Z. (2020c). Probable pangolin origin of SARS-CoV-2 associated with the COVID-19 outbreak. *Curr. Biol.* 30, 1346–1351.e2. doi: 10.1016/j.cub.2020.03.022

Zhao, Y., Zhao, Z., Wang, Y., Zhou, Y., Ma, Y., and Zuo, W. (2020). Single-cell RNA expression profiling of ACE2, the putative receptor of Wuhan 2019-nCov. *bioRxiv.* doi: 10.1101/2020.01.26.919985

Zheng, Y. Y., Ma, Y. T., Zhang, J. Y., and Xie, X. (2020). COVID-19 and the cardiovascular system. *Nat. Rev. Cardiol.* 17, 259–260. doi: 10.1038/s41569-020-0360-5

Zhou, J., Chu, H., Li, C., Wong, B. H., Cheng, Z. S., Poon, V. K., et al. (2014). Active replication of Middle East respiratory syndrome coronavirus and aberrant induction of inflammatory cytokines and chemokines in human macrophages: implications for pathogenesis. *J. Infect. Dis.* 209, 1331–1342. doi: 10.1093/infdis/jit504

Zhou, F., Yu, T., Du, R. H., Fan, G. H., Liu, Y., Liu, Z. B., et al. (2020a). Clinical course and risk factors for mortality of adult inpatients with COVID-19 in Wuhan, China: a retrospective cohort study. *Lancet* 395, 1054–1062. doi: 10.1016/S0140-6736(20)30566-3

Zhou, H., Chen, X., Hu, T., Li, J., Song, H., Liu, Y., et al. (2020b). A novel bat coronavirus closely related to SARS-CoV-2 contains natural insertions at the S1/S2 cleavage site of the spike protein. *Curr. Biol.* 30, 2196–2203.e3. doi: 10.1016/j.cub.2020.05.023

Zhou, M., Zhang, X., and Qu, J. (2020c). Coronavirus disease 2019 (COVID-19): a clinical update. *Front. Med.* 14, 126–135. doi: 10.1007/s11684-020-0767-8

Zhou, P., Yang, X.-L., Wang, X.-G., Hu, B., Zhang, L., Zhang, W., et al. (2020d). Discovery of a novel coronavirus associated with the recent pneumonia outbreak in 2 humans and its potential bat origin. *bioRxiv*. doi: 10.1038/s41586-020-2012-7

Zhou, P., Yang, X. L., Wang, X. G., Hu, B., Zhang, L., Zhang, W., et al. (2020e). A pneumonia outbreak associated with a new coronavirus of probable bat origin. *Nature* 579, 270–273.10. doi: 10.1038/s41586-020-2012-7

Ziegler, C. G. K., Allon, S. J., Nyquist, S. K., Mbano, I. M., Miao, V. N., Tzouanas, C. N., et al. (2020). SARS-CoV-2 Receptor ACE2 Is an Interferon-Stimulated Gene in Human Airway Epithelial Cells and Is Detected in Specific Cell Subsets across Tissues. *Cell* 181, 1016–1035.e19. doi: 10.1016/j.cell.2020.04.035

Zou, X., Chen, K., Zou, J., Han, P., Hao, J., and Han, Z. (2020). Single-cell RNA-seq data analysis on the receptor ACE2 expression reveals the potential risk of different human organs vulnerable to 2019-nCoV infection. *Front. Med.* 14, 185–192. doi: 10.1007/s11684-020-0754-0

Zuo, T., Zhang, F., Lui, G. C. Y., Yeoh, Y. K., Li, A. Y. L., Zhan, H., et al. (2020). Alterations in gut microbiota of patients with COVID-19 during time of hospitalization. *Gastroenterology* 159, 944–955. doi: 10.1053/j.gastro.2020.05.048

12

IgA Antibodies and IgA Deficiency in SARS-CoV-2 Infection

Isabella Quinti[1], Eva Piano Mortari[2], Ane Fernandez Salinas[1], Cinzia Milito[1] and Rita Carsetti[2]

[1] Department of Molecular Medicine, Sapienza University of Rome, Rome, Italy, [2] Department of Laboratory Medicine, Research Area Multimodal Medicine, Diagnostic Immunology and Research Unit, Bambino Gesù Children's Hospital IRCCS, Rome, Italy

***Correspondence:**
Isabella Quinti
isabella.quinti@uniroma1.it

A large repertoire of IgA is produced by B lymphocytes with T-independent and T-dependent mechanisms useful in defense against pathogenic microorganisms and to reduce immune activation. IgA is active against several pathogens, including rotavirus, poliovirus, influenza virus, and SARS-CoV-2. It protects the epithelial barriers from pathogens and modulates excessive immune responses in inflammatory diseases. An early SARS-CoV-2 specific humoral response is dominated by IgA antibodies responses greatly contributing to virus neutralization. The lack of anti-SARS-Cov-2 IgA and secretory IgA (sIgA) might represent a possible cause of COVID-19 severity, vaccine failure, and possible cause of prolonged viral shedding in patients with Primary Antibody Deficiencies, including patients with Selective IgA Deficiency. Differently from other primary antibody deficiency entities, Selective IgA Deficiency occurs in the vast majority of patients as an asymptomatic condition, and it is often an unrecognized, Studies are needed to clarify the open questions raised by possible consequences of a lack of an IgA response to SARS-CoV-2.

Keywords: IgA, secretory IgA, SARS-Cov-2, selective IgA deficiency, infectivity

HIGHLIGHTS

Lack of neutralizing anti-SARS-Cov-2 IgA and secretory IgA antibodies represents a possible cause of prolonged viral shedding in patients with Selective IgA Deficiency and in patients with Primary Antibody Deficiencies showing an increased length of SARS-CoV-2 positivity.

INTRODUCTION

IgA is the predominant immunoglobulin in the respiratory tract, the major portal of entry for many microorganisms. There are two subclasses of IgA, IgA1 and IgA2. Monomeric IgA1 predominates in serum. Dimeric and polymeric IgA1 and IgA2 - linked by a J-chain - are present on the mucosal surface where they exert a major role in protection against toxins, viruses and bacteria by neutralization, or by preventing attachment to the mucosal epithelium. IgA1 predominates in the airways and IgA2 is predominant in the colon. IgA is produced by plasma cells of the submucosa and it is transported to the apical surface of intestinal epithelial cells by the efficient mechanism involving the polymeric immunoglobulin receptor (pIgR). On the basolateral surface of mucosal epithelial cells, the pIgR binds dimeric IgA through the J chain and transports the molecule to the apical cell membrane. Here, a serine-protease (Kaetzel, 2005) cleaves off the complex leaving the secretory component fragment (SC) of the pIgR attached to the immunoglobulin, thus generating sIgA. The importance of IgA comes from studies on patients with Primary Antibody Deficiencies (PAD), where the impaired IgA production, and IgA antibody-mediated responses, are associated to the susceptibility to respiratory and gastrointestinal infections and their recurrence (Hammarström et al., 2000; Tangye et al., 2020), to upper respiratory tract colonization (Pulvirenti et al., 2020a), and to the risk to develop chronic respiratory diseases (Quinti et al., 2011). The presence of sIgA with a diverse antigen-binding repertoire is essential for maintenance of mucosal protection of the upper and lower respiratory tracts, for mucosal immune responses by its interaction with mucosal epithelial cells, and by binding to antigens and cellular receptors (Cerutti et al., 2011). IgA shows a number of unique features among the immunoglobulin classes. IgA are monomeric, dimeric, and also polymeric, displaying different functions. Both antibody affinity and avidity are important in mechanisms of protection (Terauchi et al., 2018; Saito et al., 2019).

A large repertoire of IgA is produced by B lymphocytes with T-independent and T-dependent mechanisms useful in defense against pathogenic microorganisms and to reduce immune activation. IgA class switching is the process whereby B cells acquire the expression of IgA. The T-dependent process requires at least one week to develop, a too long time in mucosal infections. Natural antibodies, mostly of IgM isotype and generated independently of previous antigen encounters, have a broad reactivity and a variable affinity. They contain the infection during the 2 weeks necessary for production of high-affinity antibodies (Ochsenbein et al., 1999; Holodick et al., 2017).

Also IgA can be rapidly produced through the faster T-independent mechanisms involving B cell activating factor (BAFF) and its receptors. We have shown that most of the IgA in the gut is generated by a T-independent mechanism involving TLR9 and TACI from IgM memory B cells. Similar to natural serum IgM, "natural IgA" may function as immediate and early protection from infection (Carsetti et al., 2020a).

IgA plays a major role in protection against several viral pathogens including RSV and other influenza viruses. BAFF is increased in the lung and it is associated with the class-switched IgA antibody responses against RSV infection (McNamara et al., 2013), and BAFF neutralization results in reduced sIgA levels and AID expression during influenza virus infection (Wang et al., 2015). Local IgA responses, in cooperation with non-specific innate factors such as muco-ciliary clearance, have been shown to protect from influenza virus natural infection without inducing a potentially deleterious inflammatory response leading to tissue damage (Pilette et al., 2011). High levels of anti-influenza virus IgA in breast milk are associated with decreased infant episodes of respiratory illness (Schlaudecker et al., 2013).

The current challenge in vaccine design is to induce long-lasting systemic and mucosal protection against the vaccine strains, but also against drifted and shifted strains. Most antiviral vaccines are now administered intramuscularly or subcutaneously, and they might not always induce a mucosal immune response (van Riet et al., 2012; Bagga et al., 2015). It has been shown that IgA antibodies on mucosal surfaces play a more relevant role than IgG for protection from influenza A virus infection and for cross-protective immunity against multiple viral hemagglutinin subtypes (Okuya et al., 2020). More recently, it has been shown in mice that immunization with MERS-CoV S1 subunit and full-length Spike protein elicited high levels of S1-specific neutralizing IgA response. However, MERS-CoV neutralizing IgA antibodies in the broncho-alveolar lavage fluid were only induced by intranasal and sublingual administration but not by intramuscular administration (Kim et al., 2019).

IgA ANTIBODIES AND SARS-CoV-2

Unless immunized, everyone is susceptible to SARS-CoV-2 infection. The variability of COVID-19 suggests that the individual immune response to SARS-CoV-2 may play a crucial role in determining the clinical course ranging from asymptomatic to mild upper respiratory tract illness, or moderate to severe disease with respiratory distress and multi-organ failure requiring intensive care and organ support (WHO, [[NoYear]]; Zhou et al., 2020). To pathogens for which there is no pre-existing immunity, our organism reacts by rapidly engaging the innate immune system with the intent of limiting the infection and giving time to adaptive immune response to generate the most specific and effective tools: high-affinity antibodies and memory B and T cells. Extensive analysis of the antibody response, showed that SARS-CoV-2 induces virus-specific antibodies, mediated by all immunoglobulin isotypes including IgM, IgG, and IgA (Long et al., 2020); all IgG subclasses were produced by individuals with COVID-19, with IgG1 being the most dominant (Goh et al., 2021). The kinetics of specific immunoglobulin production against spike-1 receptor-binding domain and nucleocapsid protein shows that the vast majority of patients produce detectable neutralizing IgG and IgA antibodies within 2-3 weeks from onset of symptoms. Then, neutralizing anti-RBD IgG and anti-NC titers increased and reached a plateau around the fourth week after symptom onset, while IgA decreased by day 28 (Sterlin et al., 2021). This might be observed also in asymptomatic SARS-CoV-2 infection as we have recently shown (Carsetti et al., 2020b).

IgA is active against several pathogens, including rotavirus, poliovirus, influenza virus, and SARS-CoV-2, it modulates excessive immune responses in inflammatory diseases and it is more effective in recruiting neutrophils for cell killing (Sterlin and Gorochov, 2021).

Peripheral expansion of IgA plasma blasts with mucosal-homing potential has been detected shortly after the onset of symptoms (Wang et al., 2020). The virus-specific antibody responses are mediated by all isotypes, but IgA contributes to virus neutralization to a greater extent compared with IgG and probably associated with protection against reinfection (Gaebler et al., 2021). During the first six months after infection, anti-SARS-CoV-2 memory B cell response evolves with accumulation of Ig somatic mutations. Sharing of VH sequences has been demonstrated between IgA and IgG, suggesting that the same B cells may generate a clone that undergoes progressive selection, specialization and class-switching (Grimsholm et al., 2020). In convalescent patients, it has been demonstrated that clones of IgM-, IgG-, and IgA-producing B cells derive from common progenitor cells. In addition, dimeric IgA was more potent than IgA monomers and IgG against the same target (Wang et al., 2020).

Being a mucosal targeted virus, SARS-CoV-2 secretory IgA plays an important role in the early defense and viral containment. As we specified above, IgA serum concentrations decreased one month after the onset of symptoms, while neutralizing IgA remained detectable in saliva for a longer time (Burgess et al., 2020). A human monoclonal IgA antibody cross-reactive with SARS-CoV and SARS-CoV-2 spike proteins was able to neutralize SARS-Cov-2 infection *in vitro* when converted to sIgA (Ejemel et al., 2020). Secretory IgA in the gut and monomeric IgA in the serum are clonally related (Iversen et al., 2017). sIgA specific for SARS-CoV-2 has been detected in the milk (Fox et al., 2020) of SARS-CoV-2 infected mothers, thus demonstrating that sIgA is produced in response to the infection and it is passed to the neonate for protection. It has been suggested that also in adults the measurement of SARS-CoV-2 sIgA might help to identify those individuals that, protected by sIgA, did not develop symptoms and disease (Burgess et al., 2020).

PRIMARY ANTIBODY DEFICIENCIES, SELECTIVE IgA DEFICIENCY AND COVID 19

The impact of the COVID-19 pandemic on patients with rare diseases is still not well defined. Inborn Errors of Immunity (IEI) encompasses a group of rare disorders characterized by congenital defects of one or more components of the immune system (Picard et al., 2018), and as such they may be considered as groups at high risk during this pandemic. Selective deficiencies of specific components of the immune response in humans might help dissect and analyze the physiologic role and the outcomes in the interactions with pathogens. The lack of antibodies associated with protection might represent a possible cause of COVID-19 severity, and vaccine failure in particular in patients with primary antibody deficiencies (PAD). We have already reported (Meyts et al., 2020; Quinti et al., 2020; Quinti et al., 2021) on patients affected by PAD lacking antibodies showing a different COVID-19 clinical course. In the most common form of symptomatic PAD - the Common Variable Immune Deficiencies, COVID-19 might have, as expected, a severe clinical course, while in patients with X-linked Agammaglobulinemia (XLA) SARS-Cov-2 infection might remain asymptomatic or have a mild disease. Both CVID and XLA have a severe hypogammaglobulinemia and a defect in antibody production. However, XLA patients only lack B cells due a BTK mutation with consequent arrest of B cell development in the bone marrow. We then speculated on a possible harmful role of B cells in COVID-19 pathogenesis and our hypothesis was further supported by the demonstration that patients under BTK inhibitors also had a mild COVID-19. However, our hypothesis was argued since other agammaglobulinemic patients later reported in the literature showed an aggressive COVID-19 disease, even if none died. This extreme variability in the context of a defective immune response may depend on various factors that need to be defined on larger cohorts of affected patients, since a low number of IEI infected patients with variable outcome has been reported until now. This low number of infected patients might be explained by the choice of most physicians involved in the management of IEI patients to inform early in the pandemic about safety measures, to switch most of them to home therapy and to remote assistance (Pulvirenti et al., 2020b). However, it should be mentioned here that each PAD patient represents a unique model in that the COVID-19 clinical expression varies also within the same immunodeficiency entity, as we knew, from many other comorbidities, patients with primary immune deficiency faced during their life.

Selective IgA Deficiency (SIgAD) is a primary immunodeficiency characterized by an undetectable level of immunoglobulin A in the blood and secretions but no other immunoglobulin deficiencies (Picard et al., 2018). The role defined for IgA antibodies in SARS-Cov-2 protection, offers the possibility to address important aspects of the interplay between SARS-CoV-2 infection and prevention in patients with SIgAD.

It has been shown that a low frequency of SIgAD has been shown to positively correlate with the lower prevalence of COVID-19 in Japan in comparison to other countries where SIgAD reaches a frequency of 1:600 inhabitants (Naito et al., 2020). However, differently from what suggested in the paper, there is not the strategy to promote the production of serum and sIgA in patients with Selective IgA deficiency, nor it is possible to use other therapeutic strategies, such as the use of convalescent plasma, in that, in patients who lack IgA there is a contraindication for the use of plasma for possible adverse reactions. Only when IgA are detectable in serum, convalescent plasma might be administered, as suggested in other forms of PAD (Ho et al., 2021).

Moreover, patients with SIgAD are prone to develop autoantibodies (Hammarström et al., 2000; Quinti et al., 2011; Tangye et al., 2020; Pulvirenti et al., 2020a). In an international study on Coronavirus disease 2019 in patients with inborn errors of immunity, one patient with Selective IgA Deficiency and IgG2 subclass deficiency and COVID died for AIHA (Meyts et al., 2020). An additional case study showed a patient affected from SIgAD since childhood who - similarly to the vast majority of Selective IgA Deficiency - was asymptomatic until a Guillain Barrè syndrome was diagnosed at the time of COVID-19, when she developed anti-ganglioside antibodies (Pfeuffer et al., 2020). The pathogenic role of autoantibodies in severe COVID-19 was further demonstrated by a study showing that clinically silent anti-IFN type I neutralizing antibodies were present in about 10% of patients who develop a severe COVID-19 and in less than 0.1% of asymptomatic patients and of healthy individuals (Bastard et al., 2020).

Lastly, PAD patients and SIgAD patients might have a very low or suboptimal response to SARS-CoV-2 immunization, lacking a major tool for systemic and mucosal protection. It has been reported that patients of PAD (Naito et al., 2020), have an increased length of SARS-CoV-2 positivity, before their swab becomes PCR negative, even if this finding may be observed even in the general population of non-immunocompromised subjects. This finding is in fact in agreement with the observation that immunocompromised patients and severe-to-critical patients may remain a source of infection to their environment (Choi et al., 2020). This prolonged viral shedding represents a potential risk for the spreading of the virus in the community, and for virus genetic changes since high rates of mutation might arise, as previously suggested in studies on patients with Primary Immune Deficiencies chronically infected with other viruses, such as chronic OPV infections (Aghamohammadi et al., 2017).

In conclusion, the strikingly different clinical course of COVID-19 in patients affected with different antibody deficiencies, including the SIgAD entity, requires in-depth studies. PAD are rare diseases while Selective IgA Deficiency is the most frequent antibody deficiency, often undiagnosed for the paucity of symptoms. We suggest to promote studies to clarify the open questions raised on possible consequences of the lack of an IgA response to SARS-CoV-2, since patients affected by primary defects of immunity might always represent a fundamental group to understand the pathogenic mechanisms underlying most infectious and inflammatory diseases.

AUTHOR CONTRIBUTIONS

IQ and RC planned and wrote the manuscript. EP, and CM reviewed the published papers on the topic. All authors contributed to the discussion of data. All authors contributed to the article and approved the submitted version.

REFERENCES

Aghamohammadi, A., Abolhassani, H., Kutukculer, N., Wassilak, SG, Pallansch, MA, Kluglein, S, et al. (2017). Patients with Primary Immunodeficiencies are a reservoir of Poliovirus and a risk to Polio eradication. *Front. Immunol.* 8, 685. doi: 10.3389/fimmu.2017.00685

Bagga, B., Cehelsky, J. E., Vaishnaw, A., Wilkinson, T, Meyers, R, Harrison, LM, et al. (2015). Effect of Preexisting Serum and Mucosal Antibody on Experimental Respiratory Syncytial Virus (RSV) Challenge and Infection of Adults. *J. Infect. Dis.* 212, 1719–1725. doi: 10.1093/infdis/jiv281

Bastard, P., Rosen, L. B., Zhang, Q., Michailidis, E, Hoffmann, HH, Zhang, Y, et al. (2020). Autoantibodies against type I IFNs in patients with life-threatening COVID-19. *Science* 370, eabd4585. doi: 10.1126/science.abd4585

Burgess, S., Ponsford, M. J., and Gill, D. (2020). Are we underestimating seroprevalence of SARS-CoV-2? *BMJ* 370:m3364. doi: 10.1136/bmj.m3364

Carsetti, R., Di Sabatino, A., Rosado, M. M., Cascioli, S, Piano Mortari, E, Milito, C, et al. (2020a). Lack of Gut Secretory Immunoglobulin A in Memory B-Cell Dysfunction-Associated Disorders: A Possible Gut-Spleen Axis. *Front. Immunol.* 10, 2937. doi: 10.3389/fimmu.2019.02937

Carsetti, R., Zaffina, S., Piano Mortari, E., Terreri, S, Corrente, F, Capponi, C, et al. (2020b). Different Innate and Adaptive Immune Responses to SARS-CoV-2 Infection of Asymptomatic, Mild, and Severe Cases. *Front. Immunol.* 11, 610300. doi: 10.3389/fimmu.2020.610300

Cerutti, A., Chen, K., and Chorny, A. (2011). Immunoglobulin responses at the mucosal interface. *Annu. Rev. Immunol.* 29, 273–293. doi: 10.1146/annurev-immunol-031210-101317

Choi, B., Choudhary, M. C., Regan, J., Sparks, J. A., Padera, R. F., Qiu, X., et al. (2020). Persistence and Evolution of SARS-CoV-2 in an Immunocompromised Host. *N. Engl. J. Med.* 383, 2291–2293. doi: 10.1056/NEJMc2031364

Ejemel, M., Li, Q., Hou, S., Schiller, ZA, Tree, JA, Wallace, A, et al. (2020). A cross reactive human IgA monoclonal antibody blocks SARS-CoV-2 spike-ACE2 interaction. *Nat. Commun.* 11, 4198. doi: 10.1038/s41467-020-18058-8

Fox, A., Marino, J., Amanat, F., Krammer, F., Hahn-Holbrook, J, Zolla-Pazner, S, et al. (2020). Robust and Specific Secretory IgA Against SARS-CoV-2 Detected in Human Milk. *iScience* 23, 101735. doi: 10.1016/j.isci.2020.101735

Gaebler, C., Wang, Z., Lorenzi, J. C. C., Muecksch, F, Finkin, S, Tokuyama, M, et al. (2021). Evolution of antibody immunity to SARS-CoV-2. *Nature.* doi: 10.1038/s41586-021-03207-w

Goh, Y. S., Chavatte, J.-M., Jieling, A. L., Lee, B., Hor, P. X., Amrun, S. N., et al. (2021). Sensitive detection of total anti-Spike antibodies and isotype switching in asymptomatic and symptomatic individuals with COVID-19. *Cell Rep. Med.* 2 (2), 100193. doi: 10.1016/j.xcrm.2021.100193

Grimsholm, O., Piano Mortari, E., Davydov, A. N., Shugay, M, Obraztsova, AS, Bocci, C, et al. (2020). The Interplay between CD27dull and CD27bright B Cells Ensures the Flexibility, Stability, and Resilience of Human B Cell Memory. *Cell Rep.* 30, 2963–2977.e625. doi: 10.1016/j.celrep.2020.02.022

Hammarström, L., Vorechovsky, I., and Webster, D. (2000). Selective IgA deficiency (SIgAD) and common variable immunodeficiency (CVID). *Clin. Exp. Immunol.* 120, 225–231. doi: 10.1046/j.1365-2249.2000.01131.x

Ho, H. E., Mathew, S., Peluso, M. J., and Cunningham-Rundles, C. (2021). Clinical outcomes and features of COVID-19 in patients with primary immunodeficiencies in New York City. *J. Allergy Clin. Immunol. Pract.* 9, 490–493.e2. doi: 10.1016/j.jaip.2020.09.052

Holodick, N. E., Rodríguez-Zhurbenko, N., and Hernández, A. M. (2017). Defining Natural Antibodies. *Front. Immunol.* 8, 872. doi: 10.3389/fimmu.2017.00872

Iversen, R., Snir, O., Stensland, M., Kroll, JE, Steinsbø, O, Korponay-Szabò, IR, et al. (2017). Strong clonal relatedness between Serum and Gut IgA despite different plasma cell origins. *Cell Rep.* 20, 2357–2367. doi: 10.1016/j.celrep.2017.08.036

Kaetzel, C. S. (2005). The polymeric immunoglobulin receptor: Bridging innate and adaptive immune responses at mucosal surfaces. *Immunol. Rev.* 206, 83–99. doi: 10.1111/j.0105-2896.2005.00278.x

Kim, M. H., Kim, H. J., and Chang, J. (2019). Superior immune responses induced by intranasal immunization with recombinant adenovirus-based vaccine expressing full-length Spike protein of Middle East respiratory syndrome coronavirus. *PloS One* 14, e0220196. doi: 10.1371/journal.pone.0220196

Long, Q.-X., Liu, B.-Z., Deng, H.-J., Wu, G.-C., Deng, K., Chen, Y.-K., et al. (2020). Antibody responses to SARS-CoV-2 in patients with COVID-19. *Nat. Med.* 26, 845–848. doi: 10.1038/s41591-020-0897-1

McNamara, P. S., Fonceca, A. M., Howarth, D., Correia, JB, Slupsky, JR, Trinick, RE, et al. (2013). Respiratory syncytial virus infection of airway epithelial cells, in vivo and in vitro, supports pulmonary antibody responses by inducing expression of the B cell differentiation factor BAFF. *Thorax* 68, 76–81. doi: 10.1136/thoraxjnl-2012-202288

Meyts, I., Bucciol, G., Quinti, I., Neven, B, Fischer, A, Seoane, E, et al. (2020). Coronavirus disease 2019 in patients with inborn errors of immunity: An international study. *J. Allergy Clin. Immunol.* 147 (2), 520–531. doi: 10.1016/j.jaci.2020.09.010

Naito, Y., Takagi, T., Yamamoto, T., and Watanabe, S. (2020). Association between selective IgA deficiency and COVID-19. *J. Clin. Biochem. Nutr.* 67, 122–125. doi: 10.3164/jcbn.20-102

Ochsenbein, A. F., Fehr, T., and Lutz, C. (1999). Control of early viral and bacterial distribution and disease by natural antibodies. *Science* 286, 2156–2159. doi: 10.1126/science.286.5447.2156

Okuya, K., Yoshida, R., Manzoor, R., Saito, S, Suzuki, T, Sasaki, M, et al. (2020). Potential role of Nonneutralizing IgA antibodies in cross-protective immunity against Influenza A viruses of multiple hemagglutinin subtypes. *J. Virol.* 94, e00408–e00420. doi: 10.1128/JVI.00408-20

Pfeuffer, S., Pawlowski, M., Joos, G. S. , Minnerup, J, Meuth, SG, Dziewas, R, et al. (2020). Autoimmunity complicating SARS-CoV-2 infection in selective IgA-deficiency. *Neurol. Neuroimmunol. Neuroinflamm.* 7, e881. doi: 10.1212/NXI.0000000000000881

Picard, C., Gaspar, H. B., Al-Herz, W., Bousfiha, A., Casanova, J. L., Chatila, T., et al. (2018). International Union of Immunological Societies: 2017 Primary Immunodeficiency Diseases Committee Report on Inborn Errors of Immunity. *J. Clin. Immunol.* 38, 96–128. doi: 10.1007/s10875-017-0464-9

Pilette, C., Ouadrhiri, Y., Godding, V., Vaerman, J. P., and Sibille, Y. (2011). Lung mucosal immunity: immunoglobulin-A revisited. *Eur. Respir. J.* 18, 571–588. doi: 10.1183/09031936.01.00228801

Pulvirenti, F., Milito, C., Cavaliere, F. M., Mezzaroma, I., Cinetto, F., and Quinti, I. (2020a). IGA Antibody Induced by Immunization With Pneumococcal Polysaccharides Is a Prognostic Tool in Common Variable Immune Deficiencies. *Front. Immunol.* 11, 1283. doi: 10.3389/fimmu.2020.01283

Pulvirenti, F., Cinetto, F., Milito, C., Bonanni, L., Pesce, A. M., Leodori, G., et al. (2020b). Health-Related Quality of Life in Common Variable Immunodeficiency Italian Patients Switched to Remote Assistance During the COVID-19 Pandemic. *J. Allergy Clin. Immunol. Pract.* 8, 1894–1899.e2. doi: 10.1016/j.jaip.2020.04.003

Quinti, I., Soresina, A., Guerra, A., Rondelli, R, Spadaro, G, Agostini, C, et al. (2011). Effectiveness of immunoglobulin replacement therapy on clinical outcome in patients with primary antibody deficiencies: results from a multicenter prospective cohort study. *J. Clin. Immunol.* 31, 315–322. doi: 10.1007/s10875-011-9511-0

Quinti, I., Lougaris, V., Milito, C., Cinetto, F., Pecoraro, A., Mezzaroma, I., et al. (2020). A possible role for B cells in COVID-19? Lesson from patients with agammaglobulinemia. *J. Allergy Clin. Immunol.* 146, 211–213.e4. doi: 10.1016/j.jaci.2020.04.013

Quinti, I., Mezzaroma, I., and Milito, C. (2021). Clinical management of patients with primary immunodeficiencies during the COVID-19 pandemic. *Expert Rev. Clin. Immunol.* 15, 1–6. doi: 10.1080/1744666X.2021.1873767

Saito, S., Sano, K., Suzuki, T., Ainai, A, Taga, Y, Ueno, T, et al. (2019). IgA tetramerization improves target breadth but not peak potency of functionality of anti-influenza virus broadly neutralizing antibody. *PloS Pathog.* 15, e1007427. doi: 10.1371/journal.ppat.1007427

Schlaudecker, E. P., Steinhoff, M. C., Omer, S. B., McNeal, MM, Roy, E, Arifeen, SE, et al. (2013). IgA and neutralizing antibodies to influenza a virus in human milk: a randomized trial of antenatal influenza immunization. *PloS One* 8, e70867. doi: 10.1371/journal.pone.0070867

Sterlin, D., and Gorochov, G. (2021). When Therapeutic IgA Antibodies Might Come of Age. *Pharmacology* 106, 9–19. doi: 10.1159/000510251

Sterlin, D., Mathian, A., Miyara, M., Mohr, A, Anna, F, Claér, L, et al. (2021). IgA dominates the early neutralizing antibody response to SARS-CoV-2. *Sci. Transl. Med.* 13 (577), eabd2223. doi: 10.1126/scitranslmed.abd2223

Tangye, S. G., Al-Herz, W., Bousfiha, A., Chatila, T, Cunningham-Rundles, C, Etzioni, A, et al. (2020). Human Inborn Errors of Immunity: 2019 Update on the Classification from the International Union of Immunological Societies Expert Committee. *J. Clin. Immunol.* 40, 24–64. doi: 10.1007/s10875-019-00737-x

Terauchi, Y., Sano, K., Ainai, A., Saito, S, Taga, Y, Ogawa-Goto, K, et al. (2018). IgA polymerization contributes to efficient virus neutralization on human upper respiratory mucosa after intranasal inactivated influenza vaccine administration. *Hum. Vaccin. Immunother.* 14, 1351–1361. doi: 10.1080/21645515.2018.1438791

van Riet, E., Ainai, A., Suzuki, T., and Hasegawa, H. (2012). Mucosal IgA responses in influenza virus infections; thoughts for vaccine design. *Vaccine* 30, 5893–5900. doi: 10.1016/j.vaccine.2012.04.109

Wang, J., Li, Q., Xie, J., and Xu, Y. (2015). Cigarette smoke inhibits BAFF expression and mucosal immunoglobulin A responses in the lung during influenza virus infection. *Respir. Res.* 16, 37. doi: 10.1186/s12931-015-0201-y

Wang, Z., Lorenzi, J. C. C., Muecksch, F., Finkin, S, Viant, C, Gaebler, C, et al. (2020). Enhanced SARS-CoV-2 neutralization by dimeric IgA. *Sci. Transl. Med.* 13, eabf1555. doi: 10.1126/scitranslmed.abf1555

WHO. https://www.who.int/emergencies/diseases/novel-coronavirus-2019/technical-guidance.

Zhou, F., Yu, T., Du, R., Fan, G., Liu, Y., Liu, Z., et al. (2020). Clinical course and risk factors for mortality of adult inpatients with COVID-19 in Wuhan, China: a retrospective cohort study. *Lancet* 395, 1054–1062. doi: 10.1016/S0140-6736(20)30566-3

13

SARS-CoV-2: Origin, Evolution and Targeting Inhibition

Shuo Ning†, Beiming Yu†, Yanfeng Wang and Feng Wang**

Key Laboratory of Molecular Medicine and Biotherapy, School of Life Science, Beijing Institute of Technology, Beijing, China

***Correspondence:**
Yanfeng Wang
yf@bit.edu.cn
Feng Wang
wfeng@bit.edu.cn

†These authors have contributed equally to this work

Severe acute respiratory syndrome coronavirus 2 (SARS-CoV-2) caused an outbreak in Wuhan city, China and quickly spread worldwide. Currently, there are no specific drugs or antibodies that claim to cure severe acute respiratory diseases. For SARS-CoV-2, the spike (S) protein recognizes and binds to the angiotensin converting enzyme 2 (ACE2) receptor, allowing viral RNA to enter the host cell. The main protease (Mpro) is involved in the proteolytic process for mature non-structural proteins, and RNA-dependent RNA polymerase (RdRp) is responsible for the viral genome replication and transcription processes. Owing to the pivotal physiological roles in viral invasion and replication, S protein, Mpro, RdRp are regarded as the main therapeutic targets for coronavirus disease 2019 (COVID-19). In this review, we carried out an evolutionary analysis of SARS-CoV-2 in comparison with other mammal-infecting coronaviruses that have sprung up in the past few decades and described the pathogenic mechanism of SARS-CoV-2. We displayed the structural details of S protein, Mpro, and RdRp, as well as their complex structures with different chemical inhibitors or antibodies. Structural comparisons showed that some neutralizing antibodies and small molecule inhibitors could inhibit S protein, Mpro, or RdRp. Moreover, we analyzed the structural differences between SARS-CoV-2 ancestral S protein and D614G mutant, which led to a second wave of infection during the recent pandemic. In this context, we outline the methods that might potentially help cure COVID-19 and provide a summary of effective chemical molecules and neutralizing antibodies.

Keywords: SARS-CoV-2, evolution, pathogenic mechanism, structure, targeting inhibition

INTRODUCTION

SARS-CoV-2 is a highly contagious virus that has led to a worldwide epidemic; it causes fever, headache, cough, myalgia, fatigue, sputum production, and hemoptysis (Chen et al., 2020; Huang et al., 2020; Coronaviridae Study Group of the International Committee on Taxonomy of V, 2020; Wong, 2020; Wu and McGoogan, 2020; Xu J. et al., 2020). Most patients infected with SARS-CoV-2 can develop acute respiratory distress syndrome (ARDS) (Zumla et al., 2020). Until April 20, 2021, there have been 142,097,799 confirmed cases and 3,029,811 deaths globally. These statistics are rising rapidly, with approximately 10,000 deaths increasing per day. Some notable SARS-CoV-2 variants probably became dominant in many countries and caused uncontrolled transmission worldwide (Korber et al., 2020; Yurkovetskiy et al., 2020; Plante et al., 2021). According to the World Health Organization's official report, SARS-CoV-2 has caused one of the worst global health emergencies in history. Until now, scientists are still struggling to prevent the spread of SARS-CoV-2 and have gained some improvements. In this review, we summarize the origin, evolution, and pathogenesis of SARS-CoV-2. In addition, we show the structures of spike protein, Mpro, and RdRp, as well as the complex structures of these three proteins with their inhibitors. In conclusion, we provide a summary of effective chemical molecules and neutralizing antibodies, which might potentially help cure COVID-19.

ORIGIN AND EVOLUTION OF SARS-COV-2

Numerous studies claim that SARS-CoV-2 belongs to the group of coronaviruses, with a single-stranded genome of about 26-32kb (+ssRNA), which is the largest genome size of RNA virus as known (Woo et al., 2012). After a year of struggles, researchers have learned more about the origin, structure, and inhibition of SARS-CoV-2. Coronaviruses belong to the order Nidovirales, family Coronaviridae and the subfamily Coronavirinae. Coronavirinae consists of α-coronavirus, β-coronavirus, γ-coronavirus and δ-coronavirus (Woo et al., 2012). Coronavirus was first isolated from chickens in 1937. It was not until the SARS outbreak in February 2003 that the coronavirus was considered highly pathogenic to humans (Fouchier et al., 2003). Before that, the coronaviruses that spread among humans mainly caused mild infections in people with a weaker immune system (Vaheri et al., 2013; Su et al., 2016; Zhou et al., 2018). Since 2002, three zoonotic outbreaks have been caused by β-coronaviruses in China, SARS-CoV in 2003 (Fouchier et al., 2003), MERS-CoV in 2012 (Zaki et al., 2012), and the latest outbreak of SARS-CoV-2 at the end of 2019 (Cauchemez et al., 2013; Cui et al., 2019; Huang et al., 2020). Apart from these, there are other four human coronaviruses: HCoV-229E, HCoV-OC43, HCoV-NL63, and HKU1. These coronaviruses could lead to mild diseases in the upper respiratory of the immune-competent hosts. Regardless, some of viruses could induce serious infections in infants, children, and the elderly (Su et al., 2016). Some people suspect that SARS-CoV-2 directly originated from SARS-CoV, while others believe that it leaked from the laboratory (Andersen et al., 2020). However, the evolutionary analysis of SARS-CoV-2, SARS-CoV, and MERS-CoV by neighbor-joining method showed that SARS-CoV-2 belongs to a new evolutionary branch of coronaviruses (**Figure 1**) (Cao et al., 2005; Chan et al., 2015; Jiang et al., 2020; Rabaan et al., 2020). Comparing the sequences of SARS-CoV and SARS-CoV-2, the homology is about 90%. Notably, the SARS-CoV-2 spike (S) protein has high sequence homology (up to 98%) with that of bat coronavirus RaTG13 (Li et al., 2003). However, the amino acid sequence homology between MERS-CoV and SARS-CoV-2 related virus is less than 90% (Chan et al., 2015). Apart from the amino acid sequence, the receptor and the host of MERS-CoV are distinct from SARS-CoV-2 and SARS-CoV (Hamming et al., 2007; Chen et al., 2013; Xia et al., 2014; Jiang et al., 2014; Forni et al., 2017; Chafekar and Fielding, 2018; Song et al., 2019; Bleibtreu et al., 2020) (**Figure 1**).

Some researchers believe that some viruses originated from rodents, such as HCoV-OC43 and HKU1; others originated from bats, which consist of HCoV-NL63, HCoV-229E SARS-CoV, and MERS-CoV (Mittal et al., 2020) (**Figure 2**). However, the origin of SARS-CoV-2 remains unknown. Some people suspect that bats might be the SARS-CoV-2's source because the RaTG13 virus isolated from bats has high sequence similarity with SARS-CoV-2 that has come from the same branch. A study reported that bat RaTG13 and SARS-CoV-2 recognize the same receptor ACE2 and have the same ability to infect cells through this receptor. These studies also identified that the ACE2 binding ridge in the bat RaTG13 receptor binding motif (RBM) contains four residues, which is the same as SARS-CoV-2. Moreover,

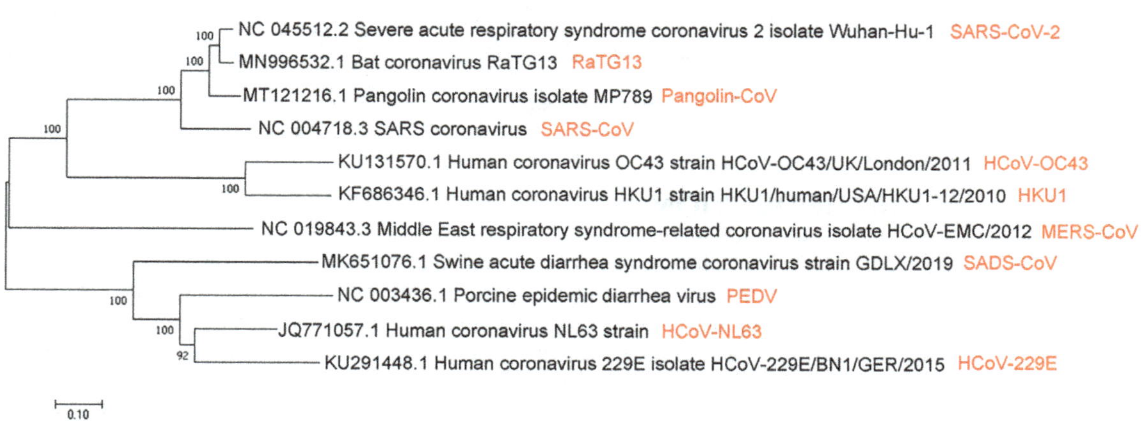

FIGURE 1 | Evolutionary relationships of SARS-CoV, MERS-CoV, SARS-CoV-2, and several viruses from α- and β-coronavirus categories by the neighbor-joining method. A coronaviruses' phylogenetic tree is shown based on the full-length genome sequence. All complete genome sequences of the coronavirus are downloaded from the NCBI reference sequence database RefSeq. The evolutionary relationship analysis involves 11 nucleotide sequences, including SARS-CoV, MERS-CoV, SARS-CoV-2, RaTG13, pangolin-CoV, HCoV-OC43, HKU1, SADS-CoV, PEDV, HCoV-NL63, and HCoV -229E. By using the neighbor-joining method, the evolutionary history was inferred. The optimal tree is shown, with the sum of branch length = 3.61257103. Next to the branches are shown the percentage of replicate trees (50 replicates) where the associated taxa are clustered together in the bootstrap test. The tree is drawn to scale, and its branch length is the same as the units used to infer the evolutionary distance of the phylogenetic tree. The phylogenetic tree is drawn by MEGA7.

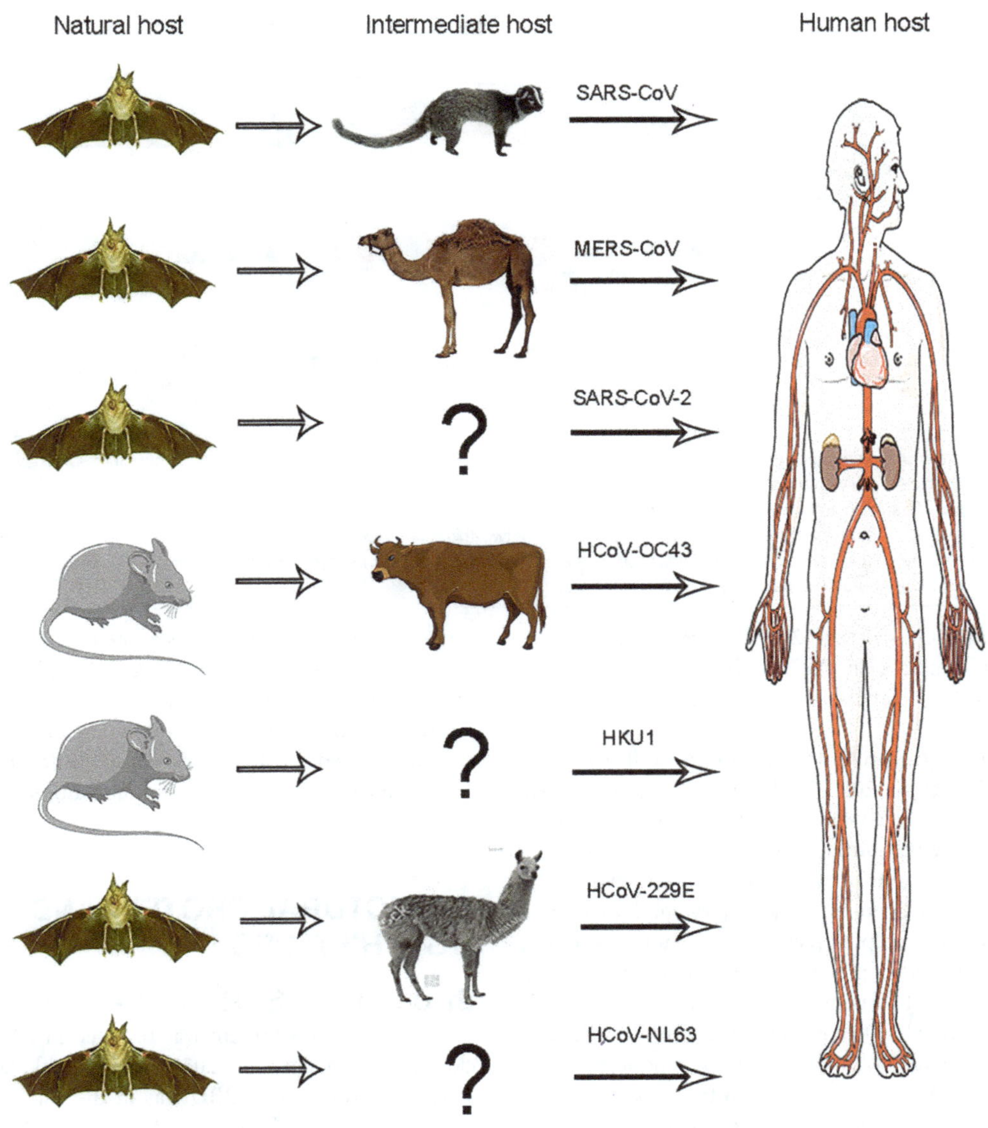

FIGURE 2 | Animal origins of human coronaviruses. SARS-CoV, MERS-CoV, and SARS-CoV-2 originated from bats; HCoV-229E and HCoV-NL63 usually lead to mild infections in immune people. The origins of these viruses have recently been found in African bats, and camelids may be intermediate hosts of HCoV-229E, HCoV-OC43, and HKU1, all of which are also harmless in humans and probably originated from rodents.

Leu455, conserved on SARS-CoV-2 and RaTG13, may contribute to the recognition of ACE2. Thus, these findings suggest that SARS-CoV-2 may be derived from RaTG13 or shares a common ancestor with RaTG13 (Li et al., 2003; Shang et al., 2020).

THE PATHOGENIC MECHANISM OF SARS-COV-2

The diameter of the SARS-CoV-2 virus particle is approximately 100 nm (**Figure 3**). It contains structural proteins (the membrane (M), envelope (E), spike (S), and nucleocapsid (N) proteins), an accessory protein, and non-structural proteins (nsps) (NSP1–16) (Cao et al., 2005; Chang et al., 2014; Lu et al., 2020; Yao et al., 2020b; Wu et al., 2020a). The SARS-CoV-2 resembles a corona because of the plenty of S proteins on the envelope. The S protein of coronaviruses, which could help to binding, fuse membrane, enter into the host cells, and induct antibody, is a type I transmembrane (TM) glycoprotein. The accessory and non-structural proteins' functions are related to virulence because those proteins are involved in viral replication and assembly (Holmes, 2003).

SARS-CoV-2 invades cells in two ways. One is interfering with target cells directly. SARS-CoV-2 occupies ACE2 on the membrane (Kuba et al., 2006; Wu et al., 2011; Hemnes et al., 2018; Gao et al., 2019), blocking signals, disturbing the renin-angiotensin (RAS) system. Another is subsequent immune

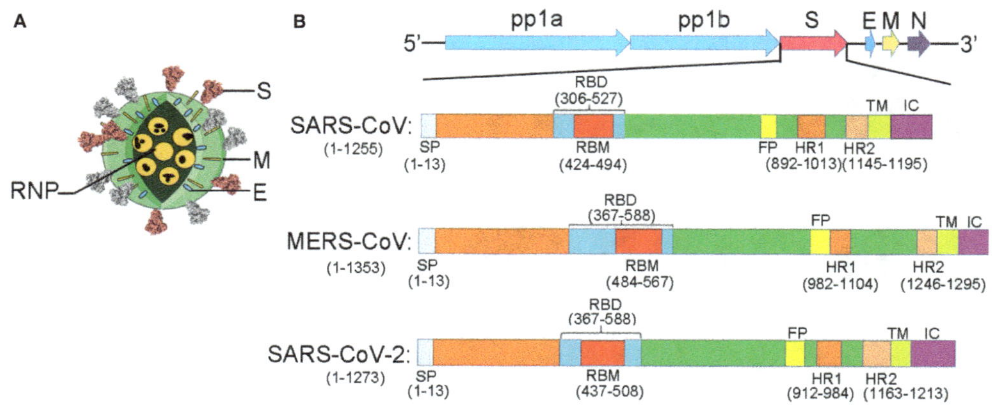

FIGURE 3 | The comparison of the structural proteins of SARS-CoV, MERS-CoV, and SARS-CoV-2. **(A)** Coronavirus virion structure. Coronaviruses, forming enveloped and spherical particles, are with a diameter of 100–160 nm. The positive-sense, single-stranded RNA (ssRNA) genome is 27–32 kb in size. RNP, ribonucleoproteins; S, spike; E, small membrane envelope; M, membrane are transmembrane proteins. **(B)** The schematic diagram for the components of the SARS-CoV, MERS-CoV, and SARS-CoV-2. A polyprotein, pp1ab, which is encoded at two-thirds of the 5′-terminal of the genome, is further cleaved into 16 non-structural proteins. These proteins are involved in transcription and replication. The structural proteins, envelope glycoproteins spike (S), envelope (E), membrane (M), and nucleocapsid (N), are encoded at the 3′ terminus.

system dysfunction (Guo et al., 2008). After SARS-CoV-2 occupies ACE2, a decrease in the number of immune cells is observed, and IL-1 levels are elevated (Chen et al., 2020) (**Figure 4**).

SARS-CoV-2 employs S protein to infect target cells by fusing the membranes (Tian et al., 2020; Walls et al., 2020; Yan et al., 2020). S protein consists of S1 and S2 subunits. An N-terminal domain (NTD), a receptor-binding domain (RBD), and a C-domain are the main domains of the S1 subunit. Moreover, RBM of the RBD, located in a C-domain's accessory subdomain, is a hypervariable region for receptor recognition. Another subunit, including two 7-valent element repeats (HR1 and HR2) and a fusion peptide (FP), could fuse to the cell membrane (Bosch et al., 2003; Belouzard et al., 2009; Burkard et al., 2014; Millet and Whittaker, 2014; Millet and Whittaker, 2015; Kirchdoerfer et al., 2016; Park et al., 2016; Walls et al., 2016). In this process, SARS-CoV-2 is more infectious than SARS-CoV because the free energy of binding between RBD and ACE2 of SARS-CoV-2 is remarkably lower than that of SARS-CoV (Wang K. et al., 2020).

After the SARS-CoV-2 entering the host cell, the viral RNA is attached to the ribosome of host, translating two large, coterminal polyproteins. Subsequently, these proteins were digested into components by proteolysis for packaging new virions. Two proteases for this proteolysis are the papain-like protease (PLpro) and the coronavirus main protease (Mpro). Like other known coronaviruses, SARS-CoV-2 also employs RNA-dependent RNA polymerase (RdRp) to replicate the genome of RNA. Above all, the four proteins, spike, Mpro, PLpro, and RdRp, are essential to virus assemble and pathogenesis (**Figure 5**) (Sheahan et al., 2020).

Given the crucial role of S protein and ACE2 in receptor recognition, as well as the critical role of Mpro and RdRp in the SARS-CoV-2's replication and transcription, interfering with their functions may provide effective antiviral strategies (Hoffmann et al., 2020). In other words, therapeutics currently targeting structural protein (S protein), non-structural proteins (Mpro, and RdRp) from SARS-CoV-2, and ACE2 from the host are potential treatment options for SARS-CoV-2. Recently, studies on the structural biology of the SARS-CoV-2 and structure-based antibody and drug discovery have appeared. We review these findings in the following sections.

STRUCTURAL PROTEIN AND ITS INHIBITORS

Structure of SARS-CoV-2 Spike Protein

The structure of S protein was resolved in two states: open and closed state (Walls et al., 2020; Wrapp et al., 2020). In the open state of S protein, one RBD was in the "up" conformation and other RBDs in the "down" conformation. The RBD domain (in "up" conformation) exhibits hinge-like conformational movement, which may be the essential determinant for binding host receptor ACE2 (**Figures 6A–C**). Meanwhile, to fuse the membranes of the virus and host cell, the S protein undergoes a drastic structural rearrangement. In the closed state of S protein, all three RBDs in the "down" conformation are at the interface among protomers (Walls et al., 2020). Compared to the "up" conformation, the "down" conformation in the close state is near the trimer's central cavity (**Figure 6D**). Thus, it is expected that the opening of the SARS-CoV-2 RBD is essential for interacting with ACE2 and triggering changes of conformation. The opening of RBD results in cleaving the S2 site, fusing membrane and entering into cells.

After the SARS-CoV-2 pandemic, 12,379 single nucleotide polymorphisms (SNPs) are downloaded in genomic data on June 25, 2020. In these SNPs, four SNPs, C3037U, C14408U, A23403G, and C241U, show high frequency. As for the A23403G, it encodes the mutant D614G in Spike protein. In

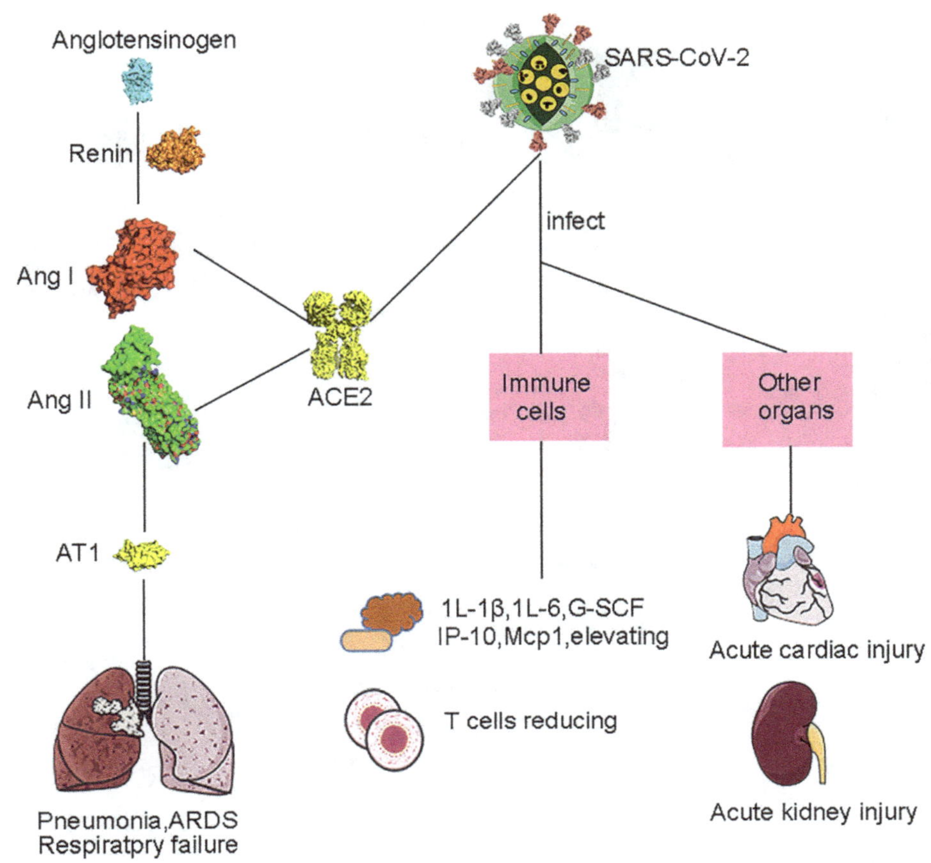

FIGURE 4 | Pathogenesis of SARS-CoV-2. By inhibiting the ACE2's function, SARS-CoV-2 could cause the injury of the lung. ACE2 plays an important role in the renin-angiotensin system (RAS). Firstly, renin converts angiotensinogen into angiotensin I (AngI), and then AngI is converted into AngII under the ACE2's action. ACE2 down-regulates the AngI's and Ang II's levels. Then, the Ang II type I (AT1) receptors are bound by Ang II, causing lung injury, which includes acute lung injury, pulmonary fibrosis, and pulmonary hypertension. At the same time, Ang II can directly induce rapid growth or proliferation of pulmonary artery smooth muscle cells through AT1, thereby causing pulmonary hypertension. Besides the intestines and lungs, the heart, kidney, esophagus, bladder, ileum, testis, and adipose tissue also could express ACE2, and its level is higher than that of the lung. In addition, tumor tissues have high ACE2 expression, making cancer patients more vulnerable than others.

late January 2020, D614G was first discovered in the viral genomes. Compared with the virus strain provided by Wuhan, Spike mutant D614G is caused by the 23,403nucleotide mutation of SARS-CoV-2. The G614 form is rare in the world, but it has attracted much attention. However, the transition of spike mutants from D614 to G614 occurred all over the world (Korber et al., 2020). Mutations that increase the chance of viral infection occurred mainly in S protein (Plante et al., 2021). With the sequencing analysis, studies showed that the S mutant D614G is a pseudo-typed virion. Because mutant D614G has association with a lower RT-PCR cycle threshold among patients, the upper respiratory tract has high viral load (Korber et al., 2020). Animal experiments also confirm these results. Hamsters infected with D614G have higher viral titers in the trachea and nasal wash than those in the lungs. This also supports the mutant D614G increase the load of virus in the Covid-19 patients' upper respiratory tract and might enhance the spread (Plante et al., 2021). Besides, the ratio of the open conformations of mutant D614G increased up to 58% and is in sharp contrast in the ancestral SARS-CoV-2 virus, in which the ratio of RBDs in the open conformation is only 18%. In comparison with the ancestral S protein in the closed state, the NTD and the INT domain of the S protein D614G shift by 4 Å and 6 Å, respectively. Moreover, the NTD of the S protein D614G has a 3Å shift in the open state (**Figure S1**) (Yurkovetskiy et al., 2020).

The structures of the S proteins between SARS-CoV-2 and SARS-CoV are similar, and the root mean square deviation (RMSD) on 959 Cα atoms is 3.8 Å. The overall structure of SARS-CoV-2 S protein resembles that of SARS-CoV S protein, with a root mean square deviation (RMSD) of 3.8 Å over 959 Cα atoms (**Figure 7A**) (Wrapp et al., 2020). For the RMSD value, the structural comparison of S2 subunits, NTDs, subdomains 1 and 2 (SD1 and SD2), and RBDs are 2.0Å, 2.6Å, 2.7Å, and 3.0Å, respectively (**Figure 7B**). The largest discrepancy exists in the RBDs "down" conformations. The "down" RBD of SARS-CoV is tightly integrated with the NTD of the neighboring chain, while that of SARS-CoV-2 is angled close to the cavity of center.

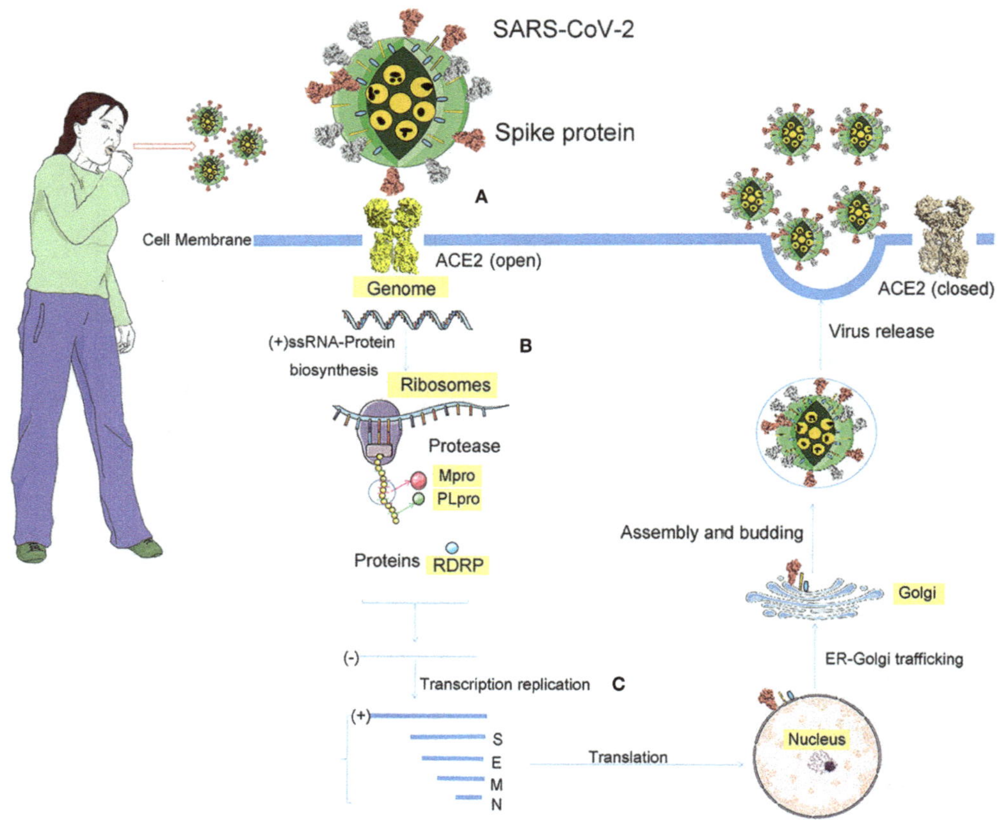

FIGURE 5 | The process of SARS-CoV-2 infection. After coughing, the infected patient will spread virus particles into the air, and people will be exposed to these virus particles. If these virions reach the cell, the infection process begins. The infection is divided into three steps. **(A)** For SARS-CoV-2, the receptor of spike protein is ACE2. The pink ball is the spike protein. **(B)** After entering the cell, the positive genomic RNA attaches to the host ribosome, translating two large coterminal polyproteins. These proteins are treated by proteolysis into components that package new virions. The two proteases involved in this proteolysis process are the major coronavirus protease (Mpro) and the papain-like protease (PLpro). **(C)** RNA-dependent RNA polymerase (RdRp), a replicase encoded by SARS-CoV-2, replicates the RNA genome.

Moreover, the HR1 domain of SARS-CoV-2 forms a six-helical bundle structure, which has higher helical stability than SARS-CoV. In addition, there are several reports suggesting that SARS-CoV-2 has a better ability to fuse membrane than SARS-CoV.

Structure of the SARS-CoV-2 S Protein and Its Binding With ACE2

Recent studies highlight that ACE2 plays a critical role in mediating SARS-CoV-2's entry. In vitro, the binding affinity of the ACE2 with SARS-CoV-2 RBD is at the nanomolar level, indicating RBD plays important roles in binding (Walls et al., 2020; Tian et al., 2020).

Compared to SARS-CoV, the SARS-CoV-2 RBM has some sequence variations, and the distal end has an obvious change of conformation. Except for that, the structure of the RBD between SARS-CoV-2 and SARS-CoV is similar, and the RMSD on 174 aligned Cα atoms is 1.2 Å (**Figures 7C, D**) (Lan et al., 2020).

The residues of SARS-CoV-2 RBD are essential for binding to ACE2. The RBD of SARS-CoV-2 forms more contacts with the ACE2's N-terminal helix, the buried area between the RBD and ACE2 is about 878.4$Å^2$, whereas, for SARS-CoV, the buried area of RBD and ACE2 is 839.45$Å^2$ (**Figure 7G**). In addition, there is a four-residue motif Gly-Val/Gln-Glu/Thr-Ser in SARS-CoV-2, instead of a three-residue motif proline-proline-alanine that is seen in SARS-CoV. Also, the Phe486, located in SARS-CoV-2 RBM, is in different directions and stays in the hydrophobic pockets, which consist of Leu79, Met82, and Tyr83 of ACE2 (Shang et al., 2020; Lan et al., 2020). Taken together, these structural changes in the SARS-CoV-2 RBM enhance the interaction for ACE2 binding.

Furthermore, more forces of interaction were formed in the joint surface between ACE2 and the RBD of SARS-CoV-2 than those in SARS-CoV. There are two virus-binding hotspots on ACE2. One hotspot is $ACE2^{Lys31}$, which forms a salt bridge with Glu35 of the RBD from SARS-CoV-2. Another hotspot is $ACE2^{Lys353,}$ which forms a salt bridge with Asp38 of the RBD from SARS-CoV-2. The Kd value of ACE2 for binding to the RBDs from SARS-CoV or SARS-CoV-2 is 44.2 nM and 185 nM, respectively. In addition, corresponding to the SARS-CoV RBM's Leu472, Phe486, located in SARS-CoV-2 RBM, has a different orientation to enhance the interactions between RBM and ACE2 (**Figures 7E, F**) (Shang et al., 2020).

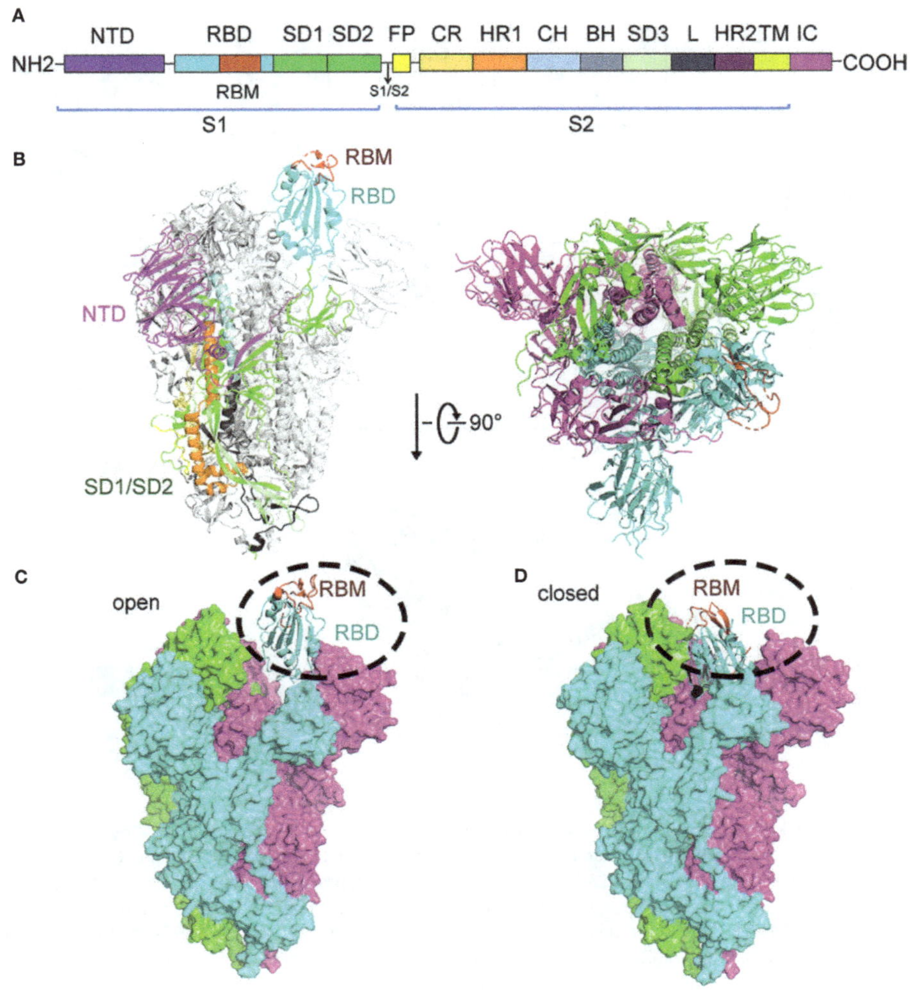

FIGURE 6 | Structure of SARS-CoV-2 spike protein. **(A)** Schematic of the SARS-CoV-2 spike protein primary structure colored by domain. NTD, N-terminal domain; RBD, receptor binding domain; RBM, receptor binding motif; SD1, subdomain 1; SD2, subdomain 2; FP, fusion peptide; CR, connecting region; HR1, heptad repeat 1; CH, central helix; BH, β-hairpin; SD3, subdomain 3; HR2, heptad repeat 2; TM, transmembrane domain; IC, cytoplasmic tail. Arrows denote protease cleavage sites. **(B)** From the side view and top view, the Cryo-EM structure of the SARS-CoV-2 spike in the prefusion conformation shows that a single RBD is in the up conformation and other RBDs are in the down conformation in either white or gray. The RBD, which in up conformation, is shown in ribbons colored corresponding to the schematic in **(A)**. **(C)** Cryo-EM structure of the SARS-CoV-2 spike in the open state. There is one open RBD domain. The three chains are depicted in green, cyan, and magnet, respectively. RBD and RBM are shown in cyan and red cartoon, respectively. **(D)** Cryo-EM structure of the SARS-CoV-2 Spike in the closed state. The three chains are depicted in green, cyan, and magnet, respectively. RBM is colored in red. RBD and RBM are shown in cyan and red cartoon, respectively. All structures are drawn by Pymol.

In conclusion, the changes of structure from SARS-CoV-2 RBM offer more favorable interactions for binding to ACE2 (Benton et al., 2020; Cao L. et al., 2020; Wu et al., 2020b). According to the known structure of SARS-CoV-2 S protein with ACE2 (Benton et al., 2020; Xu C. et al., 2020), many efforts focus on designing inhibitors to disrupt the interaction between S protein and ACE2. These strategies include competitive binding to the RBD or interference with ACE2 binding.

Inhibitors of SARS-CoV-2 S Protein

Neutralizing Antibodies

Among the inhibitors that prevent the interaction between ACE2 and the RBD, neutralizing antibodies against S protein are the most widely studied. The first reported neutralizing antibody is BD-368-2, which was selected from 14 potent neutralizing antibodies purified from patients' plasma or blood (Cao Y. et al., 2020; Long et al., 2020). The half-maximal inhibitory concentration (IC_{50}) of BD-368-2, against authentic and pseudo SARS-CoV-2, is 15 and 1.2 ng/mL, respectively. BD-368-2 could protect against SARS-CoV-2 *in vivo* experiments, providing valuable therapeutic effects. The second reported neutralizing antibody is 2B04, which could neutralize wild-type SARS-CoV-2 with remarkable potency *in vitro* (IC_{50} less than 2 ng/ml) (Alsoussi et al., 2020). 2B04 reduces the viral load of the lung, prevents systemic transmission in a murine model of SARS-CoV-2 infection, and protects challenged

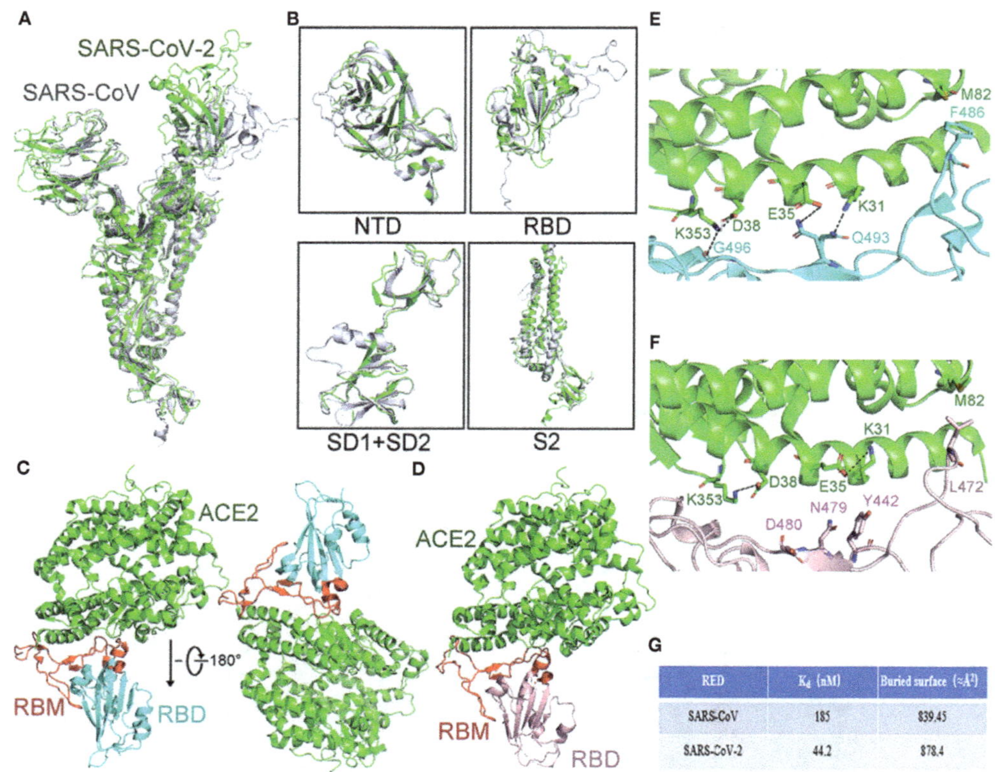

FIGURE 7 | Comparison of the S protein in SARS-CoV-2 and SARS-CoV. **(A)** Compared whole S protein between SARS-CoV-2 and SARS-CoV. SARS-CoV-2 and SARS-CoV are shown in green and gray, respectively. **(B)** Compared different domains of S protein between SARS-CoV and SARS-CoV-2. Structural domains from SARS-CoV-2 S protein have been aligned with the domain from SARS-CoV S as follows: NTD (top left), RBD (top right), SD1, and SD2 (bottom left), and S2 (bottom right). SARS-CoV and SARS-CoV-2 are shown in gray and green, respectively. **(C)** The overall structure of the SARS-CoV-2 RBD with ACE2 from the side view. ACE2 is shown in green. The SARS-CoV-2 RBD is shown in cyan and RBM in red. **(D)** The overall structure of the SARS-CoV RBD with ACE2 from the side view. The SARS-CoV RBD is shown in pink and RBM in red. ACE2 is shown in green. **(E)** The structural details of the interface between ACE2 and SARS-CoV-2 RBM. The interface between the SARS-CoV-2 RBM and ACE2 has been shown. The SARS-CoV-2 RBM is shown n cyan. ACE2 is shown in green. **(F)** The structural details of the interface between ACE2 and SARS-CoV RBM. The interface between SARS-CoV RBM and ACE2 has been shown. ACE2 is shown in green. The SARS-CoV RBM is shown in pink. **(G)** Compared Kd value and buried surface between the SARS-CoV RBD or SARS-CoV-2 RBD with ACE2. The value buried area is calculated as the average value. All structures are drawn by Pymol.

animalsfrom weight loss. Subsequently, three RBD-specific monoclonal neutralizing antibodies, P2C-1F11, P2C-1A3, and P2B-2F6, from a single B cell were reported (Ju et al., 2020). Their IC_{50} are 0.03, 0.28 and 0.41 μg/mL, respectively. These monoclonal antibodies can compete with ACE2 for RBD binding, exhibiting robust anti-SARS-CoV-2 neutralizing activity. Thereafter, a series of REGN neutralizing antibodies REGN10933 and REGN10987 showed high clinically therapeutic effects, with IC_{50} of 42.8 and 40.8 pM, respectively (Baum et al., 2020).

Structure of BD23-Fab in Complex With S Trimer

The cryogenic electron microscopy (cryo-EM)-based structure of BD-23 Fab in complex with the trimer of S protein (s trimer) was resolved at an overall resolution of 3.8 Å (Cao L. et al., 2020). In this 3D reconstruction, a single BD-23 Fab binds the "down" RBD in chain B of S trimer. As for binding to the RBD, the BD-23 Fab's heavy chain variable domain is involved. In fact, a comparison with the complex structure of RBD-ACE2 shows that BD-23 Fab competes with ACE2 for binding to RBD (**Figure 8A**).

Structure of Fab Fragments of REGN10933 and REGN10987 in Complex With RBD

In addition to acquiring antibodies from the blood of patients, many studies have attempted to obtain enough antibodies from humanized mice or other mammals and use cocktails to achieve more efficient treatments. In this way, Regeneron Pharmaceuticals developed several prospective antibodies with IC_{50} at the picomolar level (Baum et al., 2020). The complex ternary's single-particle cryo-EM with a 3.9 Å resolution displays that fab fragments of REGN10933 and REGN10987 can simultaneously bind distinct regions of the RBD. REGN10933 binds at the RBD's top. The REGN10987 epitope is located on the RBD side with little overlap with the ACE2 binding site (**Figure 8B**).

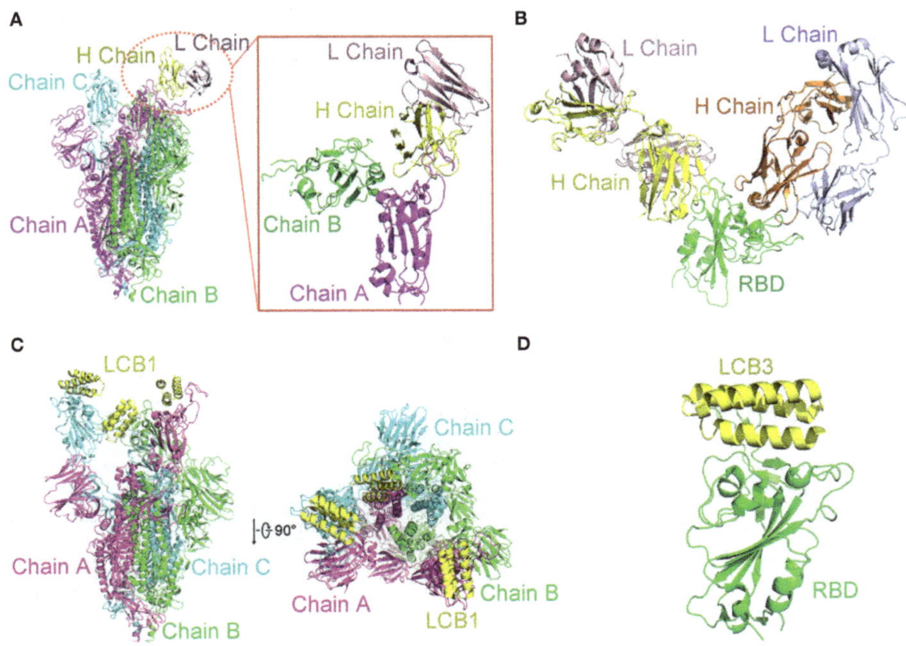

FIGURE 8 | Complex structures of SARS-CoV-2 with antibodies. **(A)** Cryo-EM structure of BD-23 Fab in complex with the spike (S) trimer. The three protomers in the S trimer are shown in green, cyan, and magenta, respectively. BD23-Fab is colored in yellow (heavy chain) and pink (light chain). The figure in the box is an amplified part of the interaction between BD-23 Fab and Chain **(B)** **(B)** Structure of REGN10933 and REGN10987 in complex with RBD. The heavy chain of REGN10933 is orange and light chain of REGN10933 is blue. The heavy chain of REGN10987 is yellow and light chain of REGN10987 is pink. RBD is shown in green. **(C)** Cryo-EM structure of LCB1 in complex with the S trimer from side view and top view. The three protomers in the S trimer are shown in green, cyan, and magenta, respectively. LCB1 is colored in yellow. **(D)** Cryo-EM structure of LCB3 in complex with the RBD. The LCB3 is shown in yellow, and RBD is colored in green. All structures are drawn by Pymol.

De Novo Protein

Interestingly, D. Baker group designed a series of *de novo* mini proteins to mimic RBD antibodies (Cao Y. et al., 2020). Applying shape and chemical complementarity strategies, they designed high-affinity mini binders that compete with ACE2 binding. Ten mini proteins (AHB1, AHB2, and LCB1-LCB8) could bind to the RBD, which affinities are ranging from 100 pM to 10 nM. These inhibitors could prevent the entry of SARS-CoV-2 into Vero E6 cells with IC_{50} from 35 pM to 35 nM. Among them, LCB1 (56 residues) and LCB3 (64 residues) showed stability and are the most potent inhibitors. Their IC_{50} values are almost six-fold that of the most effective monoclonal antibodies reported so far. Cryo-EM structures determined by the study corresponded to their computational LCB1/RBD or LCB3/RBD models (**Figures 8C, D**). In a single spike protein, three RBDs can be used simultaneously. These *de novo* hyper stable mini binders offer good points for new therapeutics of SARS-CoV-2.

Apart from those mentioned above, numerous neutralizing antibodies for SARS-CoV-2 have sprung up (**Figures S2, S3**). Structural evidence suggests that the stoichiometry of RBD with neutralizing antibodies is different (**Figure S2**). For instance, S309 Fab (Pinto et al., 2020), H104 Fab (Lv et al., 2020), and C105 Fab (Barnes et al., 2020) could bind two or three RBDs of S protein. The state of the RBD differs when it binds to different Fab fragments. S309 Fab binds RBD of S protein in the closed state (**Figures S2A, B**). However, H104 Fab and C105 Fab bind RBD of S protein in the open state (**Figures S2C–F**).

Simultaneously, some structures of neutralizing antibodies with RBD were determined. In these structures, RBD could bind one neutralizing antibody, which includes CR3022 (Yuan et al., 2020b), CC12.1, CC12.3 (Yuan et al., 2020a), and so on (**Figures S2A–H**). RBD also binds two different neutralizing antibodies (**Figures S3I–K**) and nanobody (**Figure S3M**). Here, we summarize inhibitors for S protein or RBD as follows (**Table 1**) (Toelzer et al., 2020).

Chemical Compounds

There are no effective drugs to prevent the SARS-CoV-2 spread. Thus, therapeutic agents to treat infected individuals are urgently required. Membrane fusion is a crucial step in viral infection. The previously developed coronavirus fusion inhibitors have been shown to prevent virus fusion by targeting the S2 subunit. A pan-coronavirus fusion inhibitor EK1, targeting the subunit S2's HR1 domain, could inhibit infection of SARS-CoV and MERS-CoV. Subsequently, an EK1 derivative, EK1C4, was found to inhibit the membrane fusion and pseudo-viral infection of SARS-CoV-2 with an IC_{50} of 1.3 nM and 15.8 nM, respectively (Xia et al., 2020). In addition, IPB02, a lipopeptide fusion inhibitor based on HR2 sequence, showed efficient antiviral activity (Ling et al., 2020; Zhu et al., 2020).

TABLE 1 | Summary of inhibitors for spike protein.

Type of inhibitor	Target of inhibitor	Inhibitor	IC_{50} (Pseudovirus)	IC_{50} (Authentic virus)	Kd	EC_{50}	ND_{50}	Reference
Chemical compounds	HR1 and HR2	EK1C4	15.8 nM	36.5 nM	-	-	-	(Xia et al., 2020)
	HR2	IPB02	80 nM	-	-	-	-	(Zhu et al., 2020)
	COVID-19	Glycyrrhizic acid	-	Reduces IC_{50} by about 10-fold	-	-	-	(Bailly and Vergoten, 2020)
	ACE2	Captopril	-	-	-	-	-	(Biyani et al., 2020)
		Enalapril	-	-	-	-	-	(Sharif-Askari et al., 2020)
		ARB	-	-	-	-	-	(Chung et al., 2020)
		Lisinopril	-	-	-	-	-	(Khelfaoui et al., 2020)
Neutralizing antibodies	Spike	BD-217	0.031 μg/ml	0.84 μg/ml	0.29 nM	-	-	(Cao Y. et al., 2020)
		BD-218	0.011 μg/ml	0.29 μg/ml	0.039 nM	-	-	(Cao Y. et al., 2020)
		BD-236	0.037 μg/ml	0.52 μg/ml	2.8 nM	-	-	(Cao Y. et al., 2020)
		BD-361	0.020 μg/ml	0.780 μg/ml	1.3 nM	-	-	(Cao Y. et al., 2020)
		BD-368	0.035 μg/ml	1.600 μg/ml	1.2 nM	-	-	(Cao Y. et al., 2020)
		BD-368-2	0.001.2 μg/ml	0.015 μg/ml	0.82 nM	-	-	(Cao Y. et al., 2020)
		BD-395	0.020 μg/ml	0.270 μg/ml	0.36 nM	-	-	(Cao Y. et al., 2020)
		2B04	1.46 ng/ml	-	-	-	-	(Alsoussi et al., 2020)
		CA1	-	-	4.68 ± 1.64 nM	-	0.38 μg/ml	(Shi et al., 2020)
		CB6	-	-	2.49 ± 1.65 nM	-	0.036 ± 0.007 μg/ml	(Shi et al., 2020)
		P2C-1F11	0.03 μg/ml	0.03 μg/ml	2.12 nM	-	-	(Ju et al., 2020)
		P2B-2F6	0.05 μg/ml	0.41 μg/ml	5.14 nM	-	-	(Ju et al., 2020)
		P2C-1A3	0.62 μg/ml	0.28 μg/ml	2.47 nM	-	-	(Ju et al., 2020)
		S309 Fab	-	79 ng/ml	0.81 nM	-	-	(Pinto et al., 2020)
		H11-H4-Fc	61 nM	-	5.5 nM	-	6 nM	(Huo et al., 2020)
		H11-D4-Fc	161 nM	-	10 nM	-	18 nM	(Huo et al., 2020)
		VHH72-Fc	262 nM	-	40nM	-	0.2 μg/ ml	(Huo et al., 2020)
		CR3022 Fab	347 nM	-	115 nM	-	-	(Yuan et al., 2020a)
		CR3022 IgG	-	-	1 nM	-	-	(Yuan et al., 2020a)
		H014 Fab	3 nM	38 nM	0.096 nM	0.7 nM	-	(Lv et al., 2020)
		REGN10933	42.8 pM	37.4 pM	3.37 nM	5.79 pM	-	(Baum et al., 2020)
		REGN10987	40.6 pM	42.1 pM	45.2 nM	6.33 pM	-	(Baum et al., 2020)
		REGN10989	7.23 pM	7.38 pM	3.65 nM	4.86 pM	-	(Baum et al., 2020)
		REGN10934	54.4 pM	28.3 pM	4.86 nM	2.72 pM	-	(Baum et al., 2020)
		C105 Fab	26.1 ng/mL	-	-	-	-	(Barnes et al., 2020)
		CV30	0.03 μg/mL	-	3.6 nM	-	-	(Hurlburt et al., 2020)
		EY6A	54 nM	-	2 nM	-	0.5 nM	(Zhou et al., 2020)
		CC12.1Fab	20 ng/ml	20 ng/ml	17 nM	-	-	(Yuan et al., 2020a)
		CC12.3 Fab	20 ng/ml	20 ng/ml	14 nM	-	-	(Yuan et al., 2020a)
		COVA2-39	0.036 μg/ml	0.054 μg/ml	21 nM	-	-	(Wu N. C. et al., 2020)
		COVA2-04	0.22 μg/ml	2.5 μg/ml	40 nM	-	-	(Wu N. C. et al., 2020)
		4A8	-	0.39 μg/ml	92.7 nM	0.61μg/ml	-	(Chi et al., 2020)
Nanobody		Ty1	54 nM	-	5–10 nM	-	-	(Hanke et al., 2020)

IC_{50}, half maximal inhibitory concentration; Kd, dissociation constant; EC_{50}, concentration for half of maximal effect; ND_{50}, half neutralizing dose.

Inhibitors of ACE2

Besides inhibiting the S protein, blocking ACE2 may also be a potential strategy to inhibit the coronavirus infection. Some researchers hope to interrupt the interaction between ACE2 and SARS-CoV-2 by employing existing FDA-approved ACE2 inhibitors (including captopril, enalapril, and lisinopril) (Vaduganathan et al., 2020). In fact, the application of ACE2 inhibitors brought two contradictory impacts on the patients. In some cases, ACE2 inhibitors could reduce inflammation. While in other cases, the inhibitors would improve the entry of viruses. Actually, these ACE2 inhibitors mainly act on the peptidase domain of ACE2, not on the interface for SARS-CoV-2 binding. Moreover, some adverse effects were reported, such as hypertension, heart failure, and these ACE2 inhibitors cause serious side effects in diabetic patients (Bavishi et al., 2020). Therefore, existing FDA-approved ACE2 inhibitors are not an appropriate option for treating SARS-CoV-2 patients (South et al., 2020).

Apart from that, chloroquine (CQ) and hydroxychloroquine (HCQ) were found to be potential therapeutic agents for COVID-19 (Xiu et al., 2020). CQ is a 4- aminoquinoline compound derived from quinine, which has been used to treat malaria, amoebiasis, and SARS-CoV. Studies demonstrated that CQ could increase the endosomal pH value to one which is higher than that required for cell fusion. In addition, CQ could damage the terminal glycosylation of ACE2 receptors, decreasing the interaction between viruses and their ACE2 receptor. Under cell culture conditions, CQ can prevent the interaction between the ACE2 and SARS-CoV RBD, for which ED_{50} value is 4.4 μM (Vincent et al., 2005). CQ could inhibit SARS-CoV-2, which IC_{50} value is 1.13 μM (Wang M. L. et al., 2020). HCQ is an analogue of CQ, in which one of the N-ethyl substituents of CQ is β-hydroxylated. Hydroxychloroquine has the same mechanism as CQ but shows more tolerability than CQ (Rainsford et al., 2015). The results showed that the IC_{50} value of hydroxychloroquine is 0.72 μM after 48 h of incubation (Yao X. et al., 2020).

Even though CQ and HCQ show good antiviral activity, safety, and effectiveness, studies found that they may cause QT prolongation (Stas et al., 2008), ventricular arrhythmias (Chen et al., 2006), retinopathy (Yaylali et al., 2013), and other heart-related toxicities which may be harmful to severely ill patients. Overall, the treatment with CQ and HCQ has certain limitations.

NON-STRUCTURAL PROTEIN AND ITS INHIBITORS

Structure of Mpro and Its Inhibitors

The main proteinase (Mpro or 3C-like protease) is a cysteine proteinase with a serine proteinase-like structure that can cleave the main part of the polyprotein at 11 conserved sites, releasing RdRp, helicase, and other proteins for viral RNA replication. The functional role of Mpro for the maturation of viral proteins, coupled with the human lack of closely related homology, suggests that Mpro is an attractive target designing antiviral drugs (Ziebuhr et al., 2000; Ziebuhr, 2005; Yang et al., 2005).

Structure of Mpro With N3

A Michael acceptor-based peptidomimetic inhibitor N3 designed by computer-aided drug design (CADD) can inhibit Mpro proteases in MERS-CoV and SARS-CoV (Xue et al., 2008). Consistently, N3 could also fit well inside the SARS-CoV-2's substrate-binding pocket (Jin et al., 2020). In the structure, two Mpro form dimers *via* 2-fold symmetry axes of crystallography (named protomer A and B) (**Figure 9A**). Each protomer is formed by three domains (**Figure 9B**). Antiparallel β-barrel structures are shown in domain I (residues 8–101) and domain II (residues 102–184). Domain III (residues 201–303) consists of 5 α-helices. Mpro has a Cys–His catalytic dyad, and there is a cleft between domain I and II as the N3-binding site.

The electron density indicates that the Cb of the vinyl group on N3 and the Mpro catalytic sites Cys145 form a standard 1.8 Å C–S covalent bond, confirming that the Michael addition has occurred (**Figure 9C**). Five parts from N3 inserts Mpro active sites as P1, P2, P3, P4, and P5 (Wang et al., 2017). The lactam, located on P1, inserts into the S1 subsite, forming a hydrogen bond with His163 in protomer A. At the P2 site, the Leu's side chain inserts into the hydrophobic S2 subsite. Val at P3's side chain is solvent-exposed. The P4 side Ala is encircled by Leu167's and Phe185's side chains, and the main chain of Glu189, all of which form a small hydrophobic pocket. At P5, there are van der Waals contacting with Pro168. Through plaque-reduction assay, N3 showed an inhibitory effect on SARS-CoV-2, with individual half-maximal effective concentration (EC_{50}) values of 16.77 μM (Jin et al., 2020).

Structure of Mpro With 11a and 11b

By analyzing the structure-activity relationship (SAR) of the reported inhibitor and substrate binding pocket, two compounds 11a and 11b with more effective inhibition than N3 were designed to target SARS-CoV-2 Mpro (Dai et al., 2020).

The electron density map in the complex structure clearly shows the extended conformation of compound 11a in the Mpro substrate-binding pocket (**Figure 9D**). The Mpro catalytic sites Cys145 forms a covalent bond (1.8-Å) with the aldehyde-based C of 11a (**Figure 9E**). At P1, the (S)-g-lactam ring of 11a fits well into the S1 site. At P3, the 11a indolyl group is exposed to the S4 position, and Glu166 could stabilize by a hydrogen bond. When binding 11a, multiple water molecules, named W1 to W6, play important roles. Through a 2.9 Å hydrogen bond, W1 has interaction with the amide bond of 11a. As for W2 to W6, the five molecules stabilize 11a in the binding pocket. The 11b shows a similar inhibition binding mode with 11a. (**Figure 9F**). The biggest difference in binding mode is at P2. The 3-fluorophenyl group in 11b has a downward rotation of about 42.7 degrees relative to the cyclohexyl group in 11a (Dai et al., 2020). The binding modes of 11 a and 11 b in the Mpro complex structure are similar to the previously reported N3 and other inhibitors (**Figure 9F**). More water molecules are involved in binding hydrogen bonds in 11 a and 11 b, and the functional groups on the P2 are involved in some additional interactions, which may be the reason for their enhanced inhibition (Wang et al., 2016; Zhang et al., 2020). Here we summarize inhibitors for Mpro as follows (**Table 2**).

Mpro Inhibitors From FDA Approved Library

For a medical emergency, scientists began to re-screen drugs from all protease inhibitors approved by the FDA, which could inhibit Mpro. The established FRET assay was used to identify potential SARS-CoV-2 Mpro inhibitors by screening all protease inhibitors from the Selleckchem bioactive compound library (Ma et al., 2020).

Noticeable findings are as follows: (1) Boceprevir, an FDA-approved HCV drug, inhibits the Mpro's enzymatic activity with IC_{50} of 4.13 μM and EC_{50} of 1.90 μM against the SARS-CoV-2 virus in the cellular viral cytopathogenic effect (CPE) assay. (Ma et al., 2020). (2) GC-376, an investigational veterinary drug that has the highest enzymatic inhibition against the Mpro with an IC_{50} value of 0.03 μM (Kim et al., 2016; Pedersen et al., 2018) among candidate inhibitors so far. It showed promising activity against the SARS-CoV-2 virus (EC_{50} = 3.37 μM). GC-376 can use two different configurations R and S which may explain its high binding affinity to the target Mpro. (3) Calpain/cathepsin inhibitors. Calpain inhibitors II and XII, MG-132, are three potent inhibitors of Mpro with single-digit submicromolar efficacy in the enzymatic assay. Calpain inhibitors II and XII inhibit SARS-CoV-2 with EC_{50} values of 2.07 μM and 0.49 μM, respectively. MG-132 inhibits SARS-CoV-2 with IC_{50} values of 3.90 μM (Barnard et al., 2004).

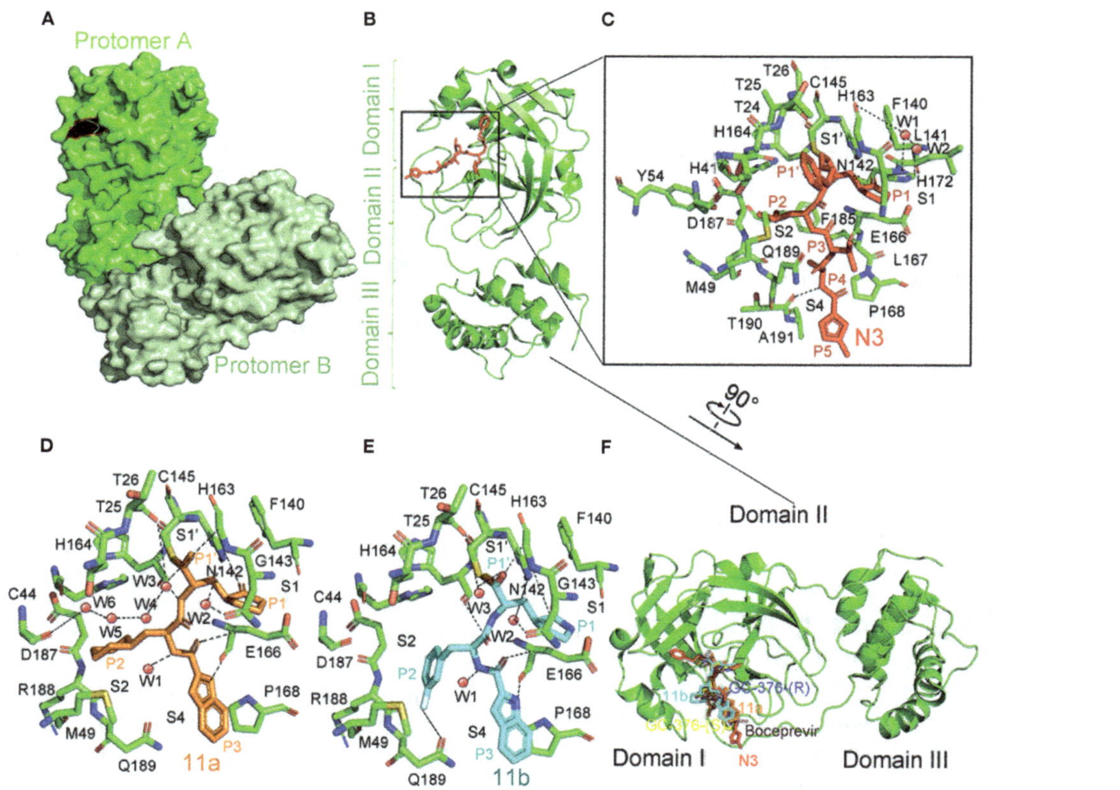

FIGURE 9 | The crystal structure of SARS-COV-2 virus Mpro in complex with inhibitors. **(A)** Surface representation of the homodimer of Mpro. Protomer A is in green, and protomer B is in pale green. **(B)** Cartoon representation of one protomer of the dimeric Mpro-inhibitor complex. The protomer is in green. N3 is in red sticks. **(C)** A zoomed view for the substrate-binding pocket. The key residues, which form the binding pocket, are shown as green sticks, the two waters, assigned as W1 and W2, are shown as red spheres. Four subsites, S1′, S1, S2, and S4, are labeled. P1, P1′, P2, P3, P4, and P5 sites of N3 are shown. Hydrogen bonds are indicated as dashed lines. **(D)** Close-up view of the 11a binding pocket. The residues involved in inhibitor binding are shown as green sticks. 11a and water molecules are shown as orange sticks and red spheres, respectively. Four subsites, S1′, S1, S2, and S4, are labeled. P1, P1′, P2, and P3 sites of 11a are indicated. Hydrogen bonds are indicated as dashed lines. **(E)** Close-up view of the 11b binding pocket. 11b and water molecules are shown as cyan sticks and red spheres, respectively. Four subsites, S1′, S1, S2, and S4, are labeled. P1, P1′, P2, and P3 sites of 11b are indicated. Hydrogen bonds are indicated as dashed lines. **(F)** Comparison of the inhibitor binding modes in SARS-CoV-2 Mpro. Two configurations (S and R) of GC-376, 11a, 11b, N3, and Boceprevir are shown in yellow, blue, orange, cyan, red, and dirty violet, respectively. All structures are drawn by Pymol.

TABLE 2 | The summary of recently reported Mpro inhibitors.

Compounds	SARS-CoV-2 Mpro inhibition (μM)	SARS-CoV-2 Antiviral activity (μM)	Development Stage
N3	Kobs/[I]=11,300 ± 800$M^{-1}S^{-1}$	EC_{50} = 16.77 ± 1.7	Preclinical; not tested in animals models
Ebselen	IC_{50} = 0.67 ± 0.09	EC_{50} = 4.67 ± 0.80	In clinical trials
11a	IC_{50} = 0.053 ± 0.005	EC_{50} = 0.53 ± 0.01	Preclinical; Favorable PK in rats and low toxicity in rats and dogs
11b	IC_{50} = 0.040 ± 0.002	EC_{50} = 0.72 ± 0.09	Preclinical; Favorable PK in rats
Boceprevir	IC_{50} = 4.13 ± 0.61 Ki=1.18	EC_{50} = 1.31 ± 0.58	FDA-approved HCV drug
GC-376	IC_{50} = 0.03 ± 0.008 K2/KI=40,800$M^{-1}S^{-1}$	EC_{50} = 3.37 ± 1.68	Preclinical; Tested in felines
MG-132	IC_{50} = 3.90 ± 1.01	NT.	Preclinical; Tested in mice
Calpain inhibitor II	IC_{50} = 0.97 ± 0.27 Ki=0.40	EC_{50} = 2.07 ± 0.76	Preclinical; not tested in animals models
Calpain inhibitor XII	IC_{50} = 0.45 ± 0.06 Ki=0.13	EC_{50} = 0.49 ± 0.18	Preclinical; not tested in animals models

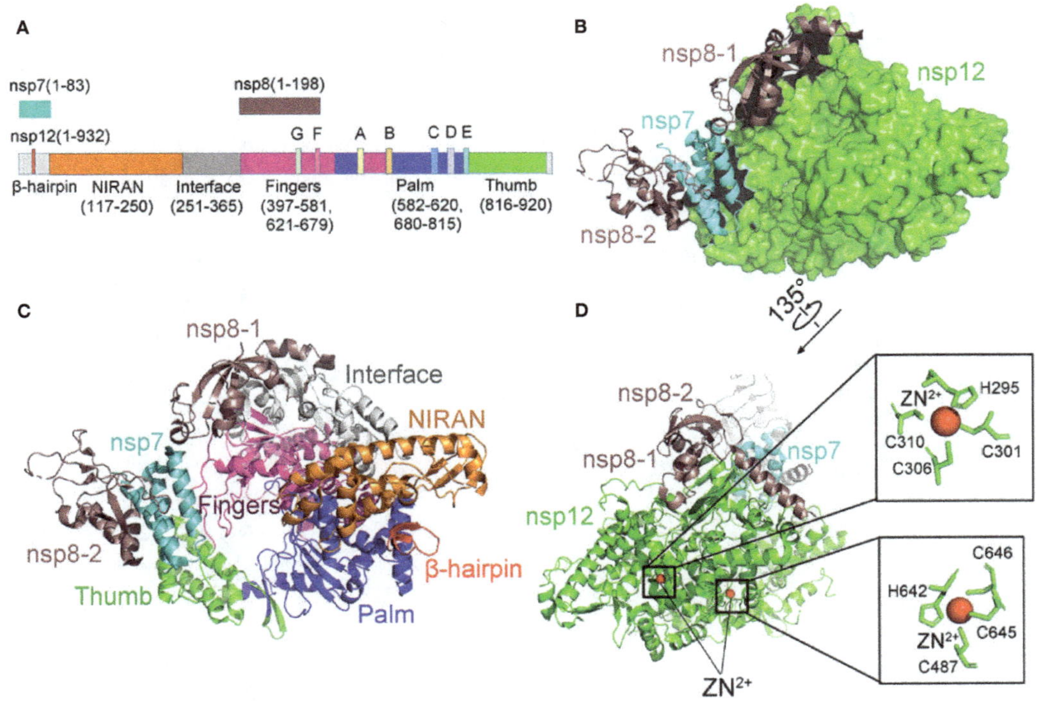

FIGURE 10 | The structure of the apo RdRp complex. **(A)** The schematic diagram for the components of the RdRp complex, which contains nsp7, nsp8, and nsp12. The polymerase motif (A-G) and β-hairpin are highlighted because it is unique to the SARS-CoV-2. **(B, C)** Two views structure of the apo nsp12-nsp7-nsp8 complex. nsp12 consists of an N-terminal β-hairpin (residues 31–50) and an extended nidovirus RdRp-associated nucleotidyl-transferase domain (NiRAN, residues 115–250). An interface domain (residues 251–365) is following the NiRAN domain. The nsp12 RdRp domain shows the canonical cupped right-handed configuration with the finger subdomain. NiRAN, Interface, Fingers, Thumb, Palm, nsp7, nsp8 are shown in orange, gray, hot pink, green, blue, cyan, and violet, respectively. **(D)** The conserved zinc-binding motifs in the apo structure rendered in ribbon are highlighted. The residues are shown as green sticks, and zinc is shown as red spheres. All structures are drawn by Pymol.

In summary, different potent SARS-CoV-2 Mpro inhibitors had been found with potent antiviral activity. Based on these hits, further development may lead to clinical application towards SARS-CoV-2 infections.

Structure of RdRp and Its Inhibitors

Remdesivir is an adenosine analogue that converts intracellularly into active drugs in the form of triphosphate (RTP), which binds to the nascent viral RNA chain, leading to premature termination (Velthuis et al., 2011; Ahn et al., 2012; Subissi et al., 2014; Kirchdoerfer and Ward, 2019; Wang M. L. et al., 2020). (including SARS/MERS/CoV/Ebola) Remdesivir is considered to be a promising antiviral drug against various RNA viruses (including SARS/MERS/Ebola virus) (Mulangu et al., 2019). Evidence showed that Remdesivir also efficiently inhibited SARS-CoV-2 infection through RdRp (van Hemert et al., 2008; Gong and Peersen, 2010; Sheahan et al., 2017).

Cryo-EM structures of RdRp provide insights into the inhibition mechanism of remdesivir (Yin et al., 2020) (**Figures 10B, C**). Different from the SARS-CoV RdRp, nsp12 of SARS-CoV-2 RdRp has an additional β-hairpin at the N-terminus (residues 31–50), as well as an extended nidovirus RdRp-associated nucleotidyl-transferase domain, which has three β-strands and seven helices (NiRAN, residues 115–250) (Lehmann et al., 2015; Gao et al., 2020). An interface domain (residues 251–365) is near the NiRAN domain (**Figures 10A, C**). The nsp12 RdRp domain displays the finger subdomain (resides 397–581 and residues 621–679), forming a closed circle with the thumb subdomain (residues 819–920). The closed conformation is stabilized by a combination of an nsp7 and an nsp8. Two zinc ions were found in the H295-C301-C306-C310 and C487-H642-C645-C646 conserved metal-binding motifs (**Figure 10D**). These zinc ions may act as conserved structural components to maintain RdRP structural integrity (Yin et al., 2020).

The structure of the template-RTP RdRp complex shows 11-base RNA in the primer strand, 14-base RNA in the template strand, and remdesivir in its monophosphate form (RMP), which is covalently linked to the primer strand (**Figures 11A–C**). Most protein–RNA interactions involve RNA ribose phosphate backbone directly linked to the 2′-OH groups, which provides the basis for distinguishing RNA from DNA. There are no base pairs in RNA from nsp12 to template-primer, indicating that the RdRP was independent of the RNA sequence. It is consistent with the fact that RdRp enzyme

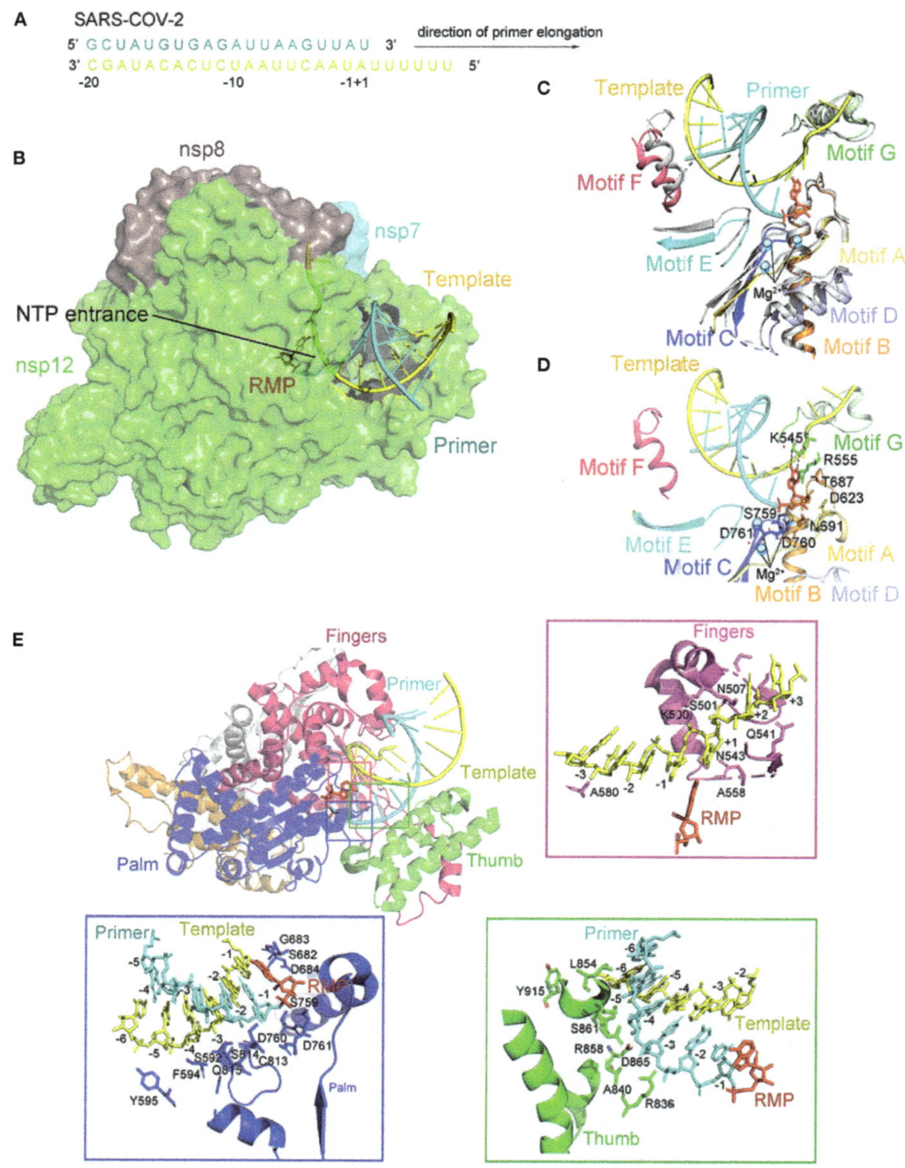

FIGURE 11 | The structure of the template-RTP RdRp complex. **(A)** The sequence of the RNA duplex with a 5′ U10 overhang as a template for extending primer and assembling the RdRp-RNA complex. **(B)** Cryo-EM Structure of the Remdesivir and RNA bound RdRp complex. Template and Primer are shown as yellow and cyan. **(C)** The conserved RdRp motifs (A to G) of the RNA-bound complex overlap with the apo structure, and color in gray, with a close view at the active site. Motifs (A to G) are shown in light orange, orange, blue, light blue, aquamarine, warm pink, and pale green, respectively. **(D)** A close view of the RdRp active site, showing the covalently bound RMP, magnesium ions, and pyrophosphate. Key residues and bases interacting with Remdesivir are shown. **(E)** Remdesivir-bound RdRp complex and protein-RNA interactions in the RNA. All structures are drawn by Pymol.

activity does not require specific sequences during the elongation step. At the 3′ end of the primer strand is RMP, covalently bound to the primer strand at the +1 position. Additional nucleotides at the +2 and +3 positions of the template strand interact with residues at the back of the finger subdomain (**Figure 11E**). As observed in the structure, only one RMP was assembled into the primer strand though the presence of excess RTP in a complex assembly (Tchesnokov et al., 2019; Gordon et al., 2020).

The RMP position is at the center of the active catalytic site (**Figure 11D**). RMP interacts with the upstream bases from the primer chains to form base stacking and forms two hydrogen bonds with the uridine groups from the template chains. In addition, RMP interacts with the side chains of K545 and R555. There were two magnesium ions near the bound RMP. Both magnesium ions interact with the diester phosphate backbone to form a part of the active catalytic site (**Figure 11D**).

Seven conserved motifs construct the active catalytic site of the nsp12 RdRp from A to G (**Figures 10C** and **11C**). Motifs ABCD are from the palm subdomain forming the active catalytic center (**Figure 11C**). Regarding the two magnesium ions in the catalytic center, both D760 and D761 are involved in the coordination (**Figure 11D**) (te Velthuis, 2014).

Interesting differences between the apo and complex structures were revealed by structural comparison (**Figure 11C**). Firstly, nsp7 moved toward the RdRp, resulting in the interface's rearrangement and lead to a weaker association of the second nsp8 in the complex. Secondly, the loop, connecting the first and second helix of the thumb subdomain, moved outward to adapt the binding of the double-stranded RNA helix. Thirdly, residues K500 and S501 from motif G moved to accommodate the template strand RNA's binding. Except for these changes, nsp12 in the apo and the RNA-complex are very similar (Venkataraman et al., 2018). In particular, the structural elements of the active catalytic site can be accurately superimposed, suggesting that RdRp is a relatively stable enzyme that can function as a replicase.

Besides remdesivir, several nucleotides, including galidesivir, ribavirin, favipiravir, and EIDD-2801, inhibit SARS-CoV-2 replication efficiently (Gordon et al., 2020). Especially, EIDD-2801 showed 3 to 10 folds more effective than remdesivir in preventing SARS-CoV-2 replication.

DISCUSSION

As the third widespread coronavirus that threatens human beings, SARS-CoV-2 has brought great disaster to the world (Yao et al., 2020a; Liang et al., 2020). Unfortunately, the SARS-CoV-2 variant D614G is more infectious than the ancestral SARS-CoV-2 (Plante et al., 2021). The analysis shows that the destruction of the interaction between D614 and T859 and the increase in the proportion of open RBD may be the reason for the increase in SARS-CoV-2 infection. Recently, other mutations, such as E484Q and L452R, have emerged and have decreased the effect of the vaccine. Fortunately, some patients who contracted SARS-CoV-2 recovered quickly after receiving cocktail therapy (Baum et al., 2020). The cocktail's formula includes Regeneron's REGN10933 and REGN10987 antibodies, zinc, vitamin D, famotidine, melatonin, and aspirin. Current drug candidates mainly inhibit S protein and some non-structural proteins (Mpro, PLpro, helicase, and RdRp). Small molecule inhibitors and neutralizing antibodies are potential therapies for SARS-CoV-2 infection.

For small molecule inhibitors, some FDA-approved compounds for clinical use have shown efficacy against SARS-CoV-2. Remdesivir, an inhibitor developed for the Ebola virus, inhibits SARS-CoV-2 by binding RNA replicase RdRp. Compared to small molecules, the neutralizing antibodies exhibit robust inhibition against SARS-CoV-2 infection. The neutralizing antibodies BD-368-2 (Cao L. et al., 2020), BD23-Fab (Cao L. et al., 2020), and P2B-2F6 (Ju et al., 2020) against S protein showed good IC_{50} values and could effectively compete with ACE2 binding. The IC_{50} values of neutralizing antibodies REGN10933 and REGN10987 can be as low as a few picomoles, which play an essential role in successful cocktail therapy. Besides this antibody cocktail, two *de novo* mini proteins designed by CADD with high affinity to S protein, LCB1and LCB3, show effective inhibition to the invasion of SARS-CoV-2 to host cells (Cao L. et al., 2020). The structure of the neutralizing antibodies and SARS-CoV-2 S protein complex provides a robust basis, further promoting the understanding of antibody-based therapy. In fact, many patients have saved their lives based on the application of antibodies.

To date, human beings have experienced several epidemic outbreaks, and each episode has had varying degrees of negative impacts on health, economy, psychology, and human behavior. When it comes to coronavirus, researchers have worked hard to discover its replication and pathogenesis and have gained some achievements in this regard. As we all know, many viruses have been present in natural reservoirs for a long time. Owing to human activities, viruses spread from natural hosts to humans or other animals. Unfortunately, people still cannot predict when the virus will arrive and what impact the virus will have. In this review, we provide the origin and evolution of SARS-CoV-2 to show that people should maintain the barrier between natural reservoirs and human society. After this worldwide epidemic, finding effective drugs or inhibitors is imminent. Although antibodies have shown positive effects, the defects are still obvious and not easy to overcome. In particular, it is impossible and costly to extract enough neutralizing antibodies from convalescent patients for countless clinical treatments. In this review, we summarize almost all the existing neutralizing antibodies or drugs and display their structures. Comparing or incorporating their characteristics is important to optimize or design more effective drugs. In the future, *de novo* recombinant protein may overcome the bottleneck of antibodies, improving the binding affinity and yield. It is theoretically feasible to minimize the effective antibodies or design *de novo* antibodies based on the structural data. In the case of Ebola, zMapp, consisting of three chimeric MBS, was successfully used to cure two Ebola patients in 2014 (Lyon et al., 2014). Therefore, the commercial antibody will bring hope to SARS-CoV-2 patients.

In addition to the above two treatments, the vaccine's clinical application will effectively prevent the spread of SARS-CoV-2 (Silveira et al., 2020). For emergency use, the whole virus inactivated vaccine and mRNA vaccine (Park et al., 2020) have shown the prospect of prevention (Calina et al., 2020). In the future, more in-depth research on SARS-CoV-2 will bring new therapeutic schemes for its prevention and treatment.

AUTHOR CONTRIBUTIONS

SN and BY were the first authors with equal contributions, and YW and FW were the corresponding authors with equal contributions. All authors contributed to the article and approved the submitted version.

FUNDING

The work was supported by National Natural Science Foundation of China (No.31770827 and 21736002), Youth Project of Beijing Natural Science Foundation 5214027, the National Key Research and Development Program of China 2016YFC0906000, Beijing Institute of Technology Innovative Talents Science and Technology Grant 3160012211907, Beijing Institute of Technology Young Backbone Teacher Start-up Fund 3160012221905, the Beijing Institute of Technology Research Fund Program for Young Scholars.

ACKNOWLEDGMENTS

We thank Dr. Qinghong from Beijing Institute of Technology for suggestions and modifications to the language.

REFERENCES

Ahn, D. G., Choi, J. K., Taylor, D. R., and Oh, J. W. (2012). Biochemical Characterization of a Recombinant SARS Coronavirus Nsp12 RNA-dependent RNA Polymerase Capable of Copying Viral RNA Templates. *Arch. Virol.* 157, 2095–2104. doi: 10.1007/s00705-012-1404-x

Alsoussi, W. B., Turner, J. S., Case, J. B., Zhao, H., Schmitz, A. J., Zhou, J. Q., et al. (2020). A Potently Neutralizing Antibody Protects Mice Against SARS-CoV-2 Infection. *J. Immunol.* 205, 915–922. doi: 10.4049/jimmunol.2000583

Andersen, K. G., Rambaut, A., Ian Lipkin, W., Holmes, E. C., and Garry, R. F. (2020). The Proximal Origin of SARS-Cov-2. *Nat. Med.* 26, 450–452. doi: 10.1038/s41591-020-0820-9

Bailly, C., and Vergoten, G. (2020). Glycyrrhizin: An Alternative Drug for the Treatment of COVID-19 Infection and the Associated Respiratory Syndrome? *Pharmacol. Ther.* 214, 1–16. doi: 10.1016/j.pharmthera.2020.107618

Barnard, D. L., Hubbard, V. D., Burton, J., Smee, D. F., Morrey, J. D., Otto, M. J., et al. (2004). Inhibition of Severe Acute Respiratory Syndrome-Associated Coronavirus (SarscoV) by Calpain Inhibitors and Beta-D-N4-Hydroxycytidine. *Antivir. Chem. Chemother.* 15, 15–22. doi: 10.1177/095632020401500102

Barnes, C. O., West, A. P.Jr., Huey-Tubman, K. E., Hoffmann, M. A. G., Sharaf, N. G., Hoffman, P. R., et al. (2020). Structures of Human Antibodies Bound to SARS-CoV-2 Spike Reveal Common Epitopes and Recurrent Features of Antibodies. *Cell* 182, 828–842. doi: 10.1016/j.cell.2020.06.025

Baum, A., Ajithdoss, D., Copin, R., Zhou, A., Lanza, K., Negron, N., et al. (2020). Regn-COV2 Antibodies Prevent and Treat SARS-CoV-2 Infection in Rhesus Macaques and Hamsters. *Science* 370, 1110–1115. doi: 10.1126/science.abe2402

Bavishi, C., Maddox, T. M., and Messerli, F. H. (2020). Coronavirus Disease 2019 (Covid-19) Infection and Renin Angiotensin System Blockers. *JAMA Cardiol.* 5, 745–747. doi: 10.1001/jamacardio.2020.1282

Belouzard, S., Chu, V. C., and Whittaker, G. R. (2009). Activation of the SARS Coronavirus Spike Protein Via Sequential Proteolytic Cleavage at Two Distinct Sites. *P Natl. Acad. Sci. U.S.A.* 106, 5871–5876. doi: 10.1073/pnas.0809524106

Benton, D. J., Wrobel, A. G., Xu, P., Roustan, C., Martin, S. R., Rosenthal, P. B., et al. (2020). Receptor Binding and Priming of the Spike Protein of SARS-CoV-2 for Membrane Fusion. *Nature* 588, 327–330. doi: 10.1038/s41586-020-2772-0

Biyani, C. S., Palit, V., and Daga, S. (2020). The Use of Captopril-Angiotensin Converting Enzyme (Ace) Inhibitor for Cystinuria During COVID-19 Pandemic. *Urology* 141, 182–183. doi: 10.1016/j.urology.2020.04.057

Bleibtreu, A., Bertine, M., Bertin, C., Houhou-Fidouh, N., and Visseaux, B. (2020). Focus on Middle East Respiratory Syndrome Coronavirus (MERS-Cov). *Med. Maladies Infect.* 50, 243–251. doi: 10.1016/j.medmal.2019.10.004

Bosch, B. J., van der Zee, R., de Haan, C. A. M., and Rottier, P. J. M. (2003). The Coronavirus Spike Protein is a Class I Virus Fusion Protein: Structural and Functional Characterization of the Fusion Core Complex. *J. Virol.* 77, 8801–8811. doi: 10.1128/Jvi.77.16.8801-8811.2003

Burkard, C., Verheije, M. H., Wicht, O., van Kasteren, S. I., van Kuppeveld, F. J., Haagmans, B. L., et al. (2014). Coronavirus Cell Entry Occurs Through the Endo-/Lysosomal Pathway in a Proteolysis-Dependent Manner. *PloS Pathog.* 10, 1–17. doi: 10.1371/journal.ppat.1004502

Calina, D., Docea, A. O., Petrakis, D., Egorov, A. M., Ishmukhametov, A. A., Gabibov, A. G., et al. (2020). Towards Effective COVID-19 Vaccines: Updates, Perspectives and Challenges (Review). *Int. J. Mol. Med.* 46, 3–16. doi: 10.3892/ijmm.2020.4596

Cao, L., Goreshnik, I., Coventry, B., Case, J. B., Miller, L., Kozodoy, L., et al. (2020). De Novo Design of Picomolar SARS-CoV-2 Miniprotein Inhibitors. *Science* 370, 426–431. doi: 10.1126/science.abd9909

Cao, Y., Su, B., Guo, X., Sun, W., Deng, Y., Bao, L., et al. (2020). Potent Neutralizing Antibodies Against SARS-CoV-2 Identified by High-Throughput Single-Cell Sequencing of Convalescent Patients' B Cells. *Cell* 182, 73–84. doi: 10.1016/j.cell.2020.05.025

Cao, S., Wang, H. H., Luhur, A., and Wong, S. M. (2005). Yeast Expression and Characterization of SARS-Cov N Protein. *J. Virol. Methods* 130, 83–88. doi: 10.1016/j.jviromet.2005.06.010

Cauchemez, S., Van Kerkhove, M. D., Riley, S., Donnelly, C. A., Fraser, C., and Ferguson, N. M. (2013). Transmission Scenarios for Middle East Respiratory Syndrome Coronavirus (Mers-CoV) and How to Tell Them Apart. *Eurosurveillance* 18, 7–13. doi: 10.1186/1475-2875-12-204

Chafekar, A., and Fielding, B. C. (2018). MERS-Cov: Understanding the Latest Human Coronavirus Threat. *Viruses-Basel* 10, 1–22. doi: 10.3390/v10020093

Chang, C. K., Hou, M. H., Chang, C. F., Hsiao, C. D., and Huang, T. H. (2014). The SARS Coronavirus Nucleocapsid Protein - Forms and Functions. *Antivir. Res.* 103, 39–50. doi: 10.1016/j.antiviral.2013.12.009

Chan, J. F. W., Lau, S. K. P., To, K. K. W., Cheng, V. C. C., Woo, P. C. Y., and Yuen, K. Y. (2015). Middle East Respiratory Syndrome Coronavirus: Another Zoonotic Betacoronavirus Causing SARS-Like Disease. *Clin. Microbiol. Rev.* 28, 465–522. doi: 10.1128/Cmr.00102-14

Chen, Y. Q., Rajashankar, K. R., Yang, Y., Agnihothram, S. S., Liu, C., Lin, Y. L., et al. (2013). Crystal Structure of the Receptor-Binding Domain From Newly Emerged Middle East Respiratory Syndrome Coronavirus. *J. Virol.* 87, 10777–10783. doi: 10.1128/Jvi.01756-13

Chen, B., Tian, E.-K., He, B., Tian, L., Han, R., Wang, S., et al. (2020). Overview of Lethal Human Coronaviruses. *Signal Transduct. Target. Ther.* 5, 89. doi: 10.1038/s41392-020-0190-2

Chen, C. Y., Wang, F. L., and Lin, C. C. (2006). Chronic Hydroxychloroquine Use Associated With QT Prolongation and Refractory Ventricular Arrhythmia. *Clin. Toxicol. (Phila)* 44, 173–175. doi: 10.1080/15563650500514558

Chi, X., Yan, R., Zhang, J., Zhang, G., Zhang, Y., Hao, M., et al. (2020). A Neutralizing Human Antibody Binds to the N-terminal Domain of the Spike Protein of SARS-Cov-2. *Science* 369, 650–655. doi: 10.1126/science.abc6952

Chung, M. K., Karnik, S., Saef, J., Bergmann, C., Barnard, J., Lederman, M. M., et al. (2020). Sars-CoV-2 and ACE2: The Biology and Clinical Data Settling the ARB and ACEI Controversy. *Ebiomedicine* 58, 1–10. doi: 10.1016/j.ebiom.2020.102907

Coronaviridae Study Group of the International Committee on Taxonomy of, V. (2020). The Species Severe Acute Respiratory Syndrome-Related Coronavirus: Classifying 2019-nCoV and Naming it SARS-Cov-2. *Nat. Microbiol.* 5, 536–544. doi: 10.1038/s41564-020-0695-z

Cui, J., Li, F., and Shi, Z. L. (2019). Origin and Evolution of Pathogenic Coronaviruses. *Nat. Rev. Microbiol.* 17, 181–192. doi: 10.1038/s41579-018-0118-9

Dai, W. H., Zhang, B., Jiang, X. M., Su, H. X., Li, J. A., Zhao, Y., et al. (2020). Structure-Based Design of Antiviral Drug Candidates Targeting the SARS-CoV-2 Main Protease. *Science* 368, 1331–1335. doi: 10.1126/science.abb4489

Forni, D., Cagliani, R., Clerici, M., and Sironi, M. (2017). Molecular Evolution of Human Coronavirus Genomes. *Trends Microbiol.* 25, 35–48. doi: 10.1016/j.tim.2016.09.001

Fouchier, R. A. M., Kuiken, T., Schutten, M., van Amerongen, G., van Doornum, J., van den Hoogen, B. G., et al. (2003). Aetiology - Koch's Postulates Fulfilled for SARS Virus. *Nature* 423, 240–240. doi: 10.1038/423240a

Gao, X. M., Xu, H., Zhang, B. N., Tao, T., Liu, Y. L., Xu, D. J., et al. (2019). Interaction of N-acetyl-seryl-aspartyl-lysyl-proline With the Angiotensin-Converting Enzyme 2-Angiotensin-(1-7)-Mas Axis Attenuates Pulmonary Fibrosis in Silicotic Rats. *Exp. Physiol.* 104, 1562–1574. doi: 10.1113/Ep087515

Gao, Y., Yan, L., Huang, Y., Liu, F., Zhao, Y., Cao, L., et al. (2020). Structure of the RNA-dependent RNA Polymerase From COVID-19 Virus. *Science* 368, 779–782. doi: 10.1126/science.abb7498

Gong, P., and Peersen, O. B. (2010). Structural Basis for Active Site Closure by the Poliovirus RNA-dependent RNA Polymerase. *Proc. Natl. Acad. Sci. U.S.A.* 10, 22505–22510. doi: 10.1073/pnas.1007626107

Gordon, C. J., Tchesnokov, E. P., Woolner, E., Perry, J. K., Feng, J. Y., Porter, D. P., et al. (2020). Remdesivir is a Direct-Acting Antiviral That Inhibits RNA-dependent RNA Polymerase From Severe Acute Respiratory Syndrome Coronavirus 2 With High Potency. *J. Biol. Chem.* 295, 6785–6797. doi: 10.1074/jbc.RA120.013679

Guo, Y., Korteweg, C., McNutt, M. A., and Gu, J. (2008). Pathogenetic Mechanisms of Severe Acute Respiratory Syndrome. *Virus Res.* 133, 4–12. doi: 10.1016/j.virusres.2007.01.022

Hamming, I., Cooper, M. E., Haagmans, B. L., Hooper, N. M., Korstanje, R., Osterhaus, A. D., et al. (2007). The Emerging Role of ACE2 in Physiology and Disease. *J. Pathol.* 212, 1–11. doi: 10.1002/path.2162

Hanke, L., Vidakovics Perez, L., Sheward, D. J., Das, H., Schulte, T., Moliner-Morro, A., et al. (2020). An Alpaca Nanobody Neutralizes SARS-CoV-2 by Blocking Receptor Interaction. *Nat. Commun.* 11, 1–9. doi: 10.1038/s41467-020-18174-5

Hemnes, A. R., Rathinasabapathy, A., Austin, E. A., Brittain, E. L., Carrier, E. J., Chen, X. P., et al. (2018). A Potential Therapeutic Role for Angiotensin-Converting Enzyme 2 in Human Pulmonary Arterial Hypertension. *Eur. Respir. J.* 51, 1–20. doi: 10.1183/13993003.02638-2017

Hoffmann, M., Kleine-Weber, H., Schroeder, S., Krüger, N., Herrler, T., Erichsen, S., et al. (2020). SARS-Cov-2 Cell Entry Depends on ACE2 and TMPRSS2 and Is Blocked by a Clinically Proven Protease Inhibitor. *Cell* 181, 271–280. doi: 10.1016/j.cell.2020.02.052

Holmes, K. V. (2003). SARS-Associated Coronavirus. *New Engl. J. Med.* 348, 1948–1951. doi: 10.1056/NEJMp030078

Huang, C., Wang, Y., Li, X., Ren, L., Zhao, J., Hu, Y., et al. (2020). Clinical Features of Patients Infected With 2019 Novel Coronavirus in Wuhan, China. *Lancet* 395, 497–506. doi: 10.1016/S0140-6736(20)30183-5

Huo, J., Le Bas, A., Ruza, R. R., Duyvesteyn, H. M. E., Mikolajek, H., Malinauskas, T., et al. (2020). Neutralizing Nanobodies Bind SARS-CoV-2 Spike RBD and Block Interaction With ACE2. *Nat. Struct. Mol. Biol.* 27, 846–854. doi: 10.1038/s41594-020-0469-6

Hurlburt, N. K., Seydoux, E., Wan, Y.-H., Edara, V. V., Stuart, A. B., Feng, J., et al. (2020). Structural Basis for Potent Neutralization of SARS-CoV-2 and Role of Antibody Affinity Maturation. *Nat. Commun.* 11, 1–7. doi: 10.1038/s41467-020-19231-9

Jiang, R. D., Liu, M. Q., Chen, Y., Shan, C., Zhou, Y. W., Shen, X. R., et al. (2020). Pathogenesis of SARS-CoV-2 in Transgenic Mice Expressing Human Angiotensin-Converting Enzyme 2. *Cell* 182, 50–58. doi: 10.1016/j.cell.2020.05.027

Jiang, L. W., Wang, N. S., Zuo, T., Shi, X. L., Poon, K. M. V., Wu, Y. K., et al. (2014). Potent Neutralization of MERS-CoV by Human Neutralizing Monoclonal Antibodies to the Viral Spike Glycoprotein. *Sci. Transl. Med.* 6, 234ra59. doi: 10.1126/scitranslmed.3008140

Jin, Z. M., Du, X. Y., Xu, Y. C., Deng, Y. Q., Liu, M. Q., Zhao, Y., et al. (2020). Structure of M-pro From SARS-CoV-2 and Discovery of its Inhibitors. *Nature* 582, 289–293. doi: 10.1038/s41586-020-2223-y

Ju, B., Zhang, Q., Ge, J. W., Wang, R. K., Sun, J., Ge, X. Y., et al. (2020). Human Neutralizing Antibodies Elicited by SARS-CoV-2 Infection. *Nature* 584, 115–119. doi: 10.1038/s41586-020-2380-z

Khelfaoui, H., Harkati, D., and Saleh, B. A. (2020). Molecular Docking, Molecular Dynamics Simulations and Reactivity, Studies on Approved Drugs Library Targeting ACE2 and SARS-CoV-2 Binding With ACE2. *J. Biomol. Struct. Dyn.* 5, 1–17. doi: 10.1080/07391102.2020.1803967

Kim, Y., Liu, H. W., Kankanamalage, A. C. G., Weerasekara, S., Hua, D. H., Groutas, W. C., et al. (2016). Reversal of the Progression of Fatal Coronavirus Infection in Cats by a Broad-Spectrum Coronavirus Protease Inhibitor. *PloS Pathog.* 12, 1–18. doi: 10.1371/journal.ppat.1005531

Kirchdoerfer, R. N., Cottrell, C. A., Wang, N. S., Pallesen, J., Yassine, H. M., Turner, H. L., et al. (2016). Pre-Fusion Structure of a Human Coronavirus Spike Protein. *Nature* 531, 118–121. doi: 10.1038/nature17200

Kirchdoerfer, R. N., and Ward, A. B. (2019). Structure of the SARS-CoV nsp12 Polymerase Bound to Nsp7 and Nsp8 Co-Factors. *Nat. Commun.* 10, 1–9. doi: 10.1038/s41467-019-10280-3

Korber, B., Fischer, W. M., Gnanakaran, S., Yoon, H., Theiler, J., Abfalterer, W., et al. (2020). Tracking Changes in SARS-CoV-2 Spike: Evidence That D614G Increases Infectivity of the COVID-19 Virus. *Cell* 182, 812–827. doi: 10.1016/j.cell.2020.06.043

Kuba, K., Imai, Y., and Penninger, J. M. (2006). Angiotensin-Converting Enzyme 2 in Lung Diseases. *Curr. Opin. Pharmacol.* 6, 271–276. doi: 10.1016/j.coph.2006.03.001

Lan, J., Ge, J., Yu, J., Shan, S., Zhou, H., Fan, S., et al. (2020). Structure of the SARS-CoV-2 Spike Receptor-Binding Domain Bound to the ACE2 Receptor. *Nature* 581, 215–220. doi: 10.1038/s41586-020-2180-5

Lehmann, K. C., Gulyaeva, A., Zevenhoven-Dobbe, J. C., Janssen, G. M. C., Ruben, M., Overkleeft, H. S., et al. (2015). Discovery of an Essential Nucleotidylating Activity Associated With a Newly Delineated Conserved Domain in the RNA Polymerase-Containing Protein of All Nidoviruses. *Nucleic Acids Res.* 43, 8416–8434. doi: 10.1093/nar/gkv838

Liang, W. H., Lin, Y. P., Bi, J. P., Li, J. F., Liang, Y., Wong, S. S., et al. (2020). Serosurvey of SARS-CoV-2 Among Hospital Visitors in China. *Cell Res.* 30, 817–818. doi: 10.1038/s41422-020-0371-0

Li, W. H., Moore, M. J., Vasilieva, N., Sui, J. H., Wong, S. K., Berne, M. A., et al. (2003). Angiotensin-Converting Enzyme 2 is a Functional Receptor for the SARS Coronavirus. *Nature* 426, 450–454. doi: 10.1038/nature02145

Ling, R., Dai, Y., Huang, B., Huang, W., Yu, J., Lu, X., et al. (2020). In Silico Design of Antiviral Peptides Targeting the Spike Protein of SARS-Cov-2. *Peptides* 130, 1–7. doi: 10.1016/j.peptides.2020.170328

Long, Q. X., Liu, B. Z., Deng, H. J., Wu, G. C., Deng, K., Chen, Y. K., et al. (2020). Antibody Responses to SARS-CoV-2 in Patients With COVID-19. *Nat. Med.* 26, 845–848. doi: 10.1038/s41591-020-0897-1

Lu, R., Zhao, X., Li, J., Niu, P., Yang, B., Wu, H., et al. (2020). Genomic Characterisation and Epidemiology of 2019 Novel Coronavirus: Implications for Virus Origins and Receptor Binding. *Lancet* 395, 565–574. doi: 10.1016/S0140-6736(20)30251-8

Lv, Z., Deng, Y. Q., Ye, Q., Cao, L., Sun, C. Y., Fan, C., et al. (2020). Structural Basis for Neutralization of SARS-CoV-2 and SARS-CoV by a Potent Therapeutic Antibody. *Science* 369, 1505–1509. doi: 10.1126/science.abc5881

Lyon, G. M., Mehta, A. K., Varkey, J. B., Brantly, K., Plyler, L., McElroy, A. K., et al. (2014). Clinical Care of Two Patients With Ebola Virus Disease in the United States. *N Engl. J. Med.* 371, 2402–2409. doi: 10.1056/NEJMoa1409838

Ma, C. L., Sacco, M. D., Hurst, B., Townsend, J. A., Hu, Y. M., Szeto, T., et al. (2020). Boceprevir, GC-376, and Calpain Inhibitors II, XII Inhibit SARS-CoV-2 Viral Replication by Targeting the Viral Main Protease. *Cell Res.* 30, 678–692. doi: 10.1038/s41422-020-0356-z

Millet, J. K., and Whittaker, G. R. (2014). Host Cell Entry of Middle East Respiratory Syndrome Coronavirus After Two-Step, Furin-Mediated Activation of the Spike Protein. *P Natl. Acad. Sci. U.S.A.* 111, 15214–15219. doi: 10.1073/pnas.1407087111

Millet, J. K., and Whittaker, G. R. (2015). Host Cell Proteases: Critical Determinants of Coronavirus Tropism and Pathogenesis. *Virus Res.* 202, 120–134. doi: 10.1016/j.virusres.2014.11.021

Mittal, A., Manjunath, K., Ranjan, R. K., Kaushik, S., Kumar, S., and Verma, V. (2020). Covid-19 Pandemic: Insights Into Structure, Function, and Hace2 Receptor Recognition by the SARS-Cov-2. *PloS Pathog.* 16, 1–19. doi: 10.20944/preprints202005.0260.v1

Mulangu, S., Dodd, L. E., Davey, R. T.Jr., Tshiani Mbaya, O., Proschan, M., Mukadi, D., et al. (2019). A Randomized, Controlled Trial of Ebola Virus Disease Therapeutics. *N Engl. J. Med.* 281, 2293–2303. doi: 10.1056/NEJMoa1910993

Park, J. E., Li, K., Barlan, A., Fehr, A. R., Perlman, S., McCray, P. B., et al. (2016). Proteolytic Processing of Middle East Respiratory Syndrome Coronavirus Spikes Expands Virus Tropism. *P Natl. Acad. Sci. U.S.A.* 113, 12262–12267. doi: 10.1073/pnas.1608147113

Park, K. S., Sun, X., Aikins, M. E., and Moon, J. J. (2020). Non-Viral COVID-19 Vaccine Delivery Systems. *Adv. Drug Delivery Rev.* 169, 137–151. doi: 10.1016/j.addr.2020.12.008

Pedersen, N. C., Kim, Y., Liu, H. W., Kankanamalage, A. C. G., Eckstrand, C., Groutas, W. C., et al. (2018). Efficacy of a 3C-Like Protease Inhibitor in Treating Various Forms of Acquired Feline Infectious Peritonitis. *J. Feline Med. Surg.* 20, 378–392. doi: 10.1177/1098612x17729626

Pinto, D., Park, Y. J., Beltramello, M., Walls, A. C., Tortorici, M. A., Bianchi, S., et al. (2020). Structural and Functional Analysis of a Potent Sarbecovirus Neutralizing Antibody. *bioRxiv* 2020.04.07.023903, 1–20. doi: 10.1101/2020.04.07.023903

Plante, J. A., Liu, Y., Liu, J., Xia, H., Johnson, B. A., Lokugamage, K. G., et al. (2021). Spike Mutation D614G Alters SARS-CoV-2 Fitness. *Nature* 592, 116–121. doi: 10.1038/s41586-020-2895-3

Rabaan, A. A., Al-Ahmed, S. H., Haque, S., Sah, R., Tiwari, R., Malik, Y. S., et al. (2020). SARS-Cov-2, SARS-CoV, and MERS-COV: A Comparative Overview. *Infez. Med.* 28, 174–184.

Rainsford, K. D., Parke, A. L., Clifford-Rashotte, M., and Kean, W. F. (2015). Therapy and Pharmacological Properties of Hydroxychloroquine and Chloroquine in Treatment of Systemic Lupus Erythematosus, Rheumatoid Arthritis and Related Diseases. *Inflammopharmacology* 5, 231–269. doi: 10.1007/s10787-015-0239-y

Shang, J., Ye, G., Shi, K., Wan, Y., Luo, C., Aihara, H., et al. (2020). Structural Basis of Receptor Recognition by SARS-Cov-2. *Nature* 581, 221–224. doi: 10.1038/s41586-020-2179-y

Sharif-Askari, N. S., Sharif-Askari, F. S., Alabed, M., Abou Tayoun, A., Loney, T., Uddin, M., et al. (2020). Effect of Common Medications on the Expression of SARS-CoV-2 Entry Receptors in Kidney Tissue. *Cts-Clin. Transl. Sci.* 13, 1048–1054. doi: 10.1111/cts.12862

Sheahan, T. P., Sims, A. C., Graham, R. L., Menachery, V. D., Gralinski, L. E., Case, J. B., et al. (2017). Broad-Spectrum Antiviral GS-5734 Inhibits Both Epidemic and Zoonotic Coronaviruses. *Sci. Transl. Med.* 9, 1–12. doi: 10.1126/scitranslmed.aal3653

Sheahan, T. P., Sims, A. C., Zhou, S., Graham, R. L., Pruijssers, A. J., Agostini, M. L., et al. (2020). An Orally Bioavailable Broad-Spectrum Antiviral Inhibits SARS-CoV-2 in Human Airway Epithelial Cell Cultures and Multiple Coronaviruses in Mice. *Sci. Transl. Med.* 12, 1–15. doi: 10.1126/scitranslmed.abb5883

Shi, R., Shan, C., Duan, X., Chen, Z., Liu, P., Song, J., et al. (2020). A Human Neutralizing Antibody Targets the Receptor-Binding Site of SARS-Cov-2. *Nature* 584, 120–124. doi: 10.1038/s41586-020-2381-y

Silveira, M. M., Moreira, G., and Mendonca, M. (2020). DNA Vaccines Against COVID-19: Perspectives and Challenges. *Life Sci.* 267, 1–7. doi: 10.1016/j.lfs.2020.118919

Song, Z. Q., Xu, Y. F., Bao, L. L., Zhang, L., Yu, P., Qu, Y. J., et al. (2019). From SARS to MERS, Thrusting Coronaviruses Into the Spotlight. *Viruses-Basel* 11, 1–28. doi: 10.3390/v11010059

South, A. M., Tomlinson, L., Edmonston, D., Hiremath, S., and Sparks, M. A. (2020). Controversies of Renin-Angiotensin System Inhibition During the COVID-19 Pandemic. *Nat. Rev. Nephrol.* 16, 305–307. doi: 10.1038/s41581-020-0279-4

Stas, P., Faes, D., and Noyens, P. (2008). Conduction Disorder and QT Prolongation Secondary to Long-Term Treatment With Chloroquine. *Int. J. Cardiol.* 2, e80–e82. doi: 10.1016/j.ijcard.2007.04.055

Subissi, L., Posthuma, C. C., Collet, A., Zevenhoven-Dobbe, J. C., Gorbalenya, A. E., Decroly, E., et al. (2014). One Severe Acute Respiratory Syndrome Coronavirus Protein Complex Integrates Processive RNA Polymerase and Exonuclease Activities. *P Natl. Acad. Sci. U.S.A.* 111, E3900–E3909. doi: 10.1073/pnas.1323705111

Su, S., Wong, G., Shi, W., Liu, J., Lai, A. C. K., Zhou, J., et al. (2016). Epidemiology, Genetic Recombination, and Pathogenesis of Coronaviruses. *Trends Microbiol.* 24, 490–502. doi: 10.1016/j.tim.2016.03.003

Tchesnokov, E. P., Feng, J. Y., Porter, D. P., and Gotte, M. (2019). Mechanism of Inhibition of Ebola Virus RNA-Dependent Rna Polymerase by Remdesivir. *Viruses* 11, 1–16. doi: 10.3390/v11040326

te Velthuis, A. J. W. (2014). Common and Unique Features of Viral RNA-dependent Polymerases. *Cell Mol. Life Sci.* 71, 4403–4420. doi: 10.1007/s00018-014-1695-z

Tian, X., Li, C., Huang, A., Xia, S., Lu, S., Shi, Z., et al. (2020). Potent Binding of 2019 Novel Coronavirus Spike Protein by a SARS Coronavirus-Specific Human Monoclonal Antibody. *Emerg. Microbes Infect.* 9, 382–385. doi: 10.1080/22221751.2020.1729069

Toelzer, C., Gupta, K., Yadav, S. K. N., Borucu, U., Davidson, A. D., Kavanagh Williamson, M., et al. (2020). Free Fatty Acid Binding Pocket in the Locked Structure of SARS-CoV-2 Spike Protein. *Science* 370, 725–730. doi: 10.1126/science.abd3255

Vaduganathan, M., Vardeny, O., Michel, T., McMurray, J. J. V., Pfeffer, M. A., and Solomon, S. D. (2020). Renin-Angiotensin-Aldosterone System Inhibitors in Patients With Covid-19. *N Engl. J. Med.* 382, 1653–1659. doi: 10.1056/NEJMsr2005760

Vaheri, A., Strandin, T., Hepojoki, J., Sironen, T., Henttonen, H., Makela, S., et al. (2013). Uncovering the Mysteries of Hantavirus Infections. *Nat. Rev. Microbiol.* 11, 539–550. doi: 10.1038/nrmicro3066

van Hemert, M. J., van den Worm, S. H., Knoops, K., Mommaas, A. M., Gorbalenya, A. E., and Snijder, E. J. (2008). SARS-Coronavirus Replication/Transcription Complexes are Membrane-Protected and Need a Host Factor for Activity In Vitro. *PloS Pathog.* 4, 1–10. doi: 10.1371/journal.ppat.1000054

Velthuis, A. J. W. T., Arnold, J. J., Cameron, C. E., van den Worm, S. H. E., and Snijder, E. J. (2011). The RNA Polymerase Activity of SARS-coronavirus nsp12 is Primer Dependent (Vol 38, Pg 203, 2010). *Nucleic Acids Res.* 39, 203–214. doi: 10.1093/nar/gkr963

Venkataraman, S., Prasad, B. V. L. S., and Selvarajan, R. (2018). Rna Dependent Rna Polymerases: Insights From Structure, Function and Evolution. *Viruses-Basel* 10, 1–23. doi: 10.3390/v10020076

Vincent, M. J., Bergeron, E., Benjannet, S., Erickson, B. R., Rollin, P. E., Ksiazek, T. G., et al. (2005). Chloroquine is a Potent Inhibitor of SARS Coronavirus Infection and Spread. *Virol. J.* 69, 1–10. doi: 10.1186/1743-422X-2-69

Walls, A. C., Park, Y. J., Tortorici, M. A., Wall, A., McGuire, A. T., and Veesler, D. (2020). Structure, Function, and Antigenicity of the SARS-CoV-2 Spike Glycoprotein. *Cell* 181, 281–292. doi: 10.1016/j.cell.2020.02.058

Walls, A. C., Tortorici, M. A., Bosch, B. J., Frenz, B., Rottier, P. J. M., DiMaio, F., et al. (2016). Cryo-Electron Microscopy Structure of a Coronavirus Spike Glycoprotein Trimer. *Nature* 531, 114–117. doi: 10.1038/nature16988

Wang, M. L., Cao, R. Y., Zhang, L. K., Yang, X. L., Liu, J., Xu, M. Y., et al. (2020). Remdesivir and Chloroquine Effectively Inhibit the Recently Emerged Novel Coronavirus, (2019-nCoV) In Vitro. *Cell Res.* 30, 269–271. doi: 10.1038/s41422-020-0282-0

Wang, F., Chen, C., Tan, W., Yang, K., and Yang, H. (2016). Structure of Main Protease From Human Coronavirus NL63: Insights for Wide Spectrum Anti-Coronavirus Drug Design. *Sci. Rep.* 6, 1–12. doi: 10.1038/srep22677

Wang, F. H., Chen, C., Yang, K. L., Xu, Y., Liu, X. M., Gao, F., et al. (2017). Michael Acceptor-Based Peptidomimetic Inhibitor of Main Protease From Porcine Epidemic Diarrhea Virus. *J. Med. Chem.* 60, 3212–3216. doi: 10.1021/acs.jmedchem.7b00103

Wang, K., Chen, W., Zhang, Z., Deng, Y., Lian, J. Q., Du, P., et al. (2020). CD147-Spike Protein is a Novel Route for SARS-CoV-2 Infection to Host Cells. *Signal Transduct. Target Ther.* 5, 1–10. doi: 10.1038/s41392-020-00426-x

Wong, R. S. Y. (2020). The SARS-CoV-2 Outbreak: An Epidemiological and Clinical Perspective. *SN Compr. Clin. Med.* 29, 1–9. doi: 10.1007/s42399-020-00546-z

Woo, P. C. Y., Lau, S. K. P., Lam, C. S. F., Lau, C. C. Y., Tsang, A. K. L., Lau, J. H. N., et al. (2012). Discovery of Seven Novel Mammalian and Avian Coronaviruses in the Genus Deltacoronavirus Supports Bat Coronaviruses as the Gene Source of Alphacoronavirus and Betacoronavirus and Avian Coronaviruses as the Gene Source of Gammacoronavirus and Deltacoronavirus. *J. Virol.* 86, 3995–4008. doi: 10.1128/Jvi.06540-11

Wrapp, D., Wang, N., Corbett, K. S., Goldsmith, J. A., Hsieh, C. L., Abiona, O., et al. (2020). Cryo-Em Structure of the 2019-Ncov Spike in the Prefusion Conformation. *Science* 367, 1260–1263. doi: 10.1126/science.abb2507

Wu, K. L., Chen, L., Peng, G. Q., Zhou, W. B., Pennell, C. A., Mansky, L. M., et al. (2011). A Virus-Binding Hot Spot on Human Angiotensin-Converting Enzyme 2 Is Critical for Binding of Two Different Coronaviruses. *J. Virol.* 85, 5331–5337. doi: 10.1128/Jvi.02274-10

Wu, Z. Y., and McGoogan, J. M. (2020). Characteristics of and Important Lessons From the Coronavirus Disease 2019 (Covid-19) Outbreak in China Summary of a Report of 72 314 Cases From the Chinese Center for Disease Control and Prevention. *Jama-J. Am. Med. Assoc.* 323, 1239–1242. doi: 10.1001/jama.2020.264810.1001/jama.2020.2648

Wu, N. C., Yuan, M., Liu, H., Lee, C. D., Zhu, X., Bangaru, S., et al. (2020). An Alternative Binding Mode of IGHV3-53 Antibodies to the SARS-CoV-2 Receptor Binding Domain. *Cell Rep.* 33, 1–8. doi: 10.1016/j.celrep.2020.108274

Wu, F., Zhao, S., Yu, B., Chen, Y.-M., Wang, W., Hu, Y., et al. (2020a). Complete Genome Characterisation of a Novel Coronavirus Associated With Severe Human Respiratory Disease in Wuhan, China. *bioRxiv* 2020, 1–33. doi: 10.1101/2020.01.24.919183

Wu, F., Zhao, S., Yu, B., Chen, Y. M., Wang, W., Song, Z. G., et al. (2020b). A New Coronavirus Associated With Human Respiratory Disease in China. *Nature* 579, 265–269. doi: 10.1038/s41586-020-2202-3

Xia, S., Liu, Q., Wang, Q., Sun, Z. W., Su, S., Dub, L. Y., et al. (2014). Middle East Respiratory Syndrome Coronavirus (MERS-CoV) Entry Inhibitors Targeting Spike Protein. *Virus Res.* 194, 200–210. doi: 10.1016/j.virusres.2014.10.007

Xia, S., Liu, M. Q., Wang, C., Xu, W., Lan, Q. S., Feng, S. L., et al. (2020). Inhibition of SARS-CoV-2 (Previously 2019-nCoV) Infection by a Highly Potent Pan-Coronavirus Fusion Inhibitor Targeting its Spike Protein That Harbors a High Capacity to Mediate Membrane Fusion. *Cell Res.* 30, 343–355. doi: 10.1038/s41422-020-0305-x

Xiu, S., Dick, A., Ju, H., Mirzaie, S., Abdi, F., Cocklin, S., et al. (2020). Inhibitors of SARS-CoV-2 Entry: Current and Future Opportunities. *J. Med. Chem.* 63, 12256–12274. doi: 10.1021/acs.jmedchem.0c00502

Xue, X. Y., Yu, H. W., Yang, H. T., Xue, F., Wu, Z. X., Shen, W., et al. (2008). Structures of Two Coronavirus Main Proteases: Implications for Substrate Binding and Antiviral Drug Design. *J. Virol.* 82, 2515–2527. doi: 10.1128/Jvi.02114-07

Xu, C., Wang, Y., Liu, C., Zhang, C., Han, W., Hong, X., et al. (2020). Conformational Dynamics of SARS-CoV-2 Trimeric Spike Glycoprotein in Complex With Receptor ACE2 Revealed by Cryo-EM. *Sci. Adv.* 7, 1–13. doi: 10.1126/sciadv.abe5575

Xu, J., Zhao, S., Teng, T., Abdalla, A. E., Zhu, W., Xie, L., et al. (2020). Systematic Comparison of Two Animal-to-Human Transmitted Human Coronaviruses: Sars-CoV-2 and SARS-Cov. *Viruses* 12, 1–17. doi: 10.3390/v12020244

Yang, H., Xie, W., Xue, X., Yang, K., Ma, J., Liang, W., et al. (2005). Design of Wide-Spectrum Inhibitors Targeting Coronavirus Main Proteases. *PloS Biol.* 3, 1742–1752. doi: 10.1371/journal.pbio.0030324

Yan, R., Zhang, Y., Li, Y., Xia, L., Guo, Y., and Zhou, Q. (2020). Structural Basis for the Recognition of SARS-CoV-2 by Full-Length Human ACE2. *Science* 367, 1444–1448. doi: 10.1126/science.abb2762

Yao, H., Lu, X., Chen, Q., Xu, K., Chen, Y., Cheng, L., et al. (2020a). Patient-Derived Mutations Impact Pathogenicity of SARS-Cov-2. *medRxiv* 2020, 1–57. doi: 10.1101/2020.04.14.20060160

Yao, H., Song, Y., Chen, Y., Wu, N., Xu, J., Sun, C., et al. (2020b). Molecular Architecture of the SARS-CoV-2 Virus. *Cell* 183, 730–738. doi: 10.1016/j.cell.2020.09.018

Yao, X., Ye, F., Zhang, M., Cui, C., Huang, B., Niu, P., et al. (2020). In Vitro Antiviral Activity and Projection of Optimized Dosing Design of Hydroxychloroquine for the Treatment of Severe Acute Respiratory Syndrome Coronavirus 2 (SARS-Cov-2). *Clin. Infect. Dis.* 15, 732–739. doi: 10.1093/cid/ciaa237

Yaylali, S. A., Sadigov, F., Erbil, H., Ekinci, A., and Akcakaya, A. A. (2013). Chloroquine and Hydroxychloroquine Retinopathy-Related Risk Factors in a Turkish Cohort. *Int. Ophthalmol.* 33, 627–634. doi: 10.1007/s10792-013-9748-0

Yin, W., Mao, C., Luan, X., Shen, D. D., Shen, Q., Su, H., et al. (2020). Structural Basis for Inhibition of the RNA-dependent RNA Polymerase From SARS-CoV-2 by Remdesivir. *Science* 368, 1499–1504. doi: 10.1126/science.abc1560

Yuan, M., Liu, H., Wu, N. C., Lee, C. D., Zhu, X., Zhao, F., et al. (2020a). Structural Basis of a Shared Antibody Response to SARS-Cov-2. *Science* 369, 1119–1123. doi: 10.1126/science.abd2321

Yuan, M., Wu, N. C., Zhu, X., Lee, C. D., So, R. T. Y., Lv, H., et al. (2020b). A Highly Conserved Cryptic Epitope in the Receptor Binding Domains of SARS-CoV-2 and SARS-Cov. *Science* 368, 630–633. doi: 10.1126/science.abb7269

Yurkovetskiy, L., Wang, X., Pascal, K. E., Tomkins-Tinch, C., Nyalile, T. P., Wang, Y., et al. (2020). Structural and Functional Analysis of the D614G SARS-Cov-2 Spike Protein Variant. *Cell* 183, 739–751. doi: 10.1016/j.cell.2020.09.032

Zaki, A. M., van Boheemen, S., Bestebroer, T. M., Osterhaus, A. D., and Fouchier, R. A. (2012). Isolation of a Novel Coronavirus From a Man With Pneumonia in Saudi Arabia. *N Engl. J. Med.* 367, 1814–1820. doi: 10.1056/NEJMoa1211721

Zhang, L. L., Lin, D. Z., Kusov, Y., Nian, Y., Ma, Q. J., Wang, J., et al. (2020). alpha-Ketoamides as Broad-Spectrum Inhibitors of Coronavirus and Enterovirus Replication: Structure-Based Design, Synthesis, and Activity Assessment. *J. Med. Chem.* 63, 4562–4578. doi: 10.1021/acs.jmedchem.9b01828

Zhou, D., Duyvesteyn, H. M. E., Chen, C. P., Huang, C. G., Chen, T. H., Shih, S. R., et al. (2020). Structural Basis for the Neutralization of SARS-CoV-2 by an Antibody From a Convalescent Patient. *Nat. Struct. Mol. Biol.* 27, 950–958. doi: 10.1038/s41594-020-0480-y

Zhou, P., Fan, H., Lan, T., Yang, X. L., Shi, W. F., Zhang, W., et al. (2018). Fatal Swine Acute Diarrhoea Syndrome Caused by an HKU2-related Coronavirus of Bat Origin. *Nature* 556, 255–258. doi: 10.1038/s41586-018-0010-9

Zhu, Y., Yu, D., Yan, H., Chong, H., and He, Y. (2020). Design of Potent Membrane Fusion Inhibitors Against SARS-CoV-2, an Emerging Coronavirus With High Fusogenic Activity. *J. Virol.* 94, 1–12. doi: 10.1128/JVI.00635-20

Ziebuhr, J. (2005). The Coronavirus Replicase. *Curr. Top. Microbiol. Immunol.* 287, 57–94. doi: 10.1007/3-540-26765-4_3

Ziebuhr, J., Snijder, E. J., and Gorbalenya, A. E. (2000). Virus-Encoded Proteinases and Proteolytic Processing in the Nidovirales. *J. Gen. Virol.* 81, 853–879. doi: 10.1099/0022-1317-81-4-853

Zumla, A., Hui, D. S., Azhar, E. I., Memish, Z. A., and Maeurer, M. (2020). Reducing Mortality From 2019-nCoV: Host-Directed Therapies Should be an Option. *Lancet* 395, e35–e36. doi: 10.1016/S0140-6736(20)30305-6

14

COVID-19 Pandemic and Vaccines Update on Challenges and Resolutions

Wajihul Hasan Khan[1,2†], Zohra Hashmi[1†], Aditya Goel[1], Razi Ahmad[3], Kanisha Gupta[1], Nida Khan[1], Iqbal Alam[4], Faheem Ahmed[5] and Mairaj Ahmed Ansari[1]*

[1] Department of Biotechnology, Host Pathogen Interaction and Molecular Immunology Laboratory, Jamia Hamdard, New Delhi, India, [2] Department of Chemical Engineering, Indian Institute of Technology Delhi, New Delhi, India, [3] Department of Chemistry, Indian Institute of Technology Delhi, New Delhi, India, [4] Department of Physiology, Hamdard Institute of Medical Sciences and Research, Jamia Hamdard, New Delhi, India, [5] Department of Community Medicine, Hamdard Institute of Medical Sciences and Research, New Delhi, India

***Correspondence:**
Mairaj Ahmed Ansari
mairaj01@gmail.com

[†]These authors have contributed equally to this work

The coronavirus disease (COVID-19) is caused by a positive-stranded RNA virus called severe acute respiratory syndrome coronavirus-2 (SARS-CoV-2), belonging to the *Coronaviridae* family. This virus originated in Wuhan City, China, and became the cause of a multiwave pandemic that has killed 3.46 million people worldwide as of May 22, 2021. The havoc intensified with the emergence of SARS-CoV-2 variants (B.1.1.7; Alpha, B.1.351; Beta, P.1; Gamma, B.1.617; Delta, B.1.617.2; Delta-plus, B.1.525; Eta, and B.1.429; Epsilon etc.) due to mutations generated during replication. More variants may emerge to cause additional pandemic waves. The most promising approach for combating viruses and their emerging variants lies in prophylactic vaccines. Several vaccine candidates are being developed using various platforms, including nucleic acids, live attenuated virus, inactivated virus, viral vectors, and protein-based subunit vaccines. In this unprecedented time, 12 vaccines against SARS-CoV-2 have been phased in following WHO approval, 184 are in the preclinical stage, and 100 are in the clinical development process. Many of them are directed to elicit neutralizing antibodies against the viral spike protein (S) to inhibit viral entry through the ACE-2 receptor of host cells. Inactivated vaccines, to the contrary, provide a wide range of viral antigens for immune activation. Being an intracellular pathogen, the cytotoxic $CD8^+$ T Cell (CTL) response remains crucial for all viruses, including SARS-CoV-2, and needs to be explored in detail. In this review, we try to describe and compare approved vaccines against SARS-CoV-2 that are currently being distributed either after phase III clinical trials or for emergency use. We discuss immune responses induced by various candidate vaccine formulations; their benefits, potential limitations, and effectiveness against variants; future challenges, such as antibody-dependent enhancement (ADE); and vaccine safety issues and their possible resolutions. Most of the current vaccines developed against SARS-CoV-2 are showing either promising or compromised efficacy against new variants. Multiple antigen-based vaccines (multivariant vaccines) should be developed on different platforms to tackle future variants. Alternatively, recombinant BCG, containing SARS-CoV-2 multiple antigens, as a live attenuated vaccine should be explored for long-term protection. Irrespective of their efficacy, all vaccines are efficient in providing protection from disease severity. We must insist on vaccine compliance for all age groups and work on vaccine hesitancy globally to achieve herd immunity and, eventually, to curb this pandemic.

Keywords: COVID-19, SARS CoV-2 variant, spike protein, mutations, immune response, vaccine, multivariant vaccines, booster dose

1. INTRODUCTION

Coronaviruses are named after the crown-like spikes present on their outer surfaces. Out of seven known human coronaviruses (HCoVs), four viruses, HCoV-229E (alphacoronavirus genus), HCoV-NL63 (alphacoronavirus genus), HCoV-OC43 (betacoronavirus genus), and HCoV-HKU1 (betacoronavirus genus), cause mild upper respiratory tract disease in adults. However, SARS-CoV and Middle East respiratory syndrome coronavirus (MERS-CoV) caused pandemic in 2002–2003 and 2012, respectively (Zeng et al., 2018; Chakraborty et al., 2020). The SARS-CoV-2, a seventh member of the HCoV family, is an etiological agent of the COVID-19 pandemic as announced by WHO on March 11, 2020 (Cucinotta and Vanelli, 2020). Surprisingly, all pandemic-causing HCoVs, including SARS-CoV-2, belong to the betacoronavirus genus and are zoonotic in nature (Mackenzie and Smith, 2020; Piret and Boivin, 2021).

In light of the evolutionary linkages of SARS-CoV-2, its genomic structures coincide with other HCoVs in the range of 65.04% to 82.45% with SARS-CoV showing the highest similarity (Gorbalenya et al., 2020; Nakagawa and Miyazawa, 2020). SARS-CoV-2 is extremely infectious and transmissible due to its high propensity for attaching to angiotensin-converting enzyme-2 (ACE-2) receptors of the host cells, resulting in its quick spread from the epicenter in Wuhan, China, to more than 200 countries worldwide. It can be transmitted directly by contacting an infected person's respiratory droplets or indirectly by coming into contact with anything used or touched by an infected person (Kanamori et al., 2020). COVID-19 symptoms include anything from a simple respiratory infection to severe pneumonia, acute respiratory distress syndrome (ARDS), hypoxia, multiorgan failure, and death. Additionally, lymphopenia is also reported in a meta-analysis study of COVID-19 patients and is linked with a higher mortality, ARDS, severe clinical symptoms, and ICU admission. It is recorded that patients who died from COVID-19 had significantly lower lymphocyte counts than survivors (Ruan et al., 2020). Because of the similitudes with SARS-CoV, the international committee on taxonomy of viruses named the novel virus SARS-CoV-2 (Gorbalenya et al., 2020; Kumar et al., 2021). SARS-CoV-2 is a spherical or pleomorphic wrapped particle containing single-stranded positive-sense RNA associated with a nucleoprotein inside a capsid (Mousavizadeh and Ghasemi, 2021). The envelope provides a platform for club-framed glycoprotein projections. Some coronaviruses additionally contain a hemagglutinin-esterase protein (HE). The RNA genome of size around 30 kb encodes 16 nonstructural proteins (Nsp1 to Nsp16) and four structural proteins named spike (S), envelope (E), membrane (M), and nucleocapsid (N) (**Figures 1A, B**). Open reading frame (ORF)1ab (265-21555 bp) encodes polyproteins PP1ab (codes for Nsp1 to Nsp16) or shorter proteins (PP1a; codes for Nsp1 to Nsp11), depending on a 1 ribosomal frameshift event. The polyproteins are cleaved either by papain-like proteinase protein (PLpro) or main protease (Mpro) to yield 16 nonstructural proteins (Gioia et al., 2020). Out of the 16 nonstructural proteins, PLpro (Nsp3), 3C-like proteinase (Nsp5, Mpro), RNA-dependent RNA polymerase (Nsp12, RdRp), helicase (Nsp13), endoRNAse (Nsp15), 2'-O-Ribose-Methyltransferase (Nsp16), and other nonstructural proteins show similarity with other coronaviruses. However, the remaining 3' genome codes for S (~180 kDa glycoprotein), E (9-12 kDa protein), M (23-35 kDa protein), and RNA binding basic N protein (~45.6 kDa). Apart from structural proteins, the 3' end also encodes nine accessory proteins, Orf3a, Orf3b, Orf6, Orf7a, Orf7b, Orf8, Orf9b, Orf9c, and Orf10, and these proteins are involved in viral replication, assembly, and egress; they also have the potential to serve as antigens (Michel et al., 2020). The S protein trimerizes to provide the viral crown structure, making it a highly exposed protein of the virus. Thus, the trimeric S antigen is a major protective antigen that elicits highly potent neutralizing antibodies (Yang et al., 2020). The spike protein is 1273 amino acid glycoprotein mainly composed of two major subunits: S1 (aa 14-685) and S2 (aa 686-1273). At the N terminal of the S1 subunit, there is a signal peptide (SP; aa 1-13); the S1 subunit contains the N terminal domain (NTD, aa 14-305) and receptor binding domain (RBD; aa 319-541), and the RBD contains RBM (aa 437-508) and a C terminal domain (CTD) (**Figure 1**). The RBD of the S1 subunit binds to the ACE-2 receptor of the host cell. However, the S2 subunit responsible for fusion and entry have fusion peptides (FP; aa 788-806), heptapeptide repeat sequence-1 (HR-1; aa 912-984), HR-2 (aa 1163-1213), transmembrane domains (TM; aa 1213-1237), and cytoplasmic tail (CP; aa 1237-1273) domains (**Figure 1B**). Based on the important role of the spike protein in viral transmission, most of the vaccines, including adenovirus-, mRNA-, and DNA-based candidates, are generating neutralizing antibodies against the spike protein to block viral entry (**Figure 1C**) (De Haan et al., 1998). On the other hand, the inactivated virus provides all the antigens; hence, the immune responses developed in vaccinated individuals are not only against the spike but against numerous viral antigens as well. Other than the S protein, the N, M, nonstructural proteins (nsps) and accessory proteins may also have antigenic potential to serve as a candidate vaccine (Blanco-Melo et al., 2020). In fact, promising antigenic determinants (epitopes) in M, N, and S proteins, 4, 8, and 13 epitopes, respectively, have been identified using an extensive immuno-informatics analysis of SARS-CoV-2 proteins. Among these, M protein (165–181 and 306–322),

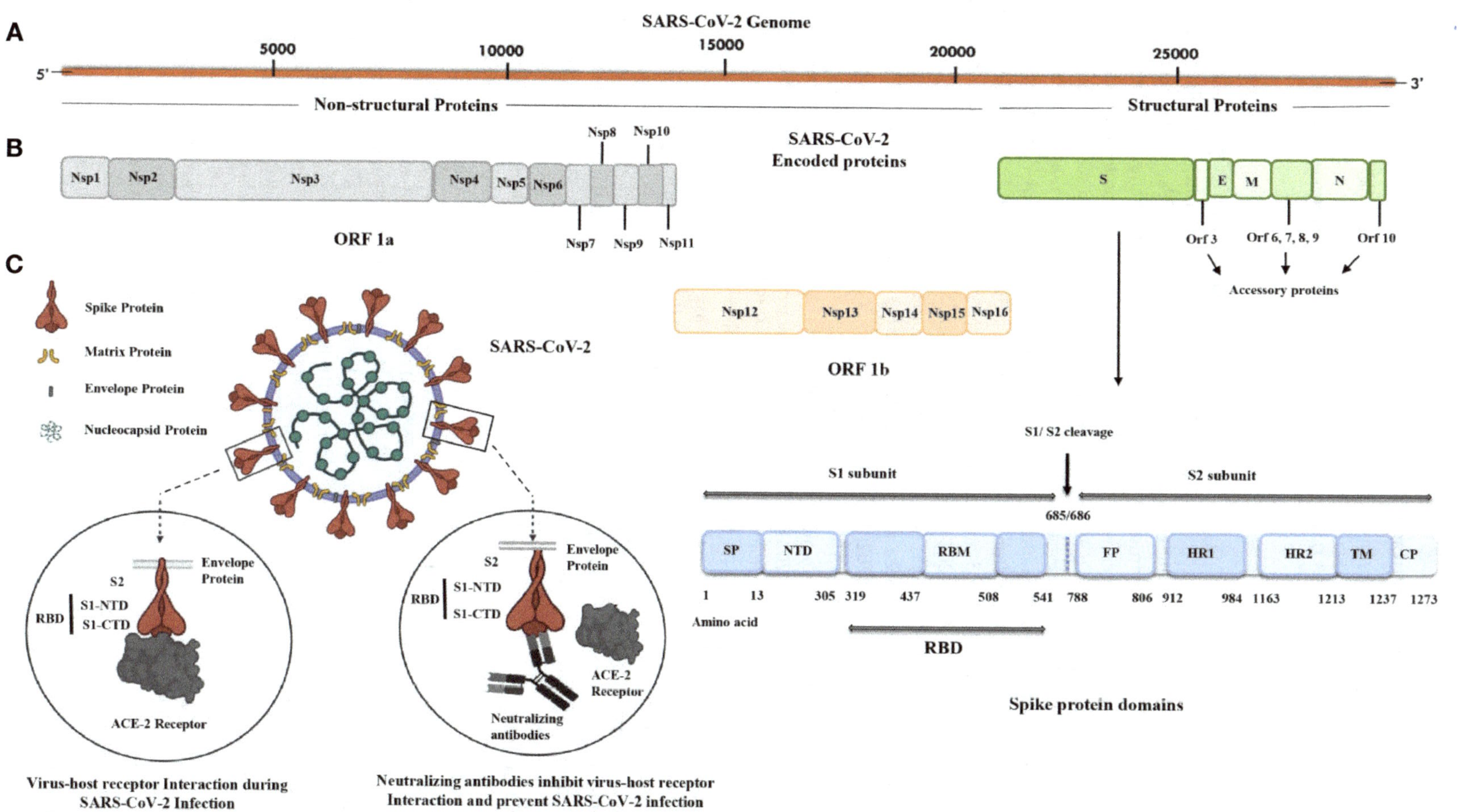

FIGURE 1 | SARS-CoV-2 genome, encoded proteins, and basic mechanism of virus fusion and entry. **(A)** Illustration of the SARS-CoV-2 genome that is around 30 kb in size and has a 5' cap and 3' poly A tail. **(B)** SARS-CoV-2 proteins: nonstructural proteins (Nsp), ORF1a, and ORF1b (Nsp1-Nsp16) and structural proteins such as spike (S), envelope (E), membrane (M), and nucleocapsid (N) with spike protein having 1273 aa (~180 kDa) containing signal peptide (SP), N-terminal domain (NTD), receptor binding motif (RBM) in receptor binding domain (RBD), fusion peptide (FP), heptad repeat (HR)-1, HR-2, transmembrane domain (TM), and cytoplasmic tail (CP) domains. There are accessory proteins Orf3; Orf6,7,8,9; and Orf10 located in between the S, E, M, and N proteins. **(C)** The spike protein subunit 1 (S1; aa 14-685) of SARS-CoV-2 consists of the RBD domain divided into two parts: S1 N-terminal domain (S1-NTD) and S1 C-terminal domain (S1-CTD) and spike protein subunit 2 (S2; aa 686-1273) containing TM and CP domains. S1-CTD interacts with the angiotensin-converting enzyme-2 (ACE-2) receptor of host cells and facilitates fusion and entry of virus. The neutralizing antibody against S1-CTD blocks the entry of the SARS-CoV-2 into host cells. ORF1a; Open reading frame 1a, ORF1b; Open reading frame 1b, aa; Amino acid.

TABLE 1 | Platform of COVID-19 Vaccine.

Platform	Type of candidate vaccine	Developer	Clinical phase trial
DNA	INO-4800+electroporation	Inovio Pharmaceuticals + International Vaccine Institute	NCT04642638 Phase II/III
	AG0301-COVID19	AnGes + Takara Bio + Osaka University	NCT04655625 Phase II/III
	nCov vaccine	Zydus Cadila	CTRI/2020/07/026352 Phase III
RNA	ARCT-021	Arcturus Therapeutics	NCT04668339 Phase II
	SARS-CoV-2 mRNA vaccine (ARCoV)	Academy of Military Science (AMS), Walvax Biotechnology and Suzhou Abogen Biosciences	NCT04847102 Phase III
	mRNA-1273.351. A lipid nanoparticle (LNP)-encapsulated mRNA-based vaccine that encodes for a full-length, prefusion stabilized S protein of the SARS-CoV-2 B.1.351 variant.	Moderna + National Institute of Allergy and Infectious Diseases (NIAID)	EUCTR2021-000930-32 Phase II
	CVnCoV Vaccine	CureVac AG	NCT04674189 Phase III
Protein Subunit	Recombinant SARS-CoV-2 vaccine (CHO Cell)	Anhui Zhifei Longcom Biopharmaceutical + Institute of Microbiology, Chinese Academy of Sciences	ChiCTR2000040153(Phase III
	VAT00002: SARS-CoV-2 S protein with adjuvant	Sanofi Pasteur + GSK	PACTR202011523101903 Phase III
	FINLAY-FR-2 anti-SARS-CoV-2 Vaccine (RBD chemically conjugated to tetanus toxoid plus adjuvant)	Instituto Finlay de Vacunas	RPCEC00000354 Phase III
	CIGB-66 (RBD+aluminum hydroxide)	Center for Genetic Engineering and Biotechnology (CIGB)	RPCEC00000359 Phase III
Non-Replicating Viral Vector	GRAd-COV2 (Replication defective Simian Adenovirus (GRAd) encoding S)	ReiThera + Leukocare + Univercells	NCT04791423 Phase II/III
Replicating Viral Vector	DelNS1-2019-nCoV-RBD-OPT1 (Intranasal flu-based-RBD)	University of Hong Kong, Xiamen University and Beijing Wantai Biological Pharmacy	Phase II ChiCTR2000039715
Inactivated	SARS-CoV-2 vaccine (vero cells)	Institute of Medical Biology + Chinese Academy of Medical Sciences	NCT04659239 Phase III
	QazCovid-in - COVID-19 inactivated vaccine	Research Institute for Biological Safety Problems, Rep of Kazakhstan	NCT04691908 Phase III
	Inactivated SARS-CoV-2 vaccine (Vero cell)	Beijing Minhai Biotechnology Co	NCT04852705 Phase III
	VLA2001	Valneva, National Institute for Health Research, United Kingdom	NCT04864561 Phase III
	COVID-19 inactivated vaccine	Shifa Pharmed Industrial Co	IRCT20201202049567N3 Phase II/III
VLP	Coronavirus-Like Particle COVID-19 (CoVLP)	Medicago Inc.	NCT04636697 Phase II/III

Platforms being used in development of vaccine against SARS CoV-2; these candidate vaccines are in either preclinical or various clinical phase trial stages and have not yet been licensed or launched by firms (WHO, 2021a).

N protein (314–330), and S protein (817–833, 891–907, 897–913, and 1182–1209) were found to be nonallergenic and nontoxic and have a low chance of producing autoimmune reactions in 87% of the world's population (Mukherjee et al., 2020). These antigens could be used for developing effective candidate vaccines against SARS-CoV-2.

In response to the outbreak, rapid diagnostics, speedy therapy, and vaccine research and development (R&D) are critical to curb the pandemic and prevent new viral outbreaks (Liu et al., 2020; Goel et al., 2021; Khan et al., 2021). Many attempts have been carried out on various platforms to develop a vaccine against SARS-CoV-2 (Callaway, 2020). Around 284 different candidate vaccines against COVID-19 are in development and are in the race to be introduced in the market after their successful phase III trials with prophylactic and safety data (WHO, 2021a). Due to the great impact on the lives of people and the economy from COVID-19, various vaccines got emergency approval after or before phase III trials (**Tables 1, 2**). Currently, various platforms, e.g., nucleic acid (RNA/DNA), attenuated live, protein subunit, viral vector, whole virus inactivated, and VLP-based vaccines are being used to develop a safe and prophylactic vaccine against SARS-CoV-2 (**Figures 2A–G**). The vaccines by Pfizer, Moderna, Oxford/AstraZeneca (Vaxzevria/Covishield), Bharat Biotech (Covaxin), Gamaleya (sputnik V), Sinopharm, and Sinovac are in the market (**Table 2**) (Bos et al., 2020; Logunov et al., 2020a;

TABLE 2 | List of marketed vaccines against SARS-CoV-2.

Developer	Vaccine Name	Vaccine Type	SARS-CoV-2 Antigen	Doses and Route	Storage	Efficacy	Status	References
Pfizer/ BioNtech	Comirnaty, tozinameran, BNT162b1 BNT162b2	mRNA encapsulated in lipid nanoparticle (LNP)	SARS-CoV-2 RBD and S protein full length in prefusion conformation for BNT162b1 and BNT162b2 respectively	Twice (3 weeks apart), I.M.	-70°C tc -80°C (6 months)	95%	Emergency use in U.S., E.U. etc., Approved in several countries	(Polack et al., 2020)
Moderna/ NIAID	mRNA-1273	mRNA encapsulated in lipid nanoparticle (LNP)	Full length S protein with prefusion conformation	Twice (4 weeks apart), I.M.	4°C (30 days), – 20°C (6 months)	94.5%	Approved in Switzerland. Emergency use in U.S., U.K., E.U., others	(Voysey et al., 2021)
Oxford University/ AstraZeneca	AZD1222/ ChAdOx1 nCoV-19 (Covishield in India)	Attenuated adenoviral vector (nonreplicating) from chimpanzee ChAd	full-length codon-optimized S protein	Twice (4 weeks apart), I.M.	2°C–8°C	70%	Emergency use in U.K., E.U., India and other countries	(Voysey et al., 2021)
Bharat Biotech/ICMR	Covaxin, BBV152 A, B, C	Whole virion Inactivated SARS-CoV-2 vaccine + adjuvant	Whole virus	Twice (2 weeks apart), I.M.	2°C–8°C	81%	Emergency use in India	(Bharat Biotech, 2021a)
Gamaleya	Sputnik V, Gam-Covid-Vac	two nonreplicating viral vectors, adenovirus type 5 (rAd5) and adenovirus type 26 (rAd26)	SARS-CoV-2 full-length glycoprotein S	Twice (3 weeks apart), I.M.	-20°C	92%	Early use in Russia. Emergency use in other countries including India	(BBC News, 2020b)
Beijing Institute of Biological Products/ Sinopharm	BBIBP-CorV	Inactivated SARS-CoV-2 vaccine (Vero cell)	Whole virus	Twice (3 weeks apart), I.M.	2°C–8°C	79%	Approved in China, U.A.E., Bahrain. Emergency use in Egypt, other countries	(BBC News, 2020a)
Sinovac	CoronaVac, PiCoVacc	Inactivated virus	Whole virus	Twice (2 weeks apart), I.M.	2°C–8°C	50%–91%	Approved in China. Emergency use in Brazil, Singapore, Malaysia, and Philippines	(BCB News, 2021)
CanSino/BIB	Convidecia, Ad5-nCoV	Adenovirus based viral vector (Ad5)-Nonreplicating	SARS-CoV-2 full length S protein	Single, I.M.	2°C–8°C	79%	Emergency use in China and Mexico	(BBC News, 2020a)
Johnson & Johnson	Ad26.COV2. S	Adenovirus based viral vector (Ad26)-Nonreplicating	SARS-CoV-2 full length S protein	Single, I.M.	-20°C (2 years), 2° C–8°C (3 months)	76.7%–85.4%	Applied for emergency use authorization in U.S.	(US FDA, 2021)
Novavax	NVX-CoV2373	S Protein adjuvanted with recombinant novavax protein	Trimeric SARS-CoV-2 full length S protein	Twice (3 weeks apart), I.M.	2°C–8°C (3 months), -20°C (2 years)	89.3% (P-3, UK), 90% (South Africa Trial)	Early use in UK and Australia	(Press release, 2021)
Vector Institute	EpiVacCorona	Chemically synthesized peptide antigens of SARS-CoV-2 proteins	Peptide Subunit Vaccine	Twice (3 weeks apart), I.M.	2°C–8°C (2 years)	100%	Early use in Russia	(Belta News, 2021)
WIBP/ Sinopharm	WIBP-CorV	Inactivated virus propagated in Vero cells	Whole virus	Twice (3 weeks apart), I.M.	2°C–8°C	72.5%	Bahrain, Jordan, Egypt, UAE	(Reuters-Staff, 2021)

Vaccines developed by several companies and institutions on multiple platforms have been introduced in most countries. Vaccine efficacy is influenced by a variety of factors, including vaccine type, proper packaging, number of dosages, and booster requirements after a certain time interval as well as the route of administration. Vaccines with the potential to boost ongoing pandemic response have been introduced in many countries, on either an approved or emergency basis (Chakraborty et al., 2021; WHO, 2021b; Yan et al., 2021).
ICMR., Indian Council of Medical Research; WIBP., Wuhan Institute of Biological Products; BIB., Beijing Institute of Biotechnology; NIAID., National Institute of Allergy and Infectious Diseases; U.S., United State, EU., European Union; U.A.E., United Arab Emirates; U.K., United Kingdom; I.M., Intramuscular, P-3 (Phase-III trial).

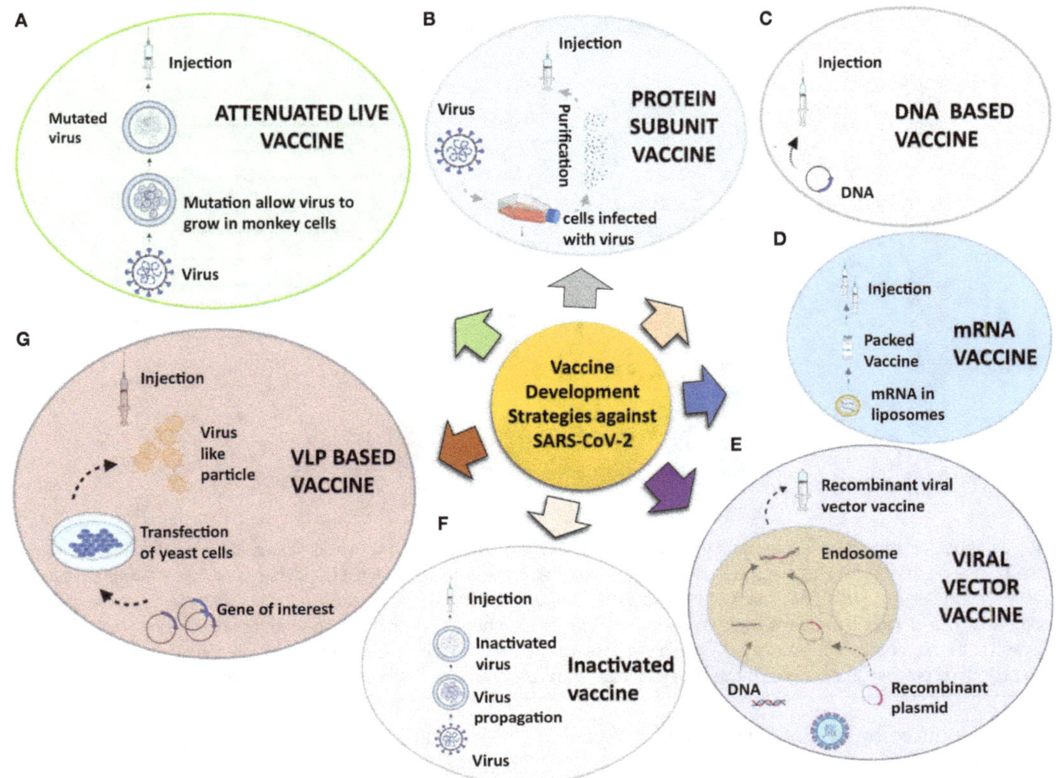

FIGURE 2 | Strategies being utilized to develop vaccine candidates against SARS-CoV-2: A concise overview of various aspects of the SARS-CoV-2 vaccine development process varying from traditional to novel platforms. **(A)** Attenuated live pathogen vaccine: A debilitated (infection incompetent) form of the live pathogen obtained by lengthy cell culture passaging in nonhuman cell lines or animals are administered. **(B)** Protein subunit vaccines are prepared from either antigen purification of pathogens replicated in cell cultures or recombinant expressed antigens. **(C, D)** Nucleic acid vaccines: mRNA **(C)** or DNA **(D)** codifying for an immunogenic protein of the pathogen express and present the antigen in antigen-presenting cells. The mRNA is mixed with nanoparticles or other stabilizing agents, and DNA is inserted in a vector. **(E)** Viral vector vaccines: Recombinant viral vectors are produced by genetic manipulation of measles or the adenoviral platform to express the antigen of interest. **(F)** Inactivated pathogen vaccines contain the whole pathogen that has been subjected to heat or chemical treatment for inactivation. **(G)** Virus-like particles vaccines: These are virus-like particles (20–200 nm) assembled and released by many baculoviruses or the mammalian expression system, e.g., recombinant yeast cells, vaccinia virus expression system, or even tobacco plants transfected with tobacco mosaic virus platform.

Logunov et al., 2020b; Baden et al., 2021; Pfizer-Biontech, 2021; Voysey et al., 2021). However, detailed phase III clinical trial-based vaccine efficacy and safety data remain elusive for some approved vaccines and many candidates that are now under clinical trials (**Figure 3** and **Table 2**).

To instigate the immune response, the protein antigens are achieved either by direct injecting protein subunit vaccines or by expression of genetic material delivered through viral or nonviral vectors into muscle cells (**Figures 4A, B**). Apart from antigens, the vaccine preparations also contain low toxic preservatives, such as 2-phenoxyethanol, to prevent vaccine contamination. The stabilizers, e.g., sugars (lactose, sucrose), amino acids (glycine), gelatin, or proteins, are used to prevent chemical reactions to achieve vaccine stability. Surfactants prevent clumping to keep the vaccine components homogeneous, and diluents (mostly distilled water) are used to achieve desired antigen concentration. Aluminum salts, such as aluminum phosphate, aluminum hydroxide, or potassium aluminum sulfate could be used as an adjuvant to enhance immune response. Vaccines may also contain traces of compounds used during vaccine manufacturing (https://www.who.int/news-room/feature-stories/detail/how-are-vaccines-developed).

Antigens in the circulatory system are recognized by antibodies on B cells, leading to isotype switching and antibody secreting plasma cell formation in germinal centers of secondary lymphoid organs. Some of the antibodies are capable of neutralizing the virus (neutralizing antibodies), which is crucial for clinical outcome (**Figures 4C, D**). Eventually, memory B cells are generated to withstand the onslaught of future infections (**Figure 4E**). The T cells, on the other hand, recognize antigens presented on (major histocompatibility complex) MHC-I or MHC-II of antigen-presenting cells (APCs) to activate $CD8^{+}T$ or $CD4^{+}T$ cells, respectively (**Figure 4F**). The activated helper T (effector $CD4^{+}T$) cells secrete Th1 or Th2 cytokines for cell-mediated or humoral immune response against the pathogen (**Figures 4G, H**). However, the activated $CD8^{+}T$ cells develop into cytotoxic T cells responsible for the killing of infected cells (**Figures 4J, K**). Both $CD4^{+}$ and $CD8^{+}$ T cells develop a central memory response (**Figures 4I, L**). Most immunizations require booster doses to strengthen the

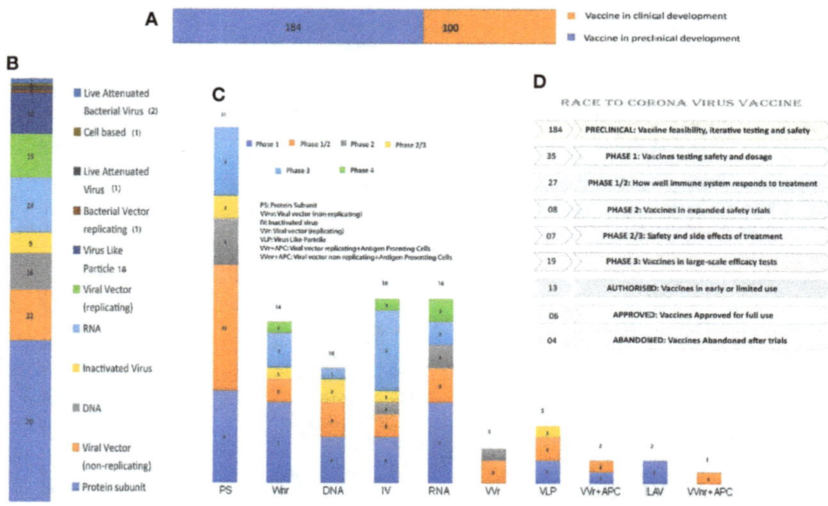

FIGURE 3 | Summary and number distribution of candidate vaccines in preclinical and clinical trials: **(A)** Clinical stages of candidate vaccines: Number of vaccines under clinical (depicted by orange color; 100) and preclinical development (depicted by blue color; 184). **(B)** Candidate vaccines of different platforms under clinical trial from bottom to top: Protein Subunit, VVnr, DNA, Inactivated Virus, RNA, VVr, VLP, BVr, LAV, Cell based and LABv with their respective candidate vaccine numbers. **(C)** Candidate vaccines of various platforms and their numbers under clinical phase 1, 2, or III: Phase-wise distribution along with the numbers in the platform used are marked in the bar graph. **(D)** Summary of various vaccines' clinical trial status is presented in the graph: Vaccine production from inception to commercialization is a prolonged process that requires multiple clinical trials, some of which have failed due to adverse effects.

immunological response induced by vaccines (**Figure 5**). A recent study suggests that S, M, and N proteins were strongly and nsp3, nsp4, and ORF8 were partially able to activate $CD4^+$ T cells. On the other hand, the SARS-CoV-2 M and S proteins were strongly recognized by $CD8^+$ T cells, and other antigens, such as nsp6, ORF3a, and the N protein, also showed significant reactivity (Grifoni et al., 2020).

The Wuhan strain of SARS-CoV-2 has undergone various mutations, resulting in B.1.1.7/alpha (United Kingdom), B.1.351/beta (South Africa), P.1/gamma (Brazil), B.1.617/delta (India), B.1.429 and B.1.427/epsilon (United States/California), B.1.525/eta (United Kingdom, Nigeria), P3/theta (Philippines), B.1.526/Iota (United States/New York), B.1.617.1/kappa (India) and C.37/lambda (Peru) lineages (https://www.gisaid.org/hcov19-variants/). The complexity in the immune response elicited during COVID-19 infection and the probability of genomic changes render a huge challenge for the scientific fraternity regarding vaccines in the market and those under development. Cutting-edge strategy needs to be adapted to achieve a prophylactic vaccine against this dreadful virus. To achieve the aim of limiting the pandemic, we address the various vaccine types, their components, immune responses against various strains, hurdles, and future challenges.

2. STRATEGIES UTILIZED IN COVID-19 VACCINE DEVELOPMENT

There are various strategies being utilized worldwide for vaccine development. An example of some of the forms of SARS-CoV-2 vaccine candidates and concepts are presented in **Figure 2**. Apart from emergency authorized vaccines for COVID-19, there are 100 candidate vaccines in the clinical evaluation phase, and 184 vaccines are in the preclinical evaluation stage (WHO, 2021a). These vaccines are being developed in various countries around the globe, including the United States, Germany, Austria, the United Kingdom, China, Australia, France, India, and Hong Kong (WHO, 2020). Development of efficacious and safe vaccines is urgently needed to curb the current pandemic. Vaccine developers must guarantee that people of all age groups, including with comorbidities, such as asthma and diabetes, can receive the COVID-19 vaccine as these categories of patients are at particularly high risk. It is, therefore, important to determine the level of safety provided by the vaccines, and patients may require more than one dose of the vaccine to preserve continued immunity to the virus. The production of a vaccine against SARS-CoV-2 is a challenging task due to many problems faced during the design phase. A variety of methods, including next-generation and traditional approaches, are being used to develop the vaccines, each one with different advantages and disadvantages (**Table 2**). The basic mechanism and details of immunological responses induced by different vaccines are shown in detail in **Figure 4**. Also, the predicted antibody response to first, second, and probable booster doses of the COVID-19 vaccination are represented in **Figure 5**. Live attenuated coronavirus vaccines provide the best protection, but their clearance is hampered by biosafety concerns. In contrast, inactivated coronavirus vaccines perform well in primate models and up to preclinical levels (Lundstrom, 2020). Because the immune systems of elderly people vary from those of healthy middle-aged adults, they sometimes do not respond equally well to immunization. Overall, there is no such thing as "one size fits all." In general, we hope that adjuvants can aid

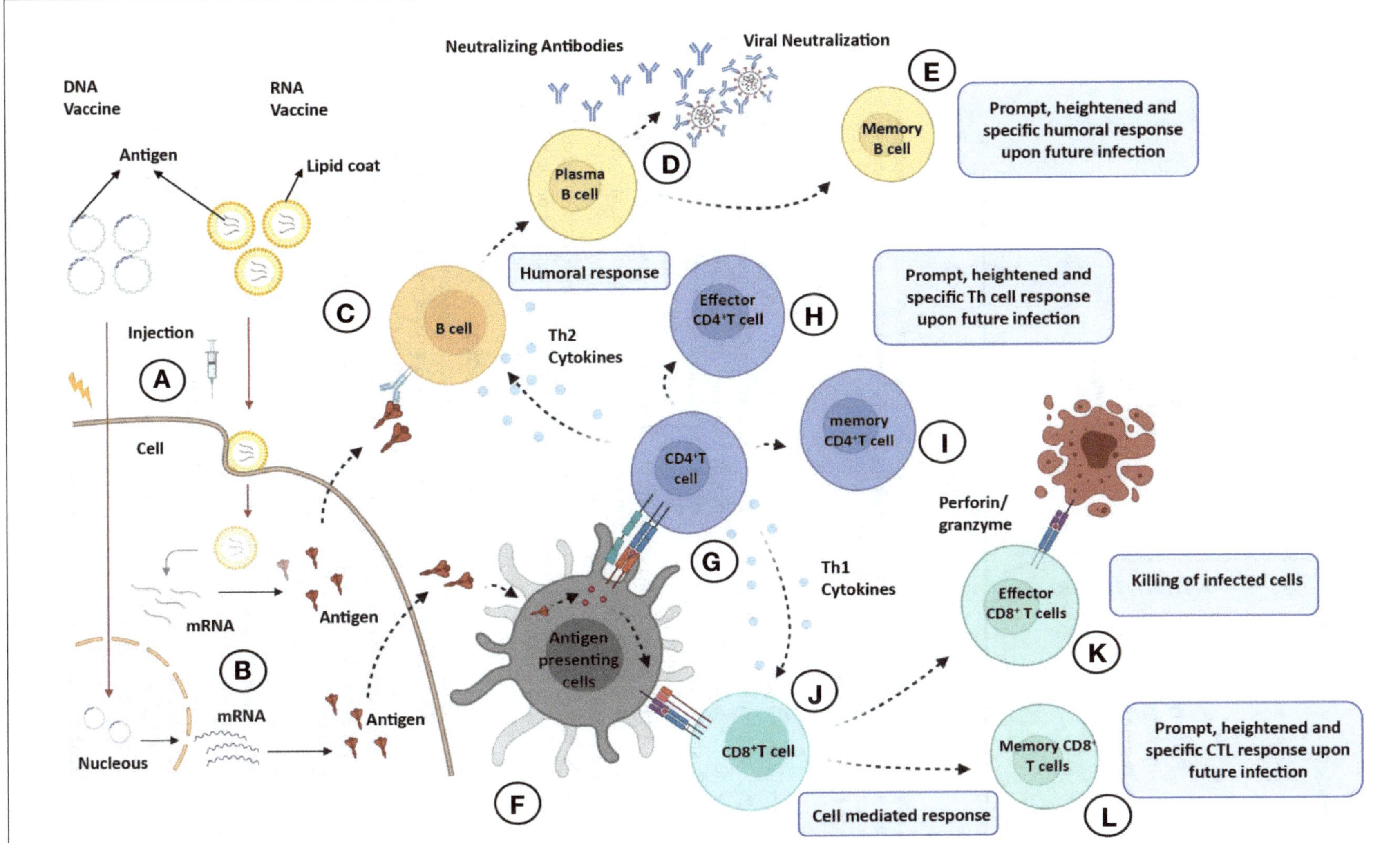

FIGURE 4 | Overview of immune response elicited by various vaccine candidates. When administered into skin or muscle cells **(A)**, the nucleic acid expresses and codes for an immunogenic protein that mimics viral infection **(B)**. **(C–E)** Humoral responses: Antigens produced by skin/muscle cells are released in blood to activate the antibody response; antigen recognition by naïve B cells **(C)** leading to clonal selection and plasma cell (antibody secreting B cells) formation **(D)** and eventually production of long-lasting memory B cells **(E)**. **(F)** Antigen processing and presentation: The antigen produced by skin/muscle cells are captured by antigen-presenting cells (APCs; dendritic cells or macrophages) for processing and presented by MHC-II or MHC-I molecules on their surface. **(G–I)** $CD4^{+}T$ helper cells effector and memory response: The presented MHC-II molecule and antigen complex on APCs recognized by TCR and CD4 molecules on $CD4^{+}$ Th cells **(G)** leading to production of effector $CD4^{+}$ Th cells **(H)**, which produce sufficient levels of cytokines (Th2 cells produce TH2 cytokines IL-4 or IL-10 for humoral response and Th1 cells produce IL-12, IFN-Y for CTL response), and eventually, long-lasting memory $CD4^{+}$ cells are generated **(I)**. **(J–L)** $CD8^{+}T$ helper cells effector and memory response: The presented antigen and MHC-II molecule complex on APCs recognized by TCR and CD8 molecules on $CD8^{+}$ T cells **(J)** leading to production of effector $CD8^{+}T$ cells also known as cytotoxic T lymphocytes (CTL), which are responsible for killing the infected or self-altered cells **(K)**, and finally, long-lasting memory $CD8^{+}T$ cells are generated **(L)**. All memory cells provide long-lasting, heightened, and antigen-specific responses upon future infections.

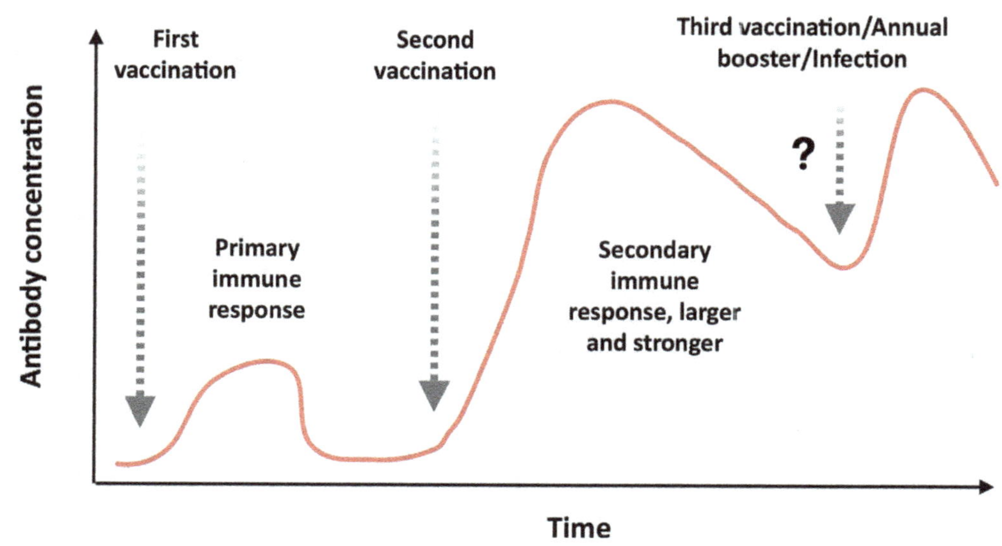

FIGURE 5 | Antibody response to first, second, and probable third/annual booster dose of COVID-19 vaccination or infection: Initially, just after the first immunization, the vaccine does not elicit sufficient neutralizing antibody to prevent the infection of SARS-CoV-2. Upon administration of the second booster dose of vaccine, the vaccine elicits a stronger neutralizing antibody response with high titer that could prevent the infection efficiently. In some cases, third or annual boosters are required to revive the immune response against the pathogen.

ongoing vaccination campaigns across the world. Adjuvants are important for eliciting a stronger, long-lasting, and broader immune response, especially in people with compromised immune systems. **Figures 3A–C** shows the number of coronavirus vaccines in the preclinical and clinical stages based on the various platforms accessible and in a phase-by-phase approach. **Figure 3D** summarizes the coronavirus vaccine and the time it takes from development and preclinical testing, need to pass through phase 1, 2, and 3 trials. Few vaccines have been dropped because of their inability to induce a robust immune response, owing to negative side effects.

2.1. Inactivated Vaccine

Various vaccines for viral and bacterial diseases, including pertussis, rabies, hepatitis A, influenza, polio, and Japanese encephalitis, are based on an inactivated form of the vaccines. Usually, they do not provide protection as strong as live vaccines and require booster shots. Sixteen inactivated vaccines of SARS-CoV-2 are in advanced clinical trials. Bharat Biotech Covaxin (BBV152) is an inactivated COVID-19 vaccine being used in India. These vaccines require a BSL-3 facility for large-scale virus propagation, rendering this platform the most time-consuming and difficult. However, the benefit of using this platform is a multiple antigen-based vaccine that remains helpful in any viral mutation on a single protein. These inactivated vaccines lead to a strong neutralizing antibody response and give a more potent $CD4^+$ T_h1 cell response as compared with $CD8^+$ T cells.

2.2. Live Attenuated Vaccine

Live vaccines are made from attenuated or weakened forms of the pathogen to stimulate a strong and long-lasting neutralizing antibody response along with both $CD4^+$ T helper and $CD8^+$ T cell mediated immunity by mimicking natural infection. However, extensive safety studies are required, and it could not be given to immunocompromised individuals. Currently, live attenuated vaccines are being used for rotavirus; chickenpox; yellow fever; and measles, mumps, and rubella. There are several benefits of a live-attenuated vaccine, including mounting an immune response to multiple virus antigens and the capacity to scale for mass production. The COVI-VAC, currently in clinical phase I trial, is a single-dose, intranasal, live-attenuated vaccine generated using Codagenix's proprietary deoptimization technology in collaboration with the Serum Institute of India.

2.3. Viral Vector

Viral vector vaccines make use of a modified version of the pathogenic virus as a vector to provide immunity. Scientists all over the world are attempting to produce a COVID-19 vaccine dependent on replicating viral vectors, such as damaged measles, while others are focusing on nonreplicating viral vectors, such as adenovirus.

2.3.1. Replicating

Three candidates from the replicating viral vector platform and two based on replicating viral vectors along with artificial APCs have reached the clinical phase. When cells are infected with the replicating viral vector vaccine, it not only produces a vaccine antigen, but it also produces more viral particles that can infect another cell. DelNS1-2019-nCoV-RBD-OPT1 is an intranasal spray vaccine based on the H1N1 influenza A virus. The dose is given twice, 28 days apart. It is currently being evaluated in a phase II clinical trial. A vaccine candidate developed by the Israel Institute for Biomedical Research makes use of recombinant vesicular stomatitis virus, in which the VSV-G protein is replaced with the SARS-CoV-2

S protein, creating a recombinant replicating virus. The candidate has reached phase I/II clinical trials for safety and efficacy evaluation.

2.3.2. Nonreplicating

Nonreplicating viral vaccines are not able to produce new viral particles and are only involved in production of the vaccine antigen. Fifteen nonreplicating viral vector vaccines and one with an artificial APC is being evaluated in human clinical trials. CanSino Biologics and the Beijing Biotechnology Institute developed the novel coronavirus vaccine (adenovirus type 5 vector) candidate (Ad5-nCoV), and it has now been authorized and made accessible as a marketed vaccine. The vaccine candidate is based on the adenovirus-based viral vector vaccine technology framework of CanSinoBIO, which was previously used to successfully produce the globally groundbreaking Ebola virus infection vaccine (Zhao et al., 2020b). The neutralizing antibody response mediated by such vaccine platforms is determined by preexisting anti-vector immunity with enhanced $CD4^+$ Th1 cell response and potent $CD8^+$ T cell response.

2.4. DNA-Based Vaccine

The DNA-based vaccine, also known as the third-generation vaccine, contains DNA encoding specific proteins or antigens of the pathogen. Ten DNA vaccine candidates are in human clinical trials, and 16 are in preclinical trials. The proteins encoded by the DNA are translated into host cells, which are identified as a foreign material by the host immune system, thus inducing an immune response. INOVIA Pharmaceuticals, a biotechnology company, is currently focused on developing a DNA vaccine, which is in phase 2/3 clinical testing in the United States for COVID-19. Using INOVIO's patented DNA medicine platform, INO-4800 was developed quickly after the genetic sequence of the coronavirus causing COVID-19 was released. A DNA-based vaccine that can be administered by a nasal spray is being produced by researchers at the University of Waterloo, Ontario, Canada. The vaccine operates using engineered bacteriophage, a process that enables the vaccine to activate the immune response in the lower respiratory tract of the nasal cavity and target tissues (WaterlooNews, 2020). DNA-based vaccines provide a sufficient neutralizing antibody response along with the $CD4^+$ Th1 cell response. However, the $CD8^+$ T cell response is less robust (Prompetchara et al., 2021).

2.5. RNA-Based Formulation

New technology is based on RNA, by which an mRNA-encoding pathogen's proteins or antigens are used to elicit an immune response. Sixteen vaccine candidates based on mRNA formulation are being tested in the clinical phase. The mRNA-1273 is a novel lipid nanoparticle (LNP)-encapsulated mRNA-based vaccine that encodes for a full-length, prefusion stabilized spike (S) protein of SARS-CoV-2. Candidates for the vaccine include nucleoside modified mRNA (modRNA), mRNA-containing uridine (uRNA), and self-amplified mRNA (saRNA). An LNP formulation is combined with any mRNA format. These vaccine candidates for COVID-19 contain either the larger spike sequence or the smaller optimized RBD of the spike protein. The vaccines based on mRNA give an adequate neutralizing antibody response although the Th1 and Th2 cell response depends on the adjuvant used.

2.6. Protein Subunit Vaccine

A protein subunit vaccine uses protein fragments of the pathogen to elicit an immune response instead of introducing the whole pathogen. Currently, it is being used for hepatitis B, human papilloma virus (HPV), whooping cough, pneumococcal disease, meningococcal disease, and shingles. These vaccines provide a strong immune response against a particular antigen of the pathogen and are safe for all recipients, including individuals with a weakened immune system. Thirty-one such candidates are being assessed in human clinical trials before being available to the general population. Although some researchers want to inject coronavirus proteins directly into the bloodstream, it is also conceivable to employ protein fragments or protein shells that look like the coronavirus's outer coat. Scientists and researchers are developing vaccines for viral protein subunits, the majority of which focus on the virus's spike protein or a central portion known as the RBD. ExpreS2ion, a biotech company, uses its clinically validated Drosophila S2 insect cell expression system, ExpreS2, to produce SARS-CoV-2 viral antigens in the clinically validated cell lines. The goal is to generate and test vaccine antigens in mice to demonstrate immunogenicity and efficacy *in vitro*. The vaccine is in preclinical trials now. Protein subunit vaccines are well recognized for eliciting a strong neutralizing antibody response; however, the Th1 and Th2 cell response is influenced by the adjuvant employed.

2.7. Virus-Like Particle Vaccine

Virus-like particles (VLPs) are protein-based vaccines that stimulate high immune responses due to VLPs' repetitive structures. These molecules mimic viruses but do not contain any viral genetic material and are not infectious. They are a very effective way of creating vaccines against diseases such as HPV, hepatitis B, malaria, and many more. There are five VLP-based vaccine candidates currently being evaluated in human clinical trials against SARS-CoV-2. The RBD SARS-CoV-2 HBsAg VLP vaccine is a subunit vaccine that uses RBD in a SARS-CoV-2 S protein conjugated with the hepatitis B surface antigen to stimulate the immune system to produce the anti-RBD antibody. The Central Committee on Research Involving Human Subjects in the Netherlands has approved an ABNCoV2 capsid virus-like particle–based COVID-19 vaccine developed by AdaptVac, a PREVENT-nCoV consortium member. The candidate vaccine is in phase I/II of study.

3. APPROVED COVID-19 VACCINES

Several COVID-19 vaccines have shown greater than 90% efficacy in preventing COVID-19 infections. A handful of vaccinations are presently authorized by both the national regulatory body and WHO. Some vaccines are in the process of being approved by WHO (WHO, 2021c).

3.1. Pfizer-BioNTech (BNT162b1 and BNT162b2)

The first time mRNA has been used as a vaccine platform was initially established by the Weissman group to develop a zika virus vaccine (Pardi et al., 2017). Pfizer-BioNTech developed BNT162b1 and BNT162b2 vaccines against SARS-CoV-2. BNT162b1 is a SARS-CoV-2 spike protein RBD encoding modified messenger RNA (mRNA) incorporating 1-methyl-pseudourine, which dampens innate immune sensing to induce mRNA translation. The RBD antigen is modified by the addition of a T4 fibritin-derived "foldon" trimerization domain to increase its immunogenicity by multivalent display (Mulligan et al., 2020). The other candidate, BNT162b2, encodes the full-length SARS-CoV-2 spike protein with two proline changes that lock it in the prefusion conformation and make it more closely mimic the intact virus to elicit prominent virus-neutralizing antibodies. Apart from mRNA (30 μg), the Pfizer-BioNTech vaccine includes lipids and cholesterol, potassium chloride, monobasic potassium phosphate, sodium chloride, dibasic sodium phosphate dihydrate, and sucrose. Storage is -70°C to -80°C; later, as an alternative, -25°C to -15°C was advised for 2 weeks (Polack et al., 2020). The European Medicines Agency (EMA) as a National Regulatory Authority (NRA) approved it, and later it was approved by WHO after evaluating the data on clinical trials (www.pfizer.com).

3.2. Moderna (mRNA1273)

The Moderna COVID-19 (mRNA1273) vaccine is a sterile, preservative-free, frozen suspension for intramuscular injection comprising the following ingredients: mRNA, lipids (SM-102, 1,2-dimyristoyl-rac-glycero tromethamine, tromethamine hydrochloride, acetic acid, sodium acetate, and sucrose), PEG2000-DMG, cholesterol, and 1,2-distearoyl-snglycero-3-phosphocholine [DSPC] (Moderna, 2021) (www.modernatx.com). The Moderna vaccine currently is licensed by EMA as well as WHO based on experimental evidence. It is a SARS-CoV-2 glycoprotein S-2P with a transmembrane anchor and an intact S1-S2 cleavage site, antigen-encoding, mRNA-based vaccine. The S2-P is stabilized in its prefusion conformation by 986 and 987 position proline substitutions at the top of the central helix in the S2 subunit. The lipid nanoparticle capsule, composed of four lipids, was formulated in a fixed ratio of mRNA and lipid. The dose is given intramuscularly in two doses 4 weeks apart. It can be stored in refrigerators for 30 days and at -20°C for 6 months. Primary efficacy analysis of the phase-III COVE study of mRNA-1273 involved 30,000 participants, including 196 cases of COVID-19, of which 30 cases were severe. Vaccine efficacy against COVID-19 was 94.1%, and vaccine efficacy against severe COVID-19 was 100%. mRNA-1273 continues to be generally well tolerated with no serious safety concerns identified to date (Baden et al., 2020).

3.3. Covaxin

Bharat Biotech's Covaxin gained certification from the Drugs Controller General of India as an NRA, and it is currently under consideration by WHO for possible approval. This vaccine is developed by Bharat Biotech, India, using a coronavirus sample isolated from an asymptomatic patient (strain: NIV-2020-770) by the National Institute of Virology, India (Bharat Biotech, 2021a). It falls under the inactivated whole virion vaccine category that uses adjuvant Alhydroxiquim-II to boost immune response for long-lasting immunity. It contains 6 μg of whole-virion inactivated SARS-CoV-2 antigen and 250 μg aluminum hydroxide gel, 15 μg TLR 7/8 agonist (imidazoquinolinone), 2.5 mg TM 2-phenoxyethanol, and phosphate buffered saline up to 0.5 ml (https://www.bharatbiotech.com). The phase I and II clinical trials were conducted on 800 subjects, and the results demonstrated that the vaccine is safe and induced a robust immune response. The phase III study enrolled 25,800 participants between 18 and 98 years of age, including 10% over the age of 60, with analysis conducted 14 days post second dose. According to phase III analysis of Covaxin on 127 symptomatic cases, the vaccine showed a point estimate of 81% vaccine efficacy against mild and moderate COVID-19 disease. The efficacy against severe COVID-19 disease was 100% with an impact on reduction in hospitalizations. The efficacy against asymptomatic COVID-19 infection was 70%, suggesting decreased transmission in Covaxin recipients (Bharat Biotech, 2021b).

3.4. Oxford-AstraZeneca (AZD1222)

The chimpanzee adenovirus vectored vaccine containing the gene for expressing spike protein ChAdOx1-nCoV-19 (AZD1222) is developed by Oxford-AstraZeneca and manufactured by the Serum Institute of India. The vaccine is administered in two separate doses of 0.5 ml each given between 4 and 12 weeks apart and can be stored at temperatures 2°C to 8°C. In India, this vaccine is named Covishield, and it includes L-histidine, L-histidine hydrochloride monohydrate, polysorbate 80, ethanol, sucrose, sodium chloride, disodium edetate dihydride (EDTA), and water for infection. Initially the booster dose was given 4 weeks postimmunization; however, due to a shortage of the vaccine, published date sets allowed the booster dose to be administered 6 to 8 weeks apart. Further studies are required to adapt the best immunization policy for this vaccine. (www.astrazeneca.com). Analysis data from four ongoing blinded, randomized, controlled trials done across the United Kingdom, Brazil, and South Africa showed an overall efficacy of 70.4%; 11,636 participants (7548 in the United Kingdom, 4088 in Brazil) were included in the interim primary efficacy analysis. Participants aged 18 years and older were randomly assigned (1:1) to the ChAdOx1 nCoV-19 vaccine or the control (Voysey et al., 2021).

3.5. Sputnik V by Gamaleya (Gam-Covid-Vac)

Also known as Gam-Covid-Vac, this vaccine was developed by the Gamaleya Research Institute, part of Russia's Ministry of Health. It is an adenoviral-based vaccine (dual viral vector) that uses a weakened virus, which, in turn, delivers small parts of the pathogen, ultimately stimulating an immune response. The gene encoding S-protein of SARS-CoV-2 is carried *via* an rAd26 vector (first dose) that provides humoral and cellular immunity, and the rAd5 vector (second dose) induces formation of memory cells. The active components are a modified replication-defective adenovirus of a different serotype modified to include the protein S-expressing gene of SARS-CoV-2. The ingredients include tris-(hydroxymethyl)-aminomethane, sodium chloride, sucrose, magnesium chloride hexahydrate, disodium EDTA dihydrate, polysorbate 80, ethanol, and water. The interim report of the phase III data include results for more than 20,000 participants aged 18 years and older, 75% of whom were assigned to receive the vaccine, and the follow up for adverse events and infection. No serious adverse events considered related to the vaccine were recorded, and vaccine efficacy, based on the numbers of confirmed COVID-19 cases from 21 days after the first dose of the vaccine, was reported as 92% (Logunov et al., 2021) (https://sputnikvaccine.com).

3.6. Sinovac (CoronaVac)

The CoronaVac vaccine was developed by Sinovac using inactive SARS-CoV-2 virus (CZ02 strain) along with aluminum hydroxide, disodium hydrogen phosphate dodecahydrate, disodium hydrogen phosphate monohydrate, and sodium chloride as adjuvant and stabilizing agents. Two doses of the vaccine about 14 to 28 days apart are administered. One main advantage associated with the vaccine developed by Sinovac is that it can be stored at 2°C–8°C. China has approved the Sinovac vaccine for emergency use since July 2020 through the National Medical Products Administration (NMPA), and later, it got approval by WHO. Other countries, such as Indonesia, Turkey, Brazil, and Chile, have also authorized emergency use of this vaccine (http://www.sinovac.com). The phase III trials conducted in Brazil and Turkey evaluated the efficacy of the vaccine candidate in healthcare workers who provide treatment to COVID-19 patients. Both trial studies were randomized, double-blind, and placebo controlled. There were 12,396 health workers over 18 years old enrolled. A total of 253 positive cases were collected during the observation period. After 14 days following vaccination with two doses of the vaccine following a 0-, 14-day schedule, the efficacy rate against diseases caused by COVID-19 was 50.65% for all cases; 83.70% for cases requiring medical treatment; and 100.00% for hospitalized, severe, and fatal cases (Palacios et al., 2020).

3.7. Sinopharm (BBIBP-CorV)

China has approved the Sinopharm multivariant vaccine (Sinopharm's BBIBP-CorV), which is a WHO approved inactivated virus vaccine. Of the three coronavirus variants obtained from patients in China, the variant that multiplied the most quickly in monkey kidney cells was chosen and was inactivated using chemical beta-propiolactone. It was then treated with an aluminum-based adjuvant to increase its immunogenicity. Unlike the Moderna and Pfizer vaccines, this vaccine is easy to transport and can be stored at 2°C–8°C (BBC News, 2020a). Being multivariant, the immune response induced by the BBIBP-CorV vaccine could not be impacted by a mutation in the virus (http://www.sinopharm.com). According to a China National Biotec Group Company study, more than 40,000 people in the United Arab Emirates and Bahrain aged 18 and above without a known history of COVID-19 participated in the trials. The vaccine showed an efficacy rate of 79% against symptomatic COVID-19 cases with rare serious adverse effects reported (Al Kaabi et al., 2021).

3.8. CanSino (Convidecia)

The CanSino vaccine from China is approved by the NMPA, China, and is in the process of getting approval from WHO. The vaccine developed by CanSino, Ad5-nCoV, is a nonreplicating human adenoviral (Ad5)-based vaccine that expresses a full-length spike glycoprotein of coronavirus. It was originally tested in mice and ferrets and was the first vaccine to enter human trials in March 2020. The phase III trial NCT04540419 with 500 participants determined a single intramuscular shot of 5×10^{10} virus particles proved to be well tolerable and immunogenic (Logunov et al., 2020a). Mexico became the first country to give emergency use approval to this vaccine developed by CanSino Biologics and People's Liberation Army scientists (http://www.cansinotech.com). CanSino Biologics conducted its phase III trials in Argentina, Chile, Mexico, Pakistan, Russia, and Saudi Arabia with 40,000 participants. The company announced that the interim analysis data of the phase III clinical trial of Convidecia shows that the vaccine candidate has an overall efficacy of 65.28% at preventing all symptomatic COVID-19 disease 28 days after single-dose vaccination and an efficacy of 90.07% at preventing severe disease 28 days after single-dose vaccination (https://www.precisionvaccinations.com/vaccines/convidicea-vaccine).

3.9. Janssen (Janssen COVID-19 Vaccine)

Janssen got licensed from EMA and approved by WHO. The vaccine developed by the Janssen and Prevention BV subsidiary of Johnson and Johnson, the Ad26.CoV.S, is based on human adenovirus Ad26 and expresses the full-length spike protein (Bos et al., 2020). The vaccine contains genetically modified organisms and ethanol derived from corn or vegetables (https://www.janssenmd.com). The vaccine can remain stable for two years at -20°C and a maximum of 3 months at temperatures of 2°C–8°C. The phase III trial was conducted across eight different countries. The U.S. Food and Drug Administration has issued emergency use authorization to this vaccine in individuals 18 years of age and older. In an international, randomized, double-blind, placebo-controlled, phase III trial, Johnson & Johnson randomly assigned adult participants in a 1:1 ratio to receive a single dose of Ad26.COV2.S (5×10^{10} viral particles) or placebo. In the per-protocol at-risk population, 468 centrally confirmed cases of symptomatic COVID-19 with an onset at least 14 days after administration were observed, of which 464 were moderate to severe–critical (116 cases in the vaccine group vs. 348 in the placebo group), which indicates a vaccine efficacy of 66.9% (Olliaro et al., 2021).

3.10. Novavax (NVX-CoV2373)

Novavax has been licensed by the EMA and is now being reviewed by WHO. The vaccine developed by Novavax is a protein subunit–based vaccine developed by using a SARS-CoV-2 spike protein subunit in its glycosylated form. The vaccine can be stored stably at 2°C–8°C and requires two doses 3 weeks apart. To increase the immune response, it is mixed with Novavax's patented saponin-based Matrix-M adjuvant (https://www.novavax.com). In the 15,000-subject UK phase III clinical trial (NCT04583995), Novavax saw 56 cases of COVID-19 in the placebo arm and six cases in the NVX-CoV2373 group at the interim analysis, resulting in an overall efficacy of 89.3%. All the cases in the vaccine cohort were mild or moderate. Twenty-seven percent of subjects were aged over 65 years. The company said that 32 of the COVID-19 cases were infected with the B.1.1.7 variant. A *post hoc* analysis put the efficacy against B.1.1.7 at 85.6% compared with an efficacy of 95.6% versus older variants. The Novavax clinical trials represent the first major controlled clinical tests of how a COVID-19 vaccine performs against the B.1.1.7 and B.1.351 variants. Overall, the results suggest NVX-CoV2373 may be as effective as any prophylactic studied to date against older variants (Shinde et al., 2021).

3.11. Vector Institute (EpiVac Corona)

EpiVac corona got approval from the Russian NRA and currently is in the process to get approval by WHO. The EpiVac corona vaccine uses chemically synthesized peptide antigens of SARS-CoV-2 along with aluminum hydroxide as an adjuvant. The vaccine is administered intramuscularly twice 21–28 days apart (Belta News, 2021). The phase I and II studies tested the safety, side effects, and immunogenicity of the potential vaccine in 100 people aged 18–60, according to the state trials register. The immunological effectiveness of the EpiVac corona vaccine was found to be 100% (Ryzhikov A.B., 2021).

3.12. WIBP/Sinopharm (WIBP-CorV)

Another vaccine by Sinopharm uses a whole inactivated virus. The double-blind, randomized, phase III trial designed by the Wuhan Institute of Biological Products Co., Ltd., and the Beijing Institute of Biological Products Co., Ltd., on 3469 participants, including adults of 18 years and older age without prior known history of SARS-CoV, SARS-CoV-2, or Middle East respiratory syndrome infection (via onsite inquiry) were enrolled, showed an efficacy rate of 72.8% against symptomatic COVID-19 cases (Al Kaabi et al., 2021).

4. CHALLENGES IN VACCINE DESIGN

Various precedented and unprecedented hurdles are encountered by designing and manufacturing agencies to develop an effective and prophylactic vaccine against novel viruses. Moreover, for a new vaccine candidate, it takes 10–15 years to be introduced for public use after rigorous and cumbersome clinical trials. Furthermore, most companies are unwilling to engage in vaccine production because vaccine profit margins are incompatible with those for drug development. Here, we discuss various challenges in SARS-CoV-2 vaccine development and propose possible solutions for respective problems (**Figure 6**).

4.1. Mutation

The novel coronavirus, like other RNA viruses, evolves by multiplying genetic material with higher rates of mutation (Raghuram et al., 2015; Islamuddin et al., 2018), resulting in greater genetic variation over time. Additionally, its capacity to shift genetic material from human to human and mutate in the human body allows it to be more transmissible (Denison et al., 2011). The rise of these variants may impact vaccine development and therapies as they spread throughout the population all over the world (**Table 3**) within a short span of time. Out of three types of possible mutations—base deletions, insertions, and substitutions—SARS-CoV-2 shows deletion and substitution mutations. Missense mutations account for 34.3%, nonsense mutations for 6.7%, and silent mutations for 0.8% of the SARS-CoV-2 genome (Pathan et al., 2020). Researchers found that a highly variable region of the spike protein in circulating viruses accounts for the top 10% of entropy (rate of mutation). A change in the amino acid in the antigenic part may hamper the neutralizing antibody functionality and could affect the degree of protection by vaccines. Importantly, to prevent the derailing of promising vaccines or antibody-based prophylactics or treatments, it is critical to understand how and whether SARS-CoV-2 may evolve to evade antibody-dependent immunity. Intriguingly, the most variable region in the coronavirus genome is the RBD of the spike protein (Zhou et al., 2020). Greaney et al. (2021b) have performed mutational scanning to detect the possible mutations in the RBD of spike protein that could affect neutralizing antibody functionality. It is, therefore, imperative to consider various clan, variants, and substrains with different mutations to reduce possibilities that will impact vaccine potential. The N439K mutation in RBD is the second most common mutation in RBD and the sixth most common mutation in the spike; it increases the binding affinity of spike with ACE-II twofold because of the salt bridge formed at the binding interface with a positively charged amino acid. This has been observed in more than 30 countries. The variant was first identified in March 2020 in Scotland, and as of January 2021, a second lineage B.1.258 has independently emerged in other European countries (**Table 3**). The N439K mutation did not change the clinical spectrum of the disease; however, in *in vivo* studies, the viral loads were increased compared with wild-type viruses with N439 residue. Also, D614G is one of the most prevalent nonsynonymous mutations of the spike protein that dominate the global pandemic (**Table 3**). The D614G mutation, like the N439K mutation, is shown to enhance viral infectivity *in vitro* and enhance viral fusion with the ACE2 receptor, but there has been no evidence of a connection between this mutation and disease severity (Hou et al., 2020; Zhang et al., 2020; Groves et al., 2021).

4.2. Global Variants of SARS-CoV-2

Various mutations, leading to rapidly spreading SARS-CoV-2 variants in the United Kingdom (B.1.1.7), South Africa (B.1.351), India (B.1.617), Brazil (P1), the United States (B1.429), and United Kingdom/Nigeria (B.1.525) strains, propagate even

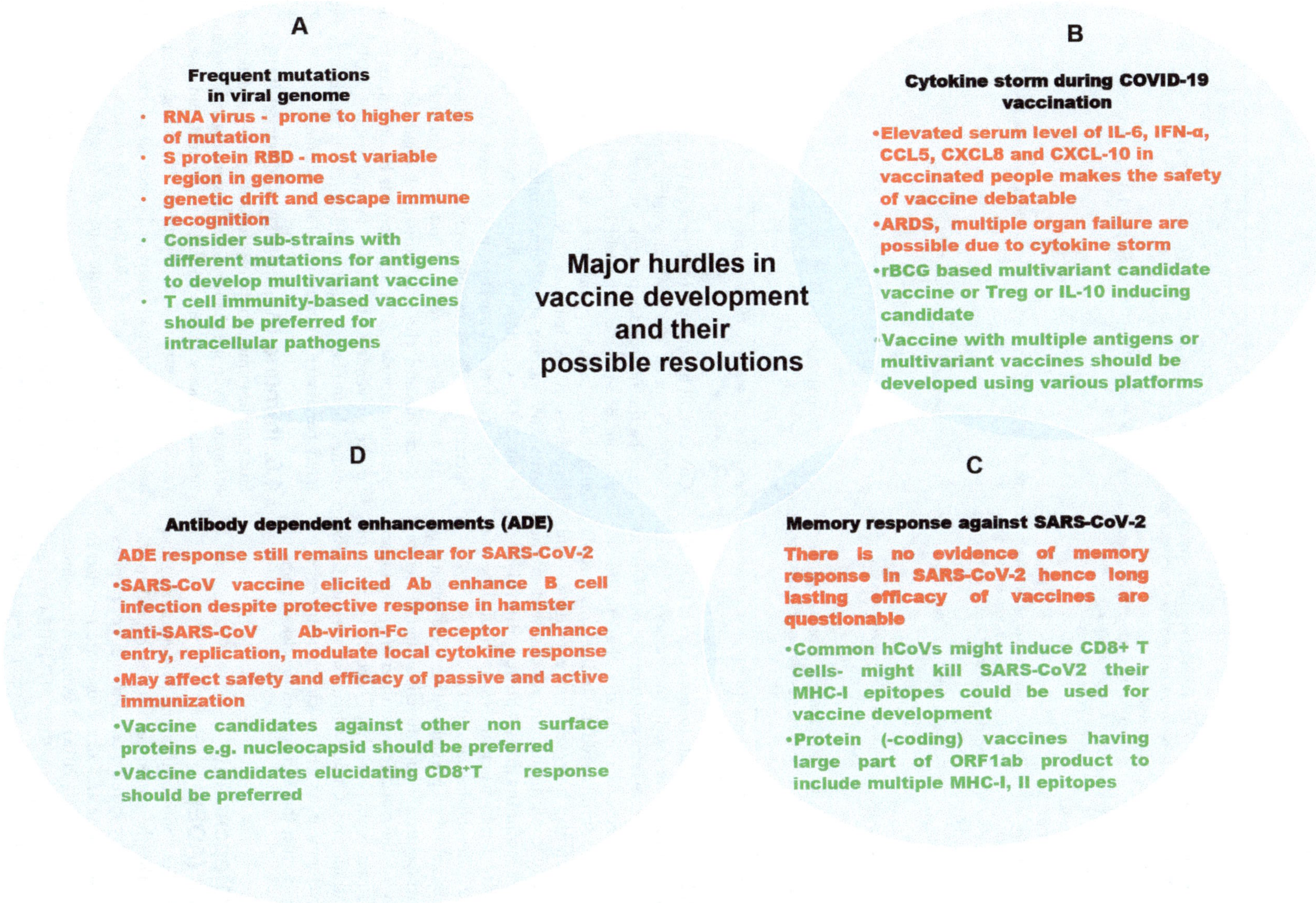

FIGURE 6 | Challenges in developing vaccines against SARS-CoV-2 (black color text), their description (red color text) and their possible resolutions (green color text). **(A)** Mutation in viral genome: The RNA viruses including SARS-CoV-2 are more prone to mutation in their genome, leading to viral immune evasion. **(B)** Cytokine storm during COVID-19 vaccination: Occasionally, the vaccination may lead to cytokine storm and other complications raised by it. **(C)** Lack of memory response: Any vaccine provides long-lasting efficacy only because of memory responses of adaptive immunity. No vaccine against SARS-CoV-2 is documented to have established memory response postvaccination. The neutralizing antibody fades away a few months post vaccination. **(D)** Antibody-dependent enhancements: There is the possibility of an antibody-mediated increase in infection called antibody dependent enhancement.

TABLE 3 | Major SARS-CoV-2 variants.

Type	First detected in country	Variation in spike	Risk and impact on vaccine efficacy	References
VOC 202012/ 01 GRY (B.1.1.7)	U.K.	N501Y 144Y del 69/70 deletion P681H, D614G	Increased risk of death compared with other variants. ~50% increased transmission, Minimal impact on neutralization by convalescent and post-vaccination sera	(Arif, 2021; CDC, 2021b; Collier et al., 2021; Edara et al., 2021; Emary et al., 2021; Galloway et al., 2021; Muik et al., 2021; Ostrov, 2021; Planas et al., 2021; Shen et al., 2021; Wang et al., 2021a; Wu et al., 2021)
VOC GH/ 501Y.V2 (B.1.351)	South Africa	Shares some mutations with B.1.1.7 K417N, E484K N501Y, D614G	No evidence to suggest that this variant has any impact on disease severity or impact on neutralizing antibodies.	(Kim et al., 2021; Planas et al., 2021; Wang et al., 2021b; Zhou et al., 2021)
VOC GR/ 501Y.V3 (P.1)	Brazil, Japan	17 unique mutations, K417T, E484K, and N501Y	The emergence of this variant raises concerns of a potential increase in transmissibility or propensity for SARS-CoV-2 re-infection of individuals.	(CDC, 2021b; Dejnirattisai et al., 2021; Hoffmann et al., 2021)
VUI G/ 484K.V3 (B.1.525)	UK, Nigeria	E484K Q677H F888L	E484K mutation associated with potential immune escape.	(Jangra et al., 2021)
VOC G/ 452R.V3 (B.1.617+)	India	L452R, E484Q, D614G	Slightly reduced neutralization by post-vaccination sera	(Greaney et al., 2021a; Yadav et al., 2021)
VUI GH/ 452R.V1 (B.1.429)	USA	S13I, W152C, L452R, D614G	~20% increased transmissibility, Reduced neutralization by convalescent and postvaccination sera	(Deng et al., 2021)

Scientists are looking into how effective a vaccination might be in protecting persons infected with SARS-CoV-2 variants. The table displays the most common variants, countries first detected in, newly identified mutations in spike protein, and the risks they bring to public health (CDC, 2021a).

more rapidly, and this could contribute to more cases of COVID-19 (**Table 3**). It is obvious that a rise in the number of cases would put pressure on healthcare infrastructure and may lead to more fatalities. Current research indicates that antibodies produced by vaccines administered to indigenous people respond to these variants; however, more evidence and research is required to confirm this. In various studies, the mutations or their combinations showed diminished neutralizing activity of serum from mRNA-vaccinated people (Diamond et al., 2021; Zeyaullah et al., 2021).

In addition, there is always a possibility that these mutations may hamper the therapeutic antibody functions and, therefore, impact the efficacy of the vaccines. Furthermore, a human infected with one strain is more likely to become immune to another variant or strain, and if it failed to do so, then it clearly necessitates the development of new vaccination strategies to produce preventive vaccines that can combat the risk of many of these variants.

4.4. Antibody Dependent Enhancements (ADE)

Virus-specific antibodies control infections by neutralizing the virus. However, in ADE, the antibodies may be helpful to the virus by facilitating its entry into the cells through Fc receptors. Some vaccines against dengue and zika viruses are reported to have ADE effects (Khandia et al., 2018). Previously, it is shown that neutralizing antibodies against RBD of MERS-CoV and SARS-CoV facilitated virus entry into Fc receptor–expressing human cells *in vitro* (Wan et al., 2020). The incidence of SARS-CoV-2 ADE has not yet been proven (Wang et al., 2014; Negro, 2020; Wan et al., 2020). An alternative target to overcome ADE may be the nonsurface proteins, such as the nucleocapsid (N) protein. Because the N protein is not on the virus surface, its antibodies cannot promote virus entry. Despite defensive responses in the hamster model, antibodies elicited by the SARS-CoV vaccine strengthened infection of B cell lines (Li et al., 2018). On the other hand, anti-nucleocapsid antibodies neither neutralized infection nor induced ADE. Therefore, the interaction with Fc receptors of virion-complexed anti-SARS-CoV antibodies can result in both increased viral cell entry and replication and clinically impactful regulation of the local cytokine response. ADE infection has become a major concern for the prevention of diseases by vaccination. ADE response studies should be included for all candidate vaccines as a major safety parameter for approval of the vaccine.

4.5. Immune Evasion by Coronavirus

Studying the immune responses to SARS-CoV-2 and its approaches to immunoevasion enhance our understanding of pathogenesis and viral clearance and lead to the development and assessment of vaccines and immune therapeutics. The subsequent immune reactions, immunopathology, and processes of immune evasion are underevaluated. SARS-CoV-2 has developed various mechanisms to avoid innate immune detection like many other viruses, including low levels of cytosine-phosphate-guanosine (CpG) in the genome, glycosylation to shield the interacting receptor to the host, RNA shielding, and viral protein generation, that effectively hinder a virus. These mechanisms together allow efficient infection and increased viral load. Innate immune evasion is enabled by cap-methylation of viral RNA, and inhibition of steps in the IFN form I/III pathways are included in such evasion. SARS-CoV-2 has established the most severe CpG deficiency of all betacoronaviruses in accordance with other viruses (Xia, 2020), thus preventing ZAP action. The processing of capping the 5' end is another technique for defending mRNA used by the host and several viruses. Capping restricts degradation and greatly inhibits identification by cytosolic pattern recognition receptors (PRRs) for both host and virus RNA. The post-translational modifications of structural and nonstructural proteins alter the target epitope, leading to compromised vaccine efficacy (Jeyanathan et al., 2020). Importantly, RNA viruses, including SARS-CoV-2, go through frequent mutation to have multiple variants that lead to immune evasion by viruses. This immune evasion makes it difficult to develop efficient vaccines, especially in the case of variants, but it allows the development of multiple epitope-based vaccine candidates, so in case one epitope does not respond, the other could take over and eventually enhance vaccine efficacy.

4.6. Cytokine Storm in COVID-19 Vaccination

Cytokine storm is a deadly, unregulated systemic inflammatory response resulting from the release of large amounts of pro-inflammatory cytokines (IFN-α, IFN-γ, IL-1β, IL-6, IL-12, IL-18, IL-33, TNF-α, etc.) and chemokines (CCL2, CCL3, CCL5, CXCL8, CXCL9, CXCL10, etc.) by immune effector cells in response to SARS-CoV-2 infection. The uncontrolled cytokine response is one of the main mechanisms for ARDS, responsible for mortality in COVID-19 patients (Williams and Chambers, 2014; Min et al., 2016). Similar ARDS-like immunopathology was observed in SARS-CoV and MERS-CoV (Williams and Chambers, 2014). Moreover, individuals with serious MERS-CoV infection display elevated serum levels of IL-6, IFN-α, and CCL-5, CXCL-8, CXCL-10 compared with those with mild-to-moderate disease, comparable to those with SARS-CoV (Coperchini et al., 2020). In extreme cases of SARS-CoV-2 infection, as is the case with SARS-CoV and MERS CoV infections, the cytokine storm forces the immune system to attack the body aggressively, causing ARDS, multiple organ failure, and eventually death. (Xu et al., 2020). The vaccines should be able to suppress cytokine storm or at least hamper its deleterious impact, e.g., the IL-10 and Th-2 cytokine could be helpful in controlling cytokine storm (Costela-Ruiz et al., 2020).

Most of the candidate vaccines for SARS-CoV-2 aim to boost the immune system as much as possible to induce strong immunization. This may lead to uncontrolled cytokine storm among some vaccinated individuals, which may lead to ARDS, one of the most common causes of death in COVID-19 patients. Vaccination in 33 African green monkeys and 200 mice induced protective immunity against SARS-Cov-2. Approximately 7% of monkeys along with 5% of experimental mice showed cytokine storm in their lungs upon post mRNA vaccination challenge by SARS-CoV-2. It seems developing a vaccine for SARS-Cov-2 that can regulate cytokine storm is needed (Farshi, 2020).

4.7. Memory Response Against SARS-CoV-2

The efficacy of a vaccine against the pathogen is confirmed by the memory response at the time of the second or subsequent attack. The reinfection in COVID-19 patients demonstrates a lack of suitable memory response after prior infection probably due to the viral immune evasion strategy. The candidate vaccines should be capable of eliciting B and T cell memory responses. Ironically, any approved vaccine does not have well-established memory response data, and it is imperative that it be deciphered for all candidate vaccines. There are some potential ways for this likely immune memory to be manipulated. For instance, it may be best to use SARS-CoV-2 genes that encode MHC-I epitopes that fit those of common coronaviruses when using RNA for immunization (Kupferschmidt and Cohen, 2020). For the most part, when considering potential strategies for SARS-CoV-2 vaccination, consideration should be given to preexisting MHC-I-based immunity resulting from previous common coronavirus infections. Common human coronaviruses can also induce some MHC-II-mediated immune memory by $CD4^+$ helper T cells with regard to SARS-CoV-2 recognition for shared epitope use by various coronaviruses. $CD4^+$ helper T cells can help stimulate cells involved in cytotoxic immune responses mediated by antibodies or cells. Recent studies also demonstrate that previously SARS-CoV infected patients show long-lasting SARS nucleoprotein (NP)-specific memory T cells displaying cross-reactivity to SARS-CoV-2 NP (Le Bert et al., 2020a). The promiscuous common T cell epitopes, which could elicit both CD4 and $CD8^+$ T cells against SARS-CoV, SARS-CoV-2, and MERS, should be taken into consideration for vaccine development. For all vaccines, the studies should be conducted on vaccine recipient individual samples for detection of long-term protection, specifically memory T and B cells. Additionally, the virus neutralization assay should be performed to detect functional antibodies in the serum of vaccine recipient individuals.

4.8. Animal Model for Vaccine Study

Animals play a crucial role in the development of COVID-19 treatments and vaccines. The race to generate and expand mice for COVID-19 research is going on in the lab. The introduction of a safe and predictable COVID-19 animal model of infection is indeed a welcome development for preliminary antiviral and vaccine evaluations, and it is likely to help researchers understand the immune evasion mechanism adopted by various strains of the virus. The hamster model is not new to corona virology, but it has the ability to offer a more stable and predictable model of infection than murine models (Roberts et al., 2005). In the murine model, hyper-accentuated immune responses after SARS-CoV-2 vaccination have previously been published (Bolles et al., 2011). In addition, transgenic animals are often employed as models in biomedical research in the lab. Genetically engineered animals, mostly mice, account for almost 95% of those utilized. They are the tools for studying the disease susceptibility, progression, and treatment response. Following the discovery of ACE-2 as the SARS-CoV host receptor, there has been a lot of interest in establishing human disease–like mouse models. This resulted in the creation of transgenic mice with human hACE2, K18-hACE2, expressed in the epithelia of tissues and organs, such as the lungs, liver, kidney, spleen, heart, and intestine (Kumar et al., 2020). They are very susceptible to SARS-CoV infection with high viral lung titers, considerable weight loss, and morbidity. The ACE-2 mouse model becomes the tool set for cardiovascular and pulmonary research and is critical to advancing medicine and technology to search for drugs and a vaccine to fight the COVID-19 pandemic (Jia et al., 2020).

4.9. Storage, Transportation, and Handling of Vaccines

Most of the vaccines, especially the mRNA vaccines, as observed, require significantly low storage temperatures that are below the freezing point, which is difficult to maintain, particularly for longer durations, and poses a huge limitation in developing countries. The vaccines developed by Pfizer, Moderna, and Johnson & Johnson require storage of vaccine vials at -70°C to -80°C, -20°C (6 months), and -20°C (2 years), respectively, thus making them extremely fragile and difficult to store and handle, especially in developing countries. Apart from the requirement of ultralow freezing temperatures, the vaccines must be protected from direct exposure to sunlight and ultraviolet light, making the handling all that more difficult. The storage and transportation requirement puts extra financial burden on the vaccine recipient. Vaccines having room temperature storage are always cost effective and ease point of care units. The advantages and disadvantages of the major vaccine platforms are mentioned in **Table 4**.

5. POSSIBLE RESOLUTIONS TO OVERCOME HURDLES IN VACCINE DEVELOPMENT AGAINST SARS COV-2

5.1. Vaccines Focused on T Cell Immunity and Memory

Most of the vaccine candidates against SARS-CoV-2 are focused on developing neutralization antibodies against the viral spike protein to diminish viral entry into host cells. However, to develop a prophylactic vaccine against intracellular pathogen-like viruses, the cytotoxic T lymphocyte (CTL) response remains indispensable (Ahmed and Akondy, 2011). A group recently suggested that the severe infection of COVID-19 provides better memory T cells than milder infection (Chen and John Wherry, 2020). Earlier studies demonstrate that only 50% of SARS survivors showed viral-specific B and T cell responses (Cao et al., 2007; Tang et al., 2011; Ng et al., 2016; Le Bert et al., 2020b). However, T cell response was long-lasting (6–17 years), associated with less severe disease, cleared the virus rapidly, and did not evolve into an ADE response. On the other hand, B cell response was short-lived (3 years), associated with severe disease (MERS survivors with higher antibody titer must stay longer in ICU), did not clear the virus rapidly, and was found to be

TABLE 4 | Advantages and disadvantages of the major vaccine platforms (Kyriakidis et al., 2021).

Vaccine Type	Advantages	Disadvantages
Nucleic acid vaccines	Scalability. Fast design and development. Extremely safe. No infectious agent handling is required. Can induce humoral and cellular responses.	Currently, few nucleic acid vaccines approved, including vaccine for SARS-CoV-2. DNA vaccines require a special delivery platform. mRNA vaccines exhibit instability and require storage at less than -20°C.
Viral-vectored vaccines[π]	Can induce robust humoral and cellular responses with a single dose. Good safety profile.	Preexisting immunity against a human viral vector can attenuate immune responses. Some candidates require storage at less than -20°C.
Protein Subunit vaccines[£]	Safety during production. Can be safely administered to immunosuppressed people. No infectious agent handling is required.	Small size of antigens diminishes their uptake by antigen-presenting cells (APCs). Low immunogenicity. Need several booster doses and adjuvants. Do not elicit cellular responses. Antigen integrity needs to be confirmed. Production limited by antigen production scalability.
Polysaccharide vaccines[¥]	Provides an alternative for vaccines against pathogens with an abundance of polysaccharide antigens (mostly bacteria).	Boost doses seldomly enhance the responses. Only IgM isotype and IgG2 subtype are induced, leading to limited antibody mediated effector functions. Poor memory responses. Works poorly on children.
Conjugate vaccines[*]	Enhances the poor immunologic responses produced by polysaccharide vaccines as it induces T-dependent responses.	Absence of cellular responses. Adjuvant and booster doses needed.
Virus-like particles vaccines[±]	They combine the efficacy of attenuated vaccines and the safety of subunit vaccines. Scalability of production. Their size makes them ideal for uptake by APCs.	The assembly of the particles is sometimes challenging.

*An example of vaccine used with this approach [πEbola; £Hep B, Hep C, Influenza, Human Papilloma Virus (HPV); ¥Pneumococcal polysaccharide vaccine (PPSV or PPV-23); *Streptococcus pneumoniae vaccine, Neisseria meningitidis conjugated vaccine (meningococcal vaccine), Typhoid vaccine, Haemophilus influenzae type b vaccine; ±HPV, Hep B].*

involved in ADE (Cao et al., 2007; Tang et al., 2011; Ng et al., 2016; Zhao et al., 2017; Liu et al., 2019; Le Bert et al., 2020b; Sekine et al., 2020; Lynch et al., 2021). A high serum level in SARS-CoV-2 infection is associated with longer stay of patients in the ICU and the need of ventilators because of severe disease condition (Cao, 2020; Zhao et al., 2020a). Thus, they may serve as candidates for designing SARS-CoV-2 vaccines. Another eight immunodominant CD4+ T cell epitopes have been suggested for use in a subunit vaccine to potentially elicit effective T and B cell responses. They are distributed across the S (232–246 and 233–247), E (55–69, 56–70, and 57–71), and M (97–111, 98–112, and 99–113) proteins. These predictions warrant further investigation and may aid in effective vaccine design against SARS-CoV-2. In addition to a strong antibody response, the coronavirus vaccines should also be capable of inducing virus-specific CD8+ T cell immunity. In addition, the focus should also be made on memory response of both humoral as well as cell-mediated responses.

5.2. Development of Multivariant Vaccines

Most viruses evolve and change over time, and SARS-CoV-2 is no exception with its composition constantly changing and raising concerns about the efficacy of existing COVID-19 vaccinations in use. With the appearance of three new strains, B.1.1.7 (United Kingdom), B.1.351 (South Africa), and P.1 (Brazil) as well as B.1.617 (India), there is a need to develop a multivariant vaccine (**Table 3**). Likewise, annual influenza vaccinations are administered to people in many countries every year. The constant mutation in the influenza virus yearly design of new vaccines is predicted on the basis of the current influenza viral strain. Both trivalent and quadrivalent vaccines targeting three and four strains of the virus, respectively, are used as flu vaccines (Rudenko et al., 2018). Gritstone Oncology, Inc., in Emeryville, California, with support from the Bill and Melinda Gates Foundation and the National Institute of Allergy and Infectious Diseases (NIAID), is working on a multivariant vaccine that targets epitopes on the spike protein as well as other areas of the virus for attack by T cells. It is an mRNA vaccine using adenovirus vectors for delivery. The Gates Foundation supported preclinical development of the vaccine, and NIAID has partnered with the company on an early stage clinical trial. Preclinical tests revealed that more regions of the SARS-CoV-2 virus elicited multiple immune responses, including high-titer neutralizing antibodies and $CD8^+$ T cell responses against the spike protein as well as a broad $CD8^+$ T cell response against epitopes from multiple viral genes beyond the spike. There are currently no approved multivariant vaccines, but efforts are underway to develop them in the future. We recommend that we proceed with the development of a SARS-CoV-2 vaccine by aiming to build a multivariant vaccine for improved protection.

5.3. BCG as a Platform for Live-Attenuated Vaccine

Recently, various reports suggest that countries with a non-BCG vaccine recipient population (Italy, Nederland, the United States) show higher case fatality rates compared with long-standing universal BCG policy-practicing countries (Hegarty et al., 2020; Miller et al., 2020). In addition, in the elderly population (Gursel and Gursel, 2020), BCG is suggestive of the notion that BCG protects the vaccinated elderly population. Its known protective immunological benefits, decreased incidences, hampered disease transmission and progression, and lowered mortality are suggestive of BCG vaccination as a potential nonspecific safe tool against COVID-19; however, various other factors make BCG efficacy against COVID-19 debatable (Dayal and Gupta, 2020; Gursel and Gursel, 2020; Hegarty et al., 2020; Hensel et al., 2020; Kirov, 2020; Miller et al., 2020).

5.3.1. BCG Vaccination Renders Nonspecific and Variable Immune Response

BCG vaccination in healthy volunteers increases IFN-γ; enhances monocyte-derived cytokines TNF and IL-1β release; and elevates activation markers CD11b and PRRs such as Toll-like receptor-4, CD-14, and scavenger receptors (Kleinnijenhuis et al., 2012; Goswami et al., 2020). BCG vaccination in infants, surprisingly, increases 11 cytokines and chemokines in response to different nonspecific innate immunity stimuli, which includes epidermal growth factor, eotaxin, IL-6, IL-7, IL-8, IL-10, IL-12p40, monocyte chemotactic protein-3, macrophage inflammatory protein-1α, soluble CD-40 ligand, and platelet-derived growth factor. Moreover, in monocytes, the heterologous production of Th1 (IFN-γ) and Th17 (IL-17 and IL-22) immune responses to non-mycobacterial stimulation remained strongly elevated even 1 year after BCG vaccination (Kleinnijenhuis et al., 2014).

The SARS-CoV-2 infection renders hyper-inflammation mediated pulmonary dysfunction due to pro-inflammatory cytokine (IL-1β, IL-4, IL-6, IL-8, MCSF, CXCL-10, and TNF-α) burst in patients (Guo et al., 2020; Li et al., 2020). Surprisingly, these elevated cytokine levels have been reported along with lymphopenia in COVID-19 patients, suggestive of a major contribution by uncontrolled innate responses. The anti-inflammatory cytokine IL-10 could be of great help in combating COVID-19 because of its anti-inflammatory nature and its capability to obstruct inflammatory cytokine production, including IFN-γ and IL-2. BCG is shown to induce T and B independent monocytes/macrophages and NK cell-mediated nonspecific trained immunity response to a secondary infection by the innate immune system to either the same or different microorganisms (Covian et al., 2019; Netea et al., 2020) in SARS-CoV-2 infection in BCG immunized individuals. Moreover, it would be imperative to compare the cytokine profiles of patients from BCG immunized and nonimmunized individuals.

Thus, BCG induces sustained changes in the immune system associated with a nonspecific response to infections that could be beneficial against COVID-19. However, the beneficial role of BCG against COVID-19 remains debatable because of the variation in testing rate, population density, median age, TB incidence, urban population, public policy, and community spread check measures in different countries (Kirov, 2020). BCG as an adjuvant is proved very efficient in producing nonspecific immune responses; in the case of COVID-19, we should perform studies to evaluate the efficacy of various adjuvants, including BCG to elicit immunoprophylactic responses by candidate vaccines. The suitable adjuvant would not only instigate immune responses, but will also facilitate memory response that could be a boon for a vaccine against this dreadful pathogen.

6. DISCUSSION AND FUTURE PROSPECTS

The most daunting threat in a century for mankind is the COVID-19 pandemic caused by SARS-CoV-2. Less than a year after COVID-19 was declared as a pandemic, several vaccine candidates were authorized for emergency use in various countries. Despite the availability of vaccinations, recent pandemic waves have created concerns about i) the effectiveness of existing vaccines against new virus variants; ii) achieving global herd immunity against COVID-19; iii) the safety of the vaccine in autoimmune disorder individuals; iv) vaccine safety for pregnant women, toddlers, and young adults; v) the possibility of cytokine storm in vaccinated people; vi) efficacy of vaccines in comorbid conditions; vii) appropriate timing of booster doses for best immune response; viii) B cell memory responses; ix) T cell immunity and memory response; x) effectiveness of vaccines in reducing viral transmission; xi) vaccine distribution to the underprivileged; xii) the effect of vaccination on infected people; xiii) vaccine hesitancy; and xiv) vaccine swapping in the absence of a second dose or improving immune response, continuing exploration of significant scientific and policy challenges (Garcia-Beltran et al., 2021; Singh et al., 2021).

Multiple waves of infection place a huge burden on the state, doctors, and scientists in establishing a successful fight against SARS-CoV-2. Some of countries have achieved a sufficient number of vaccinations to curb the pandemic. In contrast, some countries confirm lowered vaccinations either due to unavailability of vaccines as per requirement or because of vaccine hesitancy. Because of the severe impact of the pandemic in terms of infection intensity and mortality, the vaccination drives in between this pandemic have reduced vaccine hesitancy among the population, and this has contributed to achieving herd immunity. Herd immunity generally requires a protective immune response in 60%–70% of the population attained either through infection with the virus or by vaccination. Global scientific coordination and partnership is the key to successful vaccination against COVID-19. It is particularly effective because nationalistic approaches to immunization will continue to raise issues such as vaccine development and production, pricing, allocation, and deployment, and only a global resource collaboration can fulfill these goals (Voysey et al., 2021).

The vaccines used are safe, but there are reports of safety concerns with some of the vaccines, which has caused havoc and has been a source of vaccine hesitancy. Scientific evidence on vaccine safety should be established not just in the general population, but also for pregnant woman, toddlers, and teens; people with comorbid diseases such as diabetes and hypertension; and those who have been infected prior to vaccination. Because most of the vaccines are based on neutralizing antibodies against the spike protein of SARS-CoV-2, details are available for neutralizing antibodies; however, T cell immunity remains untouched for most of the vaccine candidates. Furthermore, the B and T cell memory response has not been established for most of the approved vaccines. B and T cell memory responses and T cell–mediated immunity should be deciphered for all the used vaccines with immediate attention.

Globally, the spread of different variants has worsened the situation, and we need a vaccine with prophylactic efficacy to combat COVID-19. The multivariant vaccines might be more efficient in eliciting better and stronger immune responses for better protection against virus variants. We can use various platforms to achieve multivariant vaccines. Nonetheless, the direct virus could be employed to develop live-attenuated vaccines; however, there is always the possibility of reversal. One of the major concerns during SARS-CoV-2 infection is cytokine storm, which leads to various physiological damages, including pneumonia; pulmonary embolism; and blood clotting in various organs, including brain, gastrointestinal tract, kidney, and liver; also it results in ARDS. This is suggestive that unregulated immune response due to viral immune evasion strategies renders these damages. The cytokine storm could be controlled by inducing Treg cells and IL-10 cytokine strategically. Nevertheless, BCG has been proved to elicit nonspecific controlled immune response; it would be an inclusive strategy to develop formulations of rBCG by incorporating multiple antigens of SARS-CoV-2. The live-attenuated nature of rBCG could be helpful in generating long-term protection.

Interestingly, a number of studies are currently being conducted in many parts of the world on the use of two separate vaccines for better protection against SARS-CoV-2 and its variant form. According to a German study, immunizing with AstraZeneca's ChAdOx1-nCov-19 vaccine as a first shot and BioNTech/BNT162b2 Pfizer's as a second shot 10 weeks apart boosts the immune response. BNT162b2 induced significantly higher frequencies of spike-specific CD4 and CD8 T cells and, in particular, provided high titers of neutralizing antibodies against the B.1.1.7, B.1.351, and P.1 lineage of the virus (Barros-Martins et al., 2021; Callaway, 2021). There has been speculation that using covaxin as a first shot and AstraZeneca (covishield) as a booster shot helps to protect people better. However, further research is required on the interchangeable vaccine approach.

Considering a worse hit by multiple waves, it is suggestive that individuals should take the vaccines whichever they are available at their end to curb the disease severity even if it does not provide the best protection. Importantly, prophylactic vaccines against SARS-CoV-2 have great potential to prevent future pandemics. Nonetheless, we must continue to improve the present vaccine by increasing neutralizing antibodies, and a focus on multivariant vaccines that include T cell immunity would be beneficial in combating numerous variations of this dreadful pathogen.

AUTHOR CONTRIBUTIONS

MA conceived and designed the review drafting. WH, ZH, RA, KG, AG, NK, IA, and FA contributed in writing, preparation of figure and tables, and updating the review. All authors contributed to the article and approved the submitted version.

ACKNOWLEDGMENTS

MA acknowledges the financial support from DBT-RLF and India Alliance DBT-Wellcome Trust.

REFERENCES

Ahmed, R., and Akondy, R. S. (2011). Insights Into Human CD8(+) T-Cell Memory Using the Yellow Fever and Smallpox Vaccines. *Immunol. Cell Biol.* 89, 340–345. doi: 10.1038/icb.2010.155

Al Kaabi, N., Zhang, Y., Xia, S., Yang, Y., Al Qahtani, M. M., Abdulrazzaq, N., et al. (2021). Effect of 2 Inactivated SARS-CoV-2 Vaccines on Symptomatic COVID-19 Infection in Adults: A Randomized Clinical Trial. *Jama* 326, 35–45. doi: 10.1001/jama.2021.8565

Arif, T. B. (2021). The 501.V2 and B.1.1.7 Variants of Coronavirus Disease 2019 (COVID-19): A New Time-Bomb in the Making? *Infect. Control Hosp Epidemiol.* 1–2. doi: 10.1017/ice.2020.1434

Baden, L. R., El Sahly, H. M., Essink, B., Kotloff, K., Frey, S., Novak, R., et al. (2021). Efficacy and Safety of the mRNA-1273 SARS-CoV-2 Vaccine. *New Engl. J. Med.* 384, 403–416. doi: 10.1056/NEJMoa2035389

Baden, L. R., El Sahly, H. M., Essink, B., Kotloff, K., Frey, S., Novak, R., et al. (2020). Efficacy and Safety of the mRNA-1273 SARS-CoV-2 Vaccine. *New Engl. J. Med.* 384, 403–416. doi: 10.1056/NEJMoa2035389

Barros-Martins, J., Hammerschmidt, S. I., Cossmann, A., Odak, I., Stankov, M. V., Ramos, G. M., et al. (2021). Humoral and Cellular Immune Response Against SARS-CoV-2 Variants Following Heterologous and Homologous ChAdOx1 Ncov-19/BNT162b2 Vaccination. *medRxiv.* doi: 10.1038/s41591-021-01449-9

BBC News (2020a). *BBC News. Covid-19: China Approves Sinopharm Vaccine for General Use, BBC News*, 31 December 2020. British Broadcasting Corporation.

BBC News (2020b). *Roxby, P. Russian Covid Vaccine Shows Encouraging Results. BBC News*, 11 November 2020. British Broadcasting Corporation.

BBC News (2021). *BBC News. Sinovac: Brazil Results Show Chinese Vaccine 50.4% Effective. BBC News*, 13 January 2021. British Broadcasting Corporation.

Belta News (2021). *BELTA News. Russia Reports 100% Efficacy of EpiVacCorona Vaccine, in Belarusian Telegraph Agency. BELTA News*, 19 January2021. online News site.

Bharat Biotech (2021a). *Bharat Biotech. COVAXIN®—India's First Indigenous COVID-19 Vaccine.* 2020. Available at: https://www.bharatbiotech.com/covaxin.html (Accessed 1 March 2021).

Bharat Biotech (2021b). *Bharat Biotech's Covaxin Set For Trials on Children Aged Between 2 to 18 Years.* Available at: https://www.india.com/news/india/coronavirus-vaccine-news-today-12-may-2021-bharat-biotech-covaxin-clinical-trials-on-children-between-2-to-18-years-age-group-4657989/.

Blanco-Melo, D., Nilsson-Payant, B. E., Liu, W. C., Uhl, S., Hoagland, D., Møller, R., et al. (2020). Imbalanced Host Response to SARS-CoV-2 Drives Development of COVID-19. *Cell* 181, 1036–1045.e1039. doi: 10.1016/j.cell.2020.04.026

Bolles, M., Deming, D., Long, K., Agnihothram, S., Whitmore, A., Ferris, M., et al. (2011). A Double-Inactivated Severe Acute Respiratory Syndrome Coronavirus Vaccine Provides Incomplete Protection in Mice and Induces Increased Eosinophilic Proinflammatory Pulmonary Response Upon Challenge. *J. Virol.* 85, 12201–12215. doi: 10.1128/JVI.06048-11

Bos, R., Rutten, L., van der Lubbe, J. E. M., Bakkers, M. J. G., Hardenberg, G., Wegmann, F., et al. (2020). Ad26 Vector-Based COVID-19 Vaccine Encoding a Prefusion-Stabilized SARS-CoV-2 Spike Immunogen Induces Potent Humoral and Cellular Immune Responses. *NPJ Vaccines* 5, 1–11. doi: 10.1038/s41541-020-00243-x

Callaway, E. (2020). The Race for Coronavirus Vaccines: A Graphical Guide. *Nature* 580, 576–577. doi: 10.1038/d41586-020-01221-y

Callaway, E. (2021). Mix-And-Match COVID Vaccines Trigger Potent Immune Response. *Nat. Med.* 593, 491. doi: 10.1038/d41586-021-01359-3

Cao, X. (2020). COVID-19: Immunopathology and its Implications for Therapy. *Nat. Rev. Immunol.* 20, 269–270. doi: 10.1038/s41577-020-0308-3

Cao, W. C., Liu, W., Zhang, P. H., Zhang, F., and Richardus, J. H. (2007). Disappearance of Antibodies to SARS-Associated Coronavirus After Recovery. *N Engl. J. Med.* 357, 1162–1163. doi: 10.1056/NEJMc070348

CDC (2021a). *SARS-CoV-2 Variant Classifications and Definitions.* Available at: https://www.cdc.gov/coronavirus/2019-ncov/variants/variant-info.html.

CDC (2021b). *Science Brief: Emerging SARS-CoV-2 Variants.* Available at: https://www.cdc.gov/coronavirus/2019-ncov/more/science-and-research/scientific-brief-emerging-variants.html.

Chakraborty, S., Mallajosyula, V., Tato, C. M., Tan, G. S., and Wang, T. T. (2021). SARS-CoV-2 Vaccines in Advanced Clinical Trials: Where do We Stand. *Advanced Drug Delivery Rev* 172, 314–338. doi: 10.1016/j.addr.2021.01.014

Chakraborty, C., Sharma, A. R., Sharma, G., Bhattacharya, M., and Lee, S. S. (2020). SARS-CoV-2 Causing Pneumonia-Associated Respiratory Disorder (COVID-19): Diagnostic and Proposed Therapeutic Options. *Eur. Rev. Med. Pharmacol. Sci.* 24, 4016–4026. doi: 10.26355/eurrev_202004_20871

Chen, Z., and John Wherry, E. (2020). T Cell Responses in Patients With COVID-19. *Nat. Rev. Immunol.* 20, 529–536. doi: 10.1038/s41577-020-0402-6

Collier, D. A., De Marco, A., Ferreira, I., Meng, B., Datir, R. P., Walls, A. C., et al. (2021). Sensitivity of SARS-CoV-2 B.1.1.7 to mRNA Vaccine-Elicited Antibodies. *Nature* 593, 136–141. doi: 10.1038/s41586-021-03412-7

Coperchini, F., Chiovato, L., Croce, L., Magri, F., and Rotondi, M. (2020). The Cytokine Storm in COVID-19: An Overview of the Involvement of the Chemokine/Chemokine-Receptor System. *Cytokine Growth factor Rev.* 53, 25–32. doi: 10.1016/j.cytogfr.2020.05.003

Costela-Ruiz, V. J., Illescas-Montes, R., Puerta-Puerta, J. M., Ruiz, C., and Melguizo-Rodrãguez, L. (2020). SARS-CoV-2 Infection: The Role of Cytokines in COVID-19 Disease. *Cytokine Growth factor Rev.* 54, 62–75. doi: 10.1016/j.cytogfr.2020.06.001

Covian, C., Fernandez-Fierro, A., Retamal-Diaz, A., Diaz, F. E., Vasquez, A. E., Lay, M. K., et al. (2019). BCG-Induced Cross-Protection and Development of Trained Immunity: Implication for Vaccine Design. *Front. Immunol.* 10, 2806. doi: 10.3389/fimmu.2019.02806

Cucinotta, D., and Vanelli, M. (2020). WHO Declares COVID-19 a Pandemic. *Acta BioMed.* 91, 157–160. doi: 10.23750/abm.v91i1.9397

Dayal, D., and Gupta, S. (2020). Connecting BCG Vaccination and COVID-19: Additional Data. *MedRxiv.* doi: 10.1101/2020.04.07.20053272

De Haan, C. A., Kuo, L., Masters, P. S., Vennema, H., and Rottier, P. J. (1998). Coronavirus Particle Assembly: Primary Structure Requirements of the Membrane Protein. *J. Virol.* 72, 6838–6850. doi: 10.1128/JVI.72.8.6838-6850.1998

Dejnirattisai, W., Zhou, D., Supasa, P., Liu, C., Mentzer, A. J., Ginn, H. M., et al. (2021). Antibody Evasion by the P.1 Strain of SARS-CoV-2. *Cell.* 184, 2939–2954. doi: 10.1016/j.cell.2021.03.055

Deng, X., Garcia-Knight, M. A., Khalid, M. M., Servellita, V., Wang, C., Morris, M. K., et al. (2021). Transmission, Infectivity, and Antibody Neutralization of an Emerging SARS-CoV-2 Variant in California Carrying a L452R Spike Protein Mutation. *medRxiv.* doi: 10.1101/2021.03.07.21252647

Denison, M., Graham, R., Donaldson, E., Eckerle, L., and Baric, R. (2011). An RNA Proofreading Machine Regulates Replication Fidelity and Diversity. *RNA Biol.* 8, 270–279. doi: 10.4161/rna.8.2.15013

Diamond, M., Chen, R., Xie, X., Case, J., Zhang, X., Vanblargan, L., et al. (2021). SARS-CoV-2 Variants Show Resistance to Neutralization by Many Monoclonal and Serum-Derived Polyclonal Antibodies. *Res. Square* rs. 3, rs-228079. doi: 10.21203/rs.3.rs-228079/v1

Edara, V. V., Floyd, K., Lai, L., Gardner, M., Hudson, W., Piantadosi, A., et al. (2021). Infection and mRNA-1273 Vaccine Antibodies Neutralize SARS-CoV-2 UK Variant. *medRxiv.* doi: 10.1101/2021.02.02.21250799

Emary, K. R. W., Golubchik, T., Aley, P. K., Ariani, C. V., Angus, B., Bibi, S., et al. (2021). Efficacy of ChAdOx1 Ncov-19 (AZD1222) Vaccine Against SARS-CoV-2 Variant of Concern 202012/01 (B.1.1.7): An Exploratory Analysis of a Randomised Controlled Trial. *Lancet* 397, 1351–1362. doi: 10.1016/S0140-6736(21)00628-0

Farshi, E. (2020). Cytokine Storm Response to COVID-19 Vaccinations. *J. Cytokine Biol.* 5, 2.

Galloway, S. E., Paul, P., Maccannell, D. R., Johansson, M. A., Brooks, J. T., Macneil, A., et al. (2021). Emergence of SARS-CoV-2 B.1.1.7 Lineage - United States, December 29, 2020-January 12, 2021. *MMWR Morb Mortal Wkly Rep.* 70, 95–99. doi: 10.15585/mmwr.mm7003e2

Garcia-Beltran, W. F., Lam, E. C., St Denis, K., Nitido, A. D., Garcia, Z. H., Hauser, B. M., et al. (2021). Multiple SARS-CoV-2 Variants Escape Neutralization by Vaccine-Induced Humoral Immunity. *Cell* 184, 2372–2383.e2379. doi: 10.1016/j.cell.2021.03.013

Gioia, M., Ciaccio, C., Calligari, P., De Simone, G., Sbardella, D., Tundo, G., et al. (2020). Role of Proteolytic Enzymes in the COVID-19 Infection and Promising Therapeutic Approaches. *Biochem. Pharmacol.* 182, 114225. doi: 10.1016/j.bcp.2020.114225

Goel, N., Ahmad, R., Fatima, H., and Khare, S. K. (2021). New Threatening of SARS-CoV-2 Coinfection and Strategies to Fight the Current Pandemic. *Med. Drug Discovery* 10, 100089. doi: 10.1016/j.medidd.2021.100089

Gorbalenya, A. E., Baker, S. C., Baric, R. S., De Groot, R. J., Drosten, C., Gulyaeva, A. A., et al. (2020). The Species Severe Acute Respiratory Syndrome-Related Coronavirus: Classifying 2019-Ncov and Naming it SARS-CoV-2. *Nat. Microbiol.* 5, 536–544. doi: 10.1038/s41564-020-0695-z

Goswami, R. P., Mittal, D. K., and Goswami, R. P. (2020). Interaction Between Malarial Transmission and BCG Vaccination With COVID-19 Incidence in the World Map: A Changing Landscape Human Immune System? *MedRxiv.* doi: 10.2196/preprints.19231

Greaney, A. J., Loes, A. N., Crawford, K. H. D., Starr, T. N., Malone, K. D., Chu, H. Y., et al. (2021a). Comprehensive Mapping of Mutations in the SARS-CoV-2 Receptor-Binding Domain That Affect Recognition by Polyclonal Human Plasma Antibodies. *Cell Host Microbe* 29, 463–476.e466. doi: 10.1016/j.chom.2021.02.003

Greaney, A. J., Starr, T. N., Gilchuk, P., Zost, S. J., Binshtein, E., Loes, A. N., et al. (2021b). Complete Mapping of Mutations to the SARS-CoV-2 Spike Receptor-Binding Domain That Escape Antibody Recognition. *Cell Host Microbe* 29, 44–57.e49. doi: 10.1016/j.chom.2020.11.007

Grifoni, A., Weiskopf, D., Ramirez, S. I., Mateus, J., Dan, J. M., Moderbacher, C. R., et al. (2020). Targets of T Cell Responses to SARS-CoV-2 Coronavirus in Humans With COVID-19 Disease and Unexposed Individuals. *Cell* 181, 1489–1501.e1415. doi: 10.1016/j.cell.2020.05.015

Groves, D. C., Rowland-Jones, S. L., and Angyal, A. (2021). The D614G Mutations in the SARS-CoV-2 Spike Protein: Implications for Viral Infectivity, Disease Severity and Vaccine Design. *Biochem. Biophys. Res. Commun.* 538, 104–107. doi: 10.1016/j.bbrc.2020.10.109

Guo, Y.-R., Cao, Q.-D., Hong, Z.-S., Tan, Y.-Y., Chen, S.-D., Jin, H.-J., et al. (2020). The Origin, Transmission and Clinical Therapies on Coronavirus Disease 2019 (COVID-19) Outbreak–an Update on the Status. *Military Med. Res.* 7, 1–10. doi: 10.1186/s40779-020-00240-0

Gursel, M., and Gursel, I. (2020). Is Global BCG Vaccination Coverage Relevant to the Progression of SARS-CoV-2 Pandemic? *Med. Hypotheses..* doi: 10.1016/j.mehy.2020.109707

Hegarty, P. K., Kamat, A. M., Zafirakis, H., and Dinardo, A. (2020). BCG Vaccination may be Protective Against Covid-19. *Preprint.* doi: 10.13140/RG.2.2.35948.10880

Hensel, J., Mcgrail, D. J., Mcandrews, K. M., Dowlatshahi, D., Lebleu, V. S., and Kalluri, R. (2020). Exercising Caution in Correlating COVID-19 Incidence and Mortality Rates With BCG Vaccination Policies Due to Variable Rates of SARS CoV-2 Testing. *MedRxiv.* doi: 10.1101/2020.04.08.20056051

Hoffmann, M., Arora, P., Groß, R., Seidel, A., Hörnich, B. F., Hahn, A. S., et al. (2021). SARS-CoV-2 Variants B.1.351 and P.1 Escape From Neutralizing Antibodies. *Cell* 184, 2384–2393.e2312. doi: 10.1016/j.cell.2021.03.036

Hou, Y. J., Chiba, S., Halfmann, P., Ehre, C., Kuroda, M., Dinnon, K. H.3rd, et al. (2020). SARS-CoV-2 D614G Variant Exhibits Efficient Replication Ex Vivo and Transmission In Vivo. *Science* 370, 1464–1468. doi: 10.1126/science.abe8499

Islamuddin, M., Khan, W. H., Gupta, S., Tiku, V. R., Khan, N., Akdag, A. I., et al. (2018). Surveillance and Genetic Characterization of Rotavirus Strains Circulating in Four States of North Indian Children. *Infection Genet. Evol.* 62, 253–261. doi: 10.1016/j.meegid.2018.04.030

Jangra, S., Ye, C., Rathnasinghe, R., Stadlbauer, D., Alshammary, H., Amoako, A. A., et al. (2021). SARS-CoV-2 Spike E484K Mutation Reduces Antibody Neutralisation. *Lancet Microbe* 2, 283–284. doi: 10.1016/S2666-5247(21)00068-9

Jeyanathan, M., Afkhami, S., Smaill, F., Miller, M. S., Lichty, B. D., and Xing, Z. (2020). Immunological Considerations for COVID-19 Vaccine Strategies. *Nat. Rev. Immunol.* 20, 615–632. doi: 10.1038/s41577-020-00434-6

Jia, H., Yue, X., and Lazartigues, E. (2020). ACE2 Mouse Models: A Toolbox for Cardiovascular and Pulmonary Research. *Nat. Commun.* 11, 5165. doi: 10.1038/s41467-020-18880-0

Kanamori, H., Weber, D. J., and Rutala, W. A. (2020). Role of the Healthcare Surface Environment in Severe Acute Respiratory Syndrome Coronavirus 2 (SARS-CoV-2) Transmission and Potential Control Measures. *Clin. Infect. Dis.* 72, 2052–2061. doi: 10.1093/cid/ciaa1467

Khandia, R., Munjal, A., Dhama, K., Karthik, K., Tiwari, R., Malik, Y. S., et al. (2018). Modulation of Dengue/Zika Virus Pathogenicity by Antibody-Dependent Enhancement and Strategies to Protect Against Enhancement in Zika Virus Infection. *Front. Immunol.* 9, 597. doi: 10.3389/fimmu.2018.00597

Khan, W. H., Khan, N., Mishra, A., Gupta, S., Bansode, V., Mehta, D., et al. (2021). Dimerization of SARS-CoV-2 Nucleocapsid Protein Affects Sensitivity of ELISA Based Diagnostics of COVID-19. *bioRxiv.* 2021.2005.2023.445305. doi: 10.1101/2021.05.23.445305

Kim, Y. J., Jang, U. S., Soh, S. M., Lee, J. Y., and Lee, H. R. (2021). The Impact on Infectivity and Neutralization Efficiency of SARS-CoV-2 Lineage B.1.351 Pseudovirus. *Viruses* 13, 633. doi: 10.3390/v13040633

Kirov, S. (2020). Association Between BCG Policy is Significantly Confounded by Age and is Unlikely to Alter Infection or Mortality Rates. *MedRxiv.* doi: 10.1101/2020.04.06.20055616

Kleinnijenhuis, J., Quintin, J., Preijers, F., Benn, C. S., Joosten, L. A., Jacobs, C., et al. (2014). Long-Lasting Effects of BCG Vaccination on Both Heterologous Th1/Th17 Responses and Innate Trained Immunity. *J. innate Immun.* 6, 152–158. doi: 10.1159/000355628

Kleinnijenhuis, J., Quintin, J., Preijers, F., Joosten, L. A., Ifrim, D. C., Saeed, S., et al. (2012). Bacille Calmette-Guerin Induces NOD2-Dependent Nonspecific Protection From Reinfection via Epigenetic Reprogramming of Monocytes. *Proc. Natl. Acad. Sci.* 109, 17537–17542. doi: 10.1073/pnas.1202870109

Kumar, A., Singh, R., Kaur, J., Pandey, S., Sharma, V., Thakur, L., et al. (2021). Wuhan to World: The COVID-19 Pandemic. *Front. Cell. Infection Microbiol.* 11, 242. doi: 10.3389/fcimb.2021.596201

Kumar, S., Yadav, P. K., Srinivasan, R., and Perumal, N. (2020). Selection of Animal Models for COVID-19 Research. *VirusDisease* 31, 453–458. doi: 10.1007/s13337-020-00637-4

Kupferschmidt, K., and Cohen, J. (2020). *Race to Find COVID-19 Treatments Accelerates* (American Association for the Advancement of Science) 367, 1412–1413. doi: 10.1126/science.367.6485.1412

Kyriakidis, N. C., López-Cortés, A., González, E. V., Grimaldos, A. B., and Prado, E. O. (2021). SARS-CoV-2 Vaccines Strategies: A Comprehensive Review of Phase 3 Candidates. *NPJ Vaccines* 6, 28. doi: 10.1038/s41541-021-00292-w

Le Bert, N., Tan, A. T., Kunasegaran, K., Tham, C. Y. L., Hafezi, M., Chia, A., et al. (2020a). SARS-CoV-2-Specific T Cell Immunity in Cases of COVID-19 and SARS, and Uninfected Controls. *Nature* 584, 457–462. doi: 10.1038/s41586-020-2550-z

Le Bert, N., Tan, A. T., Kunasegaran, K., Tham, C. Y. L., Hafezi, M., Chia, A., et al. (2020b). SARS-CoV-2-Specific T Cell Immunity in Cases of COVID-19 and SARS, and Uninfected Controls. *Nature* 584, 457–462. doi: 10.1038/s41586-020-2550-z

Li, G., Fan, Y., Lai, Y., Han, T., Li, Z., Zhou, P., et al. (2020). Coronavirus Infections and Immune Responses. *J. Med. Virol.* 92, 424–432. doi: 10.1002/jmv.25685

Li, J., Helal, Z. H., Karch, C. P., Mishra, N., Girshick, T., Garmendia, A., et al. (2018). A Self-Adjuvanted Nanoparticle Based Vaccine Against Infectious Bronchitis Virus. *PloS One* 13, 1–17. doi: 10.1371/journal.pone.0203771

Liu, L., Wei, Q., Lin, Q., Fang, J., Wang, H., Kwok, H., et al. (2019). Anti-Spike IgG Causes Severe Acute Lung Injury by Skewing Macrophage Responses During Acute SARS-CoV Infection. *JCI Insight* 4, 123–158. doi: 10.1172/jci.insight.123158

Liu, C., Zhou, Q., Li, Y., Garner, L. V., Watkins, S. P., Carter, L. J., et al. (2020). Research and Development on Therapeutic Agents and Vaccines for COVID-19 and Related Human Coronavirus Diseases. *ACS Cent. Sci.* 6, 315–331. doi: 10.1021/acscentsci.0c00272

Logunov, D. Y., Dolzhikova, I. V., Shcheblyakov, D. V., Tukhvatulin, A. I., Zubkova, O. V., Dzharullaeva, A. S., et al. (2020a). Safety and Efficacy of an Rad26 and Rad5 Vector-Based Heterologous Prime-Boost COVID-19 Vaccine: An Interim Analysis of a Randomised Controlled Phase 3 Trial in Russia. *Lancet* 397, 671–681. doi: 10.1016/S0140-6736(20)31866-3

Logunov, D. Y., Dolzhikova, I. V., Shcheblyakov, D. V., Tukhvatulin, A. I., Zubkova, O. V., Dzharullaeva, A. S., et al. (2021). Safety and Efficacy of an Rad26 and Rad5 Vector-Based Heterologous Prime-Boost COVID-19 Vaccine: An Interim Analysis of a Randomised Controlled Phase 3 Trial in Russia. *Lancet* 397, 671–681. doi: 10.1016/S0140-6736(21)00234-8

Logunov, D. Y., Dolzhikova, I. V., Zubkova, O. V., Tukhvatullin, A. I., Shcheblyakov, D. V., Dzharullaeva, A. S., et al. (2020b). Safety and Immunogenicity of an Rad26 and Rad5 Vector-Based Heterologous Prime-Boost COVID-19 Vaccine in Two Formulations: Two Open, non-Randomised Phase 1/2 Studies From Russia. *Lancet* 396, 887–897.

Lundstrom, K. (2020). The Current Status of COVID-19 Vaccines. *Front. Genome Editing* 2, 10. doi: 10.3389/fgeed.2020.579297

Lynch, K. L., Whitman, J. D., Lacanienta, N. P., Beckerdite, E. W., Kastner, S. A., Shy, B. R., et al. (2021). Magnitude and Kinetics of Anti-Severe Acute

Respiratory Syndrome Coronavirus 2 Antibody Responses and Their Relationship to Disease Severity. *Clin. Infect. Dis.* 72, 301–308. doi: 10.1093/cid/ciaa979

Mackenzie, J. S., and Smith, D. W. (2020). COVID-19: A Novel Zoonotic Disease Caused by a Coronavirus From China: What We Know and What We Don't. *Microbiol. Aust.*, MA20013–MA20013. doi: 10.1071/MA20013

Michel, C. J., Mayer, C., Poch, O., and Thompson, J. D. (2020). Characterization of Accessory Genes in Coronavirus Genomes. *Virol. J.* 17, 131. doi: 10.1186/s12985-020-01402-1

Miller, A., Reandelar, M. J., Fasciglione, K., Roumenova, V., Li, Y., and Otazu, G. H. (2020). Correlation Between Universal BCG Vaccination Policy and Reduced Morbidity and Mortality for COVID-19: An Epidemiological Study. *MedRxiv*. doi: 10.1101/2020.03.24.20042937

Min, C. K., Cheon, S., Ha, N. Y., Sohn, K. M., Kim, Y., Aigerim, A., et al. (2016). Comparative and Kinetic Analysis of Viral Shedding and Immunological Responses in MERS Patients Representing a Broad Spectrum of Disease Severity. *Sci. Rep.* 6, 25359. doi: 10.1038/srep25359

Moderna (2021). *Moderna Announces First Participants Dosed in Phase 2/3 Study of COVID-19 Vaccine Candidate in Pediatric Population Online from Moderna Site*, published on 16 March,2021, retrieved on 21 May, 2021.

Mousavizadeh, L., and Ghasemi, S. (2021). Genotype and Phenotype of COVID-19: Their Roles in Pathogenesis. *J. Microbiol Immunol. Infection* 54, 159–163. doi: 10.1016/j.jmii.2020.03.022

Muik, A., Wallisch, A. K., Sänger, B., Swanson, K. A., Mühl, J., Chen, W., et al. (2021). Neutralization of SARS-CoV-2 Lineage B.1.1.7 Pseudovirus by BNT162b2 Vaccine-Elicited Human Sera. *Science* 371, 1152–1153. doi: 10.1126/science.abg6105

Mukherjee, S., Tworowski, D., Detroja, R., Mukherjee, S. B., and Frenkel-Morgenstern, M. (2020). Immunoinformatics and Structural Analysis for Identification of Immunodominant Epitopes in SARS-CoV-2 as Potential Vaccine Targets. *Vaccines (Basel)* 8, 290. doi: 10.3390/vaccines8020290

Mulligan, M. J., Lyke, K. E., Kitchin, N., Absalon, J., Gurtman, A., Lockhart, S., et al. (2020). Phase I/II Study of COVID-19 RNA Vaccine BNT162b1 in Adults. *Nature* 586, 589–593. doi: 10.1038/s41586-020-2639-4

Nakagawa, S., and Miyazawa, T. (2020). Genome Evolution of SARS-CoV-2 and its Virological Characteristics. *Inflammation Regener.* 40, 17. doi: 10.1186/s41232-020-00126-7

Negro, F. (2020). Is Antibody-Dependent Enhancement Playing a Role in COVID-19 Pathogenesis? *Swiss Med. Weekly* 150, w20249–w20249. doi: 10.4414/smw.2020.20249

Netea, M. G., Domãnguez-Andres, J., Barreiro, L. B., Chavakis, T., Divangahi, M., Fuchs, E., et al. (2020). Defining Trained Immunity and its Role in Health and Disease. *Nat. Rev. Immunol.* 20, 375–388. doi: 10.1038/s41577-020-0285-6

Ng, O. W., Chia, A., Tan, A. T., Jadi, R. S., Leong, H. N., Bertoletti, A., et al. (2016). Memory T Cell Responses Targeting the SARS Coronavirus Persist Up to 11 Years Post-Infection. *Vaccine* 34, 2008–2014. doi: 10.1016/j.vaccine.2016.02.063

Olliaro, P., Torreele, E., and Vaillant, M. (2021). COVID-19 Vaccine Efficacy and Effectiveness-the Elephant (Not) in the Room. *Lancet Microbe.* 2, 279–280. doi: 10.1016/S2666-5247(21)00069-0

Ostrov, D. A. (2021). Structural Consequences of Variation in SARS-CoV-2 B.1.1.7. *J. Cell Immunol.* 3, 103–108. doi: 10.33696/immunology.3.085

Palacios, R., Patiño, E. G., De Oliveira Piorelli, R., Conde, M., Batista, A. P., Zeng, G., et al. (2020). Double-Blind, Randomized, Placebo-Controlled Phase III Clinical Trial to Evaluate the Efficacy and Safety of Treating Healthcare Professionals With the Adsorbed COVID-19 (Inactivated) Vaccine Manufactured by Sinovac - PROFISCOV: A Structured Summary of a Study Protocol for a Randomised Controlled Trial. *Trials* 21, 853. doi: 10.1186/s13063-020-04775-4

Pardi, N., Hogan, M. J., Pelc, R. S., Muramatsu, H., Andersen, H., Demaso, C. R., et al. (2017). Zika Virus Protection by a Single Low-Dose Nucleoside-Modified mRNA Vaccination. *Nature* 543, 248–251. doi: 10.1038/nature21428

Pathan, R. K., Biswas, M., and Khandaker, M. U. (2020). Time Series Prediction of COVID-19 by Mutation Rate Analysis Using Recurrent Neural Network-Based LSTM Model. *Chaos Solitons Fractals* 138, 110018. doi: 10.1016/j.chaos.2020.110018

Pfizer-Biontech (2021). *High Effectiveness of Pfizer-BioNTech COVID-19 Vaccine.* Available at: https://www.pfizer.com/news/press-release/press-release-detail/real-world-evidence-confirms-high-effectiveness-pfizer.

Piret, J., and Boivin, G. (2021). Pandemics Throughout History. *Front. Microbiol.* 11, 3594. doi: 10.3389/fmicb.2020.631736

Planas, D., Bruel, T., Grzelak, L., Guivel-Benhassine, F., Staropoli, I., Porrot, F., et al. (2021). Sensitivity of Infectious SARS-CoV-2 B.1.1.7 and B.1.351 Variants to Neutralizing Antibodies. *Nat. Med.* 27, 917–924. doi: 10.1038/s41591-021-01318-5

Polack, F. P., Thomas, S. J., Kitchin, N., Absalon, J., Gurtman, A., Lockhart, S., et al. (2020). Safety and Efficacy of the BNT162b2 mRNA Covid-19 Vaccine. *New Engl. J. Med.* 383, 2603–2615. doi: 10.1056/NEJMoa2034577

Press release (2021). Available at: https://ir.novavax.com/news-releases/news-release-details/novavax-covid-19-vaccine-demonstrates-893-efficacy-uk-phase-3.

Prompetchara, E., Ketloy, C., Tharakhet, K., Kaewpang, P., Buranapraditkun, S., Techawiwattanaboon, T., et al. (2021). DNA Vaccine Candidate Encoding SARS-CoV-2 Spike Proteins Elicited Potent Humoral and Th1 Cell-Mediated Immune Responses in Mice. *PloS One* 16, e0248007. doi: 10.1371/journal.pone.0248007

Raghuram, V. S., Khan, W. H., Deeba, F., Sullender, W., Broor, S., and Parveen, S. (2015). Retrospective Phylogenetic Analysis of Circulating BA Genotype of Human Respiratory Syncytial Virus With 60 Bp Duplication From New Delhi, India During 2007-2010. *Virusdisease* 26, 276–281. doi: 10.1007/s13337-015-0283-7

Reuters-Staff (2021). *Sinopharm's Wuhan Unit Reports 72.5% Efficacy for COVID Shot, Seeks Approval in China.* Available at: https://www.reuters.com/article/us-health-coronavirus-vaccine-sinopharm-idUSKBN2AO0WW.

Roberts, A., Vogel, L., Guarner, J., Hayes, N., Murphy, B., Zaki, S., et al. (2005). Severe Acute Respiratory Syndrome Coronavirus Infection of Golden Syrian Hamsters. *J. Virol.* 79, 503–511. doi: 10.1128/JVI.79.1.503-511.2005

Ruan, Q., Yang, K., Wang, W., Jiang, L., and Song, J. (2020). *Clinical Predictors of Mortality Due to COVID-19 Based on an Analysis of Data of 150 Patients From Wuhan, China* (Springer). *Intensive Care Med.* 46, 846–848. doi: 10.1007/s00134-020-05991-x

Rudenko, L., Kiseleva, I., Krutikova, E., Stepanova, E., Rekstin, A., Donina, S., et al. (2018). Rationale for Vaccination With Trivalent or Quadrivalent Live Attenuated Influenza Vaccines: Protective Vaccine Efficacy in the Ferret Model. *PloS One* 13, e0208028–e0208028. doi: 10.1371/journal.pone.0208028

Ryzhikov, A. B., R., E.A., Bogryantseva, M. P., Usova, S. V., Danilenko, E. D., Nechaeva, E. A., et al. (2021). A Single Blind, Placebo-Controlled Randomized Study of the Safety, Reactogenicity and Immunogenicity of the "EpiVacCorona" Vaccine for the Prevention of COVID-19, in Volunteers Aged 18–60 Years (Phase I–II). *Russian J. Infection Immun.* 11, 283–296. doi: 10.15789/2220-7619-ASB-1699

Sekine, T., Perez-Potti, A., Rivera-Ballesteros, O., Strålin, K., Gorin, J.-B., Olsson, A., et al. (2020). Robust T Cell Immunity in Convalescent Individuals With Asymptomatic or Mild COVID-19. *bioRxiv*. doi: 10.1016/j.cell.2020.08.017

Shen, X., Tang, H., Mcdanal, C., Wagh, K., Fischer, W., Theiler, J., et al. (2021). SARS-CoV-2 Variant B.1.1.7 is Susceptible to Neutralizing Antibodies Elicited by Ancestral Spike Vaccines. *Cell Host Microbe* 29, 529–539. doi: 10.1016/j.chom.2021.03.002

Shinde, V., Bhikha, S., Hoosain, Z., Archary, M., Bhorat, Q., Fairlie, L., et al. (2021). Efficacy of NVX-CoV2373 Covid-19 Vaccine Against the B.1.351 Variant. *New Engl. J. Med.* 384, 1899–1909. doi: 10.1056/NEJMoa2103055

Singh, J., Rahman, S. A., Ehtesham, N. Z., Hira, S., and Hasnain, S. E. (2021). SARS-CoV-2 Variants of Concern are Emerging in India. *Nat. Med* 27, 1131–1133. doi: 10.1038/s41591-021-01397-4

Tang, F., Quan, Y., Xin, Z. T., Wrammert, J., Ma, M. J., Lv, H., et al. (2011). Lack of Peripheral Memory B Cell Responses in Recovered Patients With Severe Acute Respiratory Syndrome: A Six-Year Follow-Up Study. *J. Immunol.* 186, 7264–7268. doi: 10.4049/jimmunol.0903490

US FDA (2021). *U.S. Food and Drug Administration. COVID-19 Vaccine Ad26.COV2.S, VAC31518 (JNJ-78436735)—Sponsor Briefing Document; FDA* (White Oak, MD, USA: U.S. Food and Drug Administration).

Voysey, M., Clemens, S. A. C., Madhi, S. A., Weckx, L. Y., Folegatti, P. M., Aley, P. K., et al. (2021). Safety and Efficacy of the ChAdOx1 Ncov-19 Vaccine (AZD1222) Against SARS-CoV-2: An Interim Analysis of Four Randomised Controlled Trials in Brazil, South Africa, and the UK. *Lancet* 397, 99–111. doi: 10.1016/S0140-6736(20)32661-1

Wang, P., Nair, M. S., Liu, L., Iketani, S., Luo, Y., Guo, Y., et al. (2021a). Antibody Resistance of SARS-CoV-2 Variants B.1.351 and B.1.1.7. *bioRxiv*. doi: 10.1101/2021.01.25.428137

Wang, P., Nair, M. S., Liu, L., Iketani, S., Luo, Y., Guo, Y., et al. (2021b). Antibody Resistance of SARS-CoV-2 Variants B.1.351 and B.1.1.7. *Nature* 593, 130–135. doi: 10.1038/s41586-021-03398-2

Wang, S. F., Tseng, S. P., Yen, C. H., Yang, J. Y., Tsao, C. H., Shen, C. W., et al. (2014). Antibody-Dependent SARS Coronavirus Infection is Mediated by Antibodies Against Spike Proteins. *Biochem. Biophys. Res. Commun.* 451, 208–214. doi: 10.1016/j.bbrc.2014.07.090

Wan, Y., Shang, J., Sun, S., Tai, W., Chen, J., Geng, Q., et al. (2020). Molecular Mechanism for Antibody-Dependent Enhancement of Coronavirus Entry. *J. Virol.* 94, 2015–2019. doi: 10.1128/JVI.02015-19

Waterloonews (2020). *University of Waterloo Developing DNA-Based COVID-19 Vaccine.* Available at: https://uwaterloo.ca/news/news/university-waterloo-developing-dna-based-covid-19-vaccine.

WHO (2020). *172 Countries and Multiple Candidate Vaccines Engaged in COVID-19 Vaccine Global Access Facility.* Available at: https://www.who.int/news/item/24-08-2020-172-countries-and-multiple-candidate-vaccines-engaged-in-covid-19-vaccine-global-access-facility.

WHO (2021a). *Draft Landscape of COVID-19 Candidate Vaccines.* Available at: https://www.who.int/who-documents-detail/draft-landscape-of-COVID-19-candidate-vaccines.

WHO (2021b). *Evidence Assessment:Sinopharm/BBIBP COVID-19 Vaccine.* World Health Organization.

WHO (2021c). *Status of COVID-19 Vaccines Within WHO EUL/PQ Evaluation Process.* Available at: https://extranet.who.int/pqweb/sites/default/files/documents/Status%20of%20COVID-19%20Vaccines%20within%20WHO%20EUL-PQ%20evaluation%20process%20-%203%20June%202021.pdf.

Williams, A. E., and Chambers, R. C. (2014). The Mercurial Nature of Neutrophils: Still an Enigma in ARDS? *Am J Physiol Lung Cell Mol Physiol*

Wu, K., Werner, A. P., Moliva, J. I., Koch, M., Choi, A., Stewart-Jones, G. B. E., et al. (2021). mRNA-1273 Vaccine Induces Neutralizing Antibodies Against Spike Mutants From Global SARS-CoV-2 Variants. *bioRxiv.* doi: 10.1101/2021.01.25.427948.

Xia, X. (2020). Extreme Genomic CpG Deficiency in SARS-CoV-2 and Evasion of Host Antiviral Defense. *Mol. Biol. Evol.* 37, 2699–2705. doi: 10.1093/molbev/msaa094

Xu, Z., Shi, L., Wang, Y., Zhang, J., Huang, L., Zhang, C., et al. (2020). Pathological Findings of COVID-19 Associated With Acute Respiratory Distress Syndrome. *Lancet Respir. Med.* 8, 420–422. doi: 10.1016/S2213-2600(20)30076-X

Yadav, P. D., Sapkal, G. N., Abraham, P., Ella, R., Deshpande, G., Patil, D. Y., et al. (2021). Neutralization of Variant Under Investigation B.1.617 With Sera of BBV152 Vaccinees. *bioRxiv.* 2021.2004.2023.441101. doi: 10.1093/cid/ciab411

Yang, Y., Xiao, Z., Ye, K., He, X., Sun, B., Qin, Z., et al. (2020). SARS-CoV-2: Characteristics and Current Advances in Research. *Virol. J.* 17, 117. doi: 10.1186/s12985-020-01369-z

Yan, Y., Pang, Y., Lyu, Z., Wang, R., Wu, X., You, C., et al. (2021). The COVID-19 Vaccines: Recent Development, Challenges and Prospects. *Vaccines* 9, 349. doi: 10.3390/vaccines9040349

Zeng, Z. Q., Chen, D. H., Tan, W. P., Qiu, S. Y., Xu, D., Liang, H. X., et al. (2018). Epidemiology and Clinical Characteristics of Human Coronaviruses OC43, 229e, NL63, and HKU1: A Study of Hospitalized Children With Acute Respiratory Tract Infection in Guangzhou, China. *Eur. J. Clin. Microbiol. Infect. Dis.* 37, 363–369. doi: 10.1007/s10096-017-3144-z

Zeyaullah, M., Alshahrani, A. M., Muzammil, K., Ahmad, I., Alam, S., Khan, W. H., et al. (2021). COVID-19 and SARS-CoV-2 Variants: Current Challenges and Health Concern. *Front. Genet.* 12, 1001. doi: 10.3389/fgene.2021.693916

Zhang, L., Jackson, C. B., Mou, H., Ojha, A., Rangarajan, E. S., Izard, T., et al. (2020). The D614G Mutation in the SARS-CoV-2 Spike Protein Reduces S1 Shedding and Increases Infectivity. *bioRxiv.* doi: 10.1101/2020.06.12.148726

Zhao, J., Alshukairi, A. N., Baharoon, S. A., Ahmed, W. A., Bokhari, A. A., Nehdi, A. M., et al. (2017). Recovery From the Middle East Respiratory Syndrome is Associated With Antibody and T-Cell Responses. *Sci. Immunol.* 2, 1–17. doi: 10.1126/sciimmunol.aan5393

Zhao, J., Yuan, Q., Wang, H., Liu, W., Liao, X., Su, Y., et al. (2020a). Antibody Responses to SARS-CoV-2 in Patients With Novel Coronavirus Disease 2019. *Clin. Infect. Dis.* 71, 2027–2034. doi: 10.1093/cid/ciaa344

Zhao, J., Zhao, S., Ou, J., Zhang, J., Lan, W., Guan, W., et al. (2020b). COVID-19: Coronavirus Vaccine Development Updates. *Front. Immunol.* 11, 3435. doi: 10.3389/fimmu.2020.602256

Zhou, D., Dejnirattisai, W., Supasa, P., Liu, C., Mentzer, A. J., Ginn, H. M., et al. (2021). Evidence of Escape of SARS-CoV-2 Variant B.1.351 From Natural and Vaccine-Induced Sera. *Cell* 184, 2348–2361.e2346. doi: 10.1016/j.cell.2021.02.037

Zhou, P., Yang, X. L., Wang, X. G., Hu, B., Zhang, L., Zhang, W., et al. (2020). A Pneumonia Outbreak Associated With a New Coronavirus of Probable Bat Origin. *Nature* 579, 270–273. doi: 10.1038/s41586-020-2012-7

15

NOX-Dependent Signaling Dysregulation in Severe COVID-19: Clues to Effective Treatments

Simona Damiano, Concetta Sozio, Giuliana La Rosa and Mariarosaria Santillo *

Dipartimento di Medicina Clinica e Chirurgia, Università di Napoli "Federico II", Napoli, Italy

Keywords: coronavirus disease 2019, severe acute respiratory syndrome coronavirus 2, NOX enzymes, angiotensin converting enzyme 2, hypertension, cardiovascular diseases, diabetes, obesity

***Correspondence:**
Mariarosaria Santillo
marsanti@unina.it

INTRODUCTION

The ongoing pandemic disease named by the World Health Organization (WHO) coronavirus disease 2019 (COVID-19), is caused by Severe Acute Respiratory Syndrome Coronavirus 2 (SARS-CoV-2), the seventh confirmed RNA single strand beta coronavirus infecting the human beings. According to the WHO, to date (November, 10th 2020), SARS-CoV-2 has affected 50,459,886 people and caused 1,257,523 deaths in the world.

Around 80% of people affected by SARS-CoV-2 infection is asymptomatic or present mild to moderate symptoms, mostly restricted to the upper and conducting airways, often including anosmia and ageusia. The other 20% develops a more critical clinical situation needing hospitalization, which progress, in 5% of cases, in a severe respiratory syndrome requiring ventilatory support and even death (Domingo et al., 2020).

SARS-CoV-2 infects predominantly endothelial cells which express Angiotensin Converting Enzyme (ACE) 2 plasma membrane protein to which the spike protein of SARS-CoV-2 binds (Wan et al., 2020). Therefore, ACE2 represents the receptor of SARS-CoV-2 and ACE2 deficiency related to viral destruction of ACE2 expressing cells, causes severe acute respiratory syndrome and other symptoms related to endothelial cells infection (See *NOX2 Activation in COVID-19*). However, endothelial cells are not the only target cells of SARS-CoV; ACE2 is also expressed in respiratory epithelium, in type II pneumocytes, and in cells of cardiovascular, gastrointestinal, renal, and central nervous systems as well as adipose tissue (Hamming et al., 2004). COVID-19 is therefore a multi-organ disease as the effects of viral infection are extended to a wide range of tissues and organs and, in many cases, death occurs from non-respiratory causes such as renal failure or ischemic episodes (Zaim et al., 2020).

Reactive oxygen species (ROS) derived from NADPH oxidase enzymes (NOXs) and oxidative stress are involved in viral pathogenesis (Khomich et al., 2018). NOX enzymes, present in cell and phagosome membranes, belong to a family of six members (NOX1-5 and DUOX1 and 2) which catalyze the dismutation of superoxide anion to hydrogen peroxide and water (Bedard and Krause, 2007). NOX-driven ROS are signaling molecules regulating numerous physiological functions (Damiano et al., 2015; Damiano et al., 2019). However, a growing body of evidence points to a connection between exceeding NOX-derived ROS and multiple chronic diseases including hypertension, diabetes, and cardiovascular disease as well as obesity (Sahoo et al., 2016).

Among patients developing the severe form COVID-19, a high percentage suffer of pre-existing pathological conditions like hypertension (57%), diabetes (34%), obesity (42%), and cardiovascular diseases (20–40%) which are also main contributing factors for COVID-19-related deaths (Zhou et al., 2020).

Highly effective therapeutics to prevent or treat the severe form of COVID-19 infection are still lacking. We believe that understanding the common denominator of COVID-19 co-existing pathological conditions and why they worsen the outcome of COVID-19 is a current need for the development of more effective interventions or even to take prevention measures to protect subjects at higher risk.

A possible common pathogenic mechanism of the main comorbidities associated with the development of the severe form of COVID-19 is the activation of the ROS generating NADPH oxidase enzymes (NOXs) and the associated oxidative stress (See *NOX Activation Is a Common Hallmark of Main Comorbidities Associated to Severe COVID-19*). Of note, endosomal NOX activation is essential for SARS-CoV cell infection and some studies have demonstrated the induction of a serum marker of NOX activation in patients affected by COVID-19 (Violi et al., 2020).

Taking into account all these evidences, we propose that a pre-existing NOX pathway dysregulation could be a determining factor in the development of the severe form of COVID-19 infection and in the onset of complications worsening the clinical outcome of disease.

NOXs AND VIRAL DISEASES

NOXs in SARS-CoV Infection

Oxidative stress is a hallmark of severe SARS-CoV infections including SARS-CoV-2 (Cecchini and Cecchini, 2020). Before the onset of COVID-19 pandemic, it has been shown that NOX2 is activated in the endosomal compartment by different types of RNA and DNA viruses employing endosomes as their primary entry mechanism (To et al., 2017). It has been proposed that the interaction between viral RNA/DNA and endosomal toll-like receptor 7 (TLR7) activates this latter which, in turn, induces NOX2, increasing ROS (To et al., 2017; DiNicolantonio and McCarty, 2020). Even if it is still unknown, it is reasonable to hypothesize that SARS-CoV-2, as well as others single stranded RNA and DNA viruses entering cells *via* endosomes, relies on the same TLR7/NOX2-dependent mechanism to infect cells and to circumvent antiviral responses inducing oxidative stress and cell injury. In viral infections, NOX derived ROS, contribute to inflammation and tissue damage (Khomich et al., 2018). However, additional functions have been attributed to NOXs in viral establishment and on the onset of complications. It has been shown that NOX enzymes play a direct role in the early events of retrovirus life cycle (Kim and Wong, 2013), while, in rhinovirus infections, they determine an impairment of epithelial barrier functions, thus facilitating bacterial transmigration (Comstock et al., 2011).

In general, as compensatory mechanism, oxidative stress induces an antioxidant response through nuclear factor E2-related factor 2 (Nrf2) pathway activation. At low levels of ROS, Nrf2 is associated in the cytoplasm with kelch-like ECH-associated protein 1 (Keap1), which targets Nrf2 to proteasomal degradation. When ROS are generated at high levels, Nrf2 dissociates from Keap1, translocates into the nucleus, and binds the antioxidant response element (ARE) of the promoters of target genes encoding mainly antioxidant enzymes like superoxide dismutases, catalase, peroxiredoxins, and glutathione peroxidases (Khomich et al., 2018).

In viral infections, oxidative cell damage can be associated to an inhibition of Nrf2 pathway (Komaravelli and Casola, 2014). Noteworthy, it has been shown that the expression of Nrf-2 related antioxidant gene expression is suppressed in biopsies obtained from COVID-19 patients (Olagnier et al., 2020) (**Figure 1**). On this basis, it has been hypothesized that antioxidant therapy, endosomal-targeted ROS inhibitors (To et al., 2017), or Nrf-2 activators could suppress pathogenicity of many viruses, including SARS-CoV-2 (Cuadrado et al., 2020).

NOX and ACE2/Ang(1-7)/Mas Receptor Signaling

About the pathogenetic mechanisms of COVID-19 and its complications, the downregulation of ACE2/Ang (1-7)/Mas axis exerts a pivotal role. ACE2 is a master regulator of the renin-angiotensin system (RAS) mainly by converting Ang (angiotensin) I and Ang II into Ang (1–9) and Ang (1–7), respectively (Wang et al., 2020). Ang (1–7), through the interaction with Mas receptor, negatively regulates AngII/AT1, thus contrasting the vasoconstrictive, proinflammatory, and prothrombotic effects of this pathway. ACE2/SARS-CoV-2 interaction results in a loss of ACE2 which is driven into the cells by endocytosis and cleaved by proteolysis. Therefore, the loss of ACE2 has two negative effects. The first is an upstream accumulation of Ang II and hyperactivation of the AngII/AT1R pathway; the second one is the downregulation of the counterregulatory Ang (1-7)/Mas receptor pathway which antagonizes AngII/AT1R. The downregulation of ACE2 ultimately can explain the severe multi-organ symptomatology subsequent to SARS-CoV-2 infection.

Interestingly, experimental data link NOXs and ACE2/Ang (1–7)/Mas receptor axis. In transgenic mouse overexpressing ACE2 in neurons, the hyperactivation of ACE2/Ang (1–7)/Mas axis has a protective effect against ischemic injury by preventing ischemia-induced NOX/ROS signaling pathway activation, especially in older animals (Zheng et al., 2014). Therefore, as opposed to ACE/AngII axis which activates NOXs, it seems that ACE2/Ang (1–7)/Mas axis activation is associated with NOXs inhibition.

NOX2 Activation in COVID-19

It has been hypothesized that oxidative stress could play a prominent role in determining cardiovascular complications in COVID-19 and that oxidative stress is linked to NOX activation (Loffredo and Violi, 2020).

Relevant experimental data are now emerging about the relationship between NOXs-dependent pathway and the course of COVID-19. NOX2 activation is associated with severe disease and thrombotic events in COVID-19 patients (Violi et al., 2020).

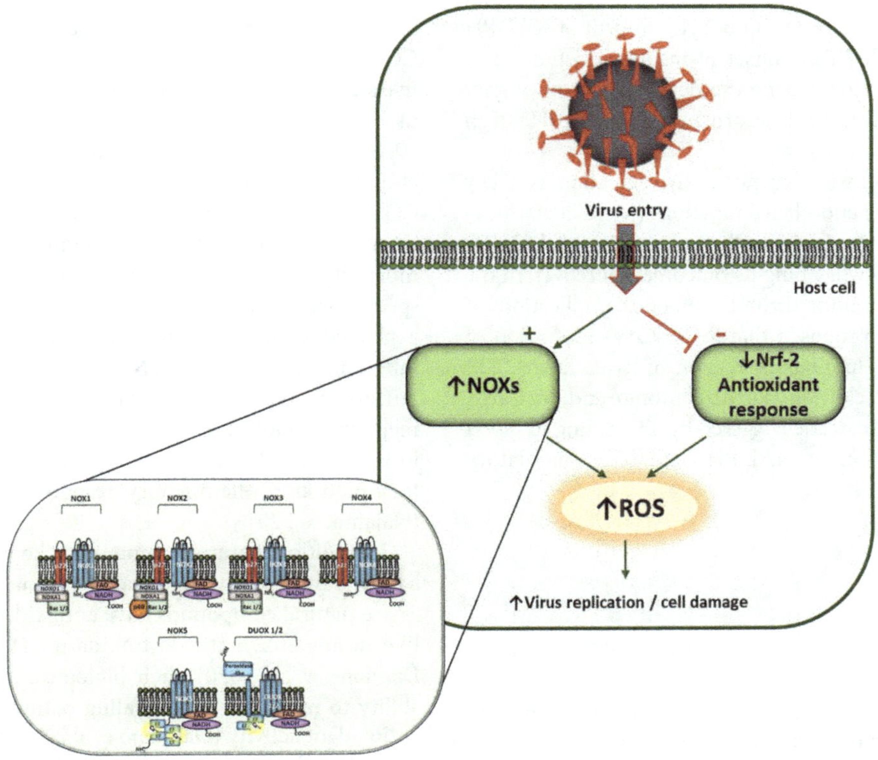

FIGURE 1 | Hypothesis of redox control of host cells in SARS-CoV-2 infection. Virus entry activates NOXs and inhibits Nrf-2 antioxidant response inducing ROS levels. NOX family members and their regulatory subunits are shown in detail on the left. NOX1-3 comprise two membrane subunits (NOX1-3 and p22phox), that represent the catalytic core of the enzyme, and different cytosolic subunits which translocate to membrane upon activation. NOX4 is constitutively active when associated with p22phox subunit. Nox5 and Duox1/2 activation involves Ca^{2+} binding to EF-hand domains.

The soluble Nox2-derived peptide (sNox2-dp), a serum marker of NOX2 activation, has been measured in 182 patients hospitalized for COVID-19. The data evidenced that sNox2-dp values were higher in COVID-19 patients compared to controls and in severe *versus* non-severe COVID-19 affected subjects.

NOX ACTIVATION IS A COMMON HALLMARK OF MAIN COMORBIDITIES ASSOCIATED TO SEVERE COVID-19

The main COVID-19 comorbidity includes hypertension, cardiovascular diseases, obesity, and diabetes, all of which are associated to NOX signaling dysregulation. Hypertension is an important risk factor for other cardiovascular diseases such as coronary artery disease, stroke, heart failure, peripheral vascular disease, chronic kidney disease, and atherosclerosis, as well as for the development of severe COVID-19. NOXs are the main source of ROS within the vascular system. Many data have shown that hypertension-associated vascular functional and structural changes are attributable to NOX-driven intravascular ROS generation. Indeed, Ang II, a well-known pro-hypertensive factor, augments blood pressure activating NOX *via* AT1 receptor (Okabe et al., 2020). Among NOX isoforms, NOX5 exerts a relevant role in blood pressure control. In support of these findings, in a recent genome-wide association study (GWAS) of 475,000 subjects, NOX5 was recognized as an important blood pressure associated gene (Kraja et al., 2017).

Diabetes mellitus, as well, has been identified as an important risk factor for severe COVID-19. A meta-analysis including 33 studies have shown that diabetes is associated with a two-fold increase in mortality and severity of COVID-19, as compared to non-diabetics (Kumar et al., 2020). Studies in type 2 diabetes (TD2) models revealed that anomalous NOX activation contributes to endothelial dysfunction. In TD2 patients hyperglycemia is coupled with inflammation and oxidative stress leading to endothelial dysfunction (Park et al., 2009). Among the endothelial cellular events triggered by hyperglycemia, NOXs are key players involved in oxidative stress generation (Feduska and Tse, 2018).

Obesity represents a high risk factor for the development of severe COVID-19 infection (Sattar et al., 2020). Experimental data mechanistically link the development of obesity with NOX activation. Obesity, along with obesity-associated conditions such as metabolic syndrome and diabetes, is associated with increased NOX-driven ROS production in key organs such as adipose tissue, skeletal muscle and vasculature. The resulting oxidative stress impairs numerous physiological processes like insulin signaling, endothelial functions, and others which overall lead to inflammation and development of pathological conditions (DeVallance et al., 2019). Is has been proposed that ROS derived by NOX4, the major adipocyte isoform of NADPH oxidase, may play a role in the onset of insulin resistance and adipose tissue inflammation during the development of obesity in mice fed a high-fat, high-sucrose diet (Den Hartigh et al., 2017).

In general, NOX pathway-dependent dysregulation is a key determinant in the loss of endothelial functions (Meza et al., 2019) which is a common feature also of other co-existing pathologies associated to COVID-19 worsening its outcome. Moreover, in the attempt to explain the common thromboembolic complications of COVID-19, it has been proposed that SARS-CoV-2 infection of endothelial cells induces luminal expression of tissue factor (TF) which activate extrinsic clotting (DiNicolantonio and McCarty, 2020). In the proteolytic cascade triggered by TF leading to blood coagulation the activation of NADPH oxidase is mandatory (Herkert et al., 2004).

DISCUSSION

The elevated number of death associated to COVID-19 arises from the inadequacy of current treatments unable to combat SARS-CoV-2 infection or to prevent severe complications and ultimately death. Therefore, exploring new treatment options interfering with signaling pathways involved in the pathogenesis of COVID-19 is an urgent need.

The data discussed in the present opinion paper suggest that reducing oxidative stress could improve the poor outcome that characterized severe COVID-19. Due to the central role exerted by NOXs pathway dysregulation and related oxidative stress in the main comorbidity associated to severe COVID-19, and considering its involvement in SARS-CoV viral infection mechanism, targeting NOX enzymes seems a promising strategy to treat COVID-19 and to prevent severe complications.

There are currently no drugs available to selectively block NOXs enzymes approved for their use in human subjects. Experimentally, it has been shown that NOX inhibitors such as diphenyleneiodonium (DPI), apocynin and 4-(2-aminoethyl) benzenesulfonyl fluoride (AEBSF), or peptidic inhibitors are effective in mitigating symptomatology in different animal models of disease (Altenhöfer et al., 2015). However, the reduction of oxidative stress by many substances used in humans is associated with downregulation of NOX signaling. Indirect evidence of the efficacy of treatments for COVID-19 influencing NOXs are represented, among others, by metformin. Contrasting data are present in literature about the association between metformin and decreased mortality in patients with COVID-19 and diabetes. However, a meta-analysis including five studies with a total of 6,937 patients showed that metformin use is associated with reduction in mortality rate from COVID-19. Similar findings are reported in a retrospective study by Luo et al. (2020). Moreover, in obese or T2DM subjects affected by COVID-19, metformin was associated with decreased mortality in women, while, among men, no significant reduction in mortality was observed (Bramante et al., 2020). This sex specific effect of metformin in protecting by COVID-19 was explained with the finding that metformin reduces the pro-inflammatory cytokine TNFalfa in female but not in male. Different hypotheses have been formulated to explain metformin molecular mechanism in protecting from severe form of COVID-19. However, importantly, metformin seems to inhibit the inflammatory response and to modulate NOX (Najafi et al., 2018).

In addition, natural compounds like polyphenols, could have a potential preventive role against the onset of severe COVID-19. These natural compounds have antioxidant properties; however, like some enzymatic antioxidants (Damiano et al., 2013; Damiano et al., 2020), their biological effects are related to the ability to modulate cell-signaling pathways rather than to their antioxidant activity (Damiano et al., 2018). Of note, polyphenols, which have been proposed to serve for prevention and therapy of COVID-19 for their anti-inflammatory properties, have an inhibitory effect on NOXs activity (Yousefian et al., 2019). The list of substances that could improve oxidative stress through inhibition of NOX-dependent pathways is broad and those reported here represent only some intriguing examples.

In conclusion, we believe that the proposed unified point of view of the clinical picture associated with the development of severe COVID-19 highlighting the role of NOXs as key molecular determinants, may provide important clues for the protection of subjects at higher risk and for the development of new targeted therapies fighting the severe forms of illness.

AUTHOR CONTRIBUTIONS

MS and SD conceived and contributed to the writing of the manuscript. CS and GLR contributed to the writing of the manuscript. All authors contributed to the article and approved the submitted version.

REFERENCES

Altenhöfer, S., Radermacher, K. A., Kleikers, P. W., Wingler, K., and Schmidt, H. H. (2015). Evolution of NADPH Oxidase Inhibitors: Selectivity and Mechanisms for Target Engagement. *Antioxid. Redox Signal* 23 (5), 406–427. doi: 10.1089/Ars.2013.5814

Bedard, K., and Krause, K. H. (2007). The NOX family of ROS-generating NADPH oxidases: physiology and pathophysiology. *Physiol. Rev.* 87 (1), 245–313. doi: 10.1152/physrev.00044.2005

Bramante, C., Ingraham, N., Murray, T., Marmor, S., Hoversten, S., Gronski, J., et al. (2020). Observational Study of Metformin and Risk of Mortality in Patients Hospitalized with Covid-19. *medRxiv*. doi: 10.1101/2020.06.19.20135095

Cecchini, R., and Cecchini, A. L. (2020). SARS-CoV-2 infection pathogenesis is related to oxidative stress as a response to aggression. *Med. Hypotheses* 143:110102. doi: 10.1016/j.mehy.2020.110102

Comstock, A. T., Ganesan, S., Chattoraj, A., Faris, A. N., Margolis, B. L., Hershenson, M. B., et al. (2011). Rhinovirus-induced barrier dysfunction in polarized airway epithelial cells is mediated by NADPH oxidase 1. *J. Virol.* 85 (13), 6795–6808. doi: 10.1128/jvi.02074-10

Cuadrado, A., Pajares, M., Benito, C., Jiménez-Villegas, J., Escoll, M., Fernández-Ginés, R., et al. (2020). Can Activation of NRF2 Be a Strategy against COVID-19? *Trends Pharmacol. Sci.* 41 (9), 598–610. doi: 10.1016/j.tips.2020.07.003

Damiano, S., Petrozziello, T., Ucci, V., Amente, S., Santillo, M., and Mondola, P. (2013). Cu-Zn superoxide dismutase activates muscarinic acetylcholine M1 receptor pathway in neuroblastoma cells. *Mol. Cell Neurosci.* 52, 31–37. doi: 10.1016/j.mcn.2012.11.001

Damiano, S., Morano, A., Ucci, V., Accetta, R., Mondola, P., Paternò, R., et al. (2015). Dual oxidase 2 generated reactive oxygen species selectively mediate the induction of mucins by epidermal growth factor in enterocytes. *Int. J. Biochem. Cell Biol.* 60, 8–18. doi: 10.1016/j.biocel.2014.12.014

Damiano, S., Sasso, A., De Felice, B., Di Gregorio, I., La Rosa, G., Lupoli, G. A., et al. (2018). Quercetin Increases MUC2 and MUC5AC Gene Expression and Secretion in Intestinal Goblet Cell-Like LS174T via PLC/PKCα/ERK1-2 Pathway. *Front. Physiol.* 9, 357. doi: 10.3389/fphys.2018.00357

Damiano, S., Muscariello, E., La Rosa, G., Di Maro, M., Mondola, P., and Santillo, M. (2019). Dual Role of Reactive Oxygen Species in Muscle Function: Can Antioxidant Dietary Supplements Counteract Age-Related Sarcopenia? *Int. J. Mol. Sci.* 20 (15), 3815. doi: 10.3390/ijms20153815

Damiano, S., Sozio, C., La Rosa, G., Guida, B., Faraonio, R., Santillo, M., et al. (2020). Metabolism Regulation and Redox State: Insight into the Role of Superoxide Dismutase 1. *Int. J. Mol. Sci.* 21 (18), 6606. doi: 10.3390/ijms21186606

Den Hartigh, L. J., Omer, M., Goodspeed, L., Wang, S., Wietecha, T., O'Brien, K. D., et al. (2017). Adipocyte-Specific Deficiency of NADPH Oxidase 4 Delays the Onset of Insulin Resistance and Attenuates Adipose Tissue Inflammation in Obesity. *Arterioscler. Thromb. Vasc. Biol.* 37 (3), 466–475. doi: 10.1161/atvbaha.116.308749

DeVallance, E., Li, Y., Jurczak, M. J., Cifuentes-Pagano, E., and Pagano, P. J. (2019). The Role of NADPH Oxidases in the Etiology of Obesity and Metabolic Syndrome: Contribution of Individual Isoforms and Cell Biology. *Antioxid. Redox Signal* 31 (10), 687–709. doi: 10.1089/ars.2018.7674

DiNicolantonio, J. J., and McCarty, M. (2020). Thrombotic complications of COVID-19 may reflect an upregulation of endothelial tissue factor expression that is contingent on activation of endosomal NADPH oxidase. *Open Heart* 7 (1), e001337. doi: 10.1136/openhrt-2020-001337

Domingo, P., Mur, I., Pomar, V., Corominas, H., Casademont, J., and de Benito, N. (2020). The four horsemen of a viral Apocalypse: The pathogenesis of SARS-CoV-2 infection (COVID-19). *EBioMedicine* 58, 102887. doi: 10.1016/j.ebiom.2020.102887

Feduska, J. M., and Tse, H. M. (2018). The proinflammatory effects of macrophage-derived NADPH oxidase function in autoimmune diabetes. *Free Radic. Biol. Med.* 125, 81–89. doi: 10.1016/j.freeradbiomed.2018.04.581

Hamming, I., Timens, W., Bulthuis, M. L., Lely, A. T., Navis, G., and van Goor, H. (2004). Tissue distribution of ACE2 protein, the functional receptor for SARS coronavirus. A first step in understanding SARS pathogenesis. *J. Pathol.* 203 (2), 631–637. doi: 10.1002/path.1570

Herkert, O., Djordjevic, T., BelAiba, R. S., and Görlach, A. (2004). Insights into the redox control of blood coagulation: role of vascular NADPH oxidase-derived reactive oxygen species in the thrombogenic cycle. *Antioxid. Redox Signal* 6 (4), 765–776. doi: 10.1089/1523086041361695

Khomich, O. A., Kochetkov, S. N., Bartosch, B., and Ivanov, A. V. (2018). Redox Biology of Respiratory Viral Infections. *Viruses* 10 (8), 392. doi: 10.3390/v10080392

Kim, S. J., and Wong, P. K. Y. (2013). ROS upregulation during the early phase of retroviral infection plays an important role in viral establishment in the host cell. *J. Gen. Virol.* 94 (Pt 10), 2309–2317. doi: 10.1099/vir.0.055228-0

Komaravelli, N., and Casola, A. (2014). Respiratory Viral Infections and Subversion of Cellular Antioxidant Defenses. *J. Pharmacogenomics Pharmacoproteomics* 5 (4), 1000141. doi: 10.4172/2153-0645.1000141

Kraja, A. T., Cook, J. P., Warren, H. R., Surendran, P., Liu, C., Evangelou, E., et al. (2017). New Blood Pressure-Associated Loci Identified in Meta-Analyses of 475 000 Individuals. *Circ. Cardiovasc. Genet.* 10 (5), e001778. doi: 10.1161/circgenetics.117.001778

Kumar, A., Arora, A., Sharma, P., Anikhindi, S. A., Bansal, N., Singla, V., et al. (2020). Is diabetes mellitus associated with mortality and severity of COVID-19? A meta-analysis. *Diabetes Metab. Syndr.* 14 (4), 535–545. doi: 10.1016/j.dsx.2020.04.044

Loffredo, L., and Violi, F. (2020). COVID-19 and cardiovascular injury: A role for oxidative stress and antioxidant treatment? *Int. J. Cardiol.* 312, 136. doi: 10.1016/j.ijcard.2020.04.066

Luo, P., Qiu, L., Liu, Y., Liu, X. L., Zheng, J. L., Xue, H. Y., et al. (2020). Metformin Treatment Was Associated with Decreased Mortality in COVID-19 Patients with Diabetes in a Retrospective Analysis. *Am. J. Trop. Med. Hyg.* 103 (1), 69–72. doi: 10.4269/ajtmh.20-0375

Meza, C. A., La Favor, J. D., Kim, D. H., and Hickner, R. C. (2019). Endothelial Dysfunction: Is There a Hyperglycemia-Induced Imbalance of NOX and NOS? *Int. J. Mol. Sci.* 20 (15), 3775. doi: 10.3390/ijms20153775

Najafi, M., Cheki, M., Rezapoor, S., Geraily, G., Motevaseli, E., Carnovale, C., et al. (2018). Metformin: Prevention of genomic instability and cancer: A review. *Mutat. Res. Genet. Toxicol. Environ. Mutagen.* 827, 1–8. doi: 10.1016/j.mrgentox.2018.01.007

Okabe, K., Matsushima, S., Ikeda, S., Ikeda, M., Ishikita, A., Tadokoro, T., et al. (2020). DPP (Dipeptidyl Peptidase)-4 Inhibitor Attenuates Ang II (Angiotensin II)-Induced Cardiac Hypertrophy via GLP (Glucagon-Like Peptide)-1-Dependent Suppression of Nox (Nicotinamide Adenine Dinucleotide Phosphate Oxidase) 4-HDAC (Histone Deacetylase) 4 Pathway. *Hypertension* 75 (4), 991–1001. doi: 10.1161/hypertensionaha.119.14400

Olagnier, D., Farahani, E., Thyrsted, J., Blay-Cadanet, J., Herengt, A., Idorn, M., et al. (2020). SARS-CoV2-mediated suppression of NRF2-signaling reveals potent antiviral and anti-inflammatory activity of 4-octyl-itaconate and dimethyl fumarate. *Nat. Commun.* 11 (1), 4938. doi: 10.1038/s41467-020-18764-3

Park, K., Gross, M., Lee, D. H., Holvoet, P., Himes, J. H., Shikany, J. M., et al. (2009). Oxidative stress and insulin resistance: the coronary artery risk development in young adults study. *Diabetes Care* 32 (7), 1302–1307. doi: 10.2337/dc09-0259

Sahoo, S., Meijles, D. N., and Pagano, P. J. (2016). NADPH oxidases: key modulators in aging and age-related cardiovascular diseases? *Clin. Sci. (Lond.)* 130 (5), 317–335. doi: 10.1042/cs20150087

Sattar, N., McInnes, I. B., and McMurray, J. J. V. (2020). Obesity Is a Risk Factor for Severe COVID-19 Infection: Multiple Potential Mechanisms. *Circulation* 142 (1), 4–6. doi: 10.1161/circulationaha.120.047659

To, E. E., Vlahos, R., Luong, R., Halls, M. L., Reading, P. C., King, P. T., et al. (2017). Endosomal NOX2 oxidase exacerbates virus pathogenicity and is a target for antiviral therapy. *Nat. Commun.* 8 (1), 69. doi: 10.1038/s41467-017-00057-x

Violi, F., Oliva, A., Cangemi, R., Ceccarelli, G., Pignatelli, P., Carnevale, R., et al. (2020). Nox2 activation in Covid-19. *Redox Biol.* 36, 101655. doi: 10.1016/j.redox.2020.101655

Wan, Y., Shang, J., Graham, R., Baric, R. S., and Li, F. (2020). Receptor Recognition by the Novel Coronavirus from Wuhan: an Analysis Based on Decade-Long Structural Studies of SARS Coronavirus. *J. Virol.* 94 (7), e00127-20. doi: 10.1128/jvi.00127-20

Wang, K., Gheblawi, M., and Oudit, G. Y. (2020). Angiotensin Converting Enzyme 2: A Double-Edged Sword. *Circulation.* 142, 426–428. doi: 10.1161/circulationaha.120.047049

Yousefian, M., Shakour, N., Hosseinzadeh, H., Hayes, A. W., Hadizadeh, F., and Karimi, G. (2019). The natural phenolic compounds as modulators of NADPH oxidases in hypertension. *Phytomedicine* 55, 200–213. doi: 10.1016/j.phymed.2018.08.002

Zaim, S., Chong, J. H., Sankaranarayanan, V., and Harky, A. (2020). COVID-19 and Multiorgan Response. *Curr. Probl. Cardiol.* 45 (8), 100618. doi: 10.1016/j.cpcardiol.2020.100618

Zheng, J. L., Li, G. Z., Chen, S. Z., Wang, J. J., Olson, J. E., Xia, H. J., et al. (2014). Angiotensin converting enzyme 2/Ang-(1-7)/mas axis protects brain from ischemic injury with a tendency of age-dependence. *CNS Neurosci. Ther.* 20 (5), 452–459. doi: 10.1111/cns.12233

Zhou, F., Yu, T., Du, R., Fan, G., Liu, Y., Liu, Z., et al. (2020). Clinical course and risk factors for mortality of adult inpatients with COVID-19 in Wuhan, China: a retrospective cohort study. *Lancet* 395 (10229), 1054–1062. doi: 10.1016/s0140-6736(20)30566-3

16

SARS-CoV-2 Nucleoprotein Enhances the Infectivity of Lentiviral Spike Particles

Tarun Mishra[1†], M. Sreepadmanabh[1†], Pavitra Ramdas[1], Amit Kumar Sahu[1], Atul Kumar[2] and Ajit Chande[1]*

[1] Molecular Virology Laboratory, Department of Biological Sciences, Indian Institute of Science Education and Research, Bhopal, India, [2] Structural Biology Laboratory, Department of Biological Sciences, Indian Institute of Science Education and Research, Bhopal, India

***Correspondence:**
Ajit Chande
ajitg@iiserb.ac.in

[†]These authors have contributed equally to this work

The establishment of SARS CoV-2 spike-pseudotyped lentiviral (LV) systems has enabled the rapid identification of entry inhibitors and neutralizing agents, alongside allowing for the study of this emerging pathogen in BSL-2 level facilities. While such frameworks recapitulate the cellular entry process in ACE2+ cells, they are largely unable to factor in supplemental contributions by other SARS CoV-2 genes. To address this, we performed an unbiased ORF screen and identified the nucleoprotein (N) as a potent enhancer of spike-pseudotyped LV particle infectivity. We further demonstrate that the spike protein is better enriched in virions when the particles are produced in the presence of N protein. This enrichment of spike renders LV particles more infectious as well as less vulnerable to the neutralizing effects of a human IgG-Fc fused ACE2 microbody. Importantly, this improvement in infectivity is observed with both wild-type spike protein as well as the D614G mutant. Our results hold important implications for the design and interpretation of similar LV pseudotyping-based studies.

Keywords: SARS-CoV-2, virus neutralization, spike lentiviral pseudotyping, nucleocapsid, ACE2-Fc

INTRODUCTION

The ongoing coronavirus disease 2019 (COVID-19) pandemic has provided a strong impetus for studies aimed at discovering and characterizing neutralizing antibodies or small molecule inhibitors targeted against the severe acute respiratory syndrome coronavirus 2 (SARS CoV-2). A major focus of these efforts has been the spike (S) glycoprotein of the virus, which mediates the viral entry into target cells by recognition and binding to the cell-surface receptor angiotensin-converting enzyme 2 (ACE2) (Huang et al., 2020; Sreepadmanabh et al., 2020).

Numerous studies have demonstrated that the spike protein may be employed to generate stably pseudotyped lentiviral, retroviral, and vesicular stomatitis virus particles (Crawford et al., 2020; Johnson et al., 2020; Plescia et al., 2020; Shang et al., 2020; Neerukonda et al., 2021). Given that live SARS CoV-2 is a biosafety level-3 agent, these pseudotyping approaches have greatly facilitated investigations undertaken within lower containment facilities. Importantly, this has also allowed for the screening and characterization of neutralizing antibodies against SARS CoV-2, as these primarily show reactivity against the spike protein (Tandon et al., 2020). Furthermore, such pseudoviruses are deployable as platforms for the large-scale screening of small molecule inhibitors and pharmacological agents which possess therapeutic potential against COVID-19 (Hu et al., 2020).

In this regard, capitalizing on the interaction of the S protein with cellular ACE2, strategies have been reported which utilize chimeric ACE2 fused to the Fc region of human IgG as a potent neutralizing agent against spike-pseudotyped viruses (Lei et al., 2020). This arsenal now includes variations such as mutations to the catalytic region of ACE2 (thereby preventing undesirable side-effects during *in vivo* administration), and modified Fc domain (Lei et al., 2020; Tada et al., 2020). However, a common feature of these studies is that they invariably adopt pseudoviruses which are enveloped by spike, but do not incorporate contributions from any other SARS CoV-2 proteins.

This point is particularly crucial in light of the manifold roles adopted by various proteins of the SARS CoV-2, as has been highlighted in recent interactome studies (Gordon et al., 2020; Khorsand et al., 2020). Indeed, the specific effects of these genes continue to be investigated and represent a wide diversity of specialized functions. Building on this, we hypothesized that specific genes of the SARS CoV-2 could play a key role in enhancing the infectivity of viral particles. To probe this, we undertook an unbiased screen of twenty-four ORFs, NSPs, and structural protein genes of the SARS CoV-2 using spike-pseudotyped lentiviral particles. Our observations implicated the N protein as an enhancer of viral infectivity for both the wild-type as well as the highly infectious D614G mutant of the spike glycoprotein. We further show that this enhancement of infectivity renders the viral particles less sensitive to ACE2-Immunoglobulin chimera-mediated neutralization.

METHODS

Cell Culture

HEK293T (from ECACC) and ACE2-positive HEK293T were cultured in DMEM containing 10% Fetal Bovine Serum (US origin certified serum), 1% penicillin-streptomycin, and 2 mM L-glutamine (complete medium), all obtained from Gibco. The ACE2 expressing stable HEK293T cell line was generated by transduction with lentiviral particles followed by selection with hygromycin until the entire non-transduced population was eliminated. Expression of ACE2 was verified as described below.

Plasmids

The list of plasmids that were used in this study is provided in the **Supplementary Information** (refer to "**Table S1**: List of Plasmids") and are available upon request. pScalps-Luciferase-Zsgreen was generated by cloning a firefly luciferase gene that was PCR amplified with primers incorporating the XhoI/EcoRI restriction sites. The resultant PCR product was digested and ligated in the pScalps Zsgreen plasmid using identical sites and the inserts were confirmed by Sanger sequencing.

ACE2 expressing lentiviral plasmid was generated by amplifying ACE2 encoding gene from the Addgene plasmid #154987 and cloning into a modified pScalps lentiviral vector carrying the hygromycin selection marker. SARS CoV2 encoding genes (detailed below in "**Table S1**: List of Plasmids") were generously provided by the Nevan Krogan Lab in the lentiviral backbone pLV-TetONE, which were further subcloned into a non-viral pcDNA based custom-designed vector for expression of these gene in transient transfection assays. After cloning, each gene of interest preserved the Strep tag in-frame.

Site-directed mutagenesis was employed to generate a D614G mutant version of the SARS CoV-2 spike glycoprotein from the available sequence (Addgene, plasmid catalog #155297). Using a pair of mutation-carrying primers (forward primer: 5'-GGTGCAATTCACGCCCTGGTACAGCAC-3' and reverse primer: 5'-GTGCTGTACCAGGGCGTGAATTGCACC-3'), the plasmid was PCR amplified. The products were processed using a PCR cleanup kit (Macherey-Nagel), digested with Dpn1 (Thermofisher Scientific) overnight, and used to transform competent XL1-blue bacterial strain. Colonies obtained were screened, plasmids were sequenced (using the primer: 5'-TCGGAAGGGACATCGCTGAT-3'), and a final clone matching the desired mutation was obtained. All the oligos for generation/sequencing of the plasmids used in this study were custom synthesized by Sigma-Aldrich.

Virus Production and Quantification

In general, lentiviral particles were produced by calcium phosphate transfection of HEK293T with 8 µg of transfer vector, 6 µg of packaging plasmid (psPAX2) and 2 µg of envelope plasmid (spike-expressing plasmid or pMD2.g). The culture medium was replaced at 16h-post transfection. Lentiviral vector-containing supernatant was collected 48h after transfection and was centrifuged and filtered through 0.22 µm syringe filters. The infectivity assay was performed after normalizing reverse transcriptase (RT) units obtained from an SGPERT assay as described earlier (Pizzato et al., 2009). Briefly, the target cells were infected in quadruplicates (or at least triplicate) with up to 125-fold dilutions and the infectivity was acquired from the dilutions in the linear range as reported previously (Chande et al., 2016). Expression of GFP or Luciferase as a quantitative measure of infection was acquired using SpectraMax-i3X plate reader (Molecular Devices, USA) or High-content imaging platform (CellInsight CX7, ThermoFisher Scientific).

The SARS CoV-2 genes' screen was performed by producing spike pseudotyped lentiviruses from HEK293T cells that were seeded in 12-well plate. Next day cells were transfected with pScalps luciferase Zsgreen (800 ng), psPax2 (600 ng), spike expression plasmid (200 ng), and either vector control or ORF carrying vector (300 ng) by the calcium phosphate method. Culture medium was replaced with fresh medium 16h after transfection. Spike pseudotyped viruses were collected after 48h of transfection. Supernatant collected was centrifuged at 1200xg for 5 min and filtered using a 0.22 µm syringe filter.

Spike pseudotyped viruses were then used to transduce ACE2 expressing HEK293T cells to check the infectivity level by either GFP positive cell count and or Luciferase assay.

To quantify the RT units, 5 µl viruses were lysed in a 5 µl lysis buffer and diluted with a core buffer to make volume 100 µl.

A 10 μl diluted viral lysate was mixed with an equal volume of 2X reaction buffer and the SGPERT assay was performed.

For immunoblotting of proteins incorporated into lentiviral particles, the lentiviral particles-containing supernatant was concentrated on sucrose cushion by ultracentrifugation at 100,000Xg for 2 hours at 4°C (Chande et al., 2016). Viral pellet obtained was resuspended in the Laemmli buffer containing 50mM TCEP as a reducing agent.

Murine Leukemia Virus (MLV)-derived vectors were produced, from HEK293T cells seeded in a 12-well plate format, by transfecting 800 ng of MLV-NCA Zsgreen plasmid with 200 ng of VSV-G envelope or spike glycoprotein encoding plasmid (200ng), either in the presence or absence of N-encoding plasmid (200ng). The reverse transcriptase units were quantified by SGPERT assay and ACE2-positive HEK293T served as target cells. The infection was quantified by counting the GFP positive cells using the SpectraMax-i3X plate reader.

Gene Expression

To check the expression of ACE2 in ACE2-transduced HEK293T cells we isolated the RNA from HEK293T and ACE2-transduced HEK293T by Trizol method. The cDNA was synthesized from 1μg of RNA using oligodT primers obtained from both the cells. To quantify the level of ACE2 expression, RT-PCR was performed using ACE2 specific primers 5'-GGGATCAGA GATCGGAAGAA-3' forward and 5'-AGGAGGTCTGAA CATCATC-3' reverse and GAPDH as control with primers 5'-TGGAGAAGGCTGGGGCTCATTTGCA-3' forward and 5'-CATACCAGGAAATGAGCTTGACAA-3'.

Quantitative real-time (qRT-PCR) for determining the expression of spike glycoprotein both in the absence and presence of N was carried out by isolating the DNA-free RNA from transfected cells as described above, and then processed for qRT-PCR using the spike-specific primers 5'- GCAACG TGACCTGGTTCCAC-3' in forward and 5'- CGATCAGC AGGCTCTGGGTC-3' in reverse.

Luciferase Assay and GFP Cell Count

Luciferase assay was performed in 96-well plates to quantify level of transduction by spike pseudotyped viral particles. Equal numbers of ACE2+ HEK293T cells were seeded in 96-well plates (10,000 cells/well) 24h before transduction and incubated with the various pseudotyped viruses for 48h. Zsgreen (GFP) cell count was first scored using the SpectraMax-i3X system (Molecular Devices). Media was aspirated from each well post-GFP acquisition and cells were lysed by treatment with 100 μl lysis buffer for 20 minutes at room temperature. Luciferase readings were measured using SpectraMax-i3X by injecting 50 μl of substrate buffer in 50 μl of cell lysate in 96-well white plates. Specifics of buffer composition may be found below in the section titled "Buffers and common reaction mixtures".

Western Blotting

For Western blot-based analysis, samples were prepared in a 4X Laemmli buffer and run on either 8%, 12.5%, or 15% tricine gels for electrophoresis depending upon the molecular weight range being detected by this method. Following this, gels were electro blotted on the PVDF membrane (Immobilon-FL, Merck-Millipore). Blocking of membranes was carried out by incubation with either a 5% BSA solution or the proprietary Odyssey Blocking Buffer (LI-COR Biosciences) for one hour, followed by both primary and secondary antibody incubations for one hour each at room temperature, each of which were followed by three washes of five minutes each.

Detection of p24, beta-actin, SARS CoV-2 spike glycoprotein, Strep-tagged SARS CoV-2 genes, and ACE2-IgFc was carried out using mouse anti-p24 (NIH ARP), rabbit anti-beta actin (LI-COR Biosciences, Cat# 926-42210, RRID: AB_1850027), mouse anti-spike (Cat# ZMS1076, Sigma Aldrich), mouse anti-Strep (Qiagen, Cat# 34850), and mouse anti-Histidine (Invitrogen, Cat# MA1-21315), respectively, as primary antibodies. Secondary antibodies used were either IR dye 680 goat anti-mouse, IR dye 800 goat mouse, or IR dye 800 goat anti-rabbit (LI-COR Biosciences Cat# 925-68070, RRID: AB_2651128, and LI-COR Biosciences Cat# 925-32211, RRID: AB_2651127).

Flow Cytometry

HEK293T cells were transfected with either pScalps Luciferase Zsgreen alone or along with N protein. Cells were harvested after 48 hours, fixed in 4% paraformaldehyde, and prepared for flow cytometry after removing the fixative. As a control, HEK293T cells were also processed in a similar manner.

ACE2-IgFc Microbody Constructs

Genomic DNA isolated from HEK293T cells using the Macherey-Nagel Nucleospin kit (#740952.50) was used as a template for PCR amplifying the Fc region of human IgG. The forward primer 5'-CAGCACCTGAACTCCTGGGGGGACCG-3' and reverse primer 5'-CCTTTGGCTTTGGAGAT GGTTTTC-3' was used to amplify the first exon encoding the Fc region. The forward primer 5'-AGGGCAGCCCCGAG AACCACAGGTG-3' and reverse primer 5'-TTTACCCGGAG ACAGGGAGAGGCT-3' was used to amplify the second exon encoding the Fc region. Both fragments were individually amplified further using the combination of forward and reverse primers as 5'-GAAAACCATCTCCAAAGCCAAAGGGCAGCC CCGAGAACCACAGGTG-'3' and 5'-TATATATTCTAGAT TAATGGTGATGGTGATGATGGCCGCCTTTACCCGG AGACAGGGA-3' for the first exon's amplicon and 5'-ATATATCTCGAGGACAAAACTCACACATGCCCACCGT GCCCAGCACCTGAACTCCTG-3' and 5'-CCTTTGGCT TTGGAGATGGTTTTC-3' for the second exon's amplicon, respectively. Finally, both these fragments were combined using the forward primer 5'-ATATATCTCGAGGAC AAAACTCACACATGCCCACCGTGCCCAGCACCTG AACTCCTG-3' and reverse primer 5'-TATATATTCTAGA TTAATGGTGATGGTGATGATGGCCGCCTTTACCCGG AGACAGGGA-3' to generate the final Fc fragment, which was cloned into pTZ57R.

Addgene (#154987) was used as template for ACE2 amplification, using the forward primer 5'-GAACAAGAATT CTTTTGTGGGA-3' and reverse primer 5'-TTTGTCCT CGAGGGAAACAGGGGGCTGGTTAG-3' a 421 bp fragment of the same was amplified and cloned into pTZ57R.

Using an EcoRI/XhoI digestion, the ACE2 fragment was combined upstream of the Fc, and the combined fragment was ligated into the ACE2 containing plasmid using a EcoRI/XbaI digestion to yield the final ACE2-IgFc construct. The construct was verified with Sanger sequencing (refer to "**Table S2**: Sequences of ACE2-IgFc").

Biochemical Characterization of ACE2-IgFc Microbody

HEK293T cells were transfected with the plasmid encoding ACE2-IgFc (5 µg plasmid in a 35 mm dish). As a control, 5 µg of pcDNA3.1BS(-) was also transfected. Media was changed twelve hours post-transfection and fresh DMEM (without FBS) was added to the dishes. Culture media was collected both 48- and 72-hours post-transfection, and samples were prepared in either 8% or 2% SDS-containing 4X Laemmli buffer (with and without TCEP added, respectively) for SDS-PAGE. 8% tricine gels were run, and analyzed using Western Blotting. The amount of ACE2 present in the supernatant was determined by comparison with standard concentrations of pure BSA as ascertained by band density analysis following silver staining of SDS-PAGE gels. For Western Blotting, the proteins were transferred to a PVDF membrane, blocked in a 5% BSA solution in TBS, and primary mouse-derived anti-Histidine antibodies were incubated with the blot in a 1:4000 dilution, followed by goat-derived anti-mouse antibodies in a 1:5000 dilution.

Pull-Down Assay Using ACE2-IgFc

Thirty microliters of protein-G Dynabeads (Thermofisher Scientific Cat #10003D) were first equilibrated by washing with 10% FBS-containing DMEM. Following this, these were incubated with gentle mixing by inversion for 15 minutes with 100 µl of ACE2-IgFc containing supernatant (equivalent of 10 µg/ml). This was split into three equal fractions of 10 µl each. The beads-containing mixtures then were immobilized on a magnetic rack, supernatant was aspirated off, and replaced with 100 µl (10mU equivalent/mL RT) of culture supernatant carrying either bald viruses or viruses pseudotyped with VSV-G or Spike glycoproteins. Mixing was carried out for a period of 15 minutes, following which these were placed back on the magnetic rack, supernatant was aspirated, and the beads washed twice with SGPERT Core Buffer - first with 500 µl and then with 100 µl. Finally, 20 µl of RT Lysis Buffer was added and the reaction was incubated at room temperature. Following this, the reaction was 10-fold diluted using core buffer. The resulting supernatant was collected after immobilizing the beads and processed for an SGPERT Assay.

Neutralization Assay

To quantify the amount of ACE2-IgFc required to inhibit the infection in ACE2+ HEK293T cells, we treated 100 µl of spike pseudotyped virus (normalized to RT units) with a variable amount of ACE2-IgFc diluted in the growth medium. The mixture was incubated for fifteen minutes at room temperature, following which each sample was used to transduce ACE2+ HEK293T cells seeded in 96-well plates. Luciferase assay was performed 48 hours post-transduction, with readings acquired using the SpectraMax-i3X plate reader.

Buffers and Common Reaction Mixtures

TBS (Tris-Buffered Saline) was prepared by mixing a 500 mM solution of Tris (pH 7.4) with water and NaCl (up to a final concentration of 1500 mM). For making TBS-T, Tween-20 (Sigma Aldrich) was added to TBS up to a final concentration of 0.01%.

For making 4X Laemmli buffer, components were mixed to achieve the final concentrations as follows: 200 mM Tris (pH 6.8), 40% glycerol (Sigma Aldrich), 50 mM Tris(2-carboxyethyl) phosphine (TCEP) (Thermo Scientific), 8% SDS (Sigma Aldrich), and water up to 50 ml. Non-reducing buffer conditions were achieved by removing TCEP from the above formula and decreasing the amount of SDS added to a final concentration of 2%.

A proprietary Odyssey Buffer for blocking of membranes and dilution of antibody stocks was used as supplied (LI-COR Biosciences).

Luciferase assay buffers were prepared as a lysis buffer and substrate buffer. Lysis buffer required a final concentration of components as 1% Triton X-100 (Sigma Aldrich), 25 mM Tricine (VWR), 15 mM of potassium phosphate (at pH 7.,8), 15 mM MgSO, 4 mM EGTA, and 1 mM DTT, with water to make up the solution. Substrate buffer required further addition of 1 mM DTT (VWR Scientific), 1 mM ATP (Sigma Aldrich), and 0.2 mM D-Luciferin (Cayman) to the aforementioned lysis buffer. All fine chemicals were procured from Sigma-Aldrich unless otherwise indicated.

Harvesting of cell samples for Western blotting was carried out using the RIPA lysis buffer (Lysis Buffer, 2017).

Software and Statistical Analysis

All graphs were generated using GraphPad Prism (version 9.0). Statistical analysis was carried out using the in-built algorithms bundled with the software. Two-tailed unpaired t-test was used to calculate the statistical significance shown for all pairwise comparisons, where **** = $p < 0.0001$, *** = $p < 0.001$, ** = $p < 0.01$, and * = $p < 0.05$. Specific portions of images were produced using Biorender. Band intensities of Western blots were calculated using the in-built analytical tools from the Image Studio Lite Ver. 5.2 (LI-COR Biosciences).

RESULTS

A custom-designed transfer vector (**Figure 1A**), termed pScalps Luciferase-Zsgreen, as well an ACE2-expressing HEK293T cell line (**Figure 1B**) were generated for this study. To investigate the effect of various SARS CoV-2 genes on viral infectivity, we undertook an unbiased screen, as outlined by the schematic in **Figure 1C**. Briefly, HEK293T producer cells were transfected with plasmids encoding the codon-optimized S protein (with a nineteen amino-acid deletion at the C terminal), the packaging plasmid psPAX2, and the pScalps Luciferase-Zsgreen reporter plasmid. Alongside this, each one of the twenty-four SARS CoV-2 genes was separately co-transfected with the above.

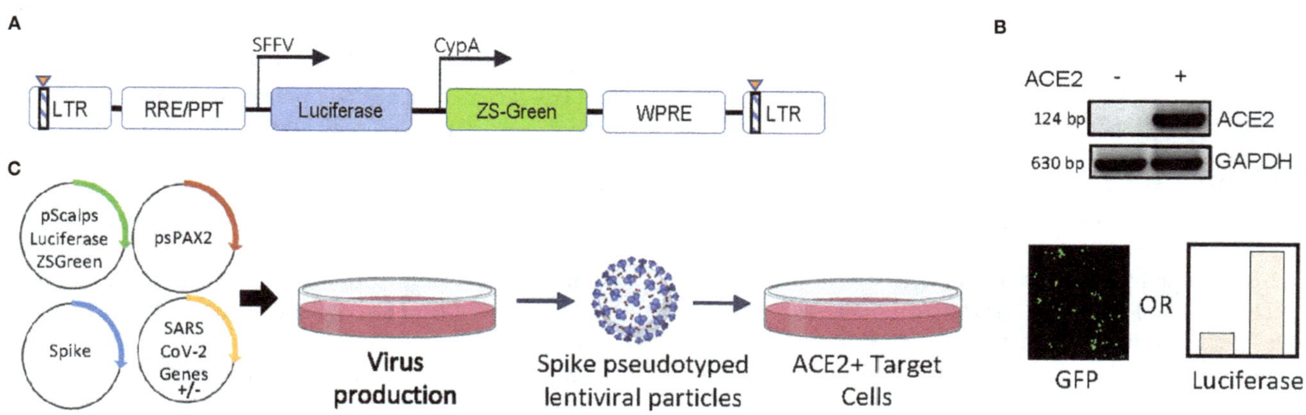

FIGURE 1 | Experimental setup and constructs. **(A)** Schematic representation of the pScalps Luciferase Zsgreen lentiviral reporter construct. **(B)** ACE2 expression from the hygromycin selected HEK293T cell line transduced with a ACE2 gene carrying lentiviral vector. **(C)** Schematic depiction of the SARS CoV-2 genes' screen. Transfection with an empty vector served as control. Readout from the screen was obtained in the form of firefly luciferase activity or GFP-positive cell count.

ACE2-expressing HEK293T cells were transduced with viruses produced in the presence of indicated SARS CoV-2 genes, and the extent of infectivity was gauged as a measure of both GFP-positive cell count and firefly luciferase activity 48 hours post-infection (**Figure 2A**). Expression of all the SARS CoV-2 genes was verified (**Supplementary Figure 1A**) and the effect of this expression was also checked on the lentiviral capsid levels by western blotting from the producer cell lysates (**Figure 2B**). While non-uniform expression pattern of a minor subset of these genes could be a limitation, we identified the nucleocapsid (N) protein as a prominent enhancer of spike-pseudovirus infectivity. We scored the effects on infectivity in conditions where the co-expression of SARS CoV-2 genes increased the infectivity without an apparent effect on the lentiviral capsid levels (**Figure 2B**). The particle infectivity enhancement by N was also discernible with a GFP reporter in the ACE2-postive target cells suggesting this assay reliably measures transduction events (**Figure 2C**). Additional control experiments were performed to exclude the influence of N protein on the reporters (**Figures 2D, E**) which helped determine that there is no significant effect of the N protein on either of these. Additionally, the infectivity-enhancement effect of N was not observed in the case of VSV-G pseudotyped lentiviral particles (**Supplementary Figure 1B**). We also employed an MLV vector to determine whether the observed phenotype was specific to HIV-1 core-based particles. While VSV-G pseudotyped MLV virions did not show any N-dependent infectivity enhancement, spike-MLV pseudovirions did mirror the enhancement in infectivity observed with the lentiviral particles (**Figure 2F** and **Supplementary Figure 1C**). Further, based on recent reports of a relatively more infectious D614G spike glycoprotein variant (Zhang et al., 2020), we decided to screen the same to assess the effect of N protein. Cellular expression of the mutant protein at levels comparable with the wild-type spike was confirmed by Western blotting (**Supplementary Figure 1D**). Consistent with previous reports, the mutant strain produced pseudoviruses which were more infectious as compared to wild-type spike-pseudovirions (**Figure 2G** and **Supplementary Figure 1E**). On top of this, inclusion of the N protein during particle production allowed for an even higher extent of infectivity, which reaffirmed its role in a manner consistent with the above results. Cumulatively, these results appear to implicate the viral N protein as an intrinsic enhancer of lentiviral spike-pseudotyped particle infectivity.

Next, we asked if such an enhancement of particle infectivity would impact the ability of neutralizing agents to block these particles from infecting host cells. Capitalizing on the interaction of the S protein with cellular ACE2, we generated a SARS CoV-2 entry receptor-based synthetic microbody consisting of a soluble ACE2 domain fused with the Fc region of human IgG (**Figure 3A**), which also carried a C-terminal 6XHistidine tag. Extracellular expression, as well as the ability of ACE2-IgFc to dimerize under the experimental conditions that retained disulphide linkage, were detected by Western blotting (**Figure 3B**). These experiments also confirmed the presence of an intact Histidine tag. Furthermore, we tested the specific interaction of the ACE2-IgFc with spike-pseudotyped LV particles by a pull-down experiment wherein the on-bead capture of viral particles using protein G-bound ACE2-IgFc resulted in a ~10,000-fold enrichment of spike pseudotyped viruses over VSV-G pseudotyped or non-enveloped (bald) lentiviral particles (**Figure 3C**). This also suggests that Fc configuration remained intact after fusion with ACE2 thereby facilitating the immobilization of the microbody on the protein G magnetic beads for virion capture. In sum, these results established that the ACE2-IgFc molecule is stably expressed and demonstrates a high affinity specifically towards the spike-laden particles.

Following this, we wished to ascertain the relative titre of ACE2-IgFc required to effectively restrict the infection of ACE2+ target cells, under the influence of the N protein. Briefly, lentiviral particles pseudotyped with spike (with and without co-transfection with N) or bald particles lacking envelope were

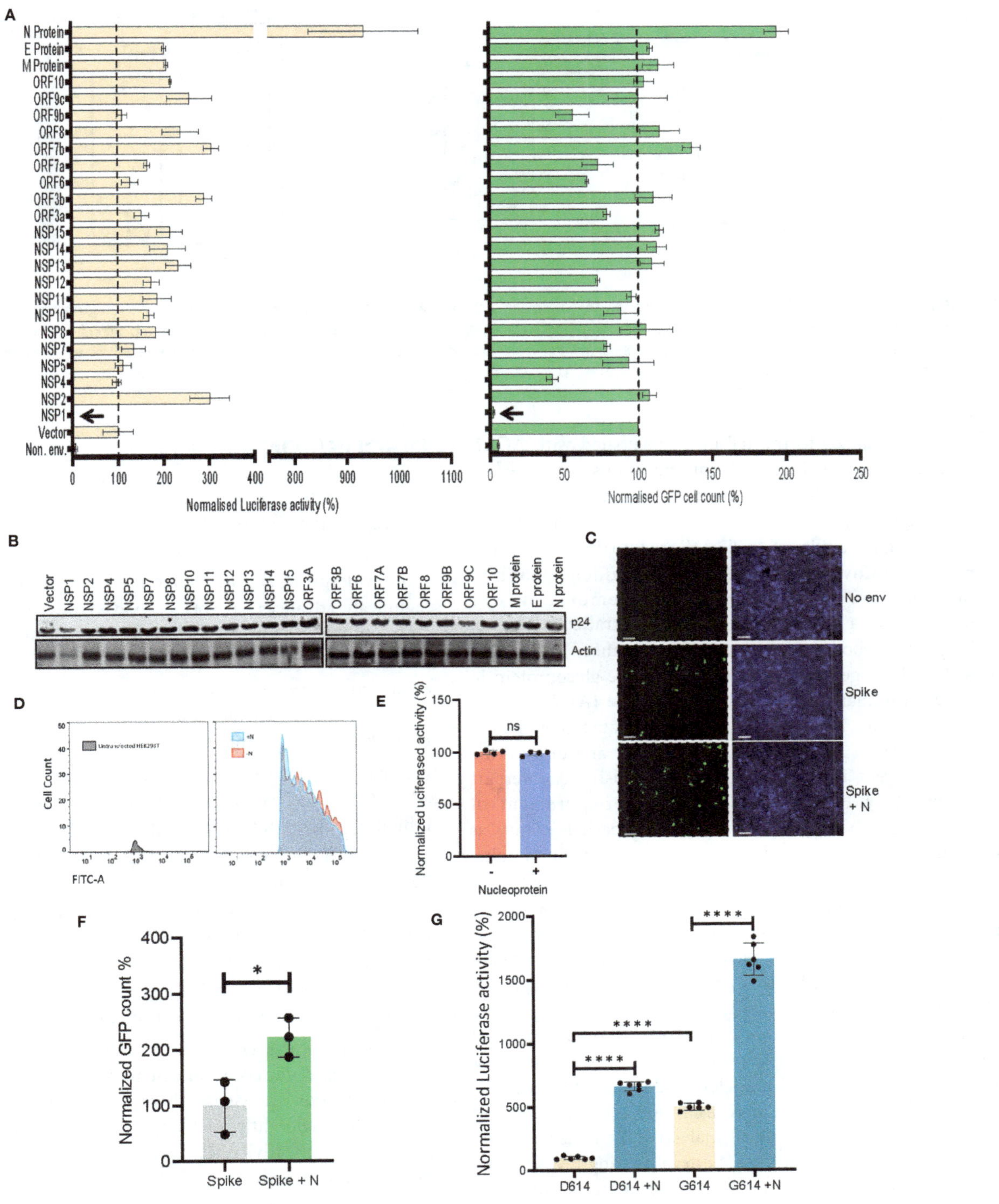

FIGURE 2 | SARS CoV-2's N protein enhances retroviral spike-pseudotyped particle infectivity. **(A)**. Results from the screen of SARS CoV-2 genes, either by quantifying luciferase activity (left panel) or GFP positive cell count (right panel). Vector normalized values for both readout methods has been shown, such as to indicate the percentage change relative to the baseline (indicated by the dotted line). Background signal levels are indicated by the non-enveloped (Non. env.) condition. n=4 ± SD. **(B)** p24 levels from the virus-producing cells for all the SARS CoV-2 genes were detected by Western blotting. Actin served as loading control. **(C)** Microscopy images for the infected cells with indicated conditions (scale 100 µm). **(D)** Representative flow cytometric analysis of the effect of N protein on Zsgreen expression, using populations transfected with either the reporter plasmid alone (red fraction) or along with the N protein (cyan fraction). **(E)** Quantification of the luciferase gene expression from the pScalps Luciferase Zsgreen reporter plasmid with and without the presence of N protein. n=4 ± SD. **(F)** Infectivity of MLV vector pseudotyped with the spike glycoprotein for both N-exclusive and N-inclusive conditions, normalized to the former. n=3 ± SD **(G)** Comparison between the infectivity of both wild-type spike and the D614G mutant, with and without N protein co-transfection, normalized to the wild-type spike-only condition n=6 ± SD. *$p < 0.05$; ****$p < 0.0001$; NS, Non significant.

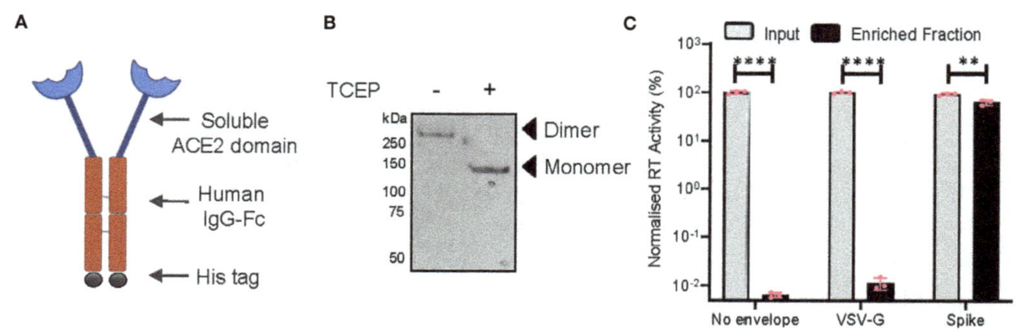

FIGURE 3 | Characterization of the ACE2-IgFc microbody. **(A)** Schematic of the ACE2-IgFc neutralizing microbody. **(B)** Effect of a reducing agent (TCEP) on the migration of ACE2-IgFc on the gel. Anti-His antibody indicating monomeric vs dimeric states of the protein visualized by western blotting from the cell culture supernatant. **(C)** Protein G-bound ACE2-IgFC and the enrichment of virus particles. The RT activity of the input VSV-G or Spike particles was normalized to the non-enveloped particles, set to 100%. n=3 ± SD. **p < 0.01; ****p < 0.0001.

generated, normalized to the RT units, incubated with ACE2-IgFc according to the indicated concentrations, and used to transduce ACE2+ HEK293T target cells. Luciferase activity assay, as a quantitative and sensitive indicator of transduction events, revealed the ability of ACE2-IgFc to impair the infectivity of spike pseudoviruses in a dose-dependent manner. Furthermore, results obtained herein demonstrate the requirement for a significantly higher neutralizing titre of ACE2-IgFc microbodies in the case of N-enhanced particles as opposed to those generated solely by the spike glycoprotein in order to elicit similar levels of inhibition (**Figure 4A**). Additional experiments using D614G mutant also indicated that the N-inclusive particles would require a higher amount of the neutralizing agent in comparison to N-exclusive counterpart (**Supplementary Figure 1F**). The higher requirement of neutralizing agent was not a result of higher particle counts as the inoculum was normalised to the reverse transcriptase units.

To better comprehend these observations, we envisaged a modification of virus particles by N that plausibly impacted the virion quality, rather than the quantity. To better understand this, we asked if N protein directly impacted the spike protein itself in order to effect infectivity enhancement. Accordingly, we first analyzed the effect of N on spike at the mRNA level using both quantitative RT-PCR and semiquantitative gel-based methods and found no significant upregulation of the same (**Figure 4B**). Next, the viral particles produced under indicated conditions were pelleted on a sucrose cushion as described earlier (Chande et al., 2016). Biochemical analysis of the virus pellet and the corresponding cell lysates by Western blotting revealed that N improved the steady-state levels of spike in the producer cell lysates. The enhancement of spike signal was noticeably more prominent from the virions (**Figures 4C, D**). The augmentary effects of N appear to be specific in nature, given that exclusively lentiviral components do not show any apparent changes in expression. Altogether, these experiments indicated that N protein likely promoted the incorporation and retainment of spike protein in the virions, thereby improving the particle quality and its infectivity.

DISCUSSION

Considering the technical difficulties associated with studying live, replication-competent native SARS CoV-2, the adoption of lentiviral or retroviral pseudotyping-based systems has enabled a more widespread and accessible investigation of this pathogen. Significant advances have been achieved in recent times, ranging from optimization of pseudotyping protocols to the application of these for screening entry inhibitors (Hu et al., 2020). The roles of structural proteins such as M, E, and N in assisting viral assembly and particle formation have also been explored (Plescia et al., 2020). Along similar lines, leading studies have deciphered the manifold cellular associations and interactions of various SARS CoV-2 genes, in processes as diverse as host translation inhibition, disruption of splicing, immune evasion, and protein trafficking, among others (Banerjee et al., 2020; Schubert et al., 2020; Xia et al., 2020; Flower et al., 2021).

In the present study, we have evaluated the potential of twenty-four SARS CoV-2 genes to elicit superior infectivity levels as compared to what may be achieved by mere pseudotyping with the spike glycoprotein. Chief among these has been the nucleocapsid (N) protein. While a previous study has established the crucial role played by N in viral genome processing and nucleocapsid assembly (Carlson et al., 2020), to the best of our knowledge there have been no prior reports specifically highlighting its ability to elevate lentiviral spike pseudovirus infectivity. It bears mentioning that similar to existent reports (Min et al., 2020; Schubert et al., 2020; Thoms et al., 2020; Lapointe et al., 2021; Zhang et al., 2021), the Nsp1 protein presumably exerts a detrimental effect on the host cell's protein translation, as indicated by the almost imperceptible extent of infectivity observed in its case (**Figure 2A**).

Our assessment of pseudoviruses generated from both N-exclusive and N-inclusive backgrounds directly implicates N as a potent enhancer of virion quality and infectivity, an effect which extends over both the wild-type spike protein as well as the

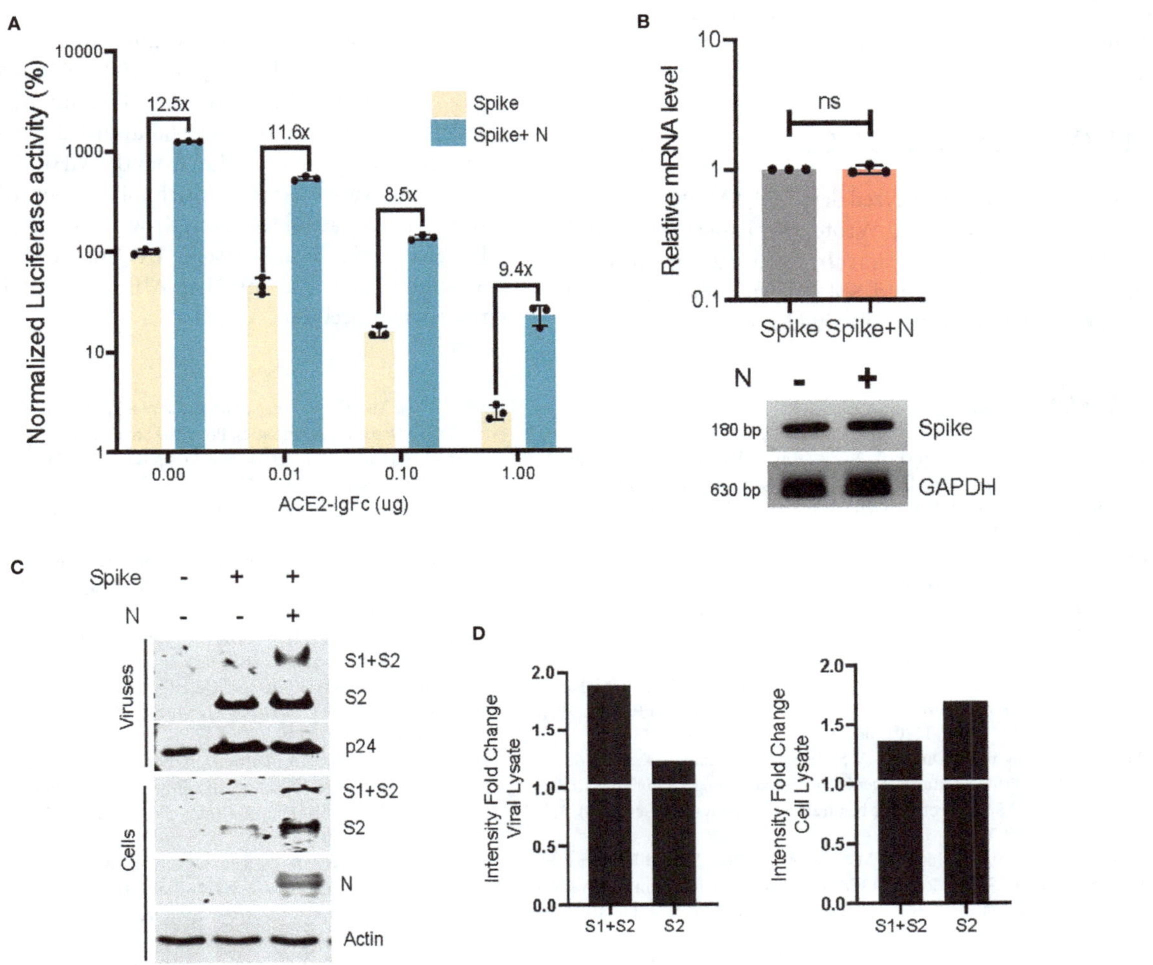

FIGURE 4 | Neutralizing effects of ACE2-IgFC on the N-enhanced spike lentiviral particles and biochemical characterization of the virions **(A)** Neutralization assay using ACE2-IgFc pre-treated lentiviral particles with indicated amount of ACE2-IgFC (on the x-axis) for the lentiviral particles produced in the presence of indicated genes. The particles were normalized to the reverse transcriptase units obtained from the SGPERT assay. Luciferase activity obtained from non-enveloped particle transduction was considered as baseline, and the data represented has been normalized to the spike-only condition without the addition of ACE2-IgFc. The lines represent extent of residual infectivity (expressed as x-fold), post-treatment of ACE2-IgFc, with respect to N-exclusive particles n=3 ± SD. **(B)** RT-PCR analysis of the mRNA fraction from cells transfected with either spike or spike + N protein. Both quantitative RT-PCR and representative semi-quantitative PCR results are shown. n=3 ± SD. **(C)** Biochemical analysis of the virus particles and the corresponding cell lysates. The viral proteins were visualized by western blotting using antibodies raised against S2 domain of SARS CoV2 spike. **(D)** Densitometric analysis of the band intensities were obtained by normalizing the S1+S2 and S2 bands to either the respective p24 levels for viral lysate or the Actin levels for cell lysate and calculating the fold change of the normalized intensities of bands in the N-inclusive condition to the spike-only condition. The N protein and p24 were detected using Anti-Strep tag and anti-p24 antibody respectively. Actin served as loading control. n=3, representative blots are shown. NS, Non significant.

D614G mutant. Similar to the proposed infectivity enhancing mechanism for the D614G variant, which relies on reduced S1 shedding and increased spike protein retainment in virions (Zhang et al., 2020), the N-dependent enrichment of spike glycoprotein within viral fractions we demonstrated lends support to this hypothesis. The identification of N in this particular role may be a telling example of how the SARS CoV-2 adopts a host of varied and as-yet incompletely explored strategies to drive its pathogenesis. Future extensions of this work may gain clinically relevant insights by including sera from vaccinated individuals or convalescent plasma from recovered patients to assess the neutralizing potential of these against similarly modified spike pseudoviral systems.

In sum, our results underscore the importance of factoring in additional contributions from the other viral genes while undertaking lentiviral vector pseudotyping with the spike glycoprotein of the SARS CoV-2. While existing studies have managed to develop and validate platforms for the screening of neutralizing antibodies and inhibitory chemical compounds, we believe that our results highlight the necessity of incorporating additional genetic elements which have been shown to boost viral infectivity. Furthermore, putative therapeutic candidates currently being scrutinized in various clinical studies would benefit from lentiviral pseudotyping assays that incorporate additional virion components during the large-scale screening stage.

AUTHOR CONTRIBUTIONS

Performed research and analyzed data: TM, SM, PR, AS, and AC. Contributed reagents: AK. Wrote the paper: AC and SM. Conceived, designed research, and supervision: AC. Contributed equally: TM and SM. All authors contributed to the article and approved the submitted version.

ACKNOWLEDGMENTS

This work was supported by the intramural funds, a Department of Biotechnology (DBT) grant (BT/PR26013/GET/119/191/2017), and the Wellcome Trust/DBT India Alliance Fellowship [grant number IA/I/18/2/504006 awarded to AC]. TM and PR are supported by a fellowship from the MHRD. AC is a recipient of the Innovative Young Biotechnologist Award from the DBT. Authors are grateful to Nevan Krogan, Massimo Pizzato, Jeremy Luban, Sonja Best, Raffaele De Francesco, Didier Trono, Sunando Datta, and the NIH AIDS Reagent Program for the reagents and cell line.

REFERENCES

Banerjee, A. K., Blanco, M. R., Bruce, E. A., Honson, D. D., Chen, L. M., Chow, A., et al. (2020). SARS-Cov-2 Disrupts Splicing, Translation, and Protein Trafficking to Suppress Host Defenses. *Cell* 183, 1325–1339.e21. doi: 10.1016/j.cell.2020.10.004

Carlson, C. R., Asfaha, J. B., Ghent, C. M., Howard, C. J., Hartooni, N., Safari, M., et al. (2020). Phosphoregulation of Phase Separation by the SARS-Cov-2 N Protein Suggests a Biophysical Basis for its Dual Functions. *Mol. Cell* 80, 1092–1103.e4. doi: 10.1016/j.molcel.2020.11.025

Chande, A., Cuccurullo, E. C., Rosa, A., Ziglio, S., Carpenter, S., and Pizzato, M. (2016). S2 From Equine Infectious Anemia Virus is an Infectivity Factor Which Counteracts the Retroviral Inhibitors SERINC5 and SERINC3. *Proc. Natl. Acad. Sci.* 113, 13197–13202. doi: 10.1073/pnas.1612044113

Crawford, K. H. D., Eguia, R, Dingens, A. S., Loes, A. N., Malone, K. D., Wolf, C. R., et al. (2020). Protocol and Reagents for Pseudotyping Lentiviral Particles With SARS-CoV-2 Spike Protein for Neutralization Assays. *Viruses* 12 (5), 513. doi: 10.3390/v12050513

Flower, T. G., Buffalo, C. Z., Hooy, R. M., Allaire, M., Ren, X., and Hurley, J. H. (2021). Structure of SARS-CoV-2 ORF8, a Rapidly Evolving Immune Evasion Protein. *Proc. Natl. Acad. Sci. U. S. A.* 118 (2), e2021785118. doi: 10.1073/pnas.2021785118

Gordon, D. E., Jang, G. M., Bouhaddou, M., Xu, J., Obernier, K., White, K. M., et al (2020). A SARS-CoV-2 Protein Interaction Map Reveals Targets for Drug Repurposing. *Nature* 583, 459–468. doi: 10.1038/s41586-020-2286-9

Huang, Y., Yang, C., Xu, X., Xu, W., and Liu, S. (2020). Structural and Functional Properties of SARS-CoV-2 Spike Protein: Potential Antivirus Drug Development for COVID-19. *Acta Pharmacol. Sin.* 41, 1141–1149. doi: 10.1038/s41401-020-0485-4

Hu, J., Gao, Q., He, C., Huang, A., Tang, N., and Wang, K. (2020). Development of Cell-Based Pseudovirus Entry Assay to Identify Potential Viral Entry Inhibitors and Neutralizing Antibodies Against SARS-Cov-2. *Genes Dis.* 7, 551–557. doi: 10.1016/j.gendis.2020.07.006

Johnson, M. C., Lyddon, T. D, Suarez, R., Salcedo, B., LePique, M., Graham, M., et al. (2020). Optimized Pseudotyping Conditions for the SARS-COV-2 Spike Glycoprotein. *J. Virol.* 94 (21), e01062–20. doi: 10.1128/JVI.01062-20

Khorsand, B., Savadi, A., and Naghibzadeh, M. (2020). Sars-CoV-2-human Protein-Protein Interaction Network. *Inform. Med. Unlocked* 20, 100413. doi: 10.1016/j.imu.2020.100413

Lapointe, C. P., Grosely, R., Johnson, A. G., Wang, J., Fernández, I. S., and Puglisi, J. D. (2021). Dynamic Competition Between SARS-CoV-2 NSP1 and mRNA on the Human Ribosome Inhibits Translation Initiation. *Proc. Natl. Acad. Sci. U. S. A.* 118 (6), e2017715118 doi: 10.1073/pnas.2017715118.

Lei, C., Qian, K., Li, T., Zhang, S., Fu, W., Ding, M., et al. (2020). Neutralization of SARS-CoV-2 Spike Pseudotyped Virus by Recombinant ACE2-Ig. *Nat. Commun.* 11, 2070. doi: 10.1038/s41467-020-16048-4

Lysis Buffer, R. I. P. A. (2017). RIPA Lysis Buffer. *Cold Spring Harb. Protoc.* 2017, pdb.rec101428 doi: 10.1101/pdb.rec101428.

Min, Y.-Q., Mo, Q., Wang, J., Deng, F., Wang, H., and Ning, Y. J. (2020). Sars-CoV-2 Nsp1: Bioinformatics, Potential Structural and Functional Features, and Implications for Drug/Vaccine Designs. *Front. Microbiol.* 11, 587317. doi: 10.3389/fmicb.2020.587317

Neerukonda, S. N., Vassell, R., Herrup, R., Liu, S., Wang, T., Takeda, K., et al. (2021). Establishment of a Well-Characterized SARS-CoV-2 Lentiviral Pseudovirus Neutralization Assay Using 293T Cells With Stable Expression of ACE2 and TMPRSS2. *PloS One* 16, e0248348. doi: 10.1371/journal.pone.0248348

Pizzato, M., Erlwein, O., Bonsall, D., Kaye, S., Muir, D., and McClure, M. O. (2009). A One-Step SYBR Green I-based Product-Enhanced Reverse Transcriptase Assay for the Quantitation of Retroviruses in Cell Culture Supernatants. *J. Virol. Methods* 156 (1-2), 1–7 doi: 10.1016/j.jviromet.2008.10.012

Plescia, C. B., David, E. A., Patra, D., Sengupta, R., Amiar, S., Su, Y., et al. (2020). SARS-CoV-2 Viral Budding and Entry can be Modeled Using BSL-2 Level Virus-Like Particles. *J. Biol. Chem.* 296, 100103. doi: 10.1074/jbc.RA120.016148

Schubert, K., Karousis, E. D., Luo, C., Scaiola, A., Echeverria, B., Gurzeler, L. A., et al. (2020). SARS-Cov-2 Nsp1 Binds the Ribosomal mRNA Channel to Inhibit Translation. *Nat. Struct. Mol. Biol.* 27, 959–966. doi: 10.1038/s41594-020-0511-8

Shang, J., Wan, Y., Ye, G., Geng, Q., Auerbach, A., Li, F., et al. (2020). Cell Entry Mechanisms of SARS-Cov-2. *Proc. Natl. Acad. Sci.* 117, 11727–11734. doi: 10.1073/pnas.2003138117

Sreepadmanabh, M., Sahu, A. K., and Chande, A. (2020). Covid-19: Advances in Diagnostic Tools, Treatment Strategies, and Vaccine Development. *J. Biosci.* 45, 148. doi: 10.1007/s12038-020-00114-6

Tada, T., Fan, C., Chen, J. S., Kaur, R., Stapleford, K. A., Gristick, H., et al. (2020). An ACE2 Microbody Containing a Single Immunoglobulin Fc Domain Is a Potent Inhibitor of SARS-Cov-2. *Cell Rep.* 33, 108528. doi: 10.1016/j.celrep.2020.108528

Tandon, R., Mitra, D., Sharma, P., McCandless, M. G., Stray, S. J., Bates, J. T., et al. (2020). Effective Screening of SARS-CoV-2 Neutralizing Antibodies in Patient Serum Using Lentivirus Particles Pseudotyped With SARS-CoV-2 Spike Glycoprotein. *Sci. Rep.* 10, 19076. doi: 10.1038/s41598-020-76135-w

Thoms, M., Buschauer, R., Ameismeier, M., Koepke, L., Denk, T., Hirschenberger, M., et al. (2020). Structural Basis for Translational Shutdown and Immune Evasion by the Nsp1 Protein of SARS-Cov-2. *Science* 369, 1249–1255. doi: 10.1126/science.abc8665

Xia, H., Cao, Z., Xie, X., Zhang, X., Chen, J. Y., Wang, H., et al. (2020). Evasion of Type I Interferon by SARS-Cov-2. *Cell Rep.* 33, 108234. doi: 10.1016/j.celrep.2020.108234

Zhang, L., Jackson, C. E., Mou, H., Ojha, A., Peng, H., Quinlan, B. D., et al. (2020). Sars-CoV-2 Spike-Protein D614G Mutation Increases Virion Spike Density and Infectivity. *Nat Commun.* 11, 6013. doi: 10.1038/s41467-020-19808-4

Zhang, K., Miorin, L., Makio, T., Dehghan, I., Gao, S., Xie, Y., et al. (2021). Nsp1 Protein of SARS-CoV-2 Disrupts the mRNA Export Machinery to Inhibit Host Gene Expression. *Sci. Adv.* 7, eabe7386. doi: 10.1126/sciadv.abe7386

17

A Saliva-Based RNA Extraction-Free Workflow Integrated with Cas13a for SARS-CoV-2 Detection

Iqbal Azmi[1†], Md Imam Faizan[1†], Rohit Kumar[2], Siddharth Raj Yadav[2], Nisha Chaudhary[1], Deepak Kumar Singh[1], Ruchika Butola[3], Aryan Ganotra[4], Gopal Datt Joshi[5], Gagan Deep Jhingan[6], Jawed Iqbal[1], Mohan C. Joshi[1*] and Tanveer Ahmad[1*]*

[1] *Multidisciplinary Centre for Advanced Research & Studies, Jamia Millia Islamia, New Delhi, India,* [2] *Department of Pulmonary Medicine and Sleep Disorders, Vardhman Mahavir Medical College, Safdarjung Hospital, New Delhi, India,* [3] *360 Diagnostic and Health Services, Noida, India,* [4] *Department of Computer Science & Engineering, Delhi Technological University, Delhi, India,* [5] *Noodle Analytics Pvt Ltd., Bangalore, India,* [6] *Valerian Chem Pvt. Ltd., New Delhi, India*

***Correspondence:**
Tanveer Ahmad
tahmad7@jmi.ac.in
Mohan C. Joshi
mjoshi@jmi.ac.in
Jawed Iqbal
jiqbal1@jmi.ac.in

†These authors have contributed equally to this work

A major bottleneck in scaling-up COVID-19 testing is the need for sophisticated instruments and well-trained healthcare professionals, which are already overwhelmed due to the pandemic. Moreover, the high-sensitive SARS-CoV-2 diagnostics are contingent on an RNA extraction step, which, in turn, is restricted by constraints in the supply chain. Here, we present CASSPIT (**C**as13 **A**ssisted **S**aliva-based & **S**martphone **I**ntegrated **T**esting), which will allow direct use of saliva samples without the need for an extra RNA extraction step for SARS-CoV-2 detection. CASSPIT utilizes CRISPR-Cas13a based SARS-CoV-2 RNA detection, and lateral-flow assay (LFA) readout of the test results. The sample preparation workflow includes an optimized chemical treatment and heat inactivation method, which, when applied to COVID-19 clinical samples, showed a 97% positive agreement with the RNA extraction method. With CASSPIT, LFA based visual limit of detection (LoD) for a given SARS-CoV-2 RNA spiked into the saliva samples was ~200 copies; image analysis-based quantification further improved the analytical sensitivity to ~100 copies. Upon validation of clinical sensitivity on RNA extraction-free saliva samples (n = 76), a 98% agreement between the lateral-flow readout and RT-qPCR data was found (Ct<35). To enable user-friendly test results with provision for data storage and online consultation, we subsequently integrated lateral-flow strips with a smartphone application. We believe CASSPIT will eliminate our reliance on RT-qPCR by providing comparable sensitivity and will be a step toward establishing nucleic acid-based point-of-care (POC) testing for COVID-19.

Keywords: COVID-19, Crispr-Cas13a, saliva, SARS-CoV-2, CRISPR Diagnostics

---

Abbreviations: CDC, Centers for Disease Control; COVID-19, Coronavirus Disease 2019; CRISPR, Clustered regularly Interspaced Short Palindromic Repeats; DETECTR, DNA Endonuclease Targeted CRISPR Trans Reporter; LAMP, Loop-mediated isothermal amplification; LFA, Lateral Flow Assay; NAC, N-acetyl Cysteine; PCR, Polymerase Chain Reaction; PK, Proteinase K; POC, Point of Care; RPA, Recombinase Polymerase Amplification; RT-LAMP, Reverse Transcription Recombinase Polymerase Amplification; RT-RPA, Reverse Transcription Loop-mediated isothermal amplification; RT-qPCR, quantitative Reverse Transcription Polymerase Chain Reaction; SARS-CoV-2, Severe acute respiratory syndrome coronavirus 2; SHERLOCK, Specific High-sensitivity Enzymatic Reporter un-LOCKing; US FDA, United States Food and Drug Administration.

INTRODUCTION

Multi-step RNA extraction is a bottleneck that impedes mass testing for COVID-19. In this direction, RNA extraction-free assays are more suitable, which also provide a practical solution to develop point-of-care (POC) devices for genetic testing (Kriegova et al., 2020; Wee et al., 2020). Recently, RNA extraction-free methods were optimized on swab samples to detect SARS-CoV-2. The results show comparable sensitivity to RNA extraction methods (Alcoba-Florez et al., 2020; Brown et al., 2020; Bruce et al., 2020; Grant et al., 2020; Hasan et al., 2020; Merindol et al., 2020; Srivatsan et al., 2020; Wee et al., 2020). Similarly, these methods were also optimized on saliva samples (Lalli et al., 2020; Ranoa et al., 2020; Vogels et al., 2020b), although contradictory reports exist regarding sensitivity based on saliva than swab samples for SARS-CoV-2 (Meyerson et al., 2020; To et al., 2020; Williams et al., 2020; Wyllie et al., 2020). Nevertheless, all these studies unanimously suggest that nucleic acid extraction-free detection of SARS-CoV-2 is feasible.

These simple assay workflows have a tremendous potential to minimize the need for laboratory set-up and trained professionals, when integrated with a similar simplified method for detection. At present, the most robust and reliable detection method is based upon RT-qPCR, which is also a gold standard for COVID-19 testing. However, PCR-based detection methods have supply chain constraints to test on a large scale, and if available, may face a shortage of well-trained professionals to conduct the assay. Though, rapid POC tests which have been developed recently can perform mass testing of SARS-CoV-2 (Döhla et al., 2020; Jung et al., 2020) but, most of these tests are based on antigen/antibody detection and thus lack the sensitivity and specificity compared to genetic testing (Döhla et al., 2020). Recent advances in isothermal amplification-based assays provide a unique opportunity to detect nucleic acids under minimal instrument settings. These approaches, like RT-LAMP or RT-RPA, were developed previously and validated recently in SARS-CoV-2 containing clinical samples (Thai et al., 2004; Piepenburg et al., 2006; Lalli et al., 2020; Xia and Chen, 2020). Likewise, these isothermal-based amplification methods also have trade-offs in non-specific amplification (Zou et al., 2020). To circumvent these limitations, more robust methods based on CRISPR-Cas technology are employed, which utilizes collateral activities of Cas12 and Cas13 enzymes (Knott and Doudna, 2018; Li et al., 2019). These methods have been successfully used to detect human pathogens in various clinical samples, such as blood, saliva, and urine (Gootenberg et al., 2017; Chen et al., 2018). Cas12a works on DNA as input sample in a technique named DNA Endonuclease-Targeted CRISPR Trans Reporter (DETECTR). Recently, this technique was optimized to detect COVID-19 in swab samples with accuracy comparable to RT-qPCR (Broughton et al., 2020). Another such technique that detects single-stranded RNA is based on Cas13a, which is validated in many biological samples including saliva, and can reliably detect bacterial and viral pathogens with both LFA and fluorescent-based readout (Gootenberg et al., 2017; Gootenberg et al., 2018; Myhrvold et al., 2018). The technique called SHERLOCK (specific high-sensitivity enzymatic reporter unlocking) has a single-base specificity and single-molecule sensitivity with precision for multiplexing in a single reaction (Gootenberg et al., 2017). The SHERLOCK based diagnostics take advantage of extensive instrument free RPA or RT-RPA based pre-amplification of the nucleic acids, which makes this approach amenable and straightforward for on-site and home testing while at the same time providing better sensitivity and specificity (Gootenberg et al., 2017; Gootenberg et al., 2018; Myhrvold et al., 2018). Recently, SHERLOCK based diagnostics has been standardized and validated for the detection of SARS-CoV-2 in clinical swab samples (Patchsung et al., 2020).

Similarly, tools like All-in-One Dual CRISPR-Cas12a (AIOD-CRISPR) or colorimetric LAMP assay using Cas12a were developed (Ding et al., 2020; Joung et al., 2020). However, optimizing these methods utilized input RNA samples obtained using commercially available kits, which adds to the test's cost and testing time. As of now, we have not come across any study which has used SHERLOCK based detection on RNA extraction-free clinical saliva samples for COVID-19 testing. In this study, we have clinically validated Cas13a integrated lateral-flow readout to detect SARS-CoV-2 in RNA extraction-free saliva samples. Further, we have developed a semi-quantitative method to provide high-sensitive test results of the lateral-flow test strip and integrated the test strip results with a smartphone application for field-deplorability and home testing.

METHODS

Patient Information and Ethical Statement

The work was indented to develop a simple workflow for SARS-CoV-2 detection. The clinical samples collected for the work were used after obtaining Institutional ethical clearance from the Safdarjung Hospital (IEC/VMMC/SJH/Project/2020-07/CC-06). The ethical clearance was also obtained from Jamia Millia Islamia (1/10/290/JMI/IEC/2020). Further, biosafety clearance was obtained from Jamia Millia Islamia (Ref.No.P1/12-21.12.2020). Patient consent was obtained to collect the samples according to the ICMR GCP guidelines.

Sample Collection

A total of 210 clinical saliva samples were collected from Safdarjung hospital from June till November 2020, New Delhi. The saliva samples were collected from the patients at the same time when swab was collected for COVID-19 testing by the hospital. The hospital provided the swab RT-qPCR confirmatory results of 201 samples, while nine samples had no corresponding confirmatory test results done in the hospital and were labeled as blind samples. Initially all the samples were collected in RNAlater solution for validation of the saliva-based detection of SARS-Cov-2 with RT-qPCR. Subsequently, samples were divided into two parts; (part 1) was collected in RNAlater solution, and (part 2) was collected in tubes containing proteinase K (1.25 mg), Triton X-100 (0.5%), and NAC (0.5%). Similarly, samples for longitudinal studies were also collected from two patents (n = 4 each). All the samples were processed in

NABL certified (MC-3486) and ICMR approved Diagnostic laboratory for COVID-19 testing following the regulatory guidelines and protocol (360 Diagnostic and Health Services, Noida, U.P., India).

Samples were collected at different time interval in the hospital and stored at −20°C until carried to the facility for further processing. The time between sample collection to processing was around 3 to 5 days.

Plasmids, Primers and Synthetic DNA Fragments

Plasmids corresponding to S and N genes were received as a gift from Krogan laboratory, Department of Cellular and Molecular Pharmacology (San Francisco, CA 94158, USA). These same plasmids are now available with Addgene (#141382 for S gene and #141391 for N gene). After propagating, plasmid DNA was isolated using commercially available DNA isolation kit (Vivantis technologies). For RT-qPCR, 1.0 ng of the DNA was used for respective genes and a set of eight primers were optimized. These primers were synthesized in-house using online primer design tools or obtained based on previously validated sequences such as N-1 primers. The list of the primers is given in **Table S1**.

Synthetic gene fragments for S gene and Orf1ab corresponding to the sequences given in **Table S1**, were obtained from Xcelris Genomics, India and Bioserve biotechnologies, India. The gene fragments were synthesized along with the T7 promoter sequence.

Viral RNA Release From Saliva Samples

Various heat-inactivation steps, chemical components and buffers were used to find the optimal assay condition for the detection of the viral RNA. Heat inactivation optimization was done at 37°C for 10 min and 95°C for 5 min. Non-ionic detergents like Triton X-100 (Sigma) and Proteinase K (Sigma, Vivantas, and Promega) were used at various combinations to find the optimal reaction composition. Optimum detection of spiked-in S gene was obtained at a concentration of 1.25 mg/ml for proteinase K and 0.5% of Triton X-100 with either two step heat-inactivation (65°C or 37°C for 10 min and 95°C for 5 min) as well as with a single heat-inactivation step (RT for 15 min and 95°C for 5 min). Further, in order to minimize the interference of the mucoprotein in saliva, mucoactive agents like sodium citrate (Sigma) and ammonium chloride (Sigma); and mucolytic agent N-acetyl cysteine (Sigma) were used at various concentrations.

RNA Extraction and RT-qPCR

RNA extraction was performed as recommended (Qiagen viral RNA extraction kit). 140 µl sample was processed according to the protocol as per manufacturer's instruction. Final elution of the RNA was done in 30 µl of the elution buffer and 2 µl of the extracted RNA/reaction was used in one-step RT-qPCR analysis using the commercially available RT-qPCR kit for SARS-CoV-2 which contains there targeting genes E, N, and RdRp along with the internal control. Similarly, we also used our in-house optimized primers/probes for validation. For RNA_ExF saliva samples, we used 4 µl of the input saliva sample per reaction. RT-qPCR was performed on Rotor gene Q (Qiagen) with the recommended reaction condition for the commercial kit (Allplex, Seegene). For SP-1 and SP-4, the following RT-qPCR conditions were used: Initial denaturation 95°C for 5 min, second cycle of the reaction include denaturation at 95°C for 30 s, annealing at 62°C for 30 s, and extension at 72°C for 30 s for 40 cycles.

Synthetic Gene Block and T7 Reverse Transcription

To determine the limit of detection (LoD), we generated synthetic gene fragments for S and Orf1ab corresponding to the regions for which crRNA has been previously validated (Zhang Lab protocol, MIT and **Table S1**). Both single stranded gene fragments were obtained commercially (Xceliris Genomics). Each (1 ng/µl) oligonucleotide fragments were first converted into double strand by end point PCR then purified (0.5 µg/µl) double stranded DNA fragment was used as a template for *in vitro* transcription reaction using *in vitro* transcription kit (T7 Ribomax, Promega, cat no P1320). The *in vitro* transcribed RNA oligonucleotide fragment was then purified using RNA cleanup kit (Vivantis, cat no-GF TR 050) and eluted in a final volume of 50 µl. The purified RNA of the respective gene fragments was used as the standard to determine LoD. Various dilutions of S gene standard RNA were made in nuclease free water corresponding to 10^0 to 10^6 copies/µl. Similarly, the standard RNA (10^5 copies/µl) was spiked into the saliva samples for optimizing various chemical and heat-inactivation conditions.

Expression and Purification of Cas13a Protein

For the expression of Cas13a protein, the pC013-Twinstrep SUMO-huLwCas13a plasmid was transformed into E. coli BL21 (DE3) cells. The transformed cells were grown overnight in 10 ml LB media containing 100 µg/ml ampicillin antibiotic at 37°C/180 rpm in incubator shaker. Next day, 5 ml of the overnight grown culture was inoculated in 1 L LB media containing 100 µg/ml Ampicillin. After reaching the growth of the culture to OD between 0.4 and 0.6, the culture was incubated at 4°C for 30 min. Before induction of the protein, 1 ml of culture was taken for SDS-PAGE analysis. Expression of the protein was induced by adding 1 ml/0.5 M IPTG and 2% glycerol to pre-chilled culture and incubated in cooling (21°C) incubator shaker for 16 h at 300 rpm. After that, the culture was harvested by centrifugation at 6000 rpm for 10 min at 4°C. supernatant was discarded and pellet was lysed in the lysis buffer.

Lysis of the Cell Pellet

The cell pellet was resuspended in lysis buffer (20 mM Tris-HCl pH 8.0, 500 mM NaCl, 1 mM DTT, 1× protease inhibitor cocktail sigma, and 0.5 mg/ml lysozyme). The cell resuspension was lysed by sonication (Sartorius Stedim) using 50% pulse amplitude (on 10 s and off 20 s) until completely lysed. The lysate was centrifuged at 12,000 rpm for 30 min at 4°C. The protein was then applied to a HiTrap SP HP column equilibrated with equilibration buffer (20 mM Tris-HCl pH 8.0, 1 mM DTT, 500 mM NaCl, 15 mM imidazole). The supernatant fraction was passed five times from the column for complete binding of the protein. After washing with the binding buffer to remove nonspecific binders, the recombinant His6–SUMO–LwaCas13a was eluted in a linear gradient (with increasing the concentration of the imidazole from 20 to 500 mM) of elution buffer. The best elution was obtained at 100 mM imidazole. Elution was done in the volume of 5 ml. For the cleavage of His tag, the eluted fraction was supplemented with 20 µl of sumoprotease (Invitrogen #125880-18,1 U/µl) and 7.5 µl of NP-40. The reaction mixture was added to the column and incubated at 4°C for overnight with gentle shaking. Next day, cleaved native LwaCas13a protein was obtained by draining the column. After draining of the column, it was washed with elution buffer containing 500 mM imidazole to ensure the complete cleavage of His-tag from LwaCas13a protein.

The drained native protein was subjected to concentration to 0.25 ml using centrifugal spin filter (50 MWCO-MERCK millipore) at 4000 rpm for 15 min at 4°C. Then 5 ml of protein storage buffer (1M Tris-HCl pH 7.5, 5M NaCl, 5% glycerol and 10 µl DTT) was added to the same filter and again centrifuged at the same condition. Storage buffer containing native Lw-Cas13a protein was diluted to 2 mg/ml in storage buffer and stored at −20°C, as described previously (Kellner et al., 2019).

RT-RPA and SHERLOCK Assay

As described previously (Gootenberg et al., 2017; Kellner et al., 2019), RT-RPA was performed using the commercially available RPA kit (TwistDx). First, each RPA tube was divided into four reaction tubes by diluting the lyophilized mix in the RPA buffer (40 µl). For LoD, forward and reverse RT-RPA primers were added 1 µl (10 µM stock) to each reaction tube along with 1 µl of reverse transcriptase enzyme (EpiScript). 4 µl of various dilutions of the standard RNA for S and Orf1ab were used as template (0 to 4000 copies/reaction). For RNA extraction-free samples, a total of 8 µl of sample input was used and the reaction components were adjusted accordingly. The reaction was initiated by adding 0.7 µl of magnesium acetate (280 mM stock). All the reagents were prepared and mixed at 4°C. Finally, the reaction mix was incubated at 42°C for 25 min and tapped in between after every 3 and 5 min. Particularly, tapping of the samples was found to exhibit better results than without and is highly recommended henceforth.

SHERLOCK assay of the above reaction mix was performed in a separate 1.5 ml Eppendorf tube which contains 1 µl of the Cas13a either from extracted pool or commercially (MCLAB, USA, Cat no. CAS13a-200) obtained source (at 63.3 µg/ml concentration), 1 µl RNase inhibitor (20 U per µl stock; Invitrogen), 0.6 µl T7 RNA polymerase (50 U per µl stock; Lucigen), 1 µl of crRNA for the respective genes (Synthego), 1 µl of $MgCl_2$ (120 mM), 0.8 µl of rNTP mix (100 mM), 2 µl of cleavage Buffer (400 mM Tris pH 7.4), and 1 µl (20 µM) reporter. 6 µl of the RPA mix from RNA extracted samples were used per reaction. The final volume of the reaction mix was adjusted to 20 µl with RNase free water. The reaction mix was incubated at 37°C for 20–25 min.

Lateral-Flow Assay Detection

The SHERLOCK reaction mix was subjected to lateral-flow assay using the commercially available test trips and buffer (Millenia Biotec). To the above reaction mix 80 µl buffer (HybriDetect assay) was added, provided with the kit. The visual readout of the test results were obtained by dipping the test strips (Milenia Biotech1T) into the respective 1.5 ml Eppendorf tubes and the reaction mix was allowed to flow for 2 min.

Analysis of the Lateral-Flow Signal to Provide a Semi-Quantitative Estimate of the Results

To provide a semi-quantitative analysis of the lateral-flow readout, we used Fiji image J software to analyze the signal in the respective T and C bands. The corresponding band intensity of the test lane (T) and control lane (C) were calculated using integrated density parameter. The image of each strip was captured using a mobile phone (width = 50, height = 220). For the quantification, the image was further cropped to image size 40 × 220 which thus removed the outliers from the image. Any background noise from the image was subtracted using the rolling ball background subtraction method by keeping radius = 50. All the images (40 × 220) were further thresholded by applying lower threshold value 0 and the upper threshold values between 240 and 245. Finally, the single band was segmented from each image in the frame size of 30 × 30 and integrated density was analyzed for the respective bands. The threshold value of T/C was calculated and found to be 0.15 above which the samples could be labeled as positive.

Smartphone Application for Lateral-Flow Test Results

The mobile application for detection and quantification of lateral-flow strips was developed using machine learning tools. The algorithm was implemented using the OpenCV package v.4.3.0 in Python 3.7.3. The Android App was developed with Android Studio v4.2 RC 2 (Google) with Java 8 and Gradle v4.1.0. To provide a clean user interface, the main screen was limited to a "COVID-19 Test" bottom tab button that opens up an in-app camera view to capture the image followed by custom image edit options. The image acquisition is only allowed through the mobile application to accurate documentation of taken images and test results. The image captured in the application is obtained as a Uri object, that is used for conversion to a byte's array. In order to obtain the image analysis outcome, the bytes array obtained is passed as an argument to the Python backend script running through Chaquopy v6.3.0 that is a software development kit used in Android development environment. The bytes array image is further processed by the integrated image analysis module of the application. In the first image pre-processing step, the acquired image is converted to grayscale and region of interest is localized in the image through adaptive thresholding and edge detection techniques. In the next step, the perspective and orientation corrections are performed on the image which are present due to un-controlled mobile imaging. The shape of the strip and marker are two primary cues used for the aforementioned corrections. The resultant image is centered around the localize region of interest and cropped to obtained the strip area image to a fixed scale. The sample and control band image regions are detected from the cropped image based on the known strip structure and darker intensity profile of the bands. The mean intensity of each band region is obtained and ratio of the sample to control band in then calculated and displayed on the mobile application to the user along with the cropped strip image. The mean intensity of the sample band region is scaled to the range of 0 to 1w.r.t a pre-defined reference point in situation when control band has weak visual appearance (signature).

The mobile application can be downloaded using the link: https://bit.ly/research-app.

Statistical Analysis

Statistical analysis of the samples was performed using GraphPad8 Prism. Spearman correlation coefficient was used for correlation analysis. Non-parametric t test was used to compare the mean difference between two data sets as mentioned in the results.

RESULTS

Optimization and Validation of SARS-CoV-2 Detection in Clinical Saliva Samples

We used plasmids containing S and N genes of SARS-CoV-2, respectively, to standardize RT-qPCR, using CDC-approved and in-house designed primers. Among a set of eight primers tested, two primer pairs for S gene (S-P-1, S-P-4) and CDC verified primer for N gene (N1) generated a single amplicon, with S gene amplification slightly better than N1 at same plasmid DNA concentration. RT-qPCR further confirmed these results (**Figure 1A; Figure S1; Table S1**). To determine the limit of detection (LoD), we generated S gene synthetic fragments containing T7 polymerase corresponding to the region flanking amplified sequence by S-P-1 primer. The synthetic DNA fragments were subsequently converted to RNA using an in-vitro transcription assay, following which the transcribed RNA was extracted, purified, and quantified (see Methods). We performed an RT-qPCR reaction with various purified RNA dilutions and plotted the corresponding Ct values against the known concentration (**Figure 1B**). Using S-P-1 primer and probe pair, we detected up to a single copy of RNA of S gene corresponding to Ct value <39.26. This LoD obtained for S gene

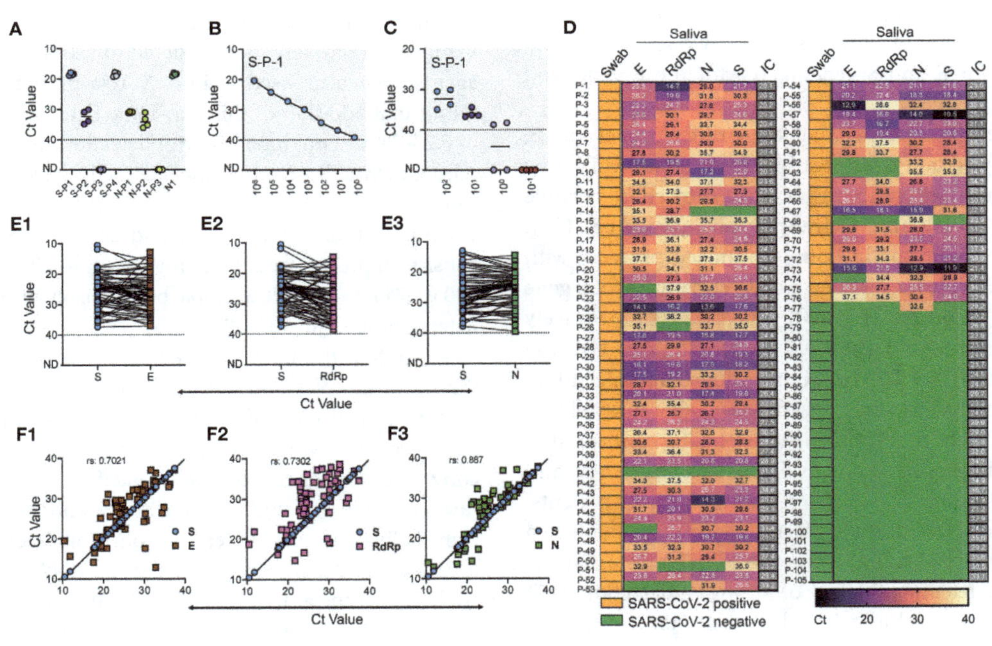

FIGURE 1 | Validation of saliva-based detection of SARS-CoV-2 in clinical samples **(A)** Standardization of SARS-CoV-2 specific primer pairs for S and N gene. Primers are labeled as S-P1 to S-P-4 for S gene and N-P1 to N-P-3 for N gene, N1 represents the CDC approved primer for N gene. Dotted line indicates lower level of detection; ND indicates not detected **(B)** Determination of limit of detection using RNA of S spiked into RNase free water with serial dilutions. **(C)** RNA extracted from four normal saliva samples was used at various copy numbers to find any interference for detection of spiked-in SARS-CoV-2 S gene RNA. **(D)** Heat map of 105 saliva samples showing RT-qPCR results represented as Ct values for E, N, RdRp and S genes respectively. The test results of these samples were validated by the hospital using swab samples, and represented as Swab. IC is the internal control. Green boxes represent the samples with Ct values not detected and were labeled as SARS-CoV-2 negative, and yellow boxes indicate swab samples positive for SARS-CoV-2. **(E1-E3)** Shows the Ct value comparison between S gene with E, RdRp, and N gene respectively. **(F1-F3)** Shows the spearman correlation of Ct values between S gene with E, RdRp, and N gene respectively.

agrees with the analytical sensitivity defined for the N gene (Vogels et al., 2020a).

Similarly, we used RNA extracted from four saliva samples of the volunteers to find any cross-reactivity. These samples were collected in 2018 for an unrelated study and stored at −80°C. Similar amplification profile and LoD was obtained with spiked-in RNA in these samples, while lack of amplification without spiked-in RNA suggests that no interference and no-cross reactivity exists with the RNA from the saliva samples (**Figure 1C**). After finding LoD, we used these same sets of primer/probes along with N1, RdRp, and E gene and performed RT-qPCR in the clinical saliva samples using a commercially available kit.

We obtained 113 clinical saliva samples from patients with matched swabs tested at Safdarjung Hospital, New Delhi. Based on the swab results for which the hospital performed the RT-qPCR, 82 samples were positive, and 31 were negative. We extracted RNA from these samples using the viral RNA extraction kit (see Methods) followed by one-step RT-qPCR analysis using the commercially available kit and compared the results with our in-house optimized protocol. Based on previous reports and the LoD derived for S gene, we set the upper limit for detection at Ct < 40 to mark the sample as positive, and samples with Ct above 40 were marked negative. In the initial screening, eight samples (six positive and two negative) showed no detectable signal for internal control and hence were eliminated for the analysis. Thus, a total of 105 saliva samples (76 positive and 29 negative) were used to perform the RT-qPCR. We found 98.7% positive agreement with swab results with at least one of the primer/probe sets tested. Individually, we found 97.4% agreement for E and S gene, 89.6% for the E gene, and 90.9% for RdRp.

Among the negative samples, all the primer/probes for E, RdRp and S showed a 100% positive agreement, while one sample with a negative swab result also showed a positive signal for the N-1 gene primer/probe (**Figure 1D**). Comparative analysis of our in-house optimized protocol with a commercially available kit revealed a close correlation of S gene with N (r = 0.887) (**Figures 1E3, F3**), which was comparatively better than comparison for S gene with E gene (**Figures 1E1, F1**) and RdRp (**Figures 1E2, F2**). Thus, our in-house optimized RT-qPCR method is in high-agreement with the CDC-approved N-1 gene-based amplification. Further, these results confirm that saliva and swab samples have a high degree of consistency, and saliva can decisively detect SARS-CoV-2 in COVID-19 patients. Our results confirm the findings of the previously published reports which have demonstrated the use of saliva as a reliable clinical sample for detecting SARS-CoV-2 with a detection limit and sensitivity comparable with the nasopharyngeal and oropharyngeal swab (hereafter swab) (Fakheran et al., 2020; Procop et al., 2020). While some other reports have shown slightly better analytical sensitivity of saliva samples (0.98 virus RNA copies/ml) than other biological fluids for SARS-CoV-2 detection (Wyllie et al., 2020), we did not perform a direct comparison.

RNA Extraction-Free Detection of SARS-CoV-2 in Clinical Saliva Samples

A major hurdle in COVID-19 testing is the need for viral RNA extraction, which poses a challenge to speed-up the testing. We envisioned to use a simple RNA extraction-free (hereafter, RNA_ExF) method and validate its analytical sensitivity on SARS-CoV-2 clinical samples. Recently, several RNA_ExF methods were employed to test their analytical sensitivity in clinical samples; however, these methods have their own benefits and limitations (Alcoba-Florez et al., 2020; Brown et al., 2020; Bruce et al., 2020; Grant et al., 2020; Hasan et al., 2020; Merindol et al., 2020; Srivatsan et al., 2020; Wee et al., 2020). Thus, we aimed to develop a more sensitive workflow for the RNA extraction-free testing of saliva samples. We initially optimized Proteinase K concentration under various heat inactivation conditions and tested by introducing 10^5 copies of the S gene into the normal saliva. We found that at a concentration of 1.25 mg and dual heat inactivation (37°C for 10 min and 95°C for 5 min), a better analytical sensitivity could be obtained in comparison to the heating of samples at 65°C or with higher concentrations of Proteinase K (**Figure 2A**). While at all concentrations tested, the detection limit was relatively less than the samples in which the S gene was spiked into RNase free water. As saliva contains mucoproteins, which may interfere with the detection, we next tried mucoactive chemicals (sodium citrate and ammonium chloride) and mucolytic agent N acetylcysteine (NAC).

Interestingly, we found that samples treated with NAC exhibited relatively better detection than other mucoactive agents. We also used Triton X-100 in the formulation and found that addition of this non-ionic detergent at concentrations of 0.25-2% did not interfere with detection, and hence may aide in release of viral RNA when applied to clinical samples (**Figure 2A**). Thus, we found an optimal heat inactivation method (37°C for 10 min and 95°C for 5 min) and chemical composition which consists of proteinase K (1.25 mg/ml), NAC (0.5%), and Triton X-100 (0.5%), to provide a simple buffer formulation for saliva-based detection of SARS-CoV-2.

To obtain the LoD, we used spiked-in S standard RNA into the saliva samples and performed chemical treatment and heat inactivation. We could accurately detect as low as 10 copies of RNA/reaction, which though slightly lesser compared to a single copy detection when RNA was spiked-in water (**Figure 2B**). We further tested this buffer's sensitivity and heat inactivation on eight saliva samples collected from volunteers in 2018 for an unrelated study. In comparison to the RNA spiked in water, we could detect the amplification in all saliva samples, while a slight increase in Ct values was observed, with a difference in the mean Ct of 2.169 ± 0.9526 (**Figures 2C1, C2**). Collectively, these results indicate that an optimized buffer and heat inactivation conditions are suitable for RNA detection in saliva samples with an RNA_ExF free workflow.

Based on the results that RNAlater solution maintains the RNA quality and detection sensitivity in clinical samples (above,

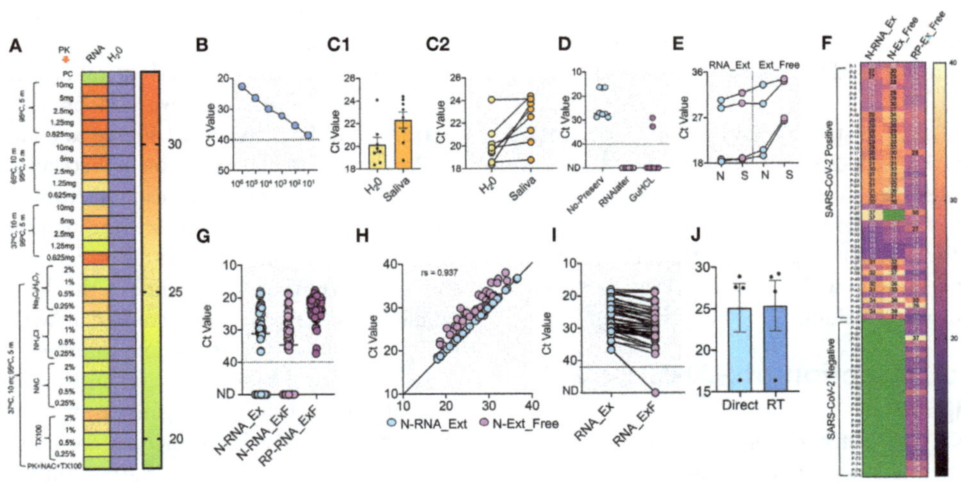

FIGURE 2 | RNA extraction-free detection of SARS-CoV-2 in saliva samples **(A)** Heat map of Ct values obtained with 10^5 copies of S gene standard RNA spiked into normal saliva and subjected to various heat inactivation and chemical treatments. PK: Proteinase K; NAC: N-acetyl cysteine and TX100: Triton X-100. Saliva samples with water was used instead of spiked-in RNA as negative control, which showed no detectable Ct value; blue boxes. **(B)** Standard curve showing various dilutions of S gene RNA spiked into normal saliva to obtain the LoD. **(C1, C2)** Comparison of Ct detected when S gene RNA was spiked into the saliva samples of eight SARS-CoV-2 negative volunteers vs the same spiked into water as control. **(D)** Optimization of various RNA storage agents like RNAlater, guanidinium hydrochloride (GuHCL) and without RNA storage agent for detection of SARS-CoV-2 in eight clinical saliva samples. **(E)** Comparison of N and S gene amplification in saliva samples after undergoing heat and chemical denaturation. **(F)** Heat map of Ct values obtained for N gene for 76 samples with RNA extraction (N-RNA_Ex) and RNA extraction-free (N-RNA_ExF) method. Human RNaseP (RP) was used as the experimental control to find the RNA integrity of the samples used. Green boxes represent the samples with not detected Ct values. **(G)** Shows the individual Ct values of N-RNA-Ex and N-RNA_ExF along with the RNaseP with dotted line indicating lower level of detection. **(H)** Correlation of Ct values between N-RNA_Ex and N-RNA_ExF method **(I)** Median of Ct values of two methods as indicated by solid lines. The dotted line represents lower Ct value below which samples were labeled as not detected (ND). **(J)** Comparison of Ct values obtained from saliva samples when stored at room temperature (RT) for 6 h with same samples processed without storage (direct).

Figure 1D), we initially used RNAlater solution and guanidine hydrochloride (GuHCL) to collect the saliva samples for validation using RNA_ExF workflow. We gave three sets of tubes for sample collection; the set-I with RNAlater, set-II with GuHCL, and set-III without any solvent. A total of eight samples collected from the same patients were obtained and used for the analysis. We found that both GuHCL and RNAlater inhibited the assay detection with our optimized chemical and heat treatment. Simultaneously, the direct use of the samples without preservatives showed better detection (**Figure 2D**). Thus, these results suggest that the collection of saliva directly into the collection tube without any chemical or RNA preservative is optimal for RNA_ExF detection of SARS-CoV-2.

Next, we used the same optimized protocol to validate the analytical sensitivity of this workflow on 83 additional clinical samples. Each collected sample was divided into two separate tubes, one containing the RNAlater solution, and in the other tube, saliva was collected without any solvent. The samples collected in RNAlater were subjected to RNA extraction using the kit-based method, while samples collected without any solvent underwent chemical treatment and heat inactivation and were directly used for RT-qPCR analysis. Initially, we tested N and S primer sensitivity with the RNA extraction-free method and performed the assay in four samples. A slightly better sensitivity was detected when we used N primer in samples with RNA extraction-free method (**Figure 2E**). This discrepancy in the sensitivity of these two genes could be due to small amplicon size of N (72 bp) than S (112 bp). So, we used N primer and the RNaseP (RP) for the subsequent screening of the clinical samples. We used RP for initial screening to qualify the sample for comparative analysis between the RNA extraction and the extraction-free method. Only those samples with a detectable Ct value for RP (76 out of 83 samples) were qualified and further used in this study.

As shown in (**Figure 2F**), 76 samples of COVID-19 were tested with RNA extraction-based method, out of which 47 tested positive, while 29 showed no detectable signal and were marked negative. With our optimized RNA extraction-free workflow, 45 out of 47 samples showed positive and 29 out of 29 showed negative results, with an overall 95.7% agreement for positive test samples and 100% agreement for the negative samples (**Figures 2F, G**). The two samples that showed no detectable signal in the RNA extraction-free method had a comparatively high Ct value obtained with the RNA extraction method (Ct: 37) (**Figure 2I**). Though the Ct values were slightly higher with the RNA extraction-free method, with a difference between the means of the two methods at 2.545 ± 1.158. Correlation analysis of Ct values reveal high degree of correlation between RNA extraction-free workflow with the RNA extraction method (spearmen coefficient, rs = 0.937) (**Figure 2H**). Overall, these results suggest that saliva can be directly used for the detection of SARS-CoV-2 without the need for costly and time-consuming

RNA extraction steps. This simple extraction free workflow thus overcomes the time-consuming and expensive RNA extraction step for SARS-CoV-2 detection and hence will eliminate the supply chain constrain and need for laboratory set-up to perform the assay.

To determine the sample stability over time, we conducted the assay on four SARS-CoV-2 saliva samples stored at room temperature. We observed no significant difference in the analytic sensitivity of the samples when stored up to 6 h (**Figure 2J**). Thus, these results suggest the feasibility of home collection of the saliva samples without technical assistance, cold storage, or viral transport medium.

Cas13a Based Detection of SARS-CoV-2 in Saliva Samples

After validating RNA_ExF detection of SARS-CoV-2 in saliva samples, we next explored detection methods, which are (1) relatively instrument-free, (2) previously validated for SARS-CoV-2, and (3) exhibit sensitivity consistent with RT-qPCR. To meet this criterion, we found the SHERLOCK-based detection method to be the most appropriate, which was also recently approved by the US FDA. SHERLOCK relies upon the collateral activity of Cas13a to cleave the colorimetric or a fluorescent reporter once the target molecule is detected (**Figure 3A**). To use this method on our optimized workflow, we obtained commercially synthesized and previously verified crRNA sequences for the S gene spanning the region for which we validated the RT-qPCR assay (**Table S1**). Similarly, we also obtained crRNA corresponding to the Orf1ab gene (Zhang lab, MIT). Cas13a was isolated from an Addgene plasmid (#90097) which was a kind gift from the Zhang Lab, MIT. The plasmid was propagated and purified based on the published protocol (Patchsung et al., 2020). Using the methodology employed by Kellner et al., we first performed SHERLOCK on standard RNA corresponding to S and Orf1ab to validate this method (Kellner et al., 2019). In addition, we also obtained the recombinant Cas13a from the commercial source to confirm the results.

Previous studies have shown that both fluorescence-based detection and lateral-flow readouts using paper-strip can be accurately used to demonstrate the working principle of this method. Considering the ease-of-use, instrument-free detection, and cost-effectiveness, we choose the lateral-flow readout to validate this method and correlated it with the corresponding RT-qPCR data. A range of various dilutions of the standard RNA spiked-in control saliva was run, and the lateral-flow readouts were labeled as positive or negative by visual detection. As shown in **Figure 3B**, a consistent increase in the positive signal in the test lane was obtained, which corresponded to the lowest RNA copy number of 200 copies/reaction for the S gene with 100% detection sensitivity with a corresponding Ct value of 35.4. In comparison, the detection limit for Orf1ab was lower at 400 copies/reaction (**Figure 3C**). The LoD for the S gene was slightly higher than the spiked-in RNA samples, which is consistent with the results from other groups (100 copies/reaction for the S gene) (Joung et al., 2020). This discrepancy is probably due to the sample processing and assay for detection. While the study by Joung et al. used spiked-in RNA samples followed by RNA extraction, and Cas12-based detection; we used RNA_ExF samples and employed Cas13-based detection. Overall, these results confirm the previous reports which show that SHERLOCK-based approach integrated with visual lateral-flow readout can be used for SARS-CoV-2 detection.

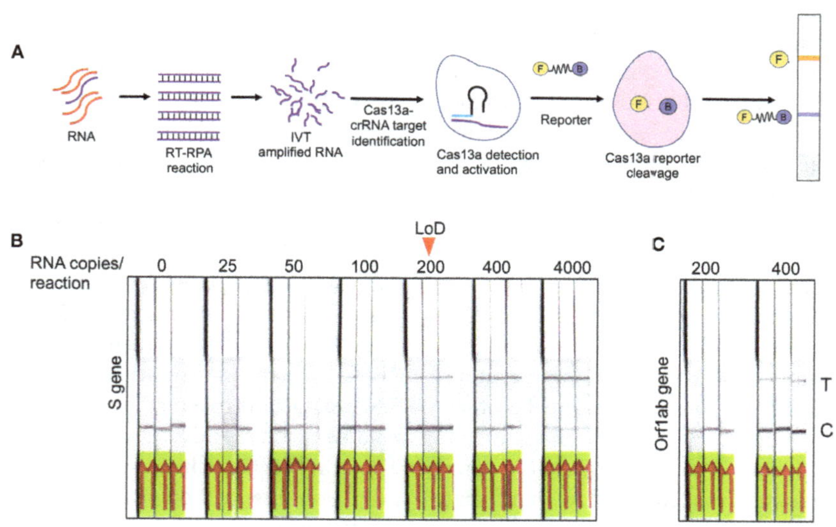

FIGURE 3 | Optimization of SHERLOCK-based detection on extraction free saliva samples **(A)** Schematic representation of various steps involved in SHERLOCK-based detection when the starting genetic material is RNA. Cas13a enzyme is used for the target recognition and reporter cleavage. For visual detection using LFA, RNA reporter molecule conjugated with 6-Carboxyfluorescein (FAM) and biotin is used. **(B)** Images of paper-strips after lateral-flow assay obtained from spiked-in saliva samples using S gene standard RNA with a range from 0 to 4, 000 copies of RNA/reaction. A consistent detection of test lane signal was obtained in all three samples with 200 copies of RNA, which was considered as LoD for visual readout. **(C)** Similarly, Orf1ab standard RNA was subjected to LFA and paper-strip images were obtained. The LoD for Orf1ab was found to be higher than S gene at 400 copies/reaction.

Validation of SHERLOCK-Based Detection on RNA Extraction-Free Saliva Samples

To make this tool affordable and accessible with a provision for field testing, we next performed SHERLOCK on the optimized RNA_ExF saliva samples. We divided the samples into four groups based on the Ct values. Group I with Ct > 25; group II with Ct between 26 and 30; group III with Ct between 31 and 35, and group IV with Ct < 36, with five samples in each group. Corroborating the RT-qPCR, 39 out of 40 positive sample also showed a positive signal with an LFA readout with Ct values below 35 (**Figure 4A** and **Supplementary Figure 2A**). Thus, SHERLOCK was in 98% agreement with the Ct values below 35, and by combining this method with RNA extraction-free saliva samples, we could obtain comparable sensitivity to the RNA extraction method for SARS-CoV-2 detection, as reported by others (Patchsung et al., 2020). To further validate the reliability of this approach, we performed a longitudinal detection analysis of the clinical samples. For this, we selected two patients who have been four times sampled (both swab and saliva) at the hospital at different time intervals after the symptom onset. We used the saliva samples and performed SHERLOCK assay, followed by lateral flow readout of the test results. We found that the SHERLOCK-based detection accurately confirmed the findings of the RT-qPCR swab results (performed in the hospital) in these test samples (**Supplementary Figures 2B1, B2**). Taken together, these results confirm that SHERLOCK-based diagnosis provides a reliable and extensive instrument free method for SARS-CoV-2, without compromising the assay's analytical sensitivity.

Semi-Quantitative Analysis of the LFA Signal With Provision for Smartphone Application

The limitation with lateral-flow readout using visual detection is that sometimes a weak signal may appear in the test lane. This usually occurs if too little or too much (High Dose Hook Effect) of the reporter molecule is used. Thus, a very precise amount of the reporter has to be added, which otherwise may interfere with test results. However, under laboratory free settings such as POCT and for home testing, the precision in handling may be challenging and it is expected that a background signal may appear in the test lane, which may sometimes be difficult to

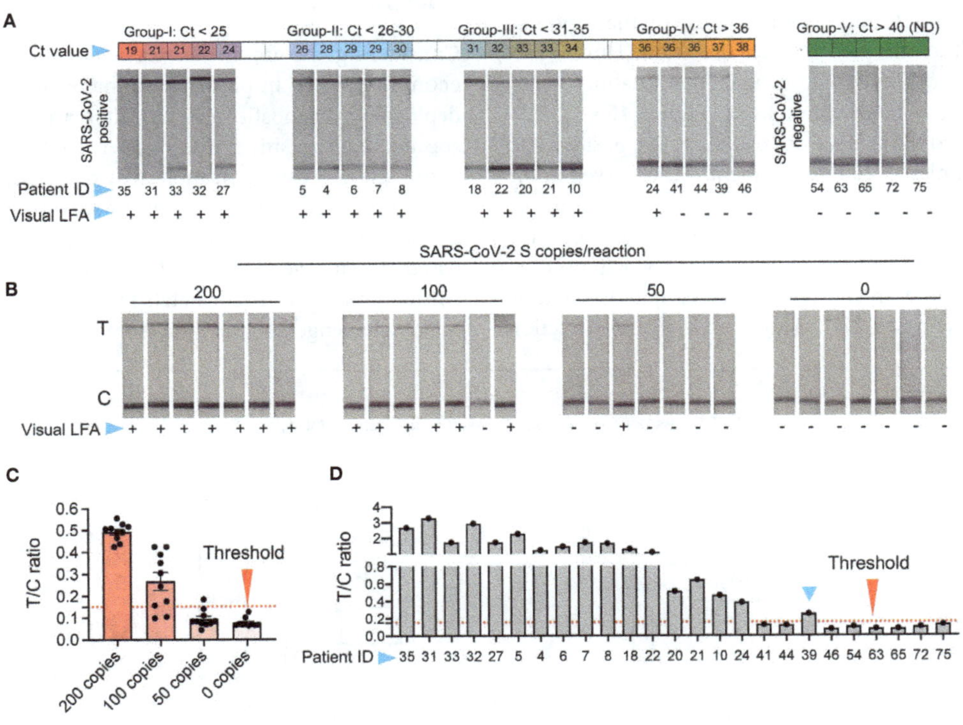

FIGURE 4 | Validation of SHERLOCK on RNA extraction-free saliva samples **(A)** RNA extraction-free samples were used for the detection with SHERLOCK-based method using visual lateral-flow. Samples were divided into five groups, based on the Ct values with Group-I Ct below 25; Group-II Ct between 26-30, Group-III Ct between 31-35, Group-IV Ct above 36, and Group-V Ct not detected (ND). The LFA images of samples with respective Ct values is shown along with the patient ID corresponding to samples in (**Figure 2**). **(B)** Representative images of the seven paperstrips with 200, 100, 50, and 0 RNA copies spiked-in to the saliva samples and subjected to SHERLOCK. **(C)** To obtain semi-quantitative analysis of the data, 10 images of paper-strips corresponding to 200, 100, 50, and 0 RNA copies as shown in **Figure 3B** and **Figure 4B**, were subjected to image quantitation. The threshold value (T/C ratio) was obtained based on the signal in the control **(C)** and test (T) lane. The T/C ratio was considered positive above the background value of 0.15. Based on T/C ratio, the detection sensitivity was found to be 80% with100 copies of RNA and 100% above 200 copies of RNA per reaction. **(D)** Similarly, visual results of paper-strips shown in **Figure 4A**, were subjected to signal quantitation and T/C ratio was calculated. One sample (blue arrow head, ID: 39), which was difficult to characterize by visual detection, was correctly characterized as positive using T/C ratio (blue arrow head).

interpret by naked eye. Further, based on our results and previously published studies (Patchsung et al., 2020), SHERLOCK with visual readout performs exceedingly well with samples at a higher copy number of the analyte. Though, the interpretation of results become difficult when samples with very low copies of analytes are present, where the signal in the test lane may be close to the background, which besides the above-mentioned issues may also in some instances appear due to non-specific probe degradation (Patchsung et al., 2020). Thus, to determine the background signal and differentiate between the noise and actual signal, we used ten replicates of negative control and samples with 50, 100, and 200 copies of RNA/reaction spiked into normal saliva and subjected to chemical treatment and heat inactivation, respectively (**Figure 4B**). The SHERLOCK assay was done and the paper-strip images were obtained and processed using Image J (see Methods). A threshold value was generated based on the ratio of signal intensity in test lane to control lane (T/C) corresponding to no RNA and three known concentrations of standard RNA. Based on the signal obtained from negative samples, we obtained a threshold value with a T/C ratio of 0.15, and below this ratio, the samples were labeled as negative (**Figure 4C**). By quantifying the signal of various dilutions, all samples with 200 copies of RNA showed T/C ratio above threshold (positive). In samples with 100 copies, nine showed positive T/C ratio, though most of these sample results were difficult to interpret by visual detection. Thus, we set this new LoD to 100 copies based on signal quantitation, which corresponded to a Ct value of about 36.32 (**Figure 4C**).

Next, we quantified the signal from the respective positive and negative clinical samples. A 100% agreement was observed in the negative samples between visual and T/C ratio. Similarly, samples with Ct > 35 also showed 100% agreement. Surprisingly, among five samples with Ct < 36, two showed T/C signal above threshold, in contrast to one sample detected by the visual readout (**Figure 4D**). Thus, while visual detection accurately detects the signal below a Ct value of 35, it suffers the detection limit in samples with very low viral RNA copy numbers. Under such circumstances, a semi-quantitative approach is more feasible, as quantitation is provided based on the ratio between the test and the control lane instead of solely relying on the signal at the test lane. Overall, these results suggest that LFA signals obtained using RNA_ExF saliva samples can be precisely quantified and correlated with Ct values to give a fair estimate of the viral load (at higher Ct) and further enhance the analytical sensitivity.

To further ease the interpretation of test results, we developed mobile application and integrated it with the lateral-flow test strips (**Figure 5**, **Video 1** and **Video 2**). The smartphone application has also provision to save the test results which can be easily accessed for research purpose. Further, the application has an online consultation option, which the patients can access to get immediate help related in performing the assay – an important development when performing home testing. The mobile application can be downloaded using the link given in the methods.

DISCUSSION

Considering the impact of COVID-19 on global health and economy, it is imperative to have at our disposal field-deployable diagnostic test kits that are robust, cost-effective, specific, and sensitive. The onset of COVID-19 pandemic has witnessed an upsurge in molecular diagnostics of SARS-CoV-2, but only a few of them have sensitivity and specificity comparable to the gold standard RT-qPCR, especially those based on nucleic acid detection such as CRISPR-Cas system (Broughton et al., 2020; Patchsung et al., 2020). However, the major challenge to use these tools as a POC device for field

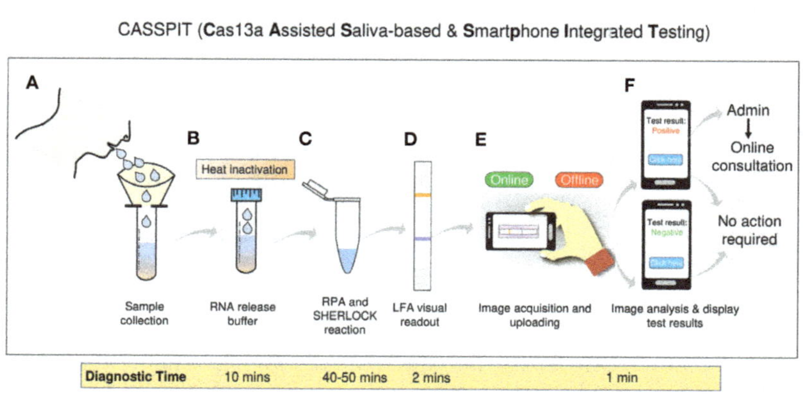

FIGURE 5 | Schematic representation of the CASSPIT workflow **(A)** Self-collection of saliva samples by the patient in a sample collection tube which contains the RNA release chemical agents. **(B)** The samples will be subjected to heat inactivation to inactivate the virus and simultaneously release the viral RNA. **(C)** Released RNA will be transferred into one-pot or two-pot SHERLOCK master mix tube to amplify the signal with RT-RPA and detect the target by Cas13a. After target detection, activated Cas13 will cleave the reporter. **(D)** Paper-strips will be immersed in the SHERLOCK reaction mix and subjected to LFA to obtain the visual results. **(E)** Using mobile phone camera, images of the paper-strip will be captured and subjected to processed using the app. Test results will be provided based on the signal detection in Test and Control lanes of the paper-strip. **(F)** Further the app will have a provision to store the images, test results and help with online assistance if needed. The overall workflow with saliva as test samples is named as **C**as13 **A**ssisted **S**aliva-based & **S**martphone **I**ntegrated **T**esting (CASSPIT).

testing or home testing persists. In addition, workflow of these methods is contingent on additional RNA extraction steps that require trained professionals and sophisticated laboratory set-up and instrumentation to perform the assay. Considering these fundamental challenges, we developed, optimized, and validated the use of a simple workflow to detect SARS-CoV-2 in saliva samples for the following reasons: (1) saliva can be self-collected with ease to minimize direct contact with the healthcare workers, and to reduce handling errors; (2) repeated sampling is feasible without incurring discomfort to the patient, with a reasonably uniform sample distribution; and (3) higher stability of the SARS-CoV-2 in saliva even when stored at room temperature (up to 7 days) (Vogels et al., 2020b).

Initially, we validated the analytical sensitivity of clinical saliva samples following RNA-extraction and RT-qPCR assay for detection, and found a close agreement with corresponding swab test results performed by the hospital. Next, we developed a simple workflow to detect SARS-CoV-2 in saliva samples without need for an extra and time-consuming RNA-extraction step. Optimization of this workflow was challenging as unlike other biological fluids, the molecular composition of saliva hinders RNA detection, besides being more amenable to RNases (Ochert et al., 1994; Ostheim et al., 2020). Also, SARS-CoV-2 being an enveloped virus, the RNA release condition had to be optimized so that its degradation is minimized. Working on various chemical treatments and heat inactivation steps, we formulated a unique buffer composition containing the optimal concentration of Proteinase K, Triton X-100, and N-acetyl cysteine, followed by heat inactivation. Together this buffer and heat condition were sufficient to cause the release SARS-CoV-2 RNA and maintain its stability. On testing this workflow on clinical samples, we found a close agreement with the kit-based RNA extraction method, which is used for detection of SARS-CoV-2. Our results were thus consistent with previous reports on the use of RNA extraction-free detection of SARS-CoV-2 (Alcoba-Florez et al., 2020; Brown et al., 2020; Bruce et al., 2020; Grant et al., 2020; Hasan et al., 2020; Merindol et al., 2020; Srivatsan et al., 2020; Vogels et al., 2020b; Wee et al., 2020).

To further simplify the diagnostic workflow, we have optimized the RNA extraction-free detection of SARS-CoV-2 with two-(step)pot SHERLOCK, which relies on the collateral activity of Cas13a—recently validated on clinical COVID-19 samples (Hou et al., 2020; Patchsung et al., 2020). Our results indicate that the two-pot SHERLOCK and RT-RPA reaction works exceedingly well in saliva samples with RNA extraction-free method, and found 98% positive agreement with the RT-qPCR data, with Ct>35, corresponding to approximately 200 copies/reaction. In view of the reports that most SARS-CoV-2 patients have a cutoff Ct values around this range (33.5 for E; 33.5 for RdRp; and 34.5 for N gene) (Uhm et al., 2020), our approach can be reliably used as an alternate to RT-qPCR with provision for RNA_ExF free workflow. The LoD which we obtained for extraction free saliva samples with a two-pot reaction is slightly lower than what others found when RNA-extraction methods were used (Patchsung et al., 2020). This could be due to: (1) High DNA, proteins, and other ions present in saliva, which interferes with the detection, irrespective of the type of detection method used, i.e., RT-qPCR or SHERLOCK (Ochert et al., 1994; Ostheim et al., 2020). (2) Ambiguity in visual detection, when the test lane signal is shallow and difficult to differentiate by the naked eye.

Thus, to further improve the detection sensitivity of these test results, we employed image-based signal quantification of lateral-flow strips. With this approach, we obtained a T/C threshold ratio, which differentiated between the positive and negative samples more precisely than visual readout, and obtained an improved LoD of 100 copies of RNA per reaction. This improved LoD based on T/C ratio is similar to the LoD obtained by Joung et al. (100 copies/reaction) with one-pot Cas12a and RT-LAMP reaction (Joung et al., 2020). Other groups have attained slightly better sensitivity with two-pot reaction. Using Cas12a and RT-LAMP, Broughton et al. achieved an LoD of 24 copies/reaction with lateral-flow readout on SARS-CoV-2 clinical samples (Broughton et al., 2020). Similarly, using Cas13a and RT-RPA, Patchsung et al. achieved an LoD of 42 copies/reaction in spiked-in saliva or nasopharyngeal samples (Patchsung et al., 2020). Thus, these studies indicate that there is scope to further improve the analytical sensitivity of RNA_ExF workflow.

Another disadvantage of paper-strip-based methods is that these test results are difficult to access for clinical studies. That includes data for survey, vaccine trials, or testing other therapeutic interventions. To overcome this challenge, we integrated the lateral-flow readout with a mobile application with provision for offline or online mode. The smartphone integrated workflow will thus provide an accurate estimate of the signal in test vs control lane, that will remove any ambiguity associated with visual detection. Further, this application will provide access to image files, patient clinical parameters, and LFA quantitative results. A video demonstration of a saliva-based workflow integrated with the mobile application is shown (**Video 1** and **Video 2**).

In summary, we provide a simple workflow for SARS-CoV-2 detection, which is a unique addition to the rapid, cost-effective, and straightforward diagnostic methods. Such user-friendly testing methods have an immediate application under the settings where trained professionals and costly instruments are limited. Further, owing to the high-sensitivity and high-specificity of Cas13a, our optimized workflow on saliva samples could provide a rapid and better alternative to the existing detection methods and speed up the testing. We envision that in coming time, CRISPR Diagnostics based on either Cas13a or a similar method which utilizes Cas12 (Broughton et al., 2020; Nguyen et al., 2020) and integrated with a smartphone-based readout (Ning et al., 2020) will be a better alternative to RT-qPCR based testing under resource limiting settings. Moreover, integrating CRISPR Diagnostics with RNA extraction-free workflow and smartphone application will provide an alternative to error-prone rapid antigen tests to scale-up COVID-19 testing across resource-constrained areas and intensify trace, test, and treat strategy for COVID-19.

The future of CRISPR Diagnostics is promising as it provides rapid, accurate, low cost, and laboratory free genetic testing. Our study has shown feasibility of this diagnostic approach with RNA extraction-free saliva samples which can be extended to home testing. There is still scope to further improve these tools, especially for use in fully instrument free settings and without pre-amplification step. While a recent study has provided an improved version of CRISPR Diagnostics, which bypasses the amplification step (Fozouni et al., 2020), more optimization is needed to provide a fully instrument-free diagnostic platform. Importantly, CRISPR Diagnostics has the provision to detect single nucleotide mismatches and hence will serve as a rapid diagnostic tool to detect any new mutations arising in the SARS-CoV-2 genome (Kirby, 2021). Some of these mutations have already been shown spreading at a higher rate and thus it is imperative to adopt and deploy CRISPR-based diagnostics to extensively screen the transmission of these new SARS-CoV-2 strains.

AUTHOR CONTRIBUTIONS

TA, MJ, and JI designed the experiments and provided financial support for the research. IA, MF, TA, DKS and NC performed experiments. RK and SY collected clinical samples. RB and GDJ facilitated experimental work. AG and GJ designed mobile app. All authors contributed to the article and approved the submitted version.

FUNDING

TA is thankful for UGC for the start-up grant support (F.4-5/2018 FRP Start-up grant). MJ is thankful to UGC-FRP startup grant (F.4.5 (236-FRP) 2015/BSR), DBT/Wellcome Trust India Alliance grant number IA/I/15/2/502086 and SERB-ECR (ECR/2017/000976) the financial support. JI is supported by the Ramalingaswami Fellowship grant (BT/RLF/Re-entry/09/2015) from Department of Biotechnology (DBT), and Early Career Research Award grant (File No. ECR/2018/002114) from Science and Engineering Research Board (SERB), Department of Science & Technology, Government of India. IA and MF acknowledge ICMR for Senior Research Fellowship.

ACKNOWLEDGMENTS

We are thankful to Dr. Arpita Rai for providing us the control saliva samples and all other faculty members of MCARS for their valuable support and discussion while preparing this manuscript. We thank Dr. Manish Kumar, BLDE university, Karnataka, for suggestions during the optimization of saliva-based workflow. We are thankful to Dr. Sushant G. Gosh and Syed Kazim Naqvi for support in establishing the molecular diagnostics facility at MCARS. We also thank Dr. Feng Zhang for the Cas13 plasmid and Dr. Nevan Krogan for SARS-CoV-2 plasmids.

SUPPLEMENTARY MATERIAL

Supplementary Video 1 | After opening the mobile application which is named as MI-SEHAT, the user will be directed to enter the details like age and name (optional). For COVID-19 test, user will click on the tab "COVID-19 test" which will open the mobile phone camera. For simplicity we have used a dummy cassette which will hold the test strip and trained the software along with the cassette. The user will select a region which should include the blue mark, and the two lines below the area where CASSPIT is written. After clicking the image, the software will display the result, which in the given example are positive, as only two bands are detected one in the control lane and another in the test lane. The user will have an option to save the test results for future use or to consult the team of experts regarding any query related to the assay. The software has also provision to provide a signal quantitation of the test results which are displayed as score. In positive samples the test score above 0.15.

Supplementary Video 2 | This is an example of a negative test result, where only one band can be seen (control lane). The test score is also displayed, which in case of negative samples will be below 0.15.

Supplementary Figure 1 | Standardization of various primers for the detection of SARS-CoV-2. **(A)** Detection of S gene amplicon by performing RT-qPCR using the S-P-1 primers. The desired amplicon size was obtained under all the annealing temperatures tested (112bp). S gene plasmid was used as template. **(B)** Similarly, S-P-4 primer for S gene amplification was used (134bp). **(C)** CDC-approved N-1 primer was used for PCR on N gene plasmid with a single amplicon (72bp) (D) PCR was performed using N-P1 primer which produced multiple amplicons. Black arrow head indicates the predicted amplicon size. The sequence of the respective primers is given in **Supplementary Table 1**.

Supplementary Figure 2 | SHERLOCK validation of saliva samples using later-flow strips and signal quantitation method. **(A1)** Paper-strip images of SARS-CoV-2 positive (left) and SARS-CoV-2 negative (right) samples which were subjected to SHERLOCK and LFA. Corresponding Ct values derived from RT-qPCR is shown above the Lateral-flow strip. The patient ID and Ct values are same as shown in *Figure 2f.* **(A2)** Corresponding T/C ratio of the images is shown. Red arrow head indicates the threshold T/C ratio **(B1)** Longitudinal test results of two patient saliva samples taken four times before the test results came negative. **(B2)** T/C ratio of the corresponding LFA images.

REFERENCES

Alcoba-Florez, J., González-Montelongo, R., Íñigo-Campos, A., De Artola, D. G.-M., Gil-Campesino, H., Team, T. M. T. S., et al. (2020). Fast SARS-CoV-2 detection by RT-qPCR in preheated nasopharyngeal swab samples. *Int. J. Infect. Dis.* 97, 66–68. doi: 10.1016/j.ijid.2020.05.099

Broughton, J. P., Deng, X., Yu, G., Fasching, C. L., Servellita, V., Singh, J., et al. (2020). CRISPR–Cas12-based detection of SARS-CoV-2. *Nat. Biotechnol.* 38, 870–874. doi: 10.1038/s41587-020-0513-4

Brown, J. R., Atkinson, L., Shah, D., and Harris, K. (2020). Validation of an extraction-free RT-PCR protocol for detection of SARS-CoV2 RNA. *medRxiv.* doi: 10.1101/2020.04.29.20085910

Bruce, E. A., Huang, M.-L., Perchetti, G. A., Tighe, S., Laaguiby, P., Hoffman, J. J., et al. (2020). Direct RT-qPCR detection of SARS-CoV-2 RNA from patient nasopharyngeal swabs without an RNA extraction step. *PLoS Biol.* 18, e3000896. doi: 10.1371/journal.pbio.3000896

Chen, J. S., Ma, E., Harrington, L. B., Da Costa, M., Tian, X., Palefsky, J. M., et al. (2018). CRISPR-Cas12a target binding unleashes indiscriminate single-stranded DNase activity. *Science* 360, 436–439 10.1126/science.aar6245. doi: 10.1126/science.aar6245

Ding, X., Yin, K., Li, Z., Lalla, R. V., Ballesteros, E., Sfeir, M. M., et al. (2020). Ultrasensitive and visual detection of SARS-CoV-2 using all-in-one dual CRISPR-Cas12a assay. *Nat. Commun.* 11, 1–10. doi: 10.1038/s41467-020-18575-6

Döhla, M., Boesecke, C., Schulte, B., Diegmann, C., Sib, E., Richter, E., et al. (2020).

Rapid point-of-care testing for SARS-CoV-2 in a community screening setting shows low sensitivity. *Public Health* 182, 170–172. doi: 10.1016/j.puhe.2020.04.009

Fakheran, O., Dehghannejad, M., and Khademi, A. (2020). Saliva as a diagnostic specimen for detection of SARS-CoV-2 in suspected patients: a scoping review. *Infect. Dis. poverty* 9, 1–7. doi: 10.1186/s40249-020-00728-w

Fozouni, P., Son, S., De León Derby, M. D., Knott, G. J., Gray, C. N., D'ambrosio, M. V., et al. (2020). Direct detection of SARS-CoV-2 using CRISPR-Cas13a and a mobile phone. *MedRxiv.* doi: 10.1101/2020.09.28.20201947

Gootenberg, J. S., Abudayyeh, O. O., Lee, J. W., Essletzbichler, P., Dy, A. J., Joung, J., et al. (2017). Nucleic acid detection with CRISPR-Cas13a/C2c2. *Science* 356, 438–442. doi: 10.1126/science.aam9321

Gootenberg, J. S., Abudayyeh, O. O., Kellner, M. J., Joung, J., Collins, J. J., and Zhang, F. (2018). Multiplexed and portable nucleic acid detection platform with Cas13, Cas12a, and Csm6. *Science* 360, 439–444. doi: 10.1126/science.aaq0179

Grant, P. R., Turner, M. A., Shin, G. Y., Nastouli, E., and Levett, L. J. (2020). Extraction-free COVID-19 (SARS-CoV-2) diagnosis by RT-PCR to increase capacity for national testing programmes during a pandemic. *BioRxiv.* doi: 10.1101/2020.04.06.028316

Hasan, M. R., Mirza, F., Al-Hail, H., Sundararaju, S., Xaba, T., Iqbal, M., et al. (2020). Correction: Detection of SARS-CoV-2 RNA by direct RT-qPCR on nasopharyngeal specimens without extraction of viral RNA. *PloS One* 15, e0240343. doi: 10.1371/journal.pone.0240343

Hou, T., Zeng, W., Yang, M., Chen, W., Ren, L., Ai, J., et al. (2020). Development and evaluation of a rapid CRISPR-based diagnostic for COVID-19. *PloS Pathog.* 16, e1008705 10.1371/journal.ppat.1008705. doi: 10.1371/journal.ppat.1008705

Joung, J., Ladha, A., Saito, M., Kim, N G., Woolley, A. E., Segel, M., et al. (2020). Detection of SARS-CoV-2 with SHERLOCK One-Pot Testing. *N. Engl. J. Med.* 383 (15), 1492–1494. doi: 10.1056/NEJMc2026172

Jung, J., Garnett, E., Jariwala, P., Pham, H., Huang, R., Benzi, E., et al. (2020). Clinical performance of a semi-quantitative assay for SARS-CoV2 IgG and SARS-CoV2 IgM antibodies. *Clin. Chim. Acta* 510, 790–795. doi: 10.1016/j.cca.2020.09.023

Kellner, M. J., Koob, J. G., Gootenberg, J. S., Abudayyeh, O. O., and Zhang, F. (2019). SHERLOCK: nucleic acid detection with CRISPR nucleases. *Nat. Protoc.* 14, 2986–3012. doi: 10.1038/s41596-019-0210-2

Kirby, T. (2021). New variant of SARS-CoV-2 in UK causes surge of COVID-19. *Lancet Respir. Med.* 9, E20–E21. doi: 10.1016/S2213-2600(21)00005-9

Knott, G. J., and Doudna, J. A. (2018). CRISPR-Cas guides the future of genetic engineering. *Science* 361, 866–869. doi: 10.1126/science.aat5011

Kriegova, E., Fillerova, R., and Kvapil, P. (2020). Direct-RT-qPCR Detection of SARS-CoV-2 without RNA Extraction as Part of a COVID-19 Testing Strategy: From Sample to Result in One Hour. *Diagnostics* 10:605. doi: 10.3390/diagnostics10080605

Lalli, M. A., Langmade, J. S., Chen, X., Fronick, C. C., Sawyer, C. S., Burcea, L. C., et al. (2020). Rapid and Extraction-Free Detection of SARS-CoV-2 from Saliva by Colorimetric Reverse-Transcription Loop-Mediated Isothermal Amplification. *Clin. Chem.* 67, 415–424. doi: 10.1093/clinchem/hvaa267

Li, Y., Li, S., Wang, J., and Liu, G. (2019). CRISPR/Cas systems towards next-generation biosensing. *Trends Biotechnol.* 37, 730–743. doi: 10.1016/j.tibtech.2018.12.005

Merindol, N., Pépin, G., Marchand, C., Rheault, M., Peterson, C., Poirier, A., et al. (2020). SARS-CoV-2 detection by direct rRT-PCR without RNA extraction. *J. Clin. Virol.* 128:104423. doi: 10.1016/j.jcv.2020.104423

Meyerson, N. R., Yang, Q., Clark, S. K., Paige, C. L., Fattor, W. T., Gilchrist, A. R., et al. (2020). A community-deployable sars-cov-2 screening test using raw saliva with 45 minutes sample-to-results turnaround. *medRxiv.* doi: 10.1101/2020.07.16.20150250

Myhrvold, C., Freije, C. A., Gootenberg, J. S., Abudayyeh, O. O., Metsky, H. C., Durbin, A. F., et al. (2018). Field-deployable viral diagnostics using CRISPR-Cas13. *Science* 360, 444–448. doi: 10.1126/science.aas8836

Nguyen, L. T., Smith, B. M., and Jain, P. K. (2020). Enhancement of trans-cleavage activity of Cas12a with engineered crRNA enables amplified nucleic acid detection. *Nat. Commun.* 11, 4906. doi: 10.1038/s41467-020-20117-z

Ning, B., Yu, T., Zhang, S., Huang, Z., Tian, D., Lin, Z., et al. (2020). A smartphone-read ultrasensitive and quantitative saliva test for COVID-19. *Sci. Adv.* 7, eabe3703. doi: 10.1126/sciadv.abe3703

Ochert, A., Boulter, A., Birnbaum, W., Johnson, N., and Teo, C. (1994). Inhibitory effect of salivary fluids on PCR: potency and removal. *PCR Methods Appl.* 3, 365–368. doi: 10.1101/gr.3.6.365

Ostheim, P., Tichý, A., Sirak, I., Davidkova, M., Stastna, M. M., Kultova, G., et al. (2020). Overcoming challenges in human saliva gene expression measurements. *Sci. Rep.* 10, 1–12. doi: 10.1038/s41598-020-67825-6

Patchsung, M., Jantarug, K., Pattama, A., Aphicho, K., Suraritdechachai, S., Meesawat, P., et al. (2020). Clinical validation of a Cas13-based assay for the detection of SARS-CoV-2 RNA. *Nat. Biomed. Eng.* 4, 1140–1149. doi: 10.1038/s41551-020-00603-x

Piepenburg, O., Williams, C. H., Stemple, D. L., and Armes, N. A. (2006). DNA detection using recombination proteins. *PloS Biol.* 4, e204. doi: 10.1128/JCM.01946-20

Procop, G. W., Shrestha, N. K., Vogel, S., Van Sickle, K., Harrington, S., Rhoads, D. D., et al. (2020). A direct comparison of enhanced saliva to nasopharyngeal swab for the detection of SARS-CoV-2 in symptomatic patients. *J. Clin. Microbiol.* 58, e01946-20. doi: 10.1128/JCM.01946-20

Ranoa, D., Holland, R., Alnaji, F. G., Green, K., Wang, L., Brooke, C., et al. (2020). Saliva-based molecular testing for SARS-CoV-2 that bypasses RNA extraction. *Biorxiv.* doi: 10.1101/2020.06.18.159434

Srivatsan, S., Han, P. D., Van Raay, K., Wolf, C. R., Mcculloch, D. J., Kim, A. E., et al. (2020). Preliminary support for a "dry swab, extraction free" protocol for SARS-CoV-2 testing via RT-qPCR. *bioRxiv.* doi: 10.1101/2020.04.22.056283

Thai, H. T. C., Le, M. Q., Vuong, C. D., Parida, M., Minekawa, H., Notomi, T., et al. (2004). Development and evaluation of a novel loop-mediated isothermal amplification method for rapid detection of severe acute respiratory syndrome coronavirus. *J. Clin. Microbiol.* 42, 1956–196110.1128/JCM.42.5.1956–1961.2004. doi: 10.1128/JCM.42.5.1956-1961.2004

To, K. K.-W., Tsang, O. T.-Y., Yip, C. C.-Y., Chan, K.-H., Wu, T.-C., Chan, J. M.-C., et al. (2020). Consistent detection of 2019 novel coronavirus in saliva. *Clin. Infect. Dis.* 71, 841–843. doi: 10.1093/cid/ciaa149

Uhm, J.-S., Ahn, J. Y., Hyun, J., Sohn, Y., Kim, J. H., Jeong, S. J., et al. (2020). Patterns of viral clearance in the natural course of asymptomatic COVID-19: Comparison with symptomatic non-severe COVID-19. *Int. J. Infect. Dis.* 99, 279–285. doi: 10.1016/j.ijid.2020.07.070

Vogels, C. B., Brito, A. F., Wyllie, A. L., Fauver, J. R., Ott, I. M., Kalinich, C. C., et al. (2020a). Analytical sensitivity and efficiency comparisons of SARS-CoV-2 RT–qPCR primer–probe sets. *Nat. Microbiol.* 5, 1299–1305. doi: 10.1038/s41564-020-0761-6

Vogels, C. B., Watkins, A. E., Harden, C. A., Brackney, D. E., Shafer, J., Wang, J., et al. (2020b). SalivaDirect: A simplified and flexible platform to enhance SARS-CoV-2 testing capacity. *Med.* doi: 10.1016/j.medj.2020.12.010

Wee, S. K., Sivalingam, S. P., and Yap, E. P. H. (2020). Rapid direct nucleic acid amplification test without RNA extraction for SARS-CoV-2 using a portable PCR thermocycler. *Genes.* 11, 664. doi: 10.3390/genes11060664

Williams, E., Bond, K., Zhang, B., Putland, M., and Williamson, D. A. (2020). Saliva as a non-invasive specimen for detection of SARS-CoV-2. *J. Clin. Microbiol.* 58, e00776-20. doi: 10.1128/JCM.00776-20

Wyllie, A. L., Fournier, J., Casanovas-Massana, A., Campbell, M., Tokuyama, M., Vijayakumar, P., et al. (2020). Saliva or nasopharyngeal swab specimens for detection of SARS-CoV-2. *N. Engl. J. Med.* 383, 1283–1286. doi: 10.1056/NEJMc2016359

Xia, S., and Chen, X. (2020). Single-copy sensitive, field-deployable, and simultaneous dual-gene detection of SARS-CoV-2 RNA via modified RT–RPA. *Cell Discovery* 6, 1–4. doi: 10.1038/s41421-020-0175-x

Zou, Y., Mason, M. G., and Botella, J. R. (2020). Evaluation and improvement of isothermal amplification methods for point-of-need plant disease diagnostics. *PloS One* 15, e0235216. doi: 10.1371/journal.pone.0235216

18

Angiotensin II Receptor Blockers (ARBs Antihypertensive Agents) Increase Replication of SARS-CoV-2 in Vero E6 Cells

Gabriel Augusto Pires de Souza [1,2†], Ikram Omar Osman [1,2†], Marion Le Bideau [1,2], Jean-Pierre Baudoin [1,2], Rita Jaafar [1,2], Christian Devaux [1,2,3] and Bernard La Scola [1,2]*

[1] Aix-Marseille Université, Institut de Recherche pour le Développement (IRD), Assistance Publique - Hôpitaux de Marseille (AP-HM), MEPHI, Marseille, France, [2] Microbes, Evolution, Phylogénie et Infection (MEPHI), IHU - Méditerranée Infection, Marseille, France, [3] Centre National de La Recherche Scientifique (CNRS), Marseille, France

***Correspondence:**
Bernard La Scola
bernard.la-scola@univ-amu.fr

[†]These authors have contributed equally to this work

Several comorbidities, including hypertension, have been associated with an increased risk of developing severe disease during SARS-CoV-2 infection. Angiotensin II receptor blockers (ARBs) are currently some of the most widely-used drugs to control blood pressure by acting on the angiotensin II type 1 receptor (AT1R). ARBs have been reported to trigger the modulation of the angiotensin I converting enzyme 2 (ACE2), the receptor used by the virus to penetrate susceptible cells, raising concern that such treatments may promote virus capture and increase their viral load in patients receiving ARBs therapy. In this *in vitro* study, we reviewed the effect of ARBs on ACE2 and AT1R expression and investigated whether treatment of permissive ACE2+/AT1R+ Vero E6 cells with ARBs alters SARS-CoV-2 replication *in vitro* in an angiotensin II-free system. After treating the cells with the ARBs, we observed an approximate 50% relative increase in SARS-CoV-2 production in infected Vero E6 cells that correlates with the ARBs-induced up-regulation of ACE2 expression. From this data, we believe that the use of ARBs in hypertensive patients infected by SARS-CoV-2 should be carefully evaluated.

Keywords: SARS-CoV-2, COVID-19, angiotensin II receptor blockers, antihypertensive, angiotensin I converting enzyme 2, Vero E6 cells

INTRODUCTION

The emergence and rapid spread of severe acute respiratory syndrome (SARS) in patients hospitalised in China in late 2019 led to the discovery of a novel coronavirus (Huang et al., 2020; Li et al., 2020; Zhou et al., 2020). The SARS-coronavirus 2 (SARS-CoV-2), which later spread across the globe and reached pandemic status, has forced several countries to adopt lockdown measures, under the threat of the health system collapsing, despite the fact that this put the economy at risk (Shang et al., 2020). Almost one-and-a-half years after the first outbreak of coronavirus disease 2019 (COVID-19) in China, the disease has caused more than three million deaths for 145 million people infected worldwide as of 25 April 2020 (https://coronavirus.jhu.edu/map.html).

SARS-CoV-2 represents one of the most severe threats to human health in more than a century. Previously, other beta coronaviruses caused outbreaks of historical significance, such as the SARS-coronavirus and the Middle East respiratory syndrome (MERS) (Drosten et al., 2003; Zaki et al., 2012; Chakravarty et al., 2020; Zhou et al., 2020). However, despite the previous experience of the SARS-CoV outbreak, much remains uncertain about SARS-CoV-2 infection and coronavirus disease 2019 (COVID-19). Some risk groups have been identified as being more likely to develop severe manifestations of the disease, such as patients with as an underlying lung injury (Yang et al., 2020). Individuals with pre-existing lung disease, diabetes mellitus, and hypertension are at particular risk for SARS-CoV-2 infection (Chen et al., 2020; Liu et al., 2020).

Hypertension is associated with the renin-angiotensin system (RAS), a cascade of vasoactive peptides that orchestrate key human physiology (Wu et al., 2020). The ACE2 monocarboxypeptidase plays a key role in this cascade by acting as a regulator of blood pressure homeostasis through its ability to catalyse the proteolysis of Angiotensin II (AngII) into Ang (Drosten et al., 2003; Zaki et al., 2012; Chakravarty et al., 2020; Huang et al., 2020; Li et al., 2020; Shang et al., 2020; Zhou et al., 2020, Wu et al., 2020). Deregulation of the RAS pathway leads to an increase in the level of AngII, which interacts with its angiotensin II type 1 receptor (AT1R), thus facilitating the activation of various intracellular pathways involved in the remodelling of the heart, vascular disease and endothelial dysfunction (Muslin, 2008; Wehbe et al., 2020).

Interestingly, ACE2 is used by SARS-CoV-2 as a receptor for cell adhesion, which is the initial stage of the virus multiplication cycle (Mostafa-Hedeab, 2020; Shang et al., 2020; Zhou et al., 2020). Once the virus finds the receptor of a permissive cell, it will penetrate it and control the cellular machinery for its replication. As ACE2 is critical to SARS-CoV-2 infection, an imbalance in the RAS, with a shift towards ACE/Ang II and suppressing ACE2/Ang- (Drosten et al., 2003; Zaki et al., 2012; Chakravarty et al., 2020; Huang et al., 2020; Li et al., 2020; Shang et al., 2020; Zhou et al., 2020), may be an important mediator of COVID-19 pathophysiology (South et al., 2020). However, many individuals with hypertension are prescribed Angiotensin II receptor blockers (ARBs) as a drug to control their blood pressure.

To date, however, there has been much debate about the relationship between the use of angiotensin-converting enzyme inhibitors (ACEi) and ARBs and the risk associated with COVID-19 (Devaux, 2020; Sama et al., 2020; Sriram and Insel, 2020; Zhang et al., 2020). Some authors suspected that treating hypertension and other cardiovascular diseases with antihypertensive drugs could increase ACE2 levels and increase the risk of SARS-CoV-2 infection and/or replication, leading to an increased risk of admission to the intensive care unit, mechanical ventilation, and, sometimes, death in patients with COVID-19 (Diaz, 2020; Fang et al., 2020; Ferrario et al., 2020). Nevertheless, in general, it is understood that there is still a long way to go to reach any conclusions in this regard (Zheng et al., 2020). In this study, we investigated whether the previous treatment of SARS-CoV-2 permissive cells with different ARBs modulates the expression of AT1R and ACE2 and impacts the virus replication in a system without Ang II.

MATERIALS AND METHODS

Cell Line Culture

The Vero E6 cell line (American type culture collection ATCC® CRL-1586 ™) were cultured in minimum essential medium (MEM. Gibco, Thermo Fischer) containing 4% foetal bovine serum (FBS. Invitrogen) and 1% l_glutamine (L-Gln. Invitrogen) at 37°C in a 5% CO_2 atmosphere using a 175 cm^2 flasks. Every two days, the medium was replenished, and the confluent culture flask was subcultured by trypsinisation.

Callu-3 cells (ATCC® HTB-55 ™) were in turn cultured in MEM containing 10% FBS and 1% L-Gln in 175 cm^2 flasks. In tests using culture plaques, the cells were prepared three days earlier and were incubated at 37°C and 5% CO_2. Caco-2 cells (ATCC® HTB-37 ™) were also cultured in 175 cm^2 flasks at 37°C and 5% CO_2, using DMEM medium supplemented with 10% FBS, 1% L-Gln, and 1% amino acids (Aa).

Drugs

Azilsartan, Eprosartan mesylate, Irbesartan, Losartan potassium, Olmesartan medoxomil, Telmisartan, and Valsartan were purchased from the Sigma Group. All ARBs were pre-diluted in DMSO according to the manufacturer's instructions.

Virus Production and Titration

The SARS-CoV-2 (strain IHUMI-3) was previously isolated from the liquid collected from a nasopharyngeal swab (Gautret et al., 2020). The isolate passed through a total of four passages in Vero E6 cells) in culture medium supplemented with 4% FBS and 1% L-Gln, incubated at 37°C in a 5% CO_2 atmosphere. Following the fourth passage in monolayers of Vero E6 cells grown in 75 cm^2 flasks, and with the almost complete cytopathic effect (about 72 hours after infection), the supernatant was collected, centrifuged at 3,000×g for 10 minutes at 4°C and then filtered through a 0.22 µm membrane. The filtrate was supplemented with 10% FBS and 1% 2- [4- (2-hydroxyethyl) piperazin-1-yl] ethanesulfonic acid (HEPES) buffer and stored at -80°C, making up the viral stock of SARS-CoV- 2. The 50% tissue culture infectious dose of the virus (TCID50) was determined using 6×10^5 Vero E6 cells/well in 96 cell plates, using eight replicate wells by dilution. The TCID50 was calculated according to the Spearman and Kärber algorithm.

Cell Viability Assay

In vitro cell viability evaluations were performed on the Vero E6, Calu-3, and Caco-2 cell lines according to the method described by Mossman, with slight modifications (Mosmann, 1983). In a 96-well plate, 6×10^5 cells were incubated, and 200 µL of the Azilsartan, Eprosartan, Irbesartan, Losartan, Olmesartan, Telmisartan, or Valsartan at different concentrations (1 mM, 500 µM, 250 µM, 125 µM, 62.5 µM, 31.25 µM, 15.62 µM, and

7.81 μM) was added to the wells, diluted in culture medium (MEM 4% FBS and 1% L-Gln for Vero E6, MEM 10% FBS and 1% L-Gln for Calu-3 and DMEM 10% FBS plus 1% Aa and 1% L-Gln for Caco-2), and incubated at 37°C in a 5% CO_2 atmosphere. Following incubation, the supernatant from each well was replaced by 100 μl of culture medium, supplemented with 10 μl of MTT solution (3-(4,5-dimethyl-2-thiazolyl)-2,5-diphenyl-2H-tetrazolium bromide, Sigma Aldrich, France) (5 mg/ml in PBS), followed by a four-hour incubation at 37°C in a 5% CO_2 atmosphere. To dissolve the formazen crystals formed by the living cells, 50μL DMSO was added to each well and incubated for 30 minutes at 37°C in a 5% CO_2 atmosphere. Absorbance was measured at 540 nm using a TECAN Infinite F200 microplate reader. The non-cytotoxic concentration was evaluated based on the percentage of viable cells compared to non-treated cell control. Concentrations that exhibited more than 90% of viable cells after five days were considered non-cytotoxic.

Ribonucleic Acid (RNA) Extraction and Quantitative-Reverse Transcription Polymerase Chain Reaction (qRT-PCR)

24-well plates were prepared with 2×10^5 cells/well of Vero E6, using MEM with 4% of FBS and 1% L-Gln. They were incubated again overnight at 37°C in a 5% CO_2 atmosphere. Cell culture supernatant was removed and replaced by drugs diluted in the culture medium. The drug concentrations tested were those previously defined as non-cytotoxic by MTT assay. Following the treatment 72 hours, the cells were infected with SARS-CoV-2 at a multiplicity of infection (MOI) of 0.1 for 24 hours at 37°C in a 5% CO_2 incubator. In accordance with the manufacturer's instructions, RNAs were extracted from cells using a RNeasy Mini Kit (QIAGEN SA) with a DNase I step to eliminate DNA contaminants. The quantity and quality of the RNA was evaluated using a Nanodrop 1000 spectrophotometer (Thermo Science). The first-strand cDNA was obtained using oligo(dT) primers and Moloney murine leukaemia virus reverse transcriptase (MMLV-RT kit; Life Technologies), using 100 ng of purified RNA. The qPCR experiments were performed using specific oligonucleotide primers and hot-start polymerase (SYBR Green Fast Master Mix; Roche Diagnostics). The amplification cycles were performed using a C1000 Touch Thermal cycler (Biorad). The specific primers used were Angiotensin Convertase Enzyme (ACE2) primers (Fwd: 5' CAG AGG GTG AAC ATA CAG TTG G 3'; Rev: 5' CAG GGA ACA GGT AGA GGA CAT 3') and Angiotensin receptor 1 (AT1R) (Fwd: 5' TGTGGACTGA ACCGACTTTTCT 3'; Rev: 5' GGAACTCTCATCTCC TGTTGCT 3'). The results of qRT-PCR were normalised using the housekeeping gene β-Actin (ACTB) (Fwd: 5' CAT GCC ATC CTG CGT CTG GA 3'; Rev: 5' CCG TGG CCA TCT CTT GCT CG 3') and expressed as relative expression ($2^{-\Delta CT}$), where ΔCT = CT (Target gene) – CT (Actin).

Western Immunoblotting Assay

Vero E6 (2x105 cells/well) were cultured in flat-bottom 24-well plates for 12 hours. Cell culture supernatant was removed and replaced by drugs diluted in the culture medium. After 72 hours of treatment, the cells were then infected with SARS-CoV-2 at a multiplicity of infection (MOI) of 0.01 for 24 hours at 37°C in a 5% CO_2 atmosphere. Following infection, the cells were immediately washed with ice-cold phosphate-buffered saline (PBS) and lysed on the plate in a 1X RIPA buffer [100 mM Tris-HCl pH7.5; 750 mM NaCl; 5mM EDTA; 5% Igepal, 0.5% sodium dodecyl sulfate (SDS); 2.5% Na Deoxycholate] supplemented with a protease cocktail inhibitor and phosphatase inhibitor (Roche, Germany). 100 μg of protein was loaded onto 10% SDS polyacrylamide gels. After being transferred onto a Nitrocellulose membrane, the blots were incubated for one hour at 4°C with a blocking solution [5% Free Fat Milk (FFM)-1XPBS-0.3% Tween 20], followed by overnight incubation with a goat ACE2 polyclonal antibody (1:1,000, MAB933, R&D Systems, Minneapolis, USA). After three washes in 1XPBS-0,3%Tween 20, the membrane was incubated with a Donkey anti-Goat IgG Horseradish peroxidase-conjugated (1:10,000 dilution with a blocking solution) for two hours at room temperature. A mouse Glyceradehyde-3-Phosphate dehydrogenase (GADPH) monoclonal antibody (1:5,000, Abnova, Taiwan), followed by incubation with a Sheep anti-mouse Horseradish peroxidase-conjugated (1:10,000 dilution with a blocking solution) (Life Technologies, France) as the loading control. The proteins were visualized using an ECL Western Blotting Substrate (Promega, USA), and images were digitized using a Fusion FX (Vilber Lourmat, France). As for the spike expression, the JessTM Simple Western system of automated Western immunoblotting was used, as previously described (Edouard et al., 2020).

Flow Cytometry

Flow cytometry was used to study the expression of ACE2 on the surface of cells. To do so, Vero E6 cells were cultured in flat-bottom six-well plates at an initial concentration of 1×10^6 cells/well and were then treated with the drugs. Cells were then detached from the solid support using 2 mM of EDTA in PBS with an incubation period of 15 minutes at 4°C, followed by centrifugation of 500 g for five minutes. The pellet was resuspended in a saturation buffer (2mM EDTA, 10% FSB in PBS) for 30 minutes. For ACE2 labelling, an anti-ACE2-PE mAb (R&D Systems, Minneapolis, USA) was incubated with cells at 4°C in the dark for 30 minutes. Fluorescence intensity was measured using a Canto II cytofluorometer (Becton Dickinson, Biosciences, Le Pont de Claix, France). The results were further analysed using a BD FACSDiva Software v.6.1.3 (Becton, Dickinson and Company, New Jersey, USA).

Immunofluorescence Assay

Vero E6 cells were cultured on sterile coverslips in 24-well plates at an initial concentration of 2×10^5 cells/mL. After 72 hours of treatment with the drugs, the cells were then infected with the SARS-CoV-2 at a multiplicity of infection (MOI) of 0.01 for 24 hours at 37°C in a 5% CO2 atmosphere. Following infection, the cells were fixed with paraformaldehyde (4%), permeabilised with 0.1% Triton X-100 for three minutes, and saturated with 3%BSA-0,1% Tween 20-PBS for 30 minutes at room temperature. For the primary labelling, a goat ACE2 polyclonal antibody (1:1,000, MAB933, R&D Systems, Minneapolis, USA), a mouse AT1R monoclonal antibody (1:1,000, MAB102441, R&D Systems,

Minneapolis, USA), and a polyclonal rabbit anti-SARS Coronavirus Spike protein (rabbit) (1:1,000, PA1-41142, Thermo Fisher, France.) were used. The 4',6'-diamino-2-fenil-indol (DAPI) (1:25,000, Life Technologies) and the Phalloidin (Alexa 488) (1:500, OZYME) were used for respectively staining the nucleus and the filamentous actin. After one hour of incubation, the slide was washed with 1XPBS-0,1% Tween 20 and incubated for 30 minutes at room temperature with a mix of Donkey anti-Goat IgG (H+L) Secondary Antibody (Alexa Fluor 555), Goat anti-Rabbit IgG (H+L) Secondary Antibody (Alexa Fluor 647) and Goat anti-Mouse IgGb (H+L) Secondary antibody (Alexa Fluor 488) (1:1,000, Thermo Fischer Scientific). The fluorescence was analysed using laser scanning confocal microscopy. Images were acquired using a confocal microscope (Zeiss LSM 800) with a 63X/1.4 oil objective, an electronic magnification of 0.5, and a resolution of 1014_1014 pixels.

Drug Testing Procedure

We prepared 96-well plates with 10^6 cells/well of Vero E6, cultured in MEM with 4% FBS and 1% L-Gln. They were incubated overnight at 37°C in a 5% CO_2 atmosphere. Cell culture supernatant was removed and replaced by drugs diluted in the culture medium. The drug concentrations tested were those previously defined as non-cytotoxic by MTT assay. After the drugs had been incubated with the cells for 72 hours, the virus suspension (SARS-CoV-2) in culture medium was added to all wells, except the negative controls (where 50 µL of the medium was added), respecting a multiplicity of infection (MOI) of 0.004. The supernatant (t=0) was immediately collected (100 µL) and 24- and 48-hours post-infection (h.p.i.), both were stored at -80°C until RNA extraction. 100 µL from each well was then collected and added to 100 µL of the ready-use VXL buffer from the QIAcube kit (Qiagen, Germany). Extraction was performed using the manual High Pure RNA Isolation Kit (Roche Life Science), following the recommended procedures. The RT-PCR was performed using the Roche RealTime PCR Ready RNA Virus Master Kit. The primers were designed against the N gene (Fwd: 5' GACCCCAAAATC AGCGAAAT 3'; Rev: 5' TCTGGTTACTGCCAGTTGAATCTG 3') using the Roche LightCycler® 480 Instrument II. Relative viral quantification was performed compared to the untreated control (viruses without drugs) using the $2^{(-\Delta CT)}$ method, where $\Delta Ct = \{[(Ct\ 48\ h.p.i)\ treated\ well] - [mean\ (Ct\ 0\ h.p.i)]\}$ (Livak and Schmittgen, 2001). We performed a statistical analysis using GraphPad Prism v9.0.0 (GraphPad Software, La Jolla, California USA). The distribution of the data did not follow a normal law. Therefore, a non-parametric Kruskal-Wallis test was used to compare each combination against positive controls using ΔCt between t48 h.p.i. and t0 h.p.i. Finally, Dunn's test was used to correct multiple comparisons. All tests were used at $p = 0.05$ parameter and were bilateral (two-sides). From the supernatant collected 24 h.p.i. of Vero E6 cells previously treated with the ARBs, TCID50 was also performed, using four replicate wells by dilution, being read in duplicate.

For this test in Caco-2 and Calu-3 cells, they were cultured in their respective culture medium in 96-well plates three days before the treatment of the cells with the non-cytotoxic concentrations of the ARBs. On treatment day, the medium was collected and replaced by the respective medium containing the respective concentrations of each of the compounds. The cells were maintained for three more days in the presence of the ARBs before being infected with SARS-CoV-2. The infection maintained the parameters of MOI (0.004) and final volume (250 µL/well), with one extra step, in which adsorption was performed by centrifugation at 2,272×g, for one hour at 37°C (Sorvall Legend XT/XF, M-20 rotor, Thermo Scientific™ 75217406/DEL). The cells were then incubated for an additional three days post-infection, when the supernatant was collected for analysis. The remaining procedures and analyses were performed as described for the Vero E6 cell above.

RESULTS

Modulation of ACE2 Gene Expression by ARBs in Vero E6 Cells

Initially, we evaluated the modulation of ACE2 and AT1R gene expression in ARBs-treated Vero E6 cells by RT-qPCR. Vero E6 cells are a common model used to evaluate the effect of drugs on coronavirus replication. The ARBs concentrations used in all *in vitro* procedures were defined from the considered non-cytotoxic concentrations by the MTT assays performed in a five-day incubation period in Vero E6 cells and two other SARS-CoV-2 susceptible cells lines (Calu-3 and Caco-2). The suitable non-toxic concentrations were 7 µM for Losartan, Telmisartan, and Valsartan, 15 µM for Azilsartan and Olmesartan Medoxomil, 30 µM for Eprosartan Mesylate, and 60 µM for Irbesartan.

Modulation was observed at the transcription of the ACE2 and AT1R genes when these cells were treated for 72 hours with the ARBs (**Figure 1**). While the expression of ACE2 mRNA increased in ARBs-treated Vero E6 (**Figure 1A**), the expression of AT1R mRNA reduced (**Figure 1B**) compared with the untreated control. However, at the protein level, the ACE2 expression increase seems more specific, being stimulated by Azilsartan, Eprosartan, Irbesartan and Telmisartan, representing four of the seven tested ARBs (**Figure 1C**).

When the percentage of positive cells for ACE2 was evaluated by flow cytometry, it was observed that treatment with ARBs does not drastically change the number of cells that are positive for the main receptor of the virus (ACE2). However, not all ARBs have the same effects, and there is a decrease in the number of positive ACE2 cells, particularly under treatment with Losartan and Telmisartan (**Supplementary Figure 1**).

When evaluating ACE2 and AT1R protein expression in Vero E6 cells treated with Azilsartan (15 µM) (**Figure 2**), it was possible to observe a wide distribution of AT1R and ACE2 in Vero E6 cells, even in the untreated control (**Figure 2A**), but also a greater fluorescence intensity at the wavelength corresponding to the ACE2 of cells treated with Azilsartan (**Figures 2A, B**). This suggests that the increase in ACE2 expression by Azilsartan is also reflected in cell surface levels. No changes were observed regarding the fluorescence intensity in the wavelength corresponding to AT1R (**Figures 2A, B**).

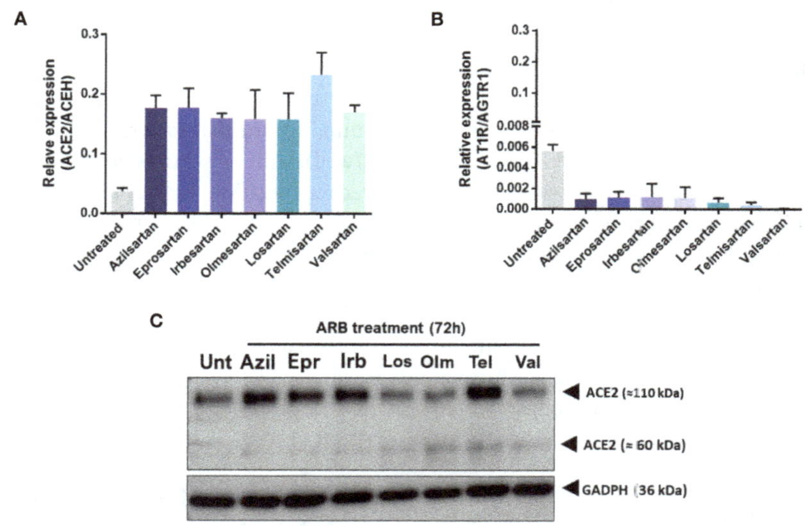

FIGURE 1 | Expression of Angiotensin II receptor type 1 (AT1R) and Angiotensin-converting enzyme 2 (ACE2) mRNAs and proteins by VERO E6 cells following 72 hours incubation with different Angiotensin II Receptor Blockers (ARBs). Non-cytotoxic concentrations of ARBs (Azil, Azilsartan 15µM; Epr, Eprosartan 30µM; Irb, Irbesartan 60µM; Los, losartan 7µM; Olm, Olmesartan 15µM; Tel, Telmisartan 7µM; Val, Valsartan 7µM) were previously defined by the MTT assay and cells were treated with the various ARBs. **(A)** Relative expression of the ACE2/ACEH gene in untreated (Unt) and ARB-treated Vero E6 cells. **(B)** Relative expression of the ATR1/AGTR1 gene in untreated versus ARB-treated Vero E6 cells. **(C)** Expression of ACE2 protein in untreated versus ARB-treated Vero E6 cells (the membrane-anchored ACE2 glycosylated protein that acts as receptor for SARS-CoV-2 is the 110kDa form of the molecule).

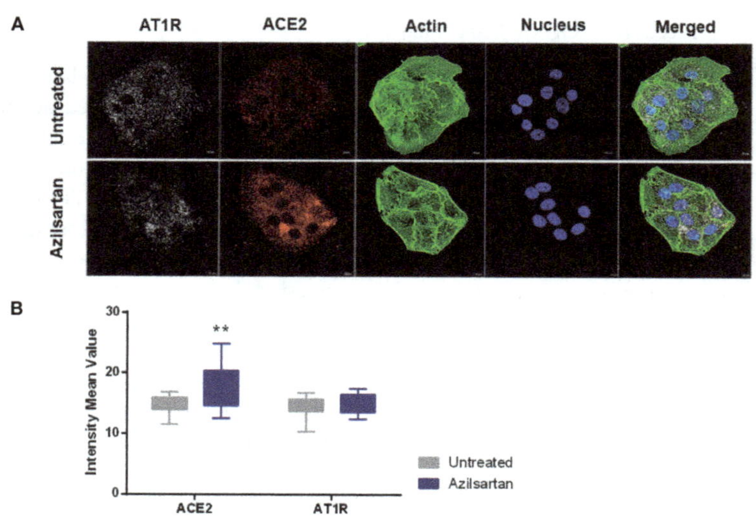

FIGURE 2 | Modulation of cell surface-expressed ATR1 and ACE2 molecules in Vero E6 cells non-infected and treated with Azilsartan (15 µM) for 72 hours by immunofluorescence microscopy. **(A)** The panel presents non-infected cells after incubation with Azilsartan (15 µM) and evaluating the fluorescence corresponding to the ATR1, ACE2, Actin, and the nucleus of the cells. The merge of the images is displayed at the right of the panel. Images were acquired using a confocal microscope (Zeiss LSM 800) with a 63X/1.4 oil objective. **(B)** Quantitative representation of Mean Fluorescence corresponding to ATR1 and ACE2 molecule expression on VERO E6 cells treated or not treated with Azilsartan. $^{**}P < 0.01$.

Modulation of SARS-CoV-2 Production by ARBs

For the drug testing procedure, Vero E6 cells were selected, as they express an ACE2 receptor compatible with SARS-CoV-2 spike binding, express the ATR1 surface molecule, with which they ARBs will interact (**Figure 2A**), and are known to allow a complete productive viral cycle.

Vero 6 cells were incubated with the different ARBs at previously defined concentrations, for 72 hours before infection with SARS-CoV-2. The relative SARS-CoV-2 replication was evaluated in the cell supernatant, 24 and 48 h.p.i. by RT-qPCR (**Figure 3A**). A significant increase in SARS-CoV-2 replication was observed for Azilsartan, Eprosartan, and Irbesartan treated Vero E6, which represented three of the seven treated groups (**Figure 3B**). This increase was also observed but with less intensity at 48 h.p.i. (data not shown).

Using Western blotting, it was also possible to detect an increase in SARS-CoV-2 spike protein expression in the groups pre-treated with Azilsartan, Eprosartan, and Irbesartan which were infected with SARS-CoV-2 (**Figure 3C**). The TCID50 of the supernatant recovered from ARBs-treated Vero E6 cells 24 h.p.i. also suggests an increase in viral multiplication. The supernatant of cells treated with Azilsartan and Irbesartan presented a TCID50 of 4.27×10^5 TCID50/mL (**Figure 3D**), which was higher than the untreated control (1.22×10^5 TCID50/mL) (**Figure 3D**). The groups treated with Eprosartan and Telmisartan displayed a moderated increase, which represents 2.40×10^5 TCID50/mL (**Figure 3D**), however, this increase was not significant according to statistical analysis. This data suggests that RNA replication and protein production are increased, as is the number of infectious particles released at 24 h.p.i. Increased detection of viral proteins in cells infected with SARS-CoV-2 (24 h.p.i.) treated with Azilsartan and therefore with increased ACE2 expression, was also observed (**Figure 4**).

DISCUSSION

Since the previous SARS-CoV outbreak, it has been established that the main receptor for this sarbecovirus/beta-coronavirus is the ACE2 receptor, which is also the main cell entry receptor for SARS-CoV-2 (Hoffmann et al., 2020; Zhou et al., 2020). It is understood that the ACE2 protein on the surface of alveolar epithelial cells in the lung allows for respiratory tract infection by SARS-CoV-2. It is assumed that ACE2 levels correlate with a susceptibility to SARS-CoV-2 infection (Devaux et al., 2020). Pre-existing comorbidities, such as respiratory diseases, diabetes and hypertension, in addition to cardiopathy, have been defined as risk factors for a higher lethality of COVID-19 (Chawla et al., 2020; Yang et al., 2020; Zhang et al., 2020).

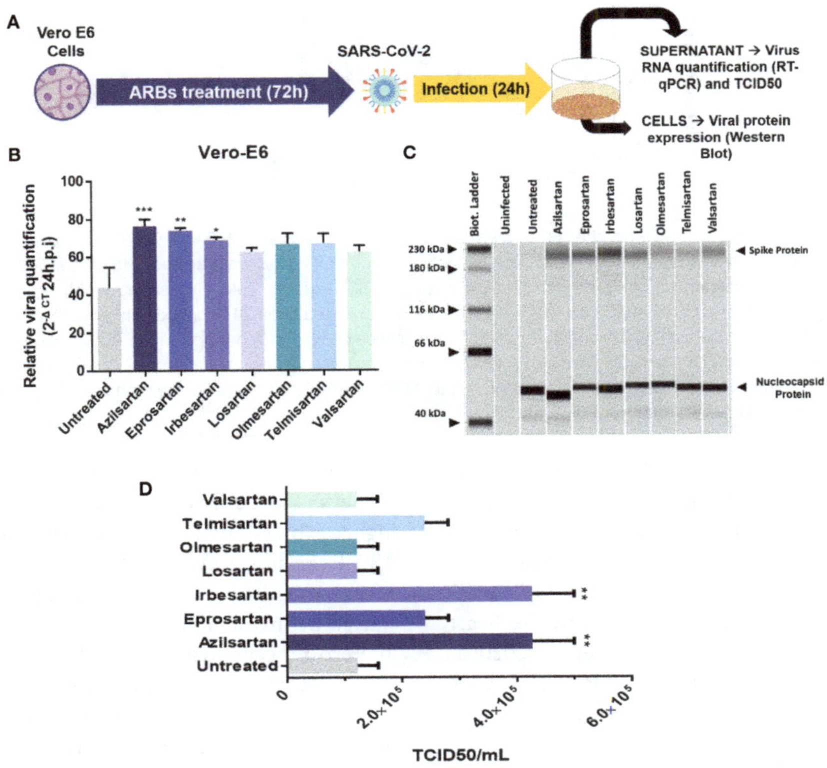

FIGURE 3 | Effects of pre-treating Vero E6 cells in cells with different ARBs on the SARS-CoV-2 production. **(A)** Schematic flow of the analysis: Vero E6 cells were treated with different non-cytotoxic concentrations of ARBs (Azilsartan 15μM; Eprosartan 30μM; Irbesartan 60μM; Losartan 7μM; Olmesartan 15μM; Telmisartan 7μM; Valsartan 7μM) were previously defined by the MTT assay and cells were treated with the different ARBs.) for 72 hours and were subsequently infected and produced virus evaluated by RT-qPCR and Western Blotting 24 hours post-infection (h.p.i.). **(B)** Relative SARS-CoV-2 genome quantification in supernatant of treated and infected Vero E6 cells by RT-qPCR: Relative viral quantification was performed compared to the untreated control (viruses without drugs) using the $2^{(-\Delta CT)}$ method, where ΔCt = {[(Ct 48 h.p.i) treated well] – [mean (Ct 0 h.p.i)]}; **(C)** Viral protein detection in treated and infected Vero E6 cells by Western Blotting performed in JessTM Simple Western system (automated Western immunoblotting), in which every column represents individual runs **(D)** TCID50 (six days post-infection) from the supernatant of the treated with different ARBs Vero E6 cells recovered 24 h.p.i. *$P < 0.05$; **$P < 0.01$; ***$P < 0.001$.

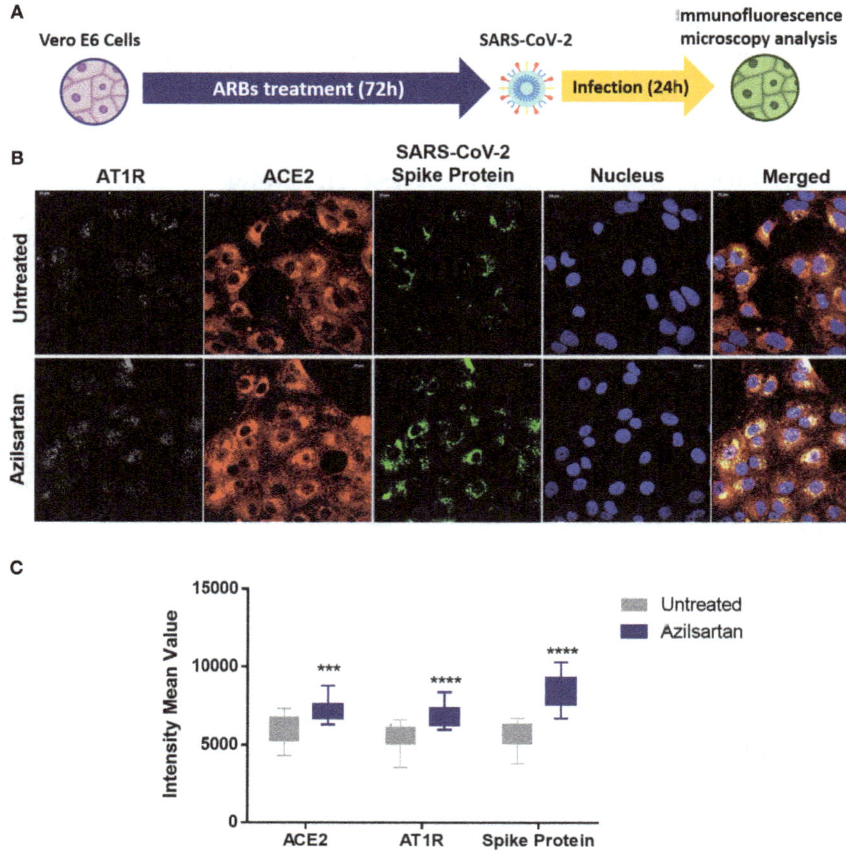

FIGURE 4 | Modulation of cell surface-expressed ATR1 and ACE2 molecules in Vero E6 cells infected with SARS-CoV-2 (24 h.p.i) and treated with Azilsartan (15 μM) for 72 hours by immunofluorescence microscopy. **(A)** Schematic flow of the analysis: Vero E6 cells were treated with various ARBs (the MTT assay previously defined non-cytotoxic concentrations: Azilosartan 15μM; Eprosartan 30μM; Irbesartan 60μM; Losartan 7μM; Olmesartan 15μM; Telmisartan 7μM; Valsartan 7μM) for 72 hours and were subsequently infected for analysis of ACE2 and ATR1 on treated and infected cells, 24 hours post-infection (h.p.i.). **(B)** The panel presents SARS-CoV-2 infected cells after incubation with Azilsartan (15 μM) and evaluation of fluorescence corresponding to the ATR1, ACE2, viral spike protein, and the nucleus of the cells. The merge of the images is displayed at the right of the panel. Images were acquired using a confocal microscope (Zeiss LSM 800) with a 63X/1.4 oil objective. **(C)** Quantitative representation of Mean Fluorescence corresponding to ATR1 and ACE2 molecules expression on VERO E6 cells treated or not treated with Azilsartan and SARS-CoV-2 in the cells. ***$P < 0.001$; ****$P < 0.0001$.

It is common for individuals with hypertension to use ARBs to control their blood pressure. As its name suggests, this type of medication works by blocking receptors for angiotensin II (AT1 receptor), which has the role of promoting the constriction of blood vessels, increasing blood pressure (Ferrario et al., 2005; Ferrario et al., 2020). These receptors are found in the heart, blood vessels, kidneys, and intestine (Gheblawi et al., 2020; Li et al., 2020; Devaux et al., 2021). Blocking the action of AngII helps to lower blood pressure and prevent damage to the heart and kidneys.

Vero E6 cells were established from kidney tissue from an African green monkey and represent a lineage of mammalian cell lines most often used for isolation and virus production, including SARS-CoV-2 (Naoki et al., 2014; Matsuyama et al., 2020). The ACE2 protein from monkeys showed very moderate polymorphism concerning the ACE2 protein from humans and could interact with the spike protein from SARS-CoV-2 (Devaux et al., 2021; Fenollar et al., 2021). One study suggested that one of the organs in which ACE2 expression levels are higher is the kidneys. The permissiveness of this cell to different viruses, the higher expression of ACE2 (Ren et al., 2006), and the presence of AT1R (**Figure 2A**) make this cell a potential for studying the effects of ARBs on SARS-CoV-2 replication. For this reason, we started by investigating the modulation of the ACE2 and AT1R in Vero E6 cells treated with different ARBs in their respective non-cytotoxic concentration in an AngII-free system. From these analyses, we could observe that ARBs increase the expression of ACE2 mRNA (**Figure 1A**). At the protein level, Azilsartan, Eprosartan, Irbesartan, and Telmisartan induce a higher expression of ACE2 in Vero E6 cells than in untreated cells (**Figure 1C**). While the expression of ACE2 increases, the expression of the receptor to which these blocking molecules bind (AT1R) reduces (**Figure 1B**).

Some animal studies indicate that the use of ARBs leads to the upregulation of ACE2 (Ishiyama et al., 2004; Ferrario et al., 2005; Igase et al., 2008; Soler et al., 2009). In Lewis rats treated for 12 days with Losartan, an increase of cardiac ACE2 mRNA and cardiac ACE2 activity was observed (Ferrario et al., 2005). In this same animal model, Losartan and Olmesartan administered *via* osmotic minipumps for 28 days after coronary artery ligation increased ACE 2 mRNA approximately three-fold (Ishiyama et al., 2004). The proposed mechanism by which these drugs increase the expression of ACE2 associates the inhibitory effect of angiotensin II on Ace2 transcription mediated with the activation of kinase 1 regulated by extracellular signal (ERK1; also known as MAPK3) and ERK2 (also known as MAPK1), after binding to AT1R (Ferrario et al., 2020). This mechanism was revealed by studies in cultured cerebellar or medullary astrocytes, obtained from rats and cardiomyocytes and cardiac fibroblasts from neonatal rats, treated with Losartan and Valsartan (Gallagher et al., 2006; Gallagher et al., 2008).

When it was understood that this modulation of ACE2 expression also occurred in Vero E6 cells, due to data that indicated a rise in the expression of ACE2 mRNA and protein (**Figure 1**), we sought to use immunofluorescence microscopy to investigate whether treatment with ARBs reflected an increase in ACE2 available on the cell surface. Azilsartan appeared to be a potent modulator of the expression of ACE2 in Vero E6 cells, both at the mRNA and protein levels, and therefore was used in this assay. In Vero E6 cells treated for 72 hours with Azilsartan, an increase in the fluorescence average in the wavelength associated with the ACE2 marker was observed (**Figure 2**). This result indicates that the expression of ACE2 would increase on the cell surface, while the superficial AT1R would not change (**Figure 2B**). Interestingly there are significant differences in the ability of ARBs to induce the overexpression of ACE2 once bound to AT1R, since some drugs at 7 μM (e.g. Telmisartan) lead to higher ACE2 increase than others when used at higher concentration (e.g. Irbesartan at 60 μM).

Flow cytometry analysis revealed that neither the number of ACE2-positive cells nor fluorescence intensity changed for most treatments (**Supplementary Figure 1**). In protein expression and in the number of positive ACE2 cells, the divergent results of Losartan are possibly related to its shortest half-life *in vivo* (Oparil, 2000). It is also known that after AngII binding, AT1R triggers ACE2 cleavage and shedding, dependent on the p38 mitogen-activated protein kinases (MAPK) pathway, resulting in reduced cell surface expression (Muslin, 2008; Wu et al., 2020). It has previously been shown that Azilsartan, Candesartan, Losartan, and Telmisartan would have opposite effects on the MAPK pathway, which, consequently, would prevent ACE2 excision (Sekine et al., 2003; Kajiya et al., 2011; Zhong et al., 2011). Therefore, it was understood that number of cells that could be susceptible to SARS-CoV-2 infection remains unchanged, even with quantitative variations in receptor expression. Nevertheless, the increased expression of ACE2 could represent a greater likelihood that the virus would bind to one of these receptors due to the increased availability of receptors on the cell surface, resulting in greater chances of infection success.

Although the adsorption step is essential, since the virus-receptor interaction orchestrates the entry of viruses into the cell, the release of the progeny virions at the end of the replication cycle determines the success of the infection (Maginnis, 2018). Therefore, we chose to evaluate whether Vero E6 cells, already characterised by expressing ACE2 modulated by the ARBs, would change the amount of viral progeny released by the infected cells when pre-treated with these ARBs. The relative production of SARS-CoV-2 was evaluated by RT-qPCR of cellular supernatant, 24 and 48 h.p.i. and after 72 hours of ARB-pre-treatment of Vero E6 cells. The increase in viral RNA expression was significant for three of the ARBs used (Azilsartan, Eprosartan, and Irbesartan) 24 h.p.i. (**Figure 3B**). Interestingly, these three ARBs were also potent positive modulators of ACE2 protein expression (**Figure 1C**).

The estimated complete replication cycle time in Vero E6 cells for SARS-CoV-2 is eight hours (Brahim Belhaouari et al., 2020), so it is challenging to observe significant changes at early stages when using a low MOI. At later stages, however, the saturation of the supernatant by viruses also makes observation difficult to interpret. This difficulty became obvious when a less significant production of SARS-CoV-2 was observed 48 h.p.i. compared to the untreated control at the same time (data not shown). However, in other cell lines, such as Caco-2 and Calu-3, both human-derived cells, this increased effect was not observed (**Supplementary Figure 2**). Previously, the treatment of Calu-3 cells with Losartan and Valsartan did not alter the gene expression of ACE2 (Baba et al., 2020). In this same study, it was suggested that one of the possible reasons for this is the low expression of AT1R, a receptor that interacts with ARBs, in human lung tissues, compared to other organs such as the kidneys (Baba et al., 2020). Therefore, these cells would not be good study models.

When we evaluated the expression of viral proteins inside cells infected with SARS-CoV-2 after treatment with ARBs, these same three compounds (Azilsartan, Eprosartan, and Irbesartan) were shown to induce increased expressions of Spike protein (S) (**Figure 3C**), reinforcing the evidence that these compounds increase the multiplication of SARS-CoV-2. A similar result was observed by immunofluorescence microscopy in cells previously treated with Azilsartan. It is possible to observe the increased detection of ACE2 and SARS-CoV-2 compared to the untreated control (**Figure 4**).

In the viral envelope, glycoprotein S is responsible for the virus attachment to host cells and penetration by membrane fusion (V'kovski et al., 2021). At the same time, the Nucleocapsid (N) of coronaviruses, in addition to playing a structural role, has already been presented as a multifunctional protein, playing a role in the initial RNA synthesis event (McBride et al., 2014). Thus, the higher expression of S protein in the treated groups compared to the untreated groups, may mean infections are established for longer, suggesting that the entry of SARS-CoV-2 may have occurred more quickly due to the increased receptor availability. That notwithstanding, the evaluation of the increased expression of RNA and protein does not necessarily reflect the number of infectious particles produced. Therefore, from the supernatant recovered from the treated and infected cells 24 h.p.i., we performed a TCID50 assay in which it was observed that the ARBs that present modulation of protein ACE2 in Vero E6

(**Figure 1C**) also increased the number of infectious particles at the end of the 24 hour cycle from 1.22×10^5 TCID50/mL (untreated) to 4.27×10^5 TCID50/mL (Azilsartan and Irbesartan) (**Figure 3D**).

Our results indicate that Vero E6 cells previously treated for 72 hours with ARBs show a relative increase of ACE2 expression and SARS-CoV-2 production. These results clearly establish a direct relationship between the use of ARBs and viral replication and suggest that when the ARBs bind to the AT1R at the surface of Vero E6 cells, they trigger AT1R-mediated intracellular signals leading to the induction of ACE2 gene expression which likely allows an increase of viral binding, uptake and/or replication. Although the Vero E6 cells model is commonly used to study coronaviruses replication and drugs effect, the relevance of this model in relation to the beneficial use of ARBs to prevent hypertension in patients during periods of high circulation of SARS-CoV-2 remains to be questioned. First, Vero E6 cells were treated with ARBs without adding AngII to the culture medium, while elevated AngII has been reported as a biomarker of severe COVID-19. Second, our experiments were performed in Vero E6 cells, a monkey cellular model. It should be emphasized that the increased SARS-CoV-2 production found in Vero E6 cells was not observed in the preliminary investigations we recently performed on two human cell lines namely Caco-2 (intestinal epithelia origin) and Calu-3 (lung epithelia origin). A wider range of human cell lines should be tested to determine whether it is possible to select an appropriated human cellular model in which ARBs could up-regulated ACE2 expression and SARS-CoV-2 production with the objective to get closer to the conditions that are encountered in human pathophysiology. Based on our current data, we believe that the beneficial use of ARBs to prevent hypertension in patients during periods of high circulation of SARS-CoV-2 should be carefully evaluated.

AUTHOR CONTRIBUTIONS

Conceptualisation: BS and CD. Methodology: BS, CD, and J-PB. Formal analysis: GP, IO, MB, and J-PB. Investigation: GP, IO, RJ, and MB. Data curation: GP, IO, and MB. Writing— original draft preparation: GP and IO. Writing—review and editing: GP, IO, BS, and CD. Supervision: BS and CD. Project administration: BS. All authors contributed to the article and approved the submitted version.

ACKNOWLEDGMENTS

Our sincere thanks to Clio Grimaldier for her help in producing the stock of viruses, to Priscilla Jardot for her assistance with molecular biology techniques, and Eloïne Bestion for donating us the antibodies against GAPDH.

SUPPLEMENTARY MATERIAL

Supplementary Figure 1 | Percentage of ACE2 positive Vero E6 cells after treatment with ARBs. The cells were treated with the ARBs for 72 hours prior to flow cytometry analysis. **(A)** Percentage of ACE2-positive cells after treatment with ARBs; **(B)** Mean Fluorescence Intensity of the cells after treatment with ARBs. Fluorescence intensity was measured using a Canto II cytofluorometer (Becton Dickinson, Biosciences, Le Pont de Claix, France) and the results were analysed using a BD FACSDiva Software v.6.1.3 (Becton, Dickinson and Company, New Jersey, United States). Non-cytotoxic concentrations were previously defined by the MTT assay: Azilsartan 15μM; Eprosartan 30μM; Irbesartan 60μM; Losartan 7μM; Olmesartan 15μM; Telmisartan 7μM; Valsartan 7μM. $^{**}P < 0.01$; $^{***}P < 0.001$.

Supplementary Figure 2 | Effects of pre-treating human secondary cells with different ARBs in the SARS-CoV-2 replication. The cells were initially treated with the drugs for 72 hours before infection and incubated in their presence for additional three days post-infection. The supernatant was collected 72 h.p.i. for RNA extraction and RT-qPCR. Relative viral quantification was performed and compared to the untreated control using the 2(−ΔCT) method. **(A)** Relative viral genome quantification of SARS-CoV-2 in the supernatant of treated and infected Caco-2 cells. **(B)** Relative SARS-CoV-2 genome quantification in the supernatant of treated and infected Calu-3 cells. Non-cytotoxic concentrations were previously defined by MTT assay. $^{*}P < 0.05$; $^{****}P < 0.0001$.

REFERENCES

Baba, R., Oki, K., Itcho, K., Kobuke, K., Nagano, G., Ohno, H., et al. (2020). Angiotensin-Converting Enzyme 2 Expression Is Not Induced by the Renin–Angiotensin System in the Lung. *ERJ Open Res.* 6 (4), 00402–02020. doi: 10.1183/23120541.00402-2020

Brahim Belhaouari, D., Fontanini, A., Baudoin, J. P., Haddad, G., Le Bideau, M., Bou Khalil, J. Y., et al. (2020). The Strengths of Scanning Electron Microscopy in Deciphering SARS-Cov-2 Infectious Cycle. *Front. Microbiol.* 11, 1–11. doi: 10.3389/fmicb.2020.02014

Chakravarty, D., Nair, S. S., Hammouda, N., Ratnani, P., Gharib, Y., Wagaskar, V., et al. (2020). Sex Differences in SARS-CoV-2 Infection Rates and the Potential Link to Prostate Cancer. *Commun. Biol.* 3 (1), 1–12. doi: 10.1038/s42003-020-1088-9

Chawla, D., Rizzo, S., Zalocusky, K., Keebler, D., Chia, J., Lindsay, L., et al. (2020). Descriptive Epidemiology of 16,780 Hospitalized COVID-19 Patients in the United States. *medRxiv* 2020. doi: 10.1101/2020.07.17.20156265

Chen, R., Liang, W., Jiang, M., Guan, W., Zhan, C., Wang, T., et al. (2020). Risk Factors of Fatal Outcome in Hospitalized Subjects With Coronavirus Disease 2019 From a Nationwide Analysis in China. *Chest* 158 (1), 97–105. doi: 10.1016/j.chest.2020.04.010

Devaux, C. A. (2020). Are ACE Inhibitors and ARBs More Beneficial Than Harmful in the Treatment of Severe COVID-19 Disease? *J. Cardiol. Cardiovasc. Med.* 7 (2), 101–103. doi: 10.17352/2455-2976.000122

Devaux, C. A., Lagier, J. C., and Raoult, D. (2021). New Insights Into the Physiopathology of COVID-19: SARS-Cov-2-Associated Gastrointestinal Illness. *Front. Med.* 8, 3–8. doi: 10.3389/fmed.2021.640073

Devaux, C. A., Pinault, L., Osman, I. O., and Raoult, D. (2021). Can ACE2 Receptor Polymorphism Predict Species Susceptibility to SARS-Cov-2? *Front. Public Health* 8, 1–12. doi: 10.3389/fpubh.2020.608765

Devaux, C. A., Rolain, J. M., and Raoult, D. (2020). ACE2 Receptor Polymorphism: Susceptibility to SARS-CoV-2, Hypertension, Multi-Organ Failure, and COVID-19 Disease Outcome. *J. Microbiol. Immunol. Infect.* 53 (3), 425–435. doi: 10.1016/j.jmii.2020.04.015

Diaz, J. H. (2020). Hypothesis: Angiotensin-Converting Enzyme Inhibitors and Angiotensin Receptor Blockers may Increase the Risk of Severe COVID-19. *J. Travel Med.* 27 (3), 1–2. doi: 10.1093/jtm/taaa041

Drosten, C., Günther, S., Preiser, W., van der Werf, S., Brodt, H. R., Becker, S., et al. (2003). Identification of a Novel Coronavirus in Patients With Severe Acute Respiratory Syndrome. *N Engl. J. Med.* 348 (20), 1967–1976. doi: 10.1056/NEJMoa030747

Edouard, S., Jaafar, R., Orain, N., Parola, P., Colson, P., la Scola, B., et al. (2020). Automated Western Immunoblotting Detection of anti-SARS-CoV-2 Serum Antibodies. *Eur J Clin Microbiol Infect Dis.* 40 (6), 1309–1317. doi: 10.3389/fmicb.2021.663815

Fang, L., Karakiulakis, G., and Roth, M. (2020). Are Patients With Hypertension and Diabetes Mellitus at Increased Risk for COVID-19 Infection? *Lancet Respir. Med.* 8 (4), e21. doi: 10.1016/S2213-2600(20)30116-8

Fenollar, F., Mediannikov, O., Maurin, M., Devaux, C., Colson, P., Levasseur, A., et al. (2021). Mink, SARS-CoV-2, and the Human-Animal Interface. *Front. Microbiol.* 12, 1–12.

Ferrario, C. M., Ahmad, S., and Groban, L. (2020). Mechanisms by Which Angiotensin-Receptor Blockers Increase ACE2 Levels. *Nat. Rev. Cardiol.* 17 (6), 378. doi: 10.1038/s41569-020-0387-7

Ferrario, C. M., Jessup, J., Chappell, M. C., Averill, D. B., Brosnihan, K. B., Tallant, E. A., et al. (2005). Effect of Angiotensin-Converting Enzyme Inhibition and Angiotensin II Receptor Blockers on Cardiac Angiotensin-Converting Enzyme 2. *Circulation* 111 (20), 2605–2610. doi: 10.1161/CIRCULATIONAHA.104.510461

Ferrario, C. M., Jessup, J., Gallagher, P. E., Averill, D. B., Brosnihan, K. B., Tallant, E. A., et al. (2005). Effects of Renin-Angiotensin System Blockade on Renal Angiotensin-(1-7) Forming Enzymes and Receptors. *Kidney Int.* 68 (5), 2189–2196. doi: 10.1111/j.1523-1755.2005.00675.x

Gallagher, P. E., Chappell, M. C., Ferrario, C. M., and Tallant, E. A. (2006). Distinct Roles for ANG II and ANG-(1-7) in the Regulation of Angiotensin-Converting Enzyme 2 in Rat Astrocytes. *Am. J. Physiol. - Cell Physiol.* 290 (2), 420–426. doi: 10.1152/ajpcell.00409.2004

Gallagher, P. E., Ferrario, C. M., and Tallant, E. A. (2008). Regulation of ACE2 in Cardiac Myocytes and Fibroblasts. *Am. J. Physiol. - Hear Circ. Physiol.* 295 (6), 2373–2379. doi: 10.1152/ajpheart.00426.2008

Gautret, P., Lagier, J. C., Parola, P., Hoang, V. T., Meddeb, L., Mailhe, M., et al. (2020). Hydroxychloroquine and Azithromycin as a Treatment of COVID-19: Results of an Open-Label Non-Randomized Clinical Trial. *Int. J. Antimicrob. Agents* 56 (1), 105949. doi: 10.1016/j.ijantimicag.2020.105949

Gheblawi, M., Wang, K., Viveiros, A., Nguyen, Q., Zhong, J. C., Turner, A. J., et al. (2020). Angiotensin-Converting Enzyme 2: SARS-CoV-2 Receptor and Regulator of the Renin-Angiotensin System: Celebrating the 20th Anniversary of the Discovery of ACE2. *Circ. Res.* 126 (10), 1456–1474. doi: 10.1161/CIRCRESAHA.120.317015

Hoffmann, M., Kleine-Weber, H., Schroeder, S., Krüger, N., Herrler, T., Erichsen, S., et al. (2020). SARS-Cov-2 Cell Entry Depends on ACE2 and TMPRSS2 and Is Blocked by a Clinically Proven Protease Inhibitor. *Cell* 181 (2), 271–280.e8. doi: 10.1016/j.cell.2020.02.052

Huang, C., Wang, Y., Li, X., Ren, L., Zhao, J., Hu, Y., et al. (2020). Clinical Features of Patients Infected With 2019 Novel Coronavirus in Wuhan, China. *Lancet* 395 (10223), 497–506. doi: 10.1016/S0140-6736(20)30183-5

Igase, M., Kohara, K., Nagai, T., Miki, T., and Ferrario, C. M. (2008). Increased Expression of Angiotensin Converting Enzyme 2 in Conjunction With Reduction of Neointima by Angiotensin II Type 1 Receptor Blockade. *Hypertens. Res.* 31 (3), 553–559. doi: 10.1291/hypres.31.553

Ishiyama, Y., Gallagher, P. E., Averill, D. B., Tallant, E. A., Brosnihan, K. B., and Ferrario, C. M. (2004). Upregulation of Angiotensin-Converting Enzyme 2 After Myocardial Infarction by Blockade of Angiotensin II Receptors. *Hypertension* 43 (5), 970–976. doi: 10.1161/01.HYP.0000124667.34652.1a

Kajiya, T., Ho, C., Wang, J., Vilardi, R., and Kurtz, T. W. (2011). Molecular and Cellular Effects of Azilsartan: A New Generation Angiotensin II Receptor Blocker. *J. Hypertens.* 29 (12), 2476–2483. doi: 10.1097/HJH.0b013e32834c46fd

Li, Q., Guan, X., Wu, P., Wang, X., Zhou, L., Tong, Y., et al. (2020). Early Transmission Dynamics in Wuhan, China, of Novel Coronavirus-Infected Pneumonia. *N Engl. J. Med.* 382 (13), 1199–1207. doi: 10.1056/NEJMoa2001316

Li, M. Y., Li, L., Zhang, Y., and Wang, X. S. (2020). Expression of the SARS-CoV-2 Cell Receptor Gene ACE2 in a Wide Variety of Human Tissues. *Infect. Dis. Poverty* 9 (1), 1–7. doi: 10.1186/s40249-020-00662-x

Liu, D., Cui, P., Zeng, S., Wang, S., Feng, X., Xu, S., et al. (2020). Risk Factors for Developing Into Critical COVID-19 Patients in Wuhan, China: A Multicenter, Retrospective, Cohort Study. *EClinicalMed* 25:100471. doi: 10.1016/j.eclinm.2020.100471

Livak, K. J., and Schmittgen, T. D. (2001). Analysis of Relative Gene Expression Data Using Real-Time Quantitative PCR and the 2-ΔΔCT Method. *Methods* 25 (4), 402–408. doi: 10.1006/meth.2001.1262

Maginnis, M. S. (2018). Virus–Receptor Interactions: The Key to Cellular Invasion. *J. Mol. Biol.* 430, 2590–2611. doi: 10.1016/j.jmb.2018.06.024

Matsuyama, S., Nao, N., Shirato, K., Kawase, M., Saito, S., Takayama, I., et al. (2020). Enhanced Isolation of SARS-CoV-2 by TMPRSS2- Expressing Cells. *Proc. Natl. Acad. Sci. U. S. A.* 117 (13), 7001–7003. doi: 10.1073/pnas.2002589117

McBride, R., van Zyl, M., and Fielding, B. C. (2014). The Coronavirus Nucleocapsid Is a Multifunctional Protein. *Viruses* 6 (8), 2991–3018. doi: 10.3390/v6082991

Mosmann, T. (1983). Rapid Colorimetric Assay for Cellular Growth and Survival: Application to Proliferation and Cytotoxicity Assays. *J. Immunol. Methods* 65 (1–2), 55–63. doi: 10.1016/0022-1759(83)90303-4

Mostafa-Hedeab, G. (2020). ACE2 as Drug Target of COVID-19 Virus Treatment, Simplified Updated Review. *Rep. Biochem. Mol. Biol.* 9 (1), 97–105. doi: 10.29252/rbmb.9.1.97

Muslin, A. J. (2008). Mapk Signaling in Cardiovascular Health and Disease: Molecular Mechanisms and Therapeutic Targets Introduction: Intracellular Signal Transduction Pathways. *Clin. Sci.* 115 (7), 203–218. doi: 10.1042/CS20070430

Naoki, O., Arihiro, K., Toshiyuki, Y., Noriko, H., Fumio, K., Suyoshi, S., et al. (2014). The Genome Landscape of the African Green Monkey Kidney-Derived Vero Cell Line. *DNA Res.* 21 (6), 673–683. doi: 10.1093/dnares/dsu029

Oparil, S. (2000). Newly Emerging Pharmacologic Differences in Angiotensin II Receptor Blockers. *Am. J. Hypertens.* 13 (1 II SUPPL.), 18–24. doi: 10.1016/S0895-7061(99)00250-2

Ren, X., Glende, J., Al-Falah, M., de Vries, V., Schwegmann-Wessels, C., Qu, X., et al. (2006). Analysis of ACE2 in Polarized Epithelial Cells: Surface Expression and Function as Receptor for Severe Acute Respiratory Syndrome-Associated Coronavirus. *J. Gen. Virol.* 87 (6), 1691–1695. doi: 10.1099/vir.0.81749-0

Sama, I. E., Ravera, A., Santema, B. T., Van Goor, H., Ter Maaten, J. M., Cleland, J. G. F., et al. (2020). Circulating Plasma Concentrations of Angiotensin-Converting Enzyme 2 Inmen and Women With Heart Failure and Effects of Renin-Angiotensin-Aldosterone Inhibitors. *Eur. Heart J.* 41 (19), 1810–1817. doi: 10.1093/eurheartj/ehaa373

Sekine, S., Nitta, K., Uchida, K., Yumura, W., and Nihei, H. (2003). Possible Involvement of Mitogen-Activated Protein Kinase in the Angiotensin II-induced Fibronectin Synthesis in Renal Interstitial Fibroblasts. *Arch. Biochem. Biophys.* 415 (1), 63–68. doi: 10.1016/S0003-9861(03)00163-2

Shang, J., Wan, Y., Luo, C., Ye, G., Geng, Q., Auerbach, A., et al. (2020). Cell Entry Mechanisms of SARS-Cov-2. *Proc. Natl. Acad. Sci. U. S. A.* 117 (21), 11727–11734. doi: 10.1073/pnas.2003138117

Soler, M. J., Ye, M., Wysocki, J., William, J., Lloveras, J., and Batlle, D. (2009). Localization of ACE2 in the Renal Vasculature: Amplification by Angiotensin II Type 1 Receptor Blockade Using Telmisartan. *Am. J. Physiol. - Ren Physiol.* 296 (2), 398–405. doi: 10.1152/ajprenal.90488.2008

South, A. M., Brady, T. M., and Flynn, J. T. (2020). Ace2 (Angiotensin-Converting Enzyme 2), COVID-19, and ACE Inhibitor and Ang II (Angiotensin II) Receptor Blocker Use During the Pandemic: The Pediatric Perspective. *Hypertension* 76 (1), 16–22. doi: 10.1161/HYPERTENSIONAHA.120.15291

Sriram, K., and Insel, P. A. (2020). Risks of ACE Inhibitor and ARB Usage in COVID-19: Evaluating the Evidence. *Clin. Pharmacol. Ther.* 108 (2), 236–241. doi: 10.1002/cpt.1863

V'kovski, P., Kratzel, A., Steiner, S., Stalder, H., and Thiel, V. (2021). Coronavirus Biology and Replication: Implications for SARS-Cov-2. *Nat. Rev. Microbiol.* 19 (3), 155–170. doi: 10.1038/s41579-020-00468-6

Wehbe, Z., Hammoud, S., Soudani, N., Zaraket, H., El-Yazbi, A., and Eid, A. H. (2020). Molecular Insights Into SARS Cov-2 Interaction With Cardiovascular Disease: Role of RAAS and MAPK Signaling. *Front. Pharmacol.* 11, 1–11. doi: 10.3389/fphar.2020.00836

Wu, C., Ye, D., Millick, A., Li, Z., Danser, A. H. J., Daughrty, A., et al. (2020). Effects of Renin-Angiotensin Inhibition on ACE2 (Angiotensin-Converting Enzyme 2) and TMPRSS2 (Transmembrane Protease Serine 2) Expression Insights. *Hypertension* 76, e29–e30. doi: 10.1161/HYPERTENSIONAHA.120.15782

Yang, X., Yu, Y., Xu, J., Shu, H., Xia, J., Liu, H., et al. (2020). Clinical Course and Outcomes of Critically Ill Patients With SARS-CoV-2 Pneumonia in Wuhan, China: A Single-Centered, Retrospective, Observational Study. *Lancet Respir. Med.* 8 (5), 475–481. doi: 10.1016/S2213-2600(20)30079-5

Zaki, A. M., Van Boheemen, S., Bestebroer, T. M., Osterhaus, A. D. M. E., and Fouchier, R. A. M. (2012). Isolation of a Novel Coronavirus From a Man With Pneumonia in Saudi Arabia. *N Engl. J. Med.* 367 (19), 1814–1820. doi: 10.1056/NEJMoa1211721

Zhang, P., Zhu, L., Cai, J., Lei, F., Qin, J. J., Xie, J., et al. (2020). Association of Inpatient Use of Angiotensin-Converting Enzyme Inhibitors and Angiotensin Ii Receptor Blockers With Mortality Among Patients With Hypertension Hospitalized With COVID-19. *Circ. Res.* 126 (12), 1671–1681. doi: 10.1161/CIRCRESAHA.120.317134

Zheng, Y. Y., Ma, Y. T., Zhang, J. Y., and Xie, X. (2020). Covid-19 and the Cardiovascular System. *Nat. Rev. Cardiol.* 17 (5), 259–260. doi: 10.1038/s41569-020-0360-5

Zhong, J. C., Ye, J. Y., Jin, H. Y., Yu, X., Yu, H. M., Zhu, D. L., et al. (2011). Telmisartan Attenuates Aortic Hypertrophy in Hypertensive Rats by the Modulation of ACE2 and Profilin-1 Expression. *Regul. Pept.* 166 (1–3), 90–97. doi: 10.1016/j.regpep.2010.09.005

Zhou, P., Lou, Y. X., XG, W., Hu, B., Zhang, L., Zhang, W., et al. (2020). A Pneumonia Outbreak Associated With a New Coronavirus of Probable Bat Origin. *Nature* 579 (7798), 270–273. doi: 10.1038/s41586-020-2012-7

19

Testosterone in COVID-19: An Adversary Bane or Comrade Boon

Hayder M. Al-kuraishy[1], *Ali I. Al-Gareeb*[1], *Hani Faidah*[2], *Athanasios Alexiou*[3,4*] *and Gaber El-Saber Batiha*[5*]

[1] *Department of Clinical Pharmacology and Medicine, College of Medicine, ALmustansiriyia University, Baghdad, Iraq,* [2] *Faculty of Medicine, Umm Al Qura University, Mecca, Saudi Arabia,* [3] *Department of Science and Engineering, Novel Global Community Educational Foundation, Hebersham, NSW, Australia,* [4] *AFNP Med Austria, Wien, Austria,* [5] *Department of Pharmacology and Therapeutics, Faculty of Veterinary Medicine, Damanhour University, Damanhour, Egypt*

Correspondence:
Athanasios Alexiou
alexiou@ngcef.net
Gaber El-Saber Batiha
gaberbatiha@gmail.com

COVID-19 is a pandemic disease caused by severe acute respiratory coronavirus 2 (SARS-CoV-2), which leads to pulmonary manifestations like acute lung injury (ALI) and acute respiratory distress syndrome (ARDS). In addition, COVID-19 may cause extra-pulmonary manifestation such as testicular injury. Both high and low levels of testosterone could affect the severity of COVID-19. Herein, there is substantial controversy regarding the potential role of testosterone in SARS-CoV-2 infection and COVID-19 severity. Therefore, the present study aimed to review and elucidate the assorted view of preponderance regarding the beneficial and harmful effects of testosterone in COVID-19. A related literature search in PubMed, Scopus, Web of Science, Google Scholar, and Science Direct was done. All published articles related to the role of testosterone and COVID-19 were included in this mini-review. The beneficial effects of testosterone in COVID-19 are through inhibition of pro-inflammatory cytokines, augmentation of anti-inflammatory cytokines, modulation of the immune response, attenuation of oxidative stress, and endothelial dysfunction. However, its harmful effects in COVID-19 are due to augmentation of transmembrane protease serine 2 (TMPRSS2), which is essential for cleaving and activating SARS-CoV-2 spike protein during acute SARS-CoV-2 infection. Most published studies illustrated that low testosterone levels are linked to COVID-19 severity. A low testosterone level in COVID-19 is mainly due to testicular injury, the primary source of testosterone.

Keywords: anti-inflammatory cytokines, COVID-19, pro-inflammatory cytokines, testosterone, TMPRSS2

INTRODUCTION

The novel coronavirus disease 19 (nCoV19), commonly known as COVID-19, is an infectious disease caused by severe acute respiratory coronavirus 2 (SARS-CoV-2), leading to acute systemic disturbances, pro-inflammatory activation, hypercytokinemia, cytokine storm, and multi-organ damage (Al-Kuraishy et al., 2020). COVID-19 affects various organs, mainly the respiratory system, presenting with pulmonary manifestations like acute lung injury (ALI) and acute respiratory distress syndrome (ARDS), and extra-pulmonary manifestations like acute cardiac, neurological disorders, pancreatic injury, acute kidney injury, and testicular injury (Al-Kuraishy et al., 2020a;

Lugnier et al., 2021). This systemic effect of COVID-19 is due to the wide distribution of angiotensin-converting enzyme 2 (AEC2), a receptor and entry point for SARS-CoV-2 (Al-Kuraishy et al., 2020b). ACE2 receptor is chiefly expressed in the lung alveolar cells type II, proximal renal tubules, and testis primarily in Sertoli and Leydig cells. Binding of SARS-CoV-2 to ACE2 leads to downregulation of these protective receptors with subsequent increment in the level of vasoconstrictors angiotensin II (Ang II) and reduction of vasodilator angiotensin (Ang 1-7) (Ang 1-9) with induction release of pro-inflammatory cytokines (Bank et al., 2021).

Since the World Health Organization (WHO) declaration of this disease as a pandemic and until late July 2021, the total confirmed cases are 194,250,977, with 4,258,789 deaths. The mortality rate ranges from 0.9% to 10.5% in COVID-19 patients without comorbidities than COVID-19 patients with comorbidities, respectively (Anjorin et al., 2021).

It has been reported that male sex is regarded as a risk factor for COVID-19 severity and had worse outcomes, which might occur due to male-specific factors that increase men's vulnerability to the SARS-CoV-2 infection compared to women (Farghaly and Makboul, 2021). One of the important male sex-specific factors is the anabolic testosterone hormone secreted mainly from testicles and to a lesser extent from the adrenal cortex (Al-Maiahy et al., 2020). Testosterone is also secreted from ovaries in females; however, the total daily testosterone production is approximately 20 times more in males than in females; thus, testosterone serum level is 8 times more in men than in women (Handelsman et al., 2018).

Testosterone serum levels are reduced on average by 2% per year after the age of 40 years, increasing the prevalence of hypogonadism in men following the age of 40 years up to 9.5%, and this prevalence is augmented in several cardiometabolic disorders (Grossmann et al., 2020). Indeed, testosterone deficiency-induced late hypogonadism is regarded as an independent risk factor for various pulmonary disorders and cardio-metabolic disturbances, including hypertension, dyslipidemia, type 2 diabetes mellitus (T2DM), endothelial dysfunction, and coagulopathy (Butanis et al., 2017; Assyov et al., 2020). Therefore, hypogonadism accounts for 53.3% of hospitalized patients with a high mortality rate due to immunosuppression and susceptibility for different viral infections (Pezzaioli et al., 2020).

During COVID-19, SARS-CoV-2 infection may affect the testicles by binding to ACE2 expressed in the Sertoli and Leydig cells, causing infertility and suppressing testosterone production (Abobaker and Raba, 2020). Schroeder et al. (2020) illustrated that low testosterone serum level is linked to SARS-CoV-2 infections and COVID-19 severity in critically ill patients due to reduced immunomodulation antiviral effects of androgen. On the other hand, Wambier et al. (2020) revealed that high testosterone and other androgens serum levels might increase the severity of COVID-19 through augmentation of the expression of transmembrane protease serine 2 (TMPRSS2), which is vital for cleaving and activation of SARS-CoV-2 spike protein during acute SARS-CoV-2 infection.

Therefore, there is substantial controversy regarding the potential role of testosterone and other androgens in SARS-CoV-2 infection and COVID-19 severity. Thus, the present study is aimed to review and elucidate the assorted view of preponderance regarding testosterone's beneficial and harmful effects in COVID-19.

METHODS AND SEARCH STRATEGY

A related literature search in PubMed, Scopus, Web of Science, Google Scholar, and Science Direct was done. All published articles related to the role of testosterone and COVID-19 were included in this mini-review. We search the international database using the medical subject heading (MeSH) to identify the relevant articles published up to 2021. The listed keywords used in this search included [COVID-19 OR SARS-CoV-2] AND [Testosterone OR Androgens], [COVID-19 OR SARS-CoV-2] AND [Hypogonadism OR Androgen sensitivity], [Hypogonadism OR Low testosterone], AND [COVID-19 severity]. The final results were mainly limited to human subjects. All types of published articles with different languages were included, and the final findings were summarized in a mini-review (**Figure 1**).

THE BENEFICIAL ROLE OF TESTOSTERONE IN COVID-19

It has been reported that testosterone serum level is reduced by aging and cardio-metabolic diseases including T2DM, obesity, dyslipidemia, heart failure, and atherosclerosis, which are common risk factors for the development of COVID-19 severity (Millar et al., 2016; Maddaloni et al., 2020).

Different studies illustrated that testosterone has a protective role in the respiratory system; it improves forced expiratory volume, vital capacity, oxygen consumption, and respiratory muscle contraction (Montano et al., 2014). Marques et al. (2020) illustrated that testosterone replacement therapy in orchiectomized male rats improves oxygenation and attenuates tissue hypoxia and hypercapnia. Thus, low testosterone serum levels in patients with hypogonadism may increase severity of obstructive pulmonary disease (Novković et al., 2019).

Testosterone and Acute Lung Injury

Testosterone has a crucial pulmo-protective effect through the modulation of lung inflammations, and a reduction of testosterone by aging may predispose the old age for chronic inflammatory pulmonary disorders and viral infections (Keilich et al., 2019). Redente et al. (2011) illustrated that testosterone's defending role against bleomycin-induced ALI is through inhibition of pro-inflammatory mediated neutrophil alveolitis. It has been observed that testosterone inhibits the production of pro-inflammatory cytokines, including IL-1β, IL-6, and TNF-α, and inflammatory adipocytokines with a cumulative effect on the anti-

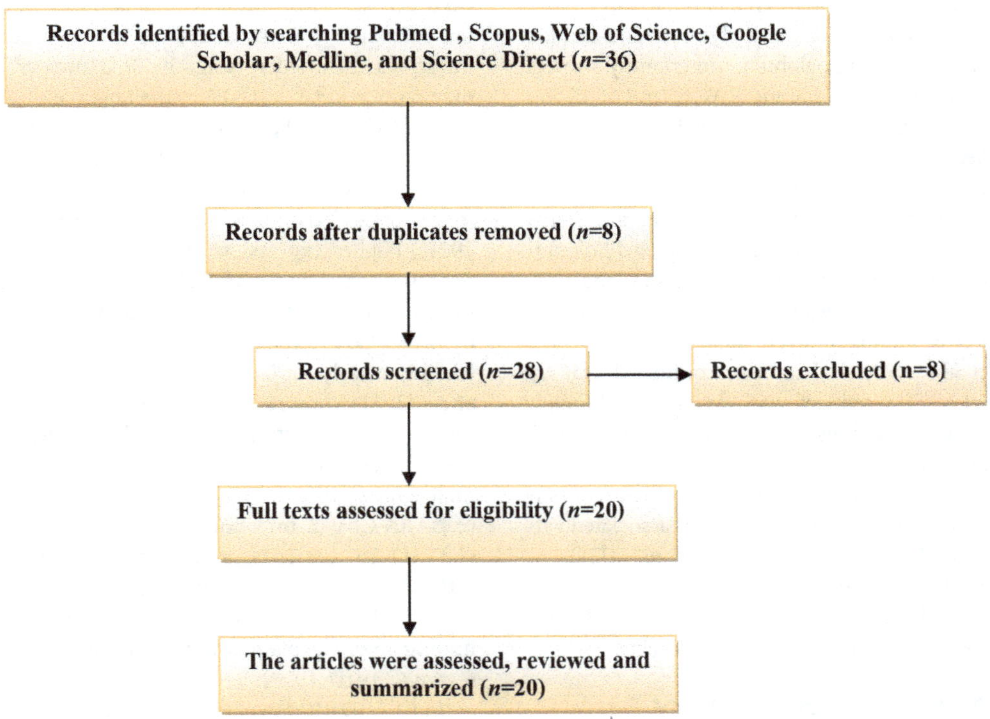

FIGURE 1 | Consort-flow diagram of the present study.

inflammatory adiponectin (Bianchi, 2019). Wang et al. (2021) revealed that testosterone therapy reduces lung inflammation and fibrosis by inhibiting nuclear respiratory factor 1 (NRF1) and the NF-κB signaling pathway.

Pro-inflammatory cytokines, mainly IL-6, are involved in the pathogenesis of ALI, ARDS, and cytokine storm-induced multi-organ damage in COVID-19 (Sun et al., 2020). Typically, testosterone inhibits the synthesis and release of IL-6 and downregulates the expression of IL-6 receptors (Sun et al., 2020). Thus, IL-6 serum level is augmented in hypogonadism patients that increase their susceptibility for COVID-19 severity (Papadopoulos et al., 2020). Besides, adiponectin, through its anti-inflammatory effects, may reduce SARS-CoV-2-induced pro-inflammatory hypercytokinemia and associated ALI (Messina et al., 2020).

Of note, activation of nod-like receptor pyrin 3 (NLRP3) inflammasome is linked to over-activation of NF-κB signaling-induced inflammatory reactions in COVID-19. Activation of NLRP3 inflammasome is also related with COVID-19 severity and associated complications like ALI and ARDS (van den Berg and Te Velde, 2020). Chen et al. (2020) in their experimental study confirmed that testosterone therapy reduces atherogenesis by suppressing NLRP3 inflammasome. However, Alves et al. (2020) showed that supra-physiological testosterone level leads to oxidative stress-induced endothelial dysfunction and vascular injury through stimulation of NLRP3 inflammasome. Previously, Vignozzi et al. (2012) disclosed that testosterone through its derivative dihydrotestosterone suppresses NF-κB signaling activation and associated pro-inflammatory activations. Therefore, testosterone therapy may improve the clinical outcomes in COVID-19 patients through NLRP3 inflammasome/NF-κB-dependent activation of anti-inflammatory cytokines and suppression of pro-inflammatory cytokines.

A prospective study involving 221 hospitalized men with COVID-19 pneumonia aged > 18 years illustrated that testosterone serum levels are reduced and correlated with COVID-19 severity and mortality (Çayan et al., 2020). Similarly, low baseline total and free testosterone in 31 COVID-19 patients recovered from ARDS in Italy are negatively correlated with inflammatory risk factors (ferritin, CRP procalcitonine, and D-dimer) and linked to COVID-19 severity (Rastrelli et al., 2020). Likewise, an observational study in Germany involving 45 COVID-19 patients revealed that 70% of them have low testosterone at the time of admission with subsequent reduction through ARDS development and admission to the intensive care unit (ICU) (Schroeder et al., 2020). Furthermore, a prospective study composed of 358 men with COVID-19 compared with 92 negative for COVID-19 illustrated that testosterone levels are reduced in COVID-19 patients and linked to poor clinical outcomes (Cinislioglu et al., 2021). In addition, a retrospective study showed that low testosterone level is connected with COVID-19 severity and risk of death (Okçelik, 2021). Low testosterone serum level is associated with reduction of body anti-inflammatory capacity with augmentation of pro-inflammatory axis. High pro-inflammatory cytokines in turn suppress release and action of testosterone in a vicious cycle manner (Bianchi, 2019).

Furthermore, the receptor for advanced glycation end-product (RAGE) is a member of immunoglobulin superfamily protein, which presents in two forms, membrane RAGE (mRAGE) and soluble RAGE (sRAGE) (Papadopoulos et al., 2020). mRAGE has an inflammatory effect through activation of NF-kB, while sRAGE has anti-inflammatory effects through upregulation of ACE2 and anti-inflammatory cytokines (Serveaux-Dancer et al., 2019). RAGE pathway is mainly expressed in lung tissue and linked to the development of acute and chronic lung injuries (Wang et al., 2018). It has been shown that SARS-CoV-2 activates mRAGE at pulmonary alveolar cells, leading to severe inflammatory reactions (Yalcin Kehribar et al., 2020). It has been confirmed that the concentration of sRAGE is reduced with aging, which might explain the susceptibility of old age to COVID-19 (Evens et al., 2020). However, in young and asymptomatic COVID-19 patients, the concentration of sRAGE is high. In severe COVID-19, sRAGE level is significantly reduced, so low sRAGE level is associated with progression of ALI and ARDS (Abbasi-Oshaghi et al., 2021).

Therefore, COVID-19-induced reduction in circulating testosterone may induce ALI due to increase of pro-inflammatory and reduction anti-inflammatory effects.

Testosterone and Testicular Injury

In COVID-19, SARS-CoV-2 may bind testicle ACE2, leading to Sertoli and Leydig cells' damage with subsequent inhibition of testicular testosterone synthesis (Illiano et al., 2020). Also, local inflammatory reaction in the testes due to SARS-CoV-2 infection and deregulation of the testicular renin–angiotensin system (RAS) may also impair testicular testosterone synthesis leading to hypogonadism (Yang et al., 2020). Analysis of testicular biopsies in patients with COVID-19 illustrated that the histopathological changes like hypoxic injury and microthrombosis are similar to that observed in COVID-19-induced ALI. However, SARS-CoV-2 was not detected in the injured testes, suggesting oxidative stress; coagulation disorders might mediate this damage as evident in COVID-19 pneumonia (Flaifel et al., 2021).

Therefore, preexistence or SARS-CoV-2-induced hypogonadism may reduce the protective effect of testosterone against SARS-CoV-2 infection, suggesting a link between testicular injury and development of ALI and ARDS in COVID-19 patients (Yang et al., 2020; Zaim et al., 2020). Moreover, high pro-inflammatory cytokines in SARS-CoV-2 infection may induce endothelial dysfunction and coagulopathy, a hallmark in COVID-19. The pro-thrombotic status and risk of thromboembolism are highly aggravated in hypogonadism (Fei et al., 2020). Local testicular thrombosis during SARS-CoV-2 infection is associated with diffuse damage of Leydig and Sertoli cells (Duarte-Neto et al., 2021). However, testosterone supplementation improves endothelial function *via* activation of nitric oxide release, inhibiting platelet activations and pro-thrombotic cascades (Hotta et al., 2019).

These clinical studies illustrated that reduction in the testosterone level is due to testicular injury with a subsequent reduction in the synthesis and release of testosterone from Leydig cells. This simple explanation is not acceptable since testicular injury is not frequently involved during SARS-CoV-2 infections (Schroeder et al., 2020). However, total testosterone may reduce in COVID-19 in the absence of testicular injury, as 90% of COVID-19 patients have a negative test for SARS-CoV-2 in the testes (Yang et al., 2020). A recent study illustrated that hypogonadism is developed in the early phase of COVID-19 due to SARS-CoV-2-induced testicular injury (Dutta and Sengupta, 2021). Higher expression of ACE2 in the testes makes them a potential target for SARS-CoV-2 with subsequent progression of male infertility. Excessive production of reactive oxygen species by SARS-CoV-2 may disrupt sperm function and morphology leading to early- or late-onset infertility (Esteves et al., 2021). Xu et al. (2021) showed that despite testicular injury during acute SARS-CoV-2 infection, male sex hormones remain unchanged even after recovery from COVID-19. Herein, extensive molecular studies are recommended to observe the implication of SARS-CoV-2 infections in reducing testosterone levels in COVID-19 patients. Zhao et al. (2016) illustrated that activation of mRAGE is correlated with inhibition of Leydig cell function with reduction of testosterone biosynthesis. This finding might explain low testosterone levels in patients with severe COVID-19.

In COVID-19, downregulation of lung ACE2 by SARS-CoV-2 is associated with high circulating AngII level, which is linked to development and progression of ALI and ARDS (Zhang et al., 2020). It has been confirmed that AngII inhibits Leydig cell function and testosterone synthesis (Reis and Reis, 2020). Add to these findings, the testes have full RAS, which is involved in the regulation function of Leydig cells and testosterone biosynthesis (Reis and Reis, 2020). Thus, systemic or testicular AngII levels are augmented due to downregulation of ACE2 in COVID-19. Local and circulating AngII activate harmful AT1R on the Leydig cells leading to the inhibition of testosterone biosynthesis (Pascolo et al., 2020). The deregulation of the protective AT2R and Mas receptors within the testes provokes inflammatory cascades that also contribute to Leydig cells' dysfunction (Aitken, 2020; Pascolo et al., 2020). From the above considerations, AngII might be the potential biomarker linking ALI and testicular injury in patients with severe COVID-19.

Testosterone and Oxidative Stress

Additional studies illustrated that SARS-CoV-2 infection leads to oxidative stress injury and oxidative storm due to membrane lipid and protein peroxidations (Ntyonga-Pono, 2020). The high neutrophil ratio in SARS-CoV-2 infection is linked to high oxidative stress due to the production of reactive oxygen species (ROS) by neutrophils. These changes provoke a cascade of immuno-biological events that the human body responds to (Ntyonga-Pono, 2020). ROS causes various pathological events related to COVID-19, such as endothelial dysfunction, erythrocyte injury, platelet activation, and thrombosis (Laforge et al., 2020). High ROS in COVID-19 promotes neutrophil extracellular traps (NETs) and induction release of pro-inflammatory cytokines (Laforge et al., 2020). NETs activate NLRP3 inflammasome, NF-κB, and induction of coagulopathy (Schönrich et al., 2020).

It has been reported that oxidative stress inhibits testosterone biosynthesis through activation of mitogen-activated protein kinase p38 (MAPK), which alter the metabolic process and gene expression (Shi and Dansen, 2020). Therefore, severe oxidative stress upregulates the p38MAPK pathway in the Leydig cells causing significant inhibition of testicular testosterone biosynthesis (Han et al., 2018). Recently, Jing et al. (2020) confirmed that oxidized low-density lipoprotein (oxLDL) inhibits testosterone synthesis through induction of p38MAPK pathway in the Leydig cells.

Oxidative stress inhibits Leydig and adrenal cells to synthesize testosterone through upregulation of cyclooxygenase 2 (COX2), induced by the p38MAPK pathway (Martin and Touaibia, 2020). Both p38MAPK pathway and COX2 are activated in COVID-19; Grimes and his colleague (Grimes and Grimes, 2020) illustrated that SARS-CoV-2 might directly or indirectly activate the p38MAPK pathway through downregulation of ACE2 and augmentation of AngII. Besides, activation of pro-inflammatory cytokines in COVID-19 induces upregulation of COX2 (Ong et al., 2020). Zhoa et al. (2019) confirmed that the NF-κB signaling pathway mediates the interaction between the p38MAPK pathway and COX2 in reducing testicular testosterone biosynthesis. In addition, activated p38MAPK provokes blood-testes barrier injury by suppressing testicular spermatogenesis and testosterone biosynthesis (Liu et al., 2018). Therefore, SARS-CoV-2 infection may reduce circulating testosterone and induces hypogonadism through activation of the p38MAPK/COX2 axis.

Into the bargain, testosterone inhibits neutrophil oxidative stress by reducing the production of superoxide anion, inhibition of lipid peroxidation, and improvement of glutathione reductase activity (Marin et al., 2010). In addition, an experimental study revealed that testosterone improves testes antioxidant potential by which it may attenuate oxidative stress-induced testicular injury (Aydilek et al., 2004).

Therefore, testosterone may reduce COVID-19 severity through mitigation of SARS-CoV-2-induced oxidative stress and associated complications.

Testosterone and Macrophage Function

Moreover, SARS-CoV-2 infection may lead to macrophage activation syndrome (MAS), which is characterized by hemophagocytosis, pancytopenia, coagulopathy, and disseminated intravascular coagulation (DIC). The MAS is developed in different viral infections including SARS-CoV-2 due to imbalanced release of pro-inflammatory cytokines (McGonagle et al., 2021). Of note, testosterone has an important regulatory role on the macrophage, monocyte, and T-cell functions. Testosterone inhibits release of pro-inflammatory and inflammatory cytokines from immune cells (Bereshchenko et al., 2018). Testosterone therapy was shown to prohibit release of pro-inflammatory cytokines from monocytes mainly in hypogonadal men compared with eugonadal one (Bianchi, 2019). In addition, testosterone decreases the expression and sensitivity of macrophage TLR4 for its ligand (Rettew et al., 2008). Of interest, TLR4 mediates early immunological interaction of SARS-CoV-2 with macrophage and other immune cells (Aboudounya and Heads, 2021). Therefore, testosterone therapy in COVID-19 patients may interrupt macrophage activation, exaggerated immune response, and development of MAS.

Furthermore, testicular macrophages (TMs) have immunoregulatory and immunotolerant functions as well as control of testicular steroidogenesis and spermatogenesis (Meinhardt et al., 2018). During sepsis and pathogen invasion, the classical type macrophage (M1) is activated and induces release of local pro-inflammatory cytokines. These cytokines impair spermatogenesis with significant inhibition of testicular steroidogenesis. The alternative type macrophage (M2) has local anti-inflammatory action supporting spermatogenesis and release of testosterone from Leydig cells (Chen et al., 2018; Meinhardt et al., 2018).

In SARS-CoV-2 infection, macrophage polarization is toward M1 phenotype resulting in testicular injury with impairment of testicular steroidogenesis and spermatogenesis (Lv et al., 2021). Becerra-Diaz et al. (2018) illustrated that testosterone and other androgens through macrophage androgenic receptor (AR) enhance M2 polarization with domination of macrophage anti-inflammatory effect. Taken together, testosterone modulates macrophage functions in general and more specifically TMs, by which it reduces the harmful effects of SARS-CoV-2 infection on the testes.

Testosterone Versus Estrogen in Men

In general, women have a robust immune system as compared to men due to the protective effect of estrogen against immunological dysregulation during different viral infections (Priyanka and Nair, 2020). It has been shown that estrogen has complex immunomodulating effects, and its effect on the inflammatory milieu in COVID-19 has been suggested (Ma et al., 2021). High estrogen serum level in premenopausal women might be a protective factor against COVID-19 severity, though older post-menopausal women are of high risk for development of COVID-19 severity compared to elderly men (Ciarambino et al., 2021). Nevertheless, reduction of estrogen level in later life in women does not appear to play a harmful role regarding COVID-19 severity in elderly women (Papadopoulos et al., 2021). In elderly men, there is significant reduction of testosterone with elevation of estrogen level due to increasing aromatization of adrenal and testicular androgens (Jardí et al., 2018). However, during sepsis in men, there is a noteworthy reduction of testosterone level with parallel increase of estrogen that reflects negative outcomes in septic men (Bech et al., 2020).

Thus, administration of estrogen in men with COVID-19 may offer a potential protective effect against COVID-19 severity (Suba, 2020). Bukowska et al. (2017) confirmed from experimental data that estrogen is able to regulate expression of the ACE/ACE2 axis, which is highly distorted in COVID-19. Also, estrogen inhibits propagation of cytokine storm and can activate B cells for antibody production. Besides, estrogen reduces expression of TMPRSS2, thereby reducing the entry of

SARS-CoV-2 to the susceptible cells (Bennink et al., 2021). So, estrogen treatment is suggested to be an effective treatment against COVID-19 (Bennink et al., 2021).

These findings highlighted the potential protective effects of testosterone against SARS-CoV-2 infection (**Table 1**). However, reduction of total testosterone level in COVID-19 is due to complex interactions between SARS-CoV-2 with oxidative stress, pro-inflammatory cytokines, and systemic and local RAS (**Figure 2**).

HARMFUL ROLE OF TESTOSTERONE IN COVID-19

Testosterone and TMPRSS2 in COVID-19

Various studies illustrated that men's higher predisposition to develop severe and serious COVID-19 complications is related to sex hormones, mainly testosterone and sociocultural factors (Lipsky and Hung, 2020). It has been confirmed that TMPRSS2 is required for proteolytic activation and priming of SARS-CoV-2 spike protein to bind ACE2 (Rahman et al., 2020). The expression of the TMPRSS2 gene is promoted by testosterone hormone, which might explain the severity of COVID-19 in men due to facilitating the entry of SARS-CoV-2 (Stopsack et al., 2020). TMPRSS2 is a cellular enzyme encoded by the human TMPRSS2 gene involved in prostatic cancer (Mehra et al., 2007) and cleaving of hemagglutinin viral antigen and infectivity of HIN1 and H7N9 influenza virus (Cheng et al., 2015). The TMPRSS2 gene is expressed in different tissues including lung and testes (Shen et al., 2020).

In addition to the androgen, nicotine smoking increases the expression of the TMPRSS2 gene, which might explain the severity of COVID-19 severity in nicotine smoker patients (Voinsky and Gurwitz, 2020). However, various studies reported the protective effect of nicotine smoking against SARS-CoV-2 due to different mechanisms, including upregulation of lung ACE2, anti-inflammatory, and immunosuppressive effects through activation of nicotinic acetylcholine receptor type 7 alpha (nAChR7α) on the macrophage (Farsalinos et al., 2020). Likewise, Donlan et al. (2020) observed that the expression of the TMPRSS2 gene is activated by IL-13, a highly expressed cytokine in COVID-19 and regarded as a predictive factor for mechanical ventilation independent of gender, age, and comorbidities. Besides, TMPRSS2 is highly co-expressed with furin, cathepsin L and B, CD209, and CD147 in men only, while co-expression with ACE2 is similar in both sexes (Piva et al., 2021). Certainly, TMPRSS2 co-expression with CD147 is important since CD147 is regarded as an entry point for SARS-CoV-2 (Radzikowska et al., 2020). Furthermore, Cao et al. (2017) in their experimental study confirmed that testosterone therapy increases the expression of CD147.

Therefore, overexpression of TMPRSS2 by androgen may implicate the testosterone in the pathogenesis of SARS-CoV-2 infection and COVID-19 severity. Thereby, TMPRSS2 inhibitors such as bromhexine, aprotinin, camostat, and nafamostat are useful in managing COVID-19 through attenuation of TMPRSS2-dependent lung inflammation, coagulopathy, and development of ARDS (Azimi, 2020; Breining et al., 2020). Indeed, the population-based study of Montopoli et al. (2020) that involved 9,280 COVID-19 patients with or without prostatic cancer illustrated that patients receiving androgen deprivation therapy (ADT) are at a lower risk for COVID-19-related complications compared to patients who did not receive ADT. This finding suggests that the anti-androgen agents reduce testosterone's activation role on the expression of TMPRSS2, and thus high testosterone level may increase COVID-19 severity. Adamowicz et al. (2020) showed that high dihydrotestosterone level is linked to poor pulmonary outcomes in COVID-19 patients, though use of 5-α reductase inhibitors may aggravate COVID-19 severity due to disturbance of intra-pulmonary androgen metabolism. However, McCoy et al. (2020) showed that using 5-α reductase inhibitors is associated with good clinical outcomes in COVID-19 patients.

Moreover, different therapeutic modalities such as dexamethasone, nitric oxide, and chloroquine, which are effective in managing COVID-19, are reported to have anti-androgenic effects and suppression of TMPRSS2 (Cronauer et al., 2007; Guo et al., 2018; Chi et al., 2020). Taken together, based on the current findings, testosterone is implicated in the facilitation of SARS-CoV-2 infection through upregulation of TMPRSS2 and androgen receptor (AR) activation.

TABLE 1 | Beneficial effects of testosterone in COVID-19.

References	Study type	Findings
Margue et al. (Marques et al., 2020)	Experimental study	Testosterone improves oxygenation and attenuates tissue hypoxia.
Wang et al. (2021)	Experimental study	Testosterone therapy reduces lung inflammation and fibrosis.
Bianch (Sun et al., 2020)	Systematic review	Testosterone inhibits the synthesis and release of IL-6.
Chen et al. (2020)	Experimental study	Testosterone therapy inhibits NLRP3 inflammasome.
Vignozzi et al. (2012)	Prospective study	Testosterone suppresses NF-κB signaling.
Cayan et al. (Çayan et al., 2020)	Cohort study	Testosterone serum levels are reduced and correlated with COVID-19 severity and mortality.
Rastrelli et al. (2020)	Cohort study	Testosterone serum level is negatively correlated with inflammatory risk factors
Schroder et al. (Rastrelli et al., 2020)	Cohort study	70% of COVID-19 patients have low testosterone at the time of admission.
Cinislioglu et al. (2021)	Prospective study	Testosterone levels are reduced in COVID-19 patients and linked to poor clinical outcomes.
Okcelik et al. (Okçelik, 2021)	Retrospective study	Low testosterone level is connected with COVID-19 severity and risk of death.
Hota et al. (Hotta et al., 2019)	Systematic review	Testosterone supplementation improves endothelial function.
Marin et al. (2010)	*In vitro* study	Testosterone inhibits oxidative stress.
Bereshchenko et al. (2018)	Systematic review	Testosterone inhibits release of pro-inflammatory and inflammatory cytokines from immune cells.

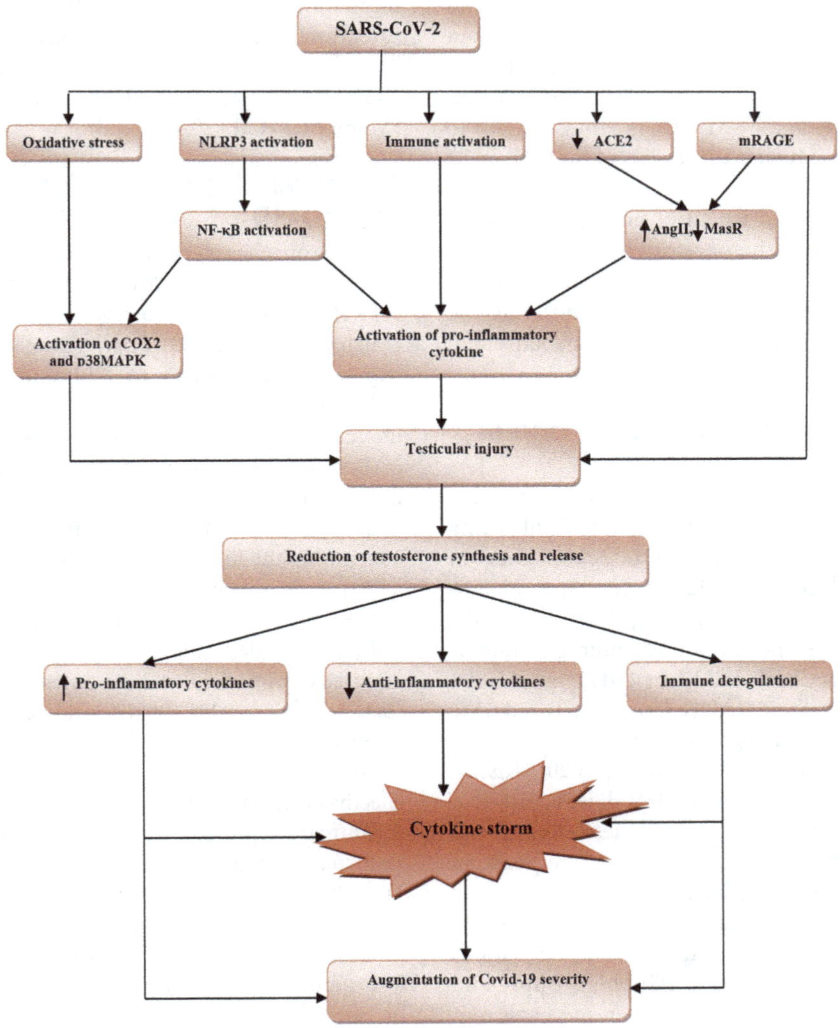

FIGURE 2 | The potential role of SARS-CoV-2 infection in the reduction of testosterone and associated COVID-19 severity. SARS-CoV-2 induces oxidative stress, activation of nod-like receptor pyrin-3 (NLRP3) inflammasome and abnormal immune activation, downregulation of angiotensin converting enzyme 2 (ACE2), and activation of receptor for advanced glycation end-product (mRAGE). Downregulation of ACE2 with activation of mRAGE increases angiotensin II (AngII) and reduces Mas receptor (MasR). Activation of NLRP3 inflammasome triggers release of nuclear factor kappa B (NF-κB) and together with cyclooxygenase-2 (COX-2) and p38 mitogen-activated protein kinase (p38MAPK) stimulate release of pro-inflammatory cytokines, which cause testicular injury. These pathophysiological changes reduce production and release of testosterone from injured testes. Reduction in the level of testosterone provokes releases of pro-inflammatory cytokines and reduces anti-inflammatory cytokines with immune deregulation. These changes lead to induction of cytokine storm with consequent augmentation of COVID-19 severity.

Androgen Sensitivity and COVID-19

The role of androgen sensitivity and polymorphism in COVID-19 is explained by different studies. It has been reported that a low mortality rate in pre-pubescent compared to the high mortality rate in adult men during the COVID-19 pandemic is due to low androgen sensitivity (Wambier et al., 2020). In addition, men with androgenic alopecia and women with polycystic ovary syndrome are at a higher risk for SARS-CoV-2 infection and COVID-19 severity due to higher androgen sensitivity. Therefore, the higher mortality rate for COVID-19 in the African American population is related to the polymorphism and higher sensitivity of androgenic receptors (Goren et al., 2020).

It has been known that the polyglutamine (poly-Q) tract of the AR affects the physiological response of circulating testosterone (Callewaert et al., 2003). Longer poly-Q of AR reduces the sensitivity to testosterone and is associated with high testosterone serum level because of impairment of negative feedback inhibition (Mohamad et al., 2018). In addition, longer poly-Q of AR is linked to activation of pro-inflammatory axis (Pierotti et al., 2010), although AR with short poly-Q has protective and anti-inflammatory roles in COVID-19 regardless of testosterone serum levels (Baldassarri et al., 2021). Therefore, testosterone may have bidirectional effects depending on the underlying length of AR poly-Q tract.

The distribution of poly-Q allele differs among diverse populations: longer in Asians, medium in Caucasians, and shorter in Africans (Ackerman et al., 2012). This might explain the high mortality in the first wave of SARS-CoV-2 infection in both China and Italy (Pereira et al., 2020). Of interest, African populations are more prone to the SARS-CoV-2 infection due to higher sensitivity of AR and higher expression of the TMPRSS2 gene (de Lusignan et al., 2020).

Therefore, AR sensitivity and length of poly-Q tract of AR seem to be more important than testosterone level in the prediction of COVID-19 severity. Besides, testosterone therapy in patients with COVID-19 may improve or worsen the clinical outcomes depending on patient AR sensitivity (Mukherjee and Pahan, 2021).

Immunological Effects of Testosterone in COVID-19

It has been reported that both adaptive and innate immune systems are crucial for contrasting viral infections and enhancing viral clearance and tissue repair (Kikkert, 2020). Giagulli et al. (2021) illustrated that circulating testosterone has immunosuppressive effects by inhibiting B and T cells, impairing immune response and immunoglobulin generations in different viral infections (Ghosh and Klein, 2017). In COVID-19, natural killer, B, and T cells are reduced; specifically reducing CD8 T cell is regarded as an independent predictor for severe COVID-19-related complications (Wang et al., 2020). Kissick et al. (2014) revealed that testosterone inhibits differentiation of CD4 T cells, providing a basis for targeting testosterone and other androgenic receptors to mitigate CD4 T-cell response in various forms of autoimmune disorders.

Several lines of evidence from various studies point to the immunosuppressive potential role of testosterone on various components of the immune system (Gubbels Bupp and Jorgensen, 2018), although the basic molecular mechanism is still not elucidated. Testosterone mediated downregulation of systemic immune response through cell-type-specific effects in many immunological disorders (LaVere et al., 2021). The precise immunological effects of testosterone and other androgens are through inhibition of antibody response to the viral infections and vaccines, suppression of macrophages and dendritic cells, promotion of immunological tolerance *via* activation of regulatory T cells, and inhibition of functions and developments of B and T cells (Trigunaite et al., 2015). Regarding these considerations, men are more vulnerable for COVID-19 severity as compared with women due to the immunosuppressive effects of testosterone (Bwire, 2020). Testosterone enhances both secretion and production of Th1-to-Th2 cytokine ratio *via* stimulated T cells and reduces humoral response and B-cell proliferation (Roved et al., 2017).

Moreover, the lysophosphatidyl serine receptor (GPR174) encoded by X-chromosome gene is highly expressed on B and T cells in women compared with men (Barnes et al., 2015). GPR174 regulates and controls the release of pro-inflammatory cytokines, B-cell migration, and macrophage polarization in septic shock and in response to chemokines (Qiu et al., 2019). These verdicts and results highlighted testosterone's potential immunosuppressive effect in the progression of SARS-CoV-2 infection and COVID-19 severity (Salonia et al., 2021). Therefore, ADT might be a therapeutic opportunity against COVID-19 by reversal of immunosuppression status (Montopoli et al., 2020).

Metabolic Effects of Testosterone in COVID-19

Testosterone has a permissive effect for circulating AngII by expressing AT1R and downregulation of ATR2 with a higher ATR1R/AT2R ratio. However, castration reverses this ratio (Mishra et al., 2019). High circulating AngII and ATR1R expression are linked to ALI and ARDS development in COVID-19 (Wu et al., 2020). Besides, a high AngII level induces testicular injury and cell apoptosis with the reduction of Leydig cells for the synthesis of testosterone (Wang et al., 2017). Thus, in SARS-CoV-2 infection, there is a vicious cycle conflict in the interaction between testosterone and AngII concerning the lung–testis axis in severe COVID-19.

To date, dipeptidyl peptidase 4 (DPP4), which is highly expressed in different tissues, mainly in lung type II alveolar cells, is regarded as an entry point for SARS-CoV-2 and is associated with poor clinical outcomes in COVID-19 patients (Solerte et al., 2020). Blauschmidt et al. (2017) observed that testosterone upregulates the expression of DPP4 receptors in women with polycystic ovary syndrome. DPP4 inhibitors effectively manage COVID-19 through modulation of the anti-inflammatory/pro-inflammatory axis (Mirani et al., 2020). Thus, testosterone may increase COVID-19 severity through the DPP4/CD26 pathway; however, there is no study related to DPP4/CD26 and testosterone in SARS-CoV-2 infection.

Moreover, obesity is associated with low circulating testosterone due to aromatization of testosterone to estrogen by adipose tissue and abnormal hypothalamic–pituitary axis (Haring et al., 2010). Obesity is regarded as an independent risk factor for COVID-19 severity despite low testosterone levels (Yang et al., 2021), although ample evidence from experimental, preclinical, and clinical studies revealed that low testosterone level promotes development of obesity (Fui et al., 2014). Testosterone improves catecholamine-induced lipolysis and inhibits uptake of triglyceride by suppressing the activity of adipose tissue lipoprotein lipase (Grossmann, 2011). It has been reported that patients with prostatic cancer on ADT had increased fat mass and visceral adipose tissue by about 22% within 6 months of established therapy (Hamilton et al., 2011). Likewise, experimental hypogonadism in young men induces obesity within 10 weeks (Mauras et al., 1998). Therefore, low testosterone-induced obesity may aggravate the clinical course of COVID-19 severity. Sarver and Wong (2021) showed that obesity increases the expression of TMPRSS2 and DPP4 with alteration of the ACE/ACE2 ratio. Thereby, obesity may increase the risk of SARS-CoV-2 infection and abnormal immune response by underlying high pro-inflammatory cytokines (Seidu et al., 2021). Therefore, testosterone's harmful effects in COVID-19 are related to TMPRSS2, ATR1, CD147, DPP4, and

AngII expression that are mutually interrelated in facilitating SARS-CoV-2 entry and associated inflammatory reactions (**Table 2** and **Figure 3**).

CONCLUSION

Testosterone hormone has diverse immunological effects; it reduces B- and T-cell activity with a noteworthy inhibitory effect on macrophage and monocyte activities. Therefore, testosterone has an immunosuppressive effect subjecting male sex for various viral infections including SARS-CoV-2. In the COVID-19 era, different reports, retrospective, and small sample size prospective studies revealed that testosterone serum might correlate with COVID-19 severity and poor clinical outcomes. However, other studies illustrated that testosterone has a protective effect against COVID-19 severity through inhibition of inflammatory signaling pathways including NF-κB, NLRP3

TABLE 2 | Harmful effects of testosterone in COVID-19.

References	Study type	Findings
Stopsack et al. (2020)	Systematic review	Testosterone promotes expression of the TMPRSS2.
Cao et al. (2017)	Experimental study	Testosterone therapy increases the expression of CD147.
Montopoli et al. (2020)	Population-based study	Androgen deprivation therapy reduces COVID-19 severity.
Adamowicz et al. (2020)	Observational study	High dihydrotestosterone level is linked to poor pulmonary outcomes in COVID-19 patients.
McCoy et al. (2020)	Observational study	5-α reductase inhibitors is associated with good clinical outcomes in COVID-19 patients.
Wambier et al. (2020)	Observational study	Low androgen sensitivity is linked to low COVID-19 mortality.
Wang et al. (2020); Bwire, (2020)	*In vitro* and review studies	Circulating testosterone has immunosuppressive effects.
Mishra et al. (2019)	Experimental study	Testosterone has a permissive effect for circulating AngII by expressing AT1R and downregulation of ATR2 with a higher ATR1R/AT2R ratio.
Blauschmidt et al. (2017)	Case-series study	Testosterone upregulates the expression of DPP4 receptors.

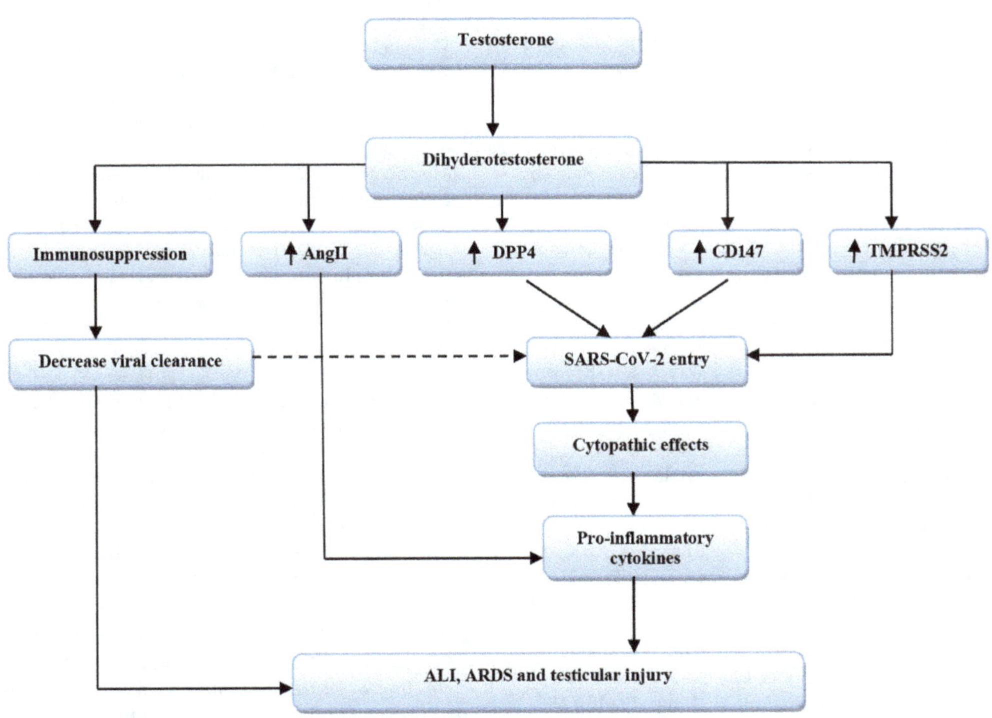

FIGURE 3 | The harmful effects of testosterone in SARS-CoV-2 infection. Dihydrotestosterone from testosterone leads to immunosuppression and increases expression of Dipeptidyl peptidase 4 (DPP4), cluster differentiation 147 (CD147), and Transmembrane protease serine 2 (TMPRSS2). Also, Dihydrotestosterone increases activity of Angiotensin II (AngII). CD147 and DPP4 increase entry of SARS-CoV-2, while TMPRSS2 facilitates SARS-CoV-2 entry. Immunosuppression reduces viral clearance that increases SARS-CoV-2 entry. These changes lead to cytopathic effects with release of pro-inflammatory cytokines with subsequent development of acute lung injury (ALI), acute respiratory distress syndrome (ARDS), and testicular injury.

inflammasomes, and p38MAPK. Also, testosterone attenuates oxidative stress-induced endothelial dysfunction and associated coagulopathy, a hallmark of COVID-19.

In the present review, depending on the recent published studies, we divided testosterone effects into beneficial and harmful effects. The beneficial effect of testosterone in COVID-19 is mediated through modulation of the pro-inflammatory/anti-inflammatory axis with inhibition of SARS-CoV-2-induced oxidative stress. Besides, testosterone attenuates development of ALI and ARDS in SARS-CoV-2 and other respiratory viral infections. The harmful effect of testosterone in COVID-19 is mediated by different unidentified mechanisms, although increased expression of TMPRSS2, DPP4, and CD147 by testosterone might be the potential mechanism. These receptors together with TMPRSS2 facilitate entry of SARS-CoV-2 to the affected cells with subsequent cytopathic effects and release of pro-inflammatory cytokines. Moreover, an increase in androgen sensitivity due to polymorphism of androgenic receptors might be a more important mechanism in the prediction of COVID-19 severity than testosterone serum levels.

On the other hand, a low testosterone serum level in COVID-19 patients might be due to direct testicular injury by SARS-CoV-2 or indirectly by the high level of pro-inflammatory cytokines. In addition, SARS-CoV-2-induced oxidative stress may affect testosterone metabolism and action. We suggest that disturbance of the hypothalamic–pituitary–gonadal axis by SARS-CoV-2 infection and associated inflammatory disorders could be the possible mechanism for low testosterone in COVID-19.

However, the assorted view of preponderance showed that low testosterone level is linked to COVID-19 severity. In addition, high inflammatory and oxidative stress burden with downregulation of ACE2 in SARS-CoV-2 infection may lead to testicular injury and reduction of testosterone biosynthesis. Despite these findings, the present study cannot conclude the beneficial or harmful effects of testosterone in COVID-19. Clinical trials and large-scale prospective studies are warranted to confirm the potential associations in this regard.

AUTHOR CONTRIBUTIONS

All authors contributed to the article and approved the submitted version.

REFERENCES

Abbasi-Oshaghi, E., Mirzaei, F., and Khodadadi, I. (2021). Letter to the Editor Regarding 'COVID-19 and Diabetes: What Does the Clinician Need to Know?'. *Prim. Care Diabetes* 15 (1), 30. doi: 10.1016/j.pcd.2020.10.010

Abobaker, A., and Raba, A. A. (2020). Does COVID-19 Affect Male Fertility? *World J. Urol.* 21, 1–2. doi: 10.1007/s00345-020-03208-w

Aboudounya, M. M., and Heads, R. J. (2021). COVID-19 and Toll-Like Receptor 4 (TLR4): SARS-CoV-2 may Bind and Activate TLR4 to Increase ACE2 Expression, Facilitating Entry and Causing Hyperinflammation. *Med. Inflamm.* 2021, 8874339. doi: 10.1155/2021/8874339

Ackerman, C. M., Lowe, L. P., Lee, H., Hayes, M. G., Dyer, A. R., Metzger, B. E., et al. (2012). Ethnic Variation in Allele Distribution of the Androgen Receptor (AR)(CAG) N Repeat. *J. Androl.* 33, 210–215. doi: 10.2164/jandrol.111.013391

Adamowicz, J., Juszczak, K., and Drewa, T. (2020). May Patients Receiving 5-Alpha-Reductase Inhibitors be in Higher Risk of COVID-19 Complications? *Med. Hypotheses* 140, 109751. doi: 10.1016/j.mehy.2020.109751

Aitken, R. J. (2020). COVID-19 and Human Spermatozoa—Potential Risks for Infertility and Sexual Transmission? *Andrology* 9 (1), 48–52. doi: 10.1111/andr.12859

Al-Kuraishy, H. M., Al-Naimi, M. S., Lungnier, C. M., and Al-Gareeb, A. I. (2020). Macrolides and COVID-19: An Optimum Premise. *Biomed. Biotechnol. Res. J. (BBRJ)* 4 (3), 189. doi: 10.4103/bbrj.bbrj_103_20

Al-Kuraishy, H. M., Hussien, N. R., Al-Naimi, M. S., Al-Buhadily, A. K., Al-Gareeb, A. I., and Lungnier, C. (2020a). Is Ivermectin–Azithromycin Combination the Next Step for COVID-19? *Biomed. Biotechnol. Res. J. (BBRJ)* 4 (5), 101. doi: 10.4103/bbrj.bbrj_103_20

Al-Kuraishy, H. M., Hussien, N. R., Al-Naimi, M. S., Al-Buhadily, A. K., Al-Gareeb, A. I., and Lungnier, C. (2020b). Renin–Angiotensin System and Fibrinolytic Pathway in COVID-19: One-Way Skepticism. *Biomed. Biotechnol. Res. J. (BBRJ)* 4 (5), 33. doi: 10.4103/bbrj.bbrj_103_20

Al-Maiahy, T. J., Al-Gareeb, A. I., and Al-kuraishy, H. M. (2020). Testosterone Is a Surrogate and Proxy Biomarker for Severity of Late-Onset Preeclampsia: A Cross-Sectional Study. *Asian Pacific J. Reprod.* 9 (1), 1. doi: 10.4103/2305-0500.275522

Alves, J. V., da Costa, R. M., Pereira, C. A., Fedoce, A. G., Silva, C. A., Carneiro, F. S., et al. (2020). Supraphysiological Levels of Testosterone Induce Vascular Dysfunction *via* Activation of the NLRP3 Inflammasome. *Front. Immunol.* 11, 1647. doi: 10.3389/fimmu.2020.01647

Anjorin, A. A., Abioye, A. I., Asowata, O. E., Soipe, A., Kazeem, M. I., Adesanya, I. O., et al. (2021). Comorbidities and the COVID-19 Pandemic Dynamics in Africa. *Trop. Med. Int. Health* 26 (1), 2–13. doi: 10.1111/tmi.13504

Assyov, Y., Gateva, A., Karamfilova, V., Gatev, T., Nedeva, I., Velikova, T., et al. (2020). Impact of Testosterone Treatment on Circulating Irisin in Men With Late-Onset Hypogonadism and Metabolic Syndrome. *Aging Male* 26, 1–7. doi: 10.1080/13685538.2020.1770721

Aydilek, N., Aksakal, M., and Karakılçık, A. Z. (2004). Effects of Testosterone and Vitamin E on the Antioxidant System in Rabbit Testis. *Andrologia* 36 (5), 277–281. doi: 10.1111/j.1439-0272.2004.00618.x

Azimi, A. (2020). TMPRSS2 Inhibitors, Bromhexine, Aprotinin, Camostat and Nafamostat as Potential Treatments for COVID-19. *Frenxiv.* doi: 10.31226/osf.io/a3rvm

Baldassarri, M., Picchiotti, N., Fava, F., Fallerini, C., Benetti, E., Daga, S., et al. (2021). Shorter Androgen Receptor polyQ Alleles Protect Against Life-Threatening COVID-19 Disease in European Males. *EBioMedicine* 65, 103246. doi: 10.1016/j.ebiom.2021.103246

Bank, S., De, S. K., Bankura, B., Maiti, S., Das, M., and Khan, G. A. (2021). ACE/ACE2 Balance Might be Instrumental to Explain the Certain Comorbidities Lead to Severe COVID-19 Cases. *Biosci. Rep.* 41 (2), BSR20202014. doi: 10.1042/BSR20202014

Barnes, M. J., Li, C. M., Xu, Y., An, J., Huang, Y., and Cyster, J. G. (2015). The Lysophosphatidylserine Receptor GPR174 Constrains Regulatory T Cell Development and Function. *J. Exp. Med.* 212 (7), 1011–1020. doi: 10.1084/jem.20141827

Becerra-Díaz, M., Strickland, A. B., Keselman, A., and Heller, N. M. (2018). Androgen and Androgen Receptor as Enhancers of M2 Macrophage Polarization in Allergic Lung Inflammation. *J. Immunol.* 201 (10), 2923–2933. doi: 10.4049/jimmunol.1800352

Bech, A., van Leeuwen, H., Telting, D., van Borren, M., and de Boer, H. (2020). Time Course of Gonadal Hormone Profiles in Male Patients With Sepsis. *Age (Years)* 72, 43–84.

Bennink, H. J., Foidart, J. M., and Debruyne, F. M. (2021). Treatment of Serious COVID-19 With Testosterone Suppression and High-Dose Estrogen Therapy. *Eur. Urol.* 6, S0302-2838(21)01865-0. doi: 10.1016/j.eururo.2021.06.024.

Bereshchenko, O., Bruscoli, S., and Riccardi, C. (2018). Glucocorticoids, Sex Hormones, and Immunity. *Front. Immunol.* 9, 1332. doi: 10.3389/fimmu.2018.01332

Bianchi, V. E. (2019). The Anti-Inflammatory Effects of Testosterone. *J. Endocr. Soc.* 3 (1), 91–107. doi: 10.1210/js.2018-00186

Blauschmidt, S., Greither, T., Lampe, K., Köller, S., Kaltwaßer, P., and Behre, H. M. (2017). Dipeptidyl Peptidase 4 Serum Activity and Concentration Are

Increased in Women With Polycystic Ovary Syndrome. *Clin. Endocrinol.* 87 (6), 741–747. doi: 10.1111/cen.13444

Breining, P., Frølund, A. L., Højen, J. F., Gunst, J. D., Staerke, N. B., Saedder, E, et al. (2020). Camostat Mesylate Against SARS-CoV-2 and COVID-19—Rationale, Dosing and Safety. *Basic Clin. Pharmacol. Toxicol.* 128 (2), 204–212. doi: 10.1111/bcpt.13533.

Bukowska, A., Spiller, L., Wolke, C., Lendeckel, U., Weinert, S., Hoffmann, J., et al. (2017). Protective Regulation of the ACE2/ACE Gene Expression by Estrogen in Human Atrial Tissue From Elderly Men. *Exp. Biol. Med.* 242 (14), 1412–1423. doi: 10.1177/1535370217718808

Butanis, J., Beckett, E., and Kabadi, U. M. (2017). Male Hypogonadism. *Primary Care Rep.* 23 (1), 23–29. doi: 10.1097/01.NPR.0000511774.51873.da

Bwire, G. M. (2020). Coronavirus: Why Men Are More Vulnerable to Covid-19 Than Women? *SN Compr. Clin. Med.* 2 (7), 874–876. doi: 10.1007/s42399-020-00341-w

Callewaert, L., Christiaens, V., Haelens, A., Verrijdt, G., Verhoeven, G., and Claessens, F. (2003). Implications of a Polyglutamine Tract in the Function of the Human Androgen Receptor. *Biochem. Biophys. Res. Commun.* 306 (1), 46–52. doi: 10.1016/S0006-291X(03)00902-1

Cao, J., Ng, M., and Felmlee, M. A. (2017). Sex Hormones Regulate Rat Hepatic Monocarboxylate Transporter Expression and Membrane Trafficking. *J. Pharm. Pharm. Sci.* 20, 435–444. doi: 10.18433/J3CH29

Çayan, S., Uğuz, M., Saylam, B., and Akbay, E. (2020). Effect of Serum Total Testosterone and Its Relationship With Other Laboratory Parameters on the Prognosis of Coronavirus Disease 2019 (COVID-19) in SARS-CoV-2 Infected Male Patients: A Cohort Study. *Aging Male* 23 (5), 1493–1503. doi: 10.1080/13685538.2020.1807930

Cheng, Z., Zhou, J., To, K. K., Chu, H., Li, C., Wang, D., et al. (2015). Identification of TMPRSS2 as a Susceptibility Gene for Severe 2009 Pandemic A (H1N1) Influenza and A (H7N9) Influenza. *J. Infect. Dis.* 212 (8), 1214–1221. doi: 10.1093/infdis/jiv246

Chen, S., Markman, J. L., Shimada, K., Crother, T. R., Lane, M., Abolhesn, A., et al. (2020). Sex-Specific Effects of the Nlrp3 Inflammasome on Atherogenesis in LDL Receptor-Deficient Mice. *Basic Trans. Sci.* 5 (6), 582–598. doi: 10.1016/j.jacbts.2020.03.016

Chen, Y., Wang, J., Chen, X., Li, D., and Han, X. (2018). Microcystin-Leucine Arginine Mediates Apoptosis and Engulfment of Leydig Cell by Testicular Macrophages Resulting in Reduced Serum Testosterone Levels. *Aquat. Toxicol.* 199, 116–126. doi: 10.1016/j.aquatox.2018.03.018

Chi, M., Shi, X., Huo, X., Wu, X., Zhang, P., and Wang, G. (2020). Dexmedetomidine Promotes Breast Cancer Cell Migration Through Rab11-Mediated Secretion of Exosomal TMPRSS2. *Ann. Trans. Med.* 8 (8), 531. doi: 10.21037/atm.2020.04.28

Ciarambino, T., Barbagelata, E., Corbi, G., Ambrosino, I., Politi, C., Lavalle, F., et al. (2021). Gender Differences in Vaccine Therapy: Where Are We in COVID-19 Pandemic? *Monaldi Arch. Chest Dis.* 8. doi: 10.4081/monaldi.2021.1669

Cinislioglu, A. E., Cinislioglu, N., Demirdogen, S. O., Sam, E., Akkas, F., Altay, M. S., et al. (2021). The Relationship of Serum Testosterone Levels With the Clinical Course and Prognosis of COVID-19 Disease in Male Patients: A Prospective Study. *Andrology.* doi: 10.1111/andr.13081

Cronauer, M. V., Ince, Y., Engers, R., Rinnab, L., Weidemann, W., Suschek, C. V., et al. (2007). Nitric Oxide-Mediated Inhibition of Androgen Receptor Activity: Possible Implications for Prostate Cancer Progression. *Oncogene* 26 (13), 1875–1884. doi: 10.1038/sj.onc.1209984

de Lusignan, S., Dorward, J., Correa, A., Jones, N., Akinyemi, O., Amirthalingam, G., et al. (2020). Risk Factors for SARS-CoV-2 Among Patients in the Oxford Royal College of General Practitioners Research and Surveillance Centre Primary Care Network: A Cross-Sectional Study. *Lancet Infect. Dis.* 20 (9), 1034–1042. doi: 10.1016/S1473-3099(20)30371-6

Donlan, A. N., Young, M., Petri, W. A., and Abhyankar, M. (2020). IL-13 Predicts the Need for Mechanical Ventilation in COVID-19 Patients. *medRxiv* 1, 2020–06. doi: 10.1101/2020.06.18.20134353

Duarte-Neto, A. N., Teixeira, T. A., Caldini, E. G., Kanamura, C. T., Gomes-Gouvêa, M. S., Dos Santos, A. B., et al. (2021). Testicular Pathology in Fatal COVID-19: A Descriptive Autopsy Study. *Andrology* 28 (1), 23–26. doi: 10.1111/andr.13073

Dutta, S., and Sengupta, P. (2021). SARS-CoV-2 and Male Infertility: Possible Multifaceted Pathology. *Reprod. Sci.* 28 (1), 23–26. doi: 10.1007/s43032-020-00261-z

Esteves, S. C., Lombardo, F., Garrido, N., Alvarez, J., Zini, A., Colpi, G. M., et al. (2021). SARS-CoV-2 Pandemic and Repercussions for Male Infertility Patients: A Proposal for the Individualized Provision of Andrological Services. *Andrology* 9 (1), 10–18. doi: 10.1111/andr.12809

Evens, L., Beliën, H., Deluyker, D., Bronckaers, A., Gervois, P., Hendrikx, M., et al. (2020). The Impact of Advanced Glycation End-Products (AGEs) on Proliferation and Apoptosis of Primary Stem Cells: A Systematic Review. *Stem Cells Int.* 14 (2020), 8886612. doi: 10.1155/2020/8886612

Farghaly, S., and Makboul, M. (2021). Correlation Between Age, Sex, and Severity of Coronavirus Disease-19 Based on Chest Computed Tomography Severity Scoring System. *Egyptian J. Radiol. Nucl. Med.* 52 (1), 1–8. doi: 10.1186/s43055-021-00408-1

Farsalinos, K., Niaura, R., Le Houezec, J., Barbouni, A., Tsatsakis, A., Kouretas, D., et al. (2020). Nicotine and SARS-CoV-2: COVID-19 may be a Disease of the Nicotinic Cholinergic System. *Toxicol. Rep.* 7, 658. doi: 10.1016/j.toxrep.2020.04.012

Fei, Y., Tang, N., Liu, H., and Cao, W. (2020). Coagulation Dysfunction: A Hallmark in COVID-19. *Arch. Pathol. Lab. Med.* 144 (10), 1223–1229. doi: 10.5858/arpa.2020-0324-SA

Flaifel, A., Guzzetta, M., Occidental, M., Najari, B. B., Melamed, J., Thomas, K. M., et al. (2021). Testicular Changes Associated With Severe Acute Respiratory Syndrome Coronavirus 2 (SARS-CoV-2). *Arch. Pathol. Lab. Med.* 145 (1), 8–9. doi: 10.5858/arpa.2020-0487-LE

Fui, M. N., Dupuis, P., and Grossmann, M. (2014). Lowered Testosterone in Male Obesity: Mechanisms, Morbidity and Management. *Asian J. Androl.* 16 (2), 223.

Ghosh, S., and Klein, R. S. (2017). Sex Drives Dimorphic Immune Responses to Viral Infections. *J. Immunol.* 198 (5), 1782–1790. doi: 10.4049/jimmunol.1601166

Giagulli, V. A., Guastamacchia, E., Magrone, T., Jirillo, E., Lisco, G., De Pergola, G., et al. (2021). Worse Progression of COVID-19 in Men: Is Testosterone a Key Factor? *Andrology* 9 (1), 53–64. doi: 10.1111/andr.12836

Goren, A., Vaño-Galván, S., Wambier, C. G., McCoy, J., Gomez-Zubiaur, A., Moreno-Arrones, O. M., et al. (2020). A Preliminary Observation: Male Pattern Hair Loss Among Hospitalized COVID-19 Patients in Spain–A Potential Clue to the Role of Androgens in COVID-19 Severity. *J. Cosmetic Dermatol.* 19 (7), 1545–1547. doi: 10.1111/jocd.13443

Grimes, J. M., and Grimes, K. V. (2020). P38 MAPK Inhibition: A Promising Therapeutic Approach for COVID-19. *J. Mol. Cell. Cardiol.* 144, 63–65. doi: 10.1016/j.yjmcc.2020.05.007

Grossmann, M. (2011). Low Testosterone in Men With Type 2 Diabetes: Significance and Treatment. *J. Clin. Endocrinol. Metab.* 96 (8), 2341–2353. doi: 10.1210/jc.2011-0118

Grossmann, M., Ng Tang Fui, M., and Cheung, A. S. (2020). Late-Onset Hypogonadism: Metabolic Impact. *Andrology* 8 (6), 1519–1529. doi: 10.1111/andr.12705

Gubbels Bupp, M. R., and Jorgensen, T. N. (2018). Androgen-Induced Immunosuppression. *Front. Immunol.* 9, 794. doi: 10.3389/fimmu.2018.00794

Guo, J., Ma, K., Xia, H. M., Chen, Q. K., Li, L., Deng, J., et al. (2018). Androgen Receptor Reverts Dexamethasone Induced Inhibition of Prostate Cancer Cell Proliferation and Migration. *Mol. Med. Rep.* 17 (4), 5887–5893. doi: 10.3892/mmr.2018.8566

Hamilton, E. J., Gianatti, E., Strauss, B. J., Wentworth, J., Lim-Joon, D., Bolton, D., et al. (2011). Increase in Visceral and Subcutaneous Abdominal Fat in Men With Prostate Cancer Treated With Androgen Deprivation Therapy. *Clin. Endocrinol.* 74 (3), 377–383. doi: 10.1111/j.1365-2265.2010.03942.x

Handelsman, D. J., Hirschberg, A. L., and Bermon, S. (2018). Circulating Testosterone as the Hormonal Basis of Sex Differences in Athletic Performance. *Endocrine Rev.* 39 (5), 803–829. doi: 10.1210/er.2018-00020

Han, A., Zou, L., Gan, X., Li, Y., Liu, F., Chang, X., et al. (2018). ROS Generation and MAPKs Activation Contribute to the Ni-Induced Testosterone Synthesis Disturbance in Rat Leydig Cells. *Toxicol. Lett.* 290, 36–45. doi: 10.1016/j.toxlet.2018.03.016

Haring, R., Ittermann, T., Völzke, H., Krebs, A., Zygmunt, M., Felix, S. B., et al. (2010). Prevalence, Incidence and Risk Factors of Testosterone Deficiency in a Population-Based Cohort of Men: Results From the Study of Health in Pomerania. *Aging Male* 13 (4), 247–257. doi: 10.3109/13685538.2010.487553

Hotta, Y., Kataoka, T., and Kimura, K. (2019). Testosterone Deficiency and Endothelial Dysfunction: Nitric Oxide, Asymmetric Dimethylarginine, and

Endothelial Progenitor Cells. *Sexual Med. Rev.* 7 (4), 661–668. doi: 10.1016/j.sxmr.2019.02.005

Illiano, E., Trama, F., and Costantini, E. (2020). Could COVID-19 Have an Impact on Male Fertility? *Andrologia* 52 (6), e13654. doi: 10.1111/and.13654

Jardí, F., Laurent, M. R., Claessens, F., and Vanderschueren, D. (2018). Estradiol and Age-Related Bone Loss in Men. *Physiol. Rev.* 98 (1), 1–. doi: 10.1152/physrev.00051.2017

Jing, J., Ding, N., Wang, D., Ge, X., Ma, J., Ma, R., et al. (2020). Oxidized-LDL Inhibits Testosterone Biosynthesis by Affecting Mitochondrial Function and the P38 MAPK/COX-2 Signaling Pathway in Leydig Cells. *Cell Death Dis.* 11 (8), 1–5. doi: 10.1038/s41419-020-02751-z

Keilich, S. R., Bartley, J. M., and Haynes, L. (2019). Diminished Immune Responses With Aging Predispose Older Adults to Common and Uncommon Influenza Complications. *Cell. Immunol.* 345, 103992. doi: 10.1016/j.cellimm.2019.103992

Kikkert, M. (2020). Innate Immune Evasion by Human Respiratory RNA Viruses. *J. Innate Immun.* 12 (1), 4–20. doi: 10.1159/000503030

Kissick, H. T., Sanda, M. G., Dunn, L. K., Pellegrini, K. L., On, S. T., Noel, J. K., et al. (2014). Androgens Alter T-Cell Immunity by Inhibiting T-Helper 1 Differentiation. *Proc. Natl. Acad. Sci.* 111 (27), 9887–9892. doi: 10.1073/pnas.1402468111

Laforge, M., Elbim, C., Frère, C., Hémadi, M., Massaad, C., Nuss, P., et al. (2020). Tissue Damage From Neutrophil-Induced Oxidative Stress in COVID-19. *Nat. Rev. Immunol.* 20 (9), 515–516. doi: 10.1038/s41577-020-0407-1

LaVere, A. A., Hamlin, H. J., Lowers, R. H., Parrott, B. B., and Ezenwa, V. O. (2021). Associations Between Testosterone and Immune Activity in Alligators Depend on Bacteria Species and Temperature. *Funct. Ecol.* 35 (5), 1018–1027. doi: 10.1111/1365-2435.13756

Lipsky, M. S., and Hung, M. (2020). Men and COVID-19: A Pathophysiologic Review. *Am. J. Men's Health* 14 (5), 1557988320954021. doi: 10.1177/1557988320954021

Liu, J., Ren, L., Wei, J., Zhang, J., Zhu, Y., Li, X., et al. (2018). Fine Particle Matter Disrupts the Blood–Testis Barrier by Activating TGF-β3/P38 MAPK Pathway and Decreasing Testosterone Secretion in Rat. *Environ. Toxicol.* 33 (7), 711–719. doi: 10.1002/tox.22556

Lugnier, C., AL-Kuraishi, H. M., and Rousseau, E. (2021). PDE4 Inhibition as a Therapeutic Strategy for Improvement of Pulmonary Dysfunctions in Covid-19 and Cigarette Smoking. *Biochem. Pharmacol.* 28, 114431. doi: 10.1016/j.bcp.2021.114431

Lv, J., Wang, Z., Qu, Y., Zhu, H., Zhu, Q., Tong, W., et al. (2021). Distinct Uptake, Amplification, and Release of SARS-CoV-2 by M1 and M2 Alveolar Macrophages. *Cell Discov.* 7 (1), 1–2. doi: 10.1038/s41421-021-00258-1

Maddaloni, E., D'Onofrio, L., Alessandri, F., Mignogna, C., Leto, G., Pascarella, G., et al. (2020). Cardiometabolic Multimorbidity Is Associated With a Worse Covid-19 Prognosis Than Individual Cardiometabolic Risk Factors: A Multicentre Retrospective Study (CoViDiab II). *Cardiovasc. Diabetol.* 19 (1), 1–1. doi: 10.1186/s12933-020-01140-2

Ma, Q., Hao, Z. W., and Wang, Y. F. (2021). The Effect of Estrogen in Coronavirus Disease 2019 (COVID-19). *Am. J. Physiol-Lung Cell. Mol. Physiol.* 321 (1), L219–L227. doi: 10.1152/ajplung.00332.2020

Marin, D. P., Bolin, A. P., de Cassia Macedo dos Santos, R., Curi, R., and Otton, R. (2010). Testosterone Suppresses Oxidative Stress in Human Neutrophils. *Cell Biochem. Funct.* 28 (5), 394–402. doi: 10.1002/cbf.1669

Marques, D. A., Patrone, L. G., Scarpellini, C. S., Bícego, K. C., Szawka, R. E., and Gargaglioni, L. H. (2020). The Role of Testosterone in the Respiratory and Thermal Responses to Hypoxia and Hypercapnia in Rats. *J. Endocrinol.* 247 (1), 101–114. doi: 10.1530/JOE-20-0257

Martin, L. J., and Touaibia, M. (2020). Improvement of Testicular Steroidogenesis Using Flavonoids and Isoflavonoids for Prevention of Late-Onset Male Hypogonadism. *Antioxidants* 9 (3), 237. doi: 10.3390/antiox9030237

Mauras, N., Hayes, V., Welch, S., Rini, A., Helgeson, K., Dokler, M., et al. (1998). Testosterone Deficiency in Young Men: Marked Alterations in Whole Body Protein Kinetics, Strength, and Adiposity. *J. Clin. Endocrinol. Metab.* 83 (6), 1886–1892. doi: 10.1210/jc.83.6.1886

McCoy, J., Cadegiani, F. A., Wambier, C. G., Herrera, S., Vaño-Galván, S., Mesinkovska, N. A., et al. (2020). 5-Alpha-Reductase Inhibitors Are Associated With Reduced Frequency of COVID-19 Symptoms in Males With Androgenetic Alopecia. *J. Eur. Acad. Dermatol. Venereol.* 35 (4), e243–e246. doi: 10.1111/jdv.17021

McGonagle, D., Ramanan, A. V., and Bridgewood, C. (2021). Immune Cartography of Macrophage Activation Syndrome in the COVID-19 Era. *Nat. Rev. Rheumatol.* 17 (3), 145–157. doi: 10.1038/s41584-020-00571-1

Mehra, R., Tomlins, S. A., Shen, R., Nadeem, O., Wang, L., Wei, J. T., et al. (2007). Comprehensive Assessment of TMPRSS2 and ETS Family Gene Aberrations in Clinically Localized Prostate Cancer. *Modern Pathol.* 20 (5), 538–544. doi: 10.1038/modpathol.3800769

Meinhardt, A., Wang, M., Schulz, C., and Bhushan, S. (2018). Microenvironmental Signals Govern the Cellular Identity of Testicular Macrophages. *J. Leukocyte Biol.* 104 (4), 757–766. doi: 10.1002/JLB.3MR0318-086RR

Messina, G., Polito, R., Monda, V., Cipolloni, L., Di Nunno, N., Di Mizio, G., et al. (2020). Functional Role of Dietary Intervention to Improve the Outcome of COVID-19: A Hypothesis of Work. *Int. J. Mol. Sci.* 21 (9), 3104. doi: 10.3390/ijms21093104

Millar, A. C., Lau, A. N., Tomlinson, G., Kraguljac, A., Simel, D. L., Detsky, A. S., et al. (2016). Predicting Low Testosterone in Aging Men: A Systematic Review. *CMAJ* 188 (13), E321–E330. doi: 10.1503/cmaj.150262

Mirani, M., Favacchio, G., Carrone, F., Betella, N., Biamonte, E., Morenghi, E., et al. (2020). Impact of Comorbidities and Glycemia at Admission and Dipeptidyl Peptidase 4 Inhibitors in Patients With Type 2 Diabetes With COVID-19: A Case Series From an Academic Hospital in Lombardy, Italy. *Diabetes Care* 43 (12), 3042–3049. doi: 10.2337/dc20-1340

Mishra, J. S., More, A. S., Gopalakrishnan, K., and Kumar, S. (2019). Testosterone Plays a Permissive Role in Angiotensin II-Induced Hypertension and Cardiac Hypertrophy in Male Rats. *Biol. Reprod.* 100 (1), 139–148. doi: 10.1093/biolre/ioy179

Mohamad, N. V., Wong, S. K., Hasan, W. N., Jolly, J. J., Nur-Farhana, M. F., Ima-Nirwana, S., et al. (2018). The Relationship Between Circulating Testosterone and Inflammatory Cytokines in Men. *Aging Male* 22 (2), 129–140. doi: 10.1080/13685538.2018.1482487

Montano, L. M., Espinoza, J., Flores-Soto, E., Chávez, J., and Perusquia, M. (2014). Androgens Are Bronchoactive Drugs That Act by Relaxing Airway Smooth Muscle and Preventing Bronchospasm. *J. Endocrinol.* 1222 (1), 1–3. doi: 10.1530/JOE-14-0074

Montopoli, M., Zumerle, S., Vettor, R., Rugge, M., Zorzi, M., Catapano, C. V., et al. (2020). Androgen-Deprivation Therapies for Prostate Cancer and Risk of Infection by SARS-CoV-2: A Population-Based Study (N= 4532). *Ann. Oncol.* 31 (8), 1040–1045. doi: 10.1016/j.annonc.2020.04.479

Mukherjee, S., and Pahan, K. (2021). Is COVID-19 Gender-Sensitive? *J. Neuroimmune Pharmacol.* 16 (1), 38–47. doi: 10.1007/s11481-020-09974-z.

Novković, L., Lazić, Z., Petrović, M., Ćupurdija, V., Vujanac, K., and Čekerevac, I. (2019). Hypogonadism in Chronic Obstructive Pulmonary Disease (COPD): Risk Factors. *Vojnosanitetski Pregled* 76 (1), 55–60. doi: 10.2298/VSP170312081N

Ntyonga-Pono, M. P. (2020). COVID-19 Infection and Oxidative Stress: An Under-Explored Approach for Prevention and Treatment? *Pan Afr. Med. J.* 35 (Suppl 2), 12. doi: 10.11604/pamj.2020.35.2.22877

Okçelik, S. (2021). COVID-19 Pneumonia Causes Lower Testosterone Levels. *Andrologia* 53 (1), e13909. doi: 10.1111/and.13909

Ong, S. W., Tan, W. Y., Chan, Y. H., Fong, S. W., Renia, L., Ng, L. F., et al. (2020). Safety and Potential Efficacy of Cyclooxygenase-2 Inhibitors in Coronavirus Disease 2019. *Clin. Trans. Immunol.* 9 (7), e1159. doi: 10.1002/cti2.1159

Papadopoulos, V., Li, L., and Samplaski, M. (2020). Why Does COVID-19 Kill More Elderly Men Than Women? Is There a Role for Testosterone? *Andrology* 22 (2), 129–140. doi: 10.1080/13685538.2018.1482487

Papadopoulos, V., Li, L., and Samplaski, M. (2021). Why Does COVID-19 Kill More Elderly Men Than Women? Is There a Role for Testosterone? *Andrology* 9 (1), 65–72. doi: 10.1111/andr.12868

Pascolo, L., Zito, G., Zupin, L., Luppi, S., Giolo, E., Martinelli, M., et al. (2020). Renin Angiotensin System, COVID-19 and Male Fertility: Any Risk for Conceiving? *Microorganisms* 8 (10), 1492. doi: 10.3390/microorganisms8101492

Pereira, M. R., Mohan, S., Cohen, D. J., Husain, S. A., Dube, G. K., Ratner, L. E., et al. (2020). COVID-19 in Solid Organ Transplant Recipients: Initial Report From the US Epicenter. *Am. J. Transplant.* 20 (7), 1800–1808. doi: 10.1111/ajt.15941

Pezzaioli, L. C., Quiros-Roldan, E., Paghera, S., Porcelli, T., Maffezzoni, F., Delbarba, A., et al. (2020). The Importance of SHBG and Calculated Free Testosterone for the Diagnosis of Symptomatic Hypogonadism in HIV-Infected Men: A Single-Centre Real-Life Experience. *Infection* 49 (2), 295–303. doi: 10.1007/s15010-020-01558-6

Pierotti, S., Lolli, F., Lauretta, R., Graziadio, C., Di Dato, C., Sbardella, E., et al. (2010). Androgen Modulation of Pro-Inflammatory and Anti-Inflammatory Cytokines During Preadipocyte Differentiation. *Horm. Mol. Biol. Clin. Invest.* 4 (1), 483–488. doi: 10.1515/HMBCI.2010.059

Piva, F., Sabanovic, B., Cecati, M., and Giulietti, M. (2021). Expression and Co-Expression Analyses of TMPRSS2, a Key Element in COVID-19. *Eur. J. Clin. Microbiol. Infect. Dis.* 40 (2), 451–455. doi: 10.1007/s10096-020-04089-y

Priyanka, H. P., and Nair, R. S. (2020). Neuroimmunomodulation by Estrogen in Health and Disease. *AIMS Neurosci.* 7 (4), 401. doi: 10.3934/Neuroscience.2020025

Qiu, D., Chu, X., Hua, L., Yang, Y., Li, K., Han, Y., et al. (2019). Gpr174-Deficient Regulatory T Cells Decrease Cytokine Storm in Septic Mice. *Cell Death Dis.* 10 (3), 1–4. doi: 10.1038/s41419-019-1462-z

Radzikowska, U., Ding, M., Tan, G., Zhakparov, D., Peng, Y., Wawrzyniak, P., et al. (2020). Distribution of ACE2, CD147, CD26, and Other SARS-CoV-2 Associated Molecules in Tissues and Immune Cells in Health and in Asthma, COPD, Obesity, Hypertension, and COVID-19 Risk Factors. *Allergy* 75 (11), 2829–2845. doi: 10.1111/all.14429

Rahman, N., Basharat, Z., Yousuf, M., Castaldo, G., Rastrelli, L., and Khan, H. (2020). Virtual Screening of Natural Products Against Type II Transmembrane Serine Protease (TMPRSS2), the Priming Agent of Coronavirus 2 (SARS-CoV-2). *Molecules* 25 (10), 2271. doi: 10.3390/molecules25102271

Rastrelli, G., Di Stasi, V., Inglese, F., Beccaria, M., Garuti, M., Di Costanzo, D., et al. (2020). Low Testosterone Levels Predict Clinical Adverse Outcomes in SARS-CoV-2 Pneumonia Patients. *Andrology* 9 (1), 88–98. doi: 10.1111/andr.12821

Redente, E. F., Jacobsen, K. M., Solomon, J. J., Lara, A. R., Faubel, S., Keith, R. C., et al. (2011). Age and Sex Dimorphisms Contribute to the Severity of Bleomycin-Induced Lung Injury and Fibrosis. *Am. J. Physiol-Lung Cell. Mol. Physiol.* 301 (4), L510–L518. doi: 10.1152/ajplung.00122.2011

Reis, F. M., and Reis, A. M. (2020). Angiotensin-Converting Enzyme 2 (ACE2), Angiotensin-(1-7) and Mas Receptor in Gonadal and Reproductive Functions. *Clin. Sci.* 134 (22), 2929–2941. doi: 10.1042/CS20200865

Rettew, J. A., Huet-Hudson, Y. M., and Marriott, I. (2008). Testosterone Reduces Macrophage Expression in the Mouse of Toll-Like Receptor 4, A Trigger for Inflammation and Innate Immunity. *Biol. Reprod.* 78 (3), 432–437. doi: 10.1095/biolreprod.107.063545

Roved, J., Westerdahl, H., and Hasselquist, D. (2017). Sex Differences in Immune Responses: Hormonal Effects, Antagonistic Selection, and Evolutionary Consequences. *Horm. Behav.* 88, 95–105. doi: 10.1016/j.yhbeh.2016.11.017

Salonia, A., Corona, G., Giwercman, A., Maggi, M., Minhas, S., Nappi, R. E., et al. (2021). SARS-CoV-2, Testosterone and Frailty in Males (PROTEGGIMI): A Multidimensional Research Project. *Andrology* 9 (1), 19–22. doi: 10.1111/andr.12811

Sarver, D. C., and Wong, G. W. (2021). Obesity Alters Ace2 and Tmprss2 Expression in Lung, Trachea, and Esophagus in a Sex-Dependent Manner: Implications for COVID-19. *Biochem. Biophys. Res. Commun.* 538, 92–96. doi: 10.1016/j.bbrc.2020.10.066

Schönrich, G., Raftery, M. J., and Samstag, Y. (2020). Devilishly Radical NETwork in COVID-19: Oxidative Stress, Neutrophil Extracellular Traps (NETs), and T Cell Suppression. *Adv. Biol. Regul.* 77, 100741. doi: 10.1016/j.jbior.2020.100741

Schroeder, M., Tuku, B., Jarczak, D., Nierhaus, A., Bai, T., Jacobsen, H., et al. (2020). The Majority of Male Patients With COVID-19 Present Low Testosterone Levels on Admission to Intensive Care in Hamburg, Germany: A Retrospective Cohort Study. *medRxiv*. doi: 10.1101/2020.05.07.20073817

Seidu, S., Gillies, C., Zaccardi, F., Kunutsor, S. K., Hartmann-Boyce, J., Yates, T., et al. (2021). The Impact of Obesity on Severe Disease and Mortality in People With SARS-CoV-2: A Systematic Review and Meta-Analysis. *Endocrinol. Diabetes Metab.* 4 (1), e00176. doi: 10.1002/edm2.176

Serveaux-Dancer, M., Jabaudon, M., Creveaux, I., Belville, C., Blondonnet, R., Gross, C., et al. (2019). Pathological Implications of Receptor for Advanced Glycation End-Product (AGER) Gene Polymorphism. *Dis. Markers* 2019, 2067353. doi: 10.1155/2019/2067353

Shen, L. W., Qian, M. Q., Yu, K., Narva, S., Yu, F., Wu, Y. L., et al. (2020). Inhibition of Influenza A Virus Propagation by Benzoselenoxanthenes Stabilizing TMPRSS2 Gene G-Quadruplex and Hence Down-Regulating TMPRSS2 Expression. *Sci. Rep.* 10 (1), 1–2. doi: 10.1038/s41598-020-64368-8

Shi, T., and Dansen, T. B. (2020). Reactive Oxygen Species Induced P53 Activation: DNA Damage, Redox Signaling, or Both? *Antioxid. Redox Signal.* 33 (12), 839–859. doi: 10.1089/ars.2020.8074

Solerte, S. B., Di Sabatino, A., Galli, M., and Fiorina, P. (2020). Dipeptidyl Peptidase-4 (DPP4) Inhibition in COVID-19. *Acta Diabetol.* 57, 779–783. doi: 10.1007/s00592-020-01539-z

Stopsack, K. H., Mucci, L. A., Antonarakis, E. S., Nelson, P. S., and Kantoff, P. W. (2020). TMPRSS2 and COVID-19: Serendipity or Opportunity for Intervention? *Cancer Discov.* 10 (6), 779–782. doi: 10.1158/2159-8290.CD-20-0451

Suba, Z. (2020). Prevention and Therapy of COVID-19 *via* Exogenous Estrogen Treatment for Both Male and Female Patients: Prevention and Therapy of COVID-19. *J. Pharm. Pharm. Sci.* 23, 75–85. doi: 10.18433/jpps31069

Sun, X., Wang, T., Cai, D., Hu, Z., Liao, H., Zhi, L., et al. (2020). Cytokine Storm Intervention in the Early Stages of COVID-19 Pneumonia. *Cytokine Growth Factor Rev.* 53, 38–42. doi: 10.1016/j.cytogfr.2020.04.002

Trigunaite, A., Dimo, J., and Jørgensen, T. N. (2015). Suppressive Effects of Androgens on the Immune System. *Cell. Immunol.* 294 (2), 87–94. doi: 10.1016/j.cellimm.2015.02.004

van den Berg, D. F., and Te Velde, A. A. (2020). Severe COVID-19: NLRP3 Inflammasome Dysregulated. *Front. Immunol.* 11, 1580. doi: 10.3389/fimmu.2020.01580

Vignozzi, L., Cellai, I., Santi, R., Lombardelli, L., Morelli, A., Comeglio, P., et al. (2012). Antiinflammatory Effect of Androgen Receptor Activation in Human Benign Prostatic Hyperplasia Cells. *J. Endocrinol.* 214 (1), 31. doi: 10.1530/JOE-12-0142.

Voinsky, I., and Gurwitz, D. (2020). Smoking and COVID-19: Similar Bronchial ACE2 and TMPRSS2 Expression and Higher TMPRSS4 Expression in Current Versus Never Smokers. *Drug Dev. Res.* 81 (8), 1073–1080. doi: 10.1002/ddr.21729

Wambier, C. G., Goren, A., Vaño-Galván, S., Ramos, P. M., Ossimetha, A., Nau, G., et al. (2020). Androgen Sensitivity Gateway to COVID-19 Disease Severity. *Drug Dev. Res.* 81 (7), 771–776. doi: 10.1002/ddr.21688

Wang, X., Huang, L., Jiang, S., Cheng, K., Wang, D., Luo, Q., et al. (2021). Testosterone Attenuates Pulmonary Epithelial Inflammation in Male Rats of COPD Model Through Preventing NRF1-Derived NF-κb Signaling. *J. Mol. Cell Biol.* 13 (2), 128–140. doi: 10.1093/jmcb/mjaa079

Wang, F., Nie, J., Wang, H., Zhao, Q., Xiong, Y., Deng, L., et al. (2020). Characteristics of Peripheral Lymphocyte Subset Alteration in COVID-19 Pneumonia. *J. Infect. Dis.* 221 (11), 1762–1769. doi: 10.1093/infdis/jiaa150

Wang, H., Wang, T., Yuan, Z., Cao, Y., Zhou, Y., He, J., et al. (2018). Role of Receptor for Advanced Glycation End Products in Regulating Lung Fluid Balance in Lipopolysaccharide-Induced Acute Lung Injury and Infection-Related Acute Respiratory Distress Syndrome. *Shock* 50 (4), 472–482. doi: 10.1097/SHK.0000000000001032

Wang, Y., Wu, H., Xin, Y., Bai, Y., Kong, L., Tan, Y., et al. (2017). Sulforaphane Prevents Angiotensin II-Induced Testicular Cell Death *via* Activation of NRF2. *Oxid. Med. Cell. Longev.* 2017, 5374897. doi: 10.1155/2017/5374897

Wu, Z., Hu, R., Zhang, C., Ren, W., Yu, A., and Zhou, X. (2020). Elevation of Plasma Angiotensin II Level Is a Potential Pathogenesis for the Critically Ill COVID-19 Patients. *Crit. Care* 24, 1–3. doi: 10.1186/s13054-020-03015-0

Xu, H., Wang, Z., Feng, C., Yu, W., Chen, Y., Zeng, X., et al. (2021). Effects of SARS-CoV-2 Infection on Male Sex-Related Hormones in Recovering Patients. *Andrology* 9 (1), 107–114. doi: 10.1111/andr.12942

Yalcin Kehribar, D., Cihangiroglu, M., Sehmen, E., Avci, B., Capraz, A., Yildirim Bilgin, A., et al. (2020). The Receptor for Advanced Glycation End Product (RAGE) Pathway in COVID-19. *Biomarkers* 7, 1–7. doi: 10.1080/1354750X.2020.1861099

Yang, M., Chen, S., Huang, B., Zhong, J. M., Su, H., Chen, Y. J., et al. (2020). Pathological Findings in the Testes of COVID-19 Patients: Clinical Implications. *Eur. Urol. Focus* 6 (5), 1124–1129. doi: 10.1016/j.euf.2020.05.009

Yang, J., Hu, J., and Zhu, C. (2021). Obesity Aggravates COVID-19: A Systematic Review and Meta-Analysis. *J. Med. Virol.* 93 (1), 257–261. doi: 10.1002/jmv.26237

Zaim, S., Chong, J. H., Sankaranarayanan, V., and Harky, A. (2020). COVID-19 and Multi-Organ Response. *Curr. Problems Cardiol.* 28, 100618. doi: 10.1016/j.cpcardiol.2020.100618

Zhang, X., Li, S., and Niu, S. (2020). ACE2 and COVID-19 and the Resulting ARDS. *Postgrad. Med. J.* 96 (1137), 403–407. doi: 10.1136/postgradmedj-2020-137935

Zhao, Y., Liu, X., Qu, Y., Wang, L., Geng, D., Chen, W., et al. (2019). The Roles of P38 MAPK→ COX2 and NF-κb→ COX2 Signal Pathways in Age-Related Testosterone Reduction. *Sci. Rep.* 9 (1), 10556. doi: 10.1038/s41598-019-46794-5

Zhao, Y. T., Qi, Y. W., Hu, C. Y., Chen, S. H., and Liu, Y. (2016). Advanced Glycation End Products Inhibit Testosterone Secretion by Rat Leydig Cells by Inducing Oxidative Stress and Endoplasmic Reticulum Stress. *Int. J. Mol. Med.* 38 (2), 659–665. doi: 10.3892/ijmm.2016.2645

Permissions

All chapters in this book were first published by Frontiers; hereby published with permission under the Creative Commons Attribution License or equivalent. Every chapter published in this book has been scrutinized by our experts. Their significance has been extensively debated. The topics covered herein carry significant findings which will fuel the growth of the discipline. They may even be implemented as practical applications or may be referred to as a beginning point for another development.

The contributors of this book come from diverse backgrounds, making this book a truly international effort. This book will bring forth new frontiers with its revolutionizing research information and detailed analysis of the nascent developments around the world.

We would like to thank all the contributing authors for lending their expertise to make the book truly unique. They have played a crucial role in the development of this book. Without their invaluable contributions this book wouldn't have been possible. They have made vital efforts to compile up to date information on the varied aspects of this subject to make this book a valuable addition to the collection of many professionals and students.

This book was conceptualized with the vision of imparting up-to-date information and advanced data in this field. To ensure the same, a matchless editorial board was set up. Every individual on the board went through rigorous rounds of assessment to prove their worth. After which they invested a large part of their time researching and compiling the most relevant data for our readers.

The editorial board has been involved in producing this book since its inception. They have spent rigorous hours researching and exploring the diverse topics which have resulted in the successful publishing of this book. They have passed on their knowledge of decades through this book. To expedite this challenging task, the publisher supported the team at every step. A small team of assistant editors was also appointed to further simplify the editing procedure and attain best results for the readers.

Apart from the editorial board, the designing team has also invested a significant amount of their time in understanding the subject and creating the most relevant covers. They scrutinized every image to scout for the most suitable representation of the subject and create an appropriate cover for the book.

The publishing team has been an ardent support to the editorial, designing and production team. Their endless efforts to recruit the best for this project, has resulted in the accomplishment of this book. They are a veteran in the field of academics and their pool of knowledge is as vast as their experience in printing. Their expertise and guidance has proved useful at every step. Their uncompromising quality standards have made this book an exceptional effort. Their encouragement from time to time has been an inspiration for everyone.

The publisher and the editorial board hope that this book will prove to be a valuable piece of knowledge for researchers, students, practitioners and scholars across the globe.

List of Contributors

Mariana Guilger-Casagrande
Institute of Science and Technology, São Paulo State University–UNESP, Sorocaba, Brazil
Laboratory for Evaluation of the Bioactivity and Toxicology of Nanomaterials, University of Sorocaba-UNISO, Sorocaba, Brazil

Cecilia T. de Barros, Vitória A. N. Antunes and Renata Lima
Laboratory for Evaluation of the Bioactivity and Toxicology of Nanomaterials, University of Sorocaba-UNISO, Sorocaba, Brazil

Daniele R. de Araujo
Human and Natural Sciences Center, Federal University of ABC, Santo André, Brazil

Manu N. Capoor
Laboratory of Bacterial Pathogenesis and Immunology, Rockefeller University, New York, NY, United States
Executive Office, MMF Systems, Inc., New York, NY, United States

Fahad S. Ahmed
Data Science and Engineering, MyMedicalFiles (MMF) Systems, Inc., New York, NY, United States

Andrew McDowell
Nutrition Innovation Centre for Food and Health (NICHE), School of Biomedical Sciences, Ulster University, Coleraine, United Kingdom

Ondrej Slaby
Central European Institute of Technology (CEITEC), Masaryk University, Brno, Czechia
Department of Biology, Faculty of Medicine, Masaryk University, Brno, Czechia

Obdulio García-Nicolás, Philip V'kovski, Gert Zimmer, Volker Thiel and Artur Summerfield
Institute of Virology and Immunology (IVI), Bern, Switzerland
Department of Infectious Diseases and Pathobiology, Vetsuisse Faculty, University of Bern, Bern, Switzerland

Ferdinand Zettl
Institute of Virology and Immunology (IVI), Bern, Switzerland

Elisa B. Prestes
Institut Necker Enfants Malades, Université Paris Descartes, Paris, France

Julia C. P. Bruno and Leticia A. M. Carneiro
Laboratório de Inflamação e Imunidade, Instituto de Microbiologia Paulo de Goes, Universidade Federal do Rio de Janeiro, Rio de Janeiro, Brazil

Leonardo H. Travassos
Laboratório de Imunoreceptores e Sinalização Celular, Instituto de Biofísica Carlos Chagas Filho, Universidade Federal do Rio de Janeiro, Rio de Janeiro, Brazil

Johannes J. Kovarik, Anna K. Kämpf, Fabian Gasser, Markus Wahrmann and Susanne Haindl
Department of Internal Medicine III, Division of Nephrology and Dialysis Medical University Vienna, Vienna, Austria

Anna N. Herdina, Monika Breuer and Robert Strassl
Department of Laboratory Medicine, Institute of Clinical Virology, Medical University of Vienna, Vienna, Austria

Christopher C. Kaltenecker
Department of Pathology, Medical University Vienna, Vienna, Austria

Florian Mayer and Klaus G. Schmetterer
Department of Laboratory Medicine, Medical University of Vienna, Vienna, Austria

Ludwig Traby, Manuel Kussmann and Oliver Robak
Department of Internal Medicine I, Medical University of Vienna, Vienna, Austria

Veronique Touzeau-Roemer
Department of Dermatology, Medical University Vienna, Vienna, Austria

Katharina Grabmeier-Pfistershammer
Department of Dermatology, Medical University Vienna, Vienna, Austria
Institute of Immunology, Center for Pathophysiology, Infectiology and Immunology, Medical University Vienna, Vienna, Austria

Harald Willschke and Care Ay
Department of Anaesthesia, Intensive Care Medicine and Pain Medicine, Medical University of Vienna, Vienna, Austria

Marcus D. Säemann
6th Medical Department With Nephrology and Dialysis, Wilhelminen Hospital, Vienna, Austria
Sigmund Freud University, Vienna, Austria

Jitender Sharma
Department of Biochemistry, All India Institute of Medical Sciences, Bathinda, India

Roopali Rajput and Vikas Sood
Department of Biochemistry, School of Chemical and Life Sciences, Jamia Hamdard, New Delhi, India

Manika Bhatia and Pooja Arora
Department of Zoology, Hansraj College, University of Delhi, Delhi, India

Francisco Javier Gil-Etayo, Oscar Cabrera-Marante, Daniel Arroyo, Laura Naranjo and Daniel E Pleguezuelo
Department of Immunology, Hospital Universitario 12 de Octubre, Madrid, Spain

Patricia Suàrez-Fernández and Sara Garcinuño
Departamento de Inmunologá, Instituto de Investigación, Sanitaria Hospital 12 de Octubre (imas12), Madrid, Spain

Luis M Allende and Esther Mancebo
Department of Immunology, Hospital Universitario 12 de Octubre, Madrid, Spain
Departamento de Inmunologá, Instituto de Investigación, Sanitaria Hospital 12 de Octubre (imas12), Madrid, Spain

Antonio Lalueza
Departamento de Inmunologá, Instituto de Investigación, Sanitaria Hospital 12 de Octubre (imas12), Madrid, Spain
Department of Internal Medicine, Hospital Universitario 12 de Octubre, Madrid, Spain
Departamento de Medicina, Facultad de Medicina, Universidad Complutense de Madrid, Madrid, Spain

Raquel Díaz-Simón
Department of Internal Medicine, Hospital Universitario 12 de Octubre, Madrid, Spain

Estela Paz-Artal
Department of Immunology, Hospital Universitario 12 de Octubre, Madrid, Spain
Departamento de Inmunologá, Instituto de Investigación, Sanitaria Hospital 12 de Octubre (imas12), Madrid, Spain
Departamento de Inmunología, Oftalmología y Otorrinolaringología, Facultad de Medicina, Universidad Complutense de Madrid, Madrid, Spain

Antonio Serrano
Department of Immunology, Hospital Universitario 12 de Octubre, Madrid, Spain
Departamento de Inmunologá, Instituto de Investigación, Sanitaria Hospital 12 de Octubre (imas12), Madrid, Spain
Department of Epidemiology, Biomedical Research Centre Network for Epidemiology and Public Health (CIBERESP), Madrid, Spain

Akira Nakazono, Yuji Nakamaru, Shogo Kimura, Aya Honma, Masanobu Suzuki and Akihiro Homma
Department of Otolaryngology-Head and Neck Surgery, Faculty of Medicine and Graduate School of Medicine, Hokkaido University, Sapporo, Japan

Mahnaz Ramezanpour, P. J. Wormald and Sarah Vreugde
Department of Surgery–Otorhinolaryngology Head and Neck Surgery, Central Adelaide Local Health Network and the University of Adelaide, Adelaide, SA, Australia

Takeshi Kondo, Masashi Watanabe and Shigetsugu Hatakeyama
Department of Biochemistry, Faculty of Medicine and Graduate School of Medicine, Hokkaido University, Sapporo, Japan

Mei-Yue Wang, Rong Zhao, Li-Juan Gao, Xue-Fei Gao, De-Ping Wang and Ji-Min Cao
Key Laboratory of Cellular Physiology at Shanxi Medical University, Ministry of Education, Key Laboratory of Cellular Physiology of Shanxi Province, and the Department of Physiology, Shanxi Medical University, Taiyuan, China

Syairah Hanan Shaharuddin, Victoria Wang, Roberta S. Santos and Andrew Gross
Board of Governors Regenerative Medicine Institute, Cedars-Sinai Medical Center, Los Angeles, CA, United States
Cedars-Sinai Biomanufacturing Center, Cedars-Sinai Medical Center, Los Angeles, CA, United States

Yizhou Wang
Department of Biomedical Sciences, Cedars-Sinai Medical Center, Los Angeles, CA, United States
Genomics Core, Cedars-Sinai Medical Center, Los Angeles, CA, United States

Harneet Jawanda and Yi Zhang
Biobank and Translational Research Core, Samuel Oschin Comprehensive Cancer Institute (SOCCI), Cedars-Sinai Medical Center, Los Angeles, CA, United States

Wohaib Hasan
Department of Biomedical Sciences, Cedars-Sinai Medical Center, Los Angeles, CA, United States
Biobank and Translational Research Core, Samuel Oschin Comprehensive Cancer Institute (SOCCI), Cedars-Sinai Medical Center, Los Angeles, CA, United States
Department of Pathology and Laboratory Medicine, Cedars-Sinai Medical Center, Los Angeles, CA, United States

Gustavo GarciaJr.
Department of Molecular and Medical Pharmacology, David Geffen School of Medicine, University of California, Los Angeles, Los Angeles, CA, United States

Vaithilingaraja Arumugaswami
Department of Molecular and Medical Pharmacology, David Geffen School of Medicine, University of California, Los Angeles, Los Angeles, CA, United States
Eli and Edythe Broad Center of Regenerative Medicine and Stem Cell Research, University of California, Los Angeles, Los Angeles, CA, United States

Dhruv Sareen
Board of Governors Regenerative Medicine Institute, Cedars-Sinai Medical Center, Los Angeles, CA, United States
Cedars-Sinai Biomanufacturing Center, Cedars-Sinai Medical Center, Los Angeles, CA, United States
Department of Biomedical Sciences, Cedars-Sinai Medical Center, Los Angeles, CA, United States
iPSC Core, David and Janet Polak Foundation Stem Cell Core Laboratory, Cedars-Sinai Medical Center, Los Angeles, CA, United States

Xiaomin Chen, Kun Pang, Xin Xu and Jinyu Wu
Institute of Genomic Medicine, Wenzhou Medical University, Wenzhou, China

Yutong Kang
Wenzhou Key Laboratory of Sanitary Microbiology, Ministry of Education, Wenzhou, China
Key Laboratory of Laboratory Medicine, Ministry of Education, Wenzhou, China
School of Laboratory Medicine and Life Sciences, Wenzhou Medical University, Wenzhou, China

Jing Luo
Rheumatology Department, The First Affiliated Hospital of Wenzhou Medical University, Wenzhou, China

Xiaokun Li
Chemical Biology Research Center, School of Pharmaceutical Sciences, Wenzhou Medical University, Wenzhou, China

Shengwei Jin
Department of Anesthesia and Critical Care, Second Affiliated Hospital of Wenzhou Medical University, Wenzhou, China

Isabella Quinti, Ane Fernandez Salinas and Cinzia Milito
Department of Molecular Medicine, Sapienza University of Rome, Rome, Italy

Eva Piano Mortari and Rita Carsetti
Department of Laboratory Medicine, Research Area Multimodal Medicine, Diagnostic Immunology and Research Unit, Bambino Gesù Children's Hospital IRCCS, Rome, Italy

Shuo Ning, Beiming Yu, Yanfeng Wang and Feng Wang
Key Laboratory of Molecular Medicine and Biotherapy, School of Life Science, Beijing Institute of Technology, Beijing, China

Wajihul Hasan Khan
Department of Biotechnology, Host Pathogen Interaction and Molecular Immunology Laboratory, Jamia Hamdard, New Delhi, India
Department of Chemical Engineering, Indian Institute of Technology Delhi, New Delhi, India

Zohra Hashmi, Aditya Goel, Kanisha Gupta, Nida Khan and Mairaj Ahmed Ansari
Department of Biotechnology, Host Pathogen Interaction and Molecular Immunology Laboratory, Jamia Hamdard, New Delhi, India

Razi Ahmad
Department of Chemistry, Indian Institute of Technology Delhi, New Delhi, India

Iqbal Alam
Department of Physiology, Hamdard Institute of Medical Sciences and Research, Jamia Hamdard, New Delhi, India

Faheem Ahmed
Department of Community Medicine, Hamdard Institute of Medical Sciences and Research, New Delhi, India

Simona Damiano, Concetta Sozio, Giuliana La Rosa and Mariarosaria Santillo
Dipartimento di Medicina Clinica e Chirurgia, Università di Napoli "Federico II", Napoli, Italy

Tarun Mishra, M. Sreepadmanabh, Pavitra Ramdas, Amit Kumar Sahu and Ajit Chande
Molecular Virology Laboratory, Department of Biological Sciences, Indian Institute of Science Education and Research, Bhopal, India

Atul Kumar
Structural Biology Laboratory, Department of Biological Sciences, Indian Institute of Science Education and Research, Bhopal, India

Iqbal Azmi, Md Imam Faizan, Jawed Iqbal, Mohan C. Joshi, Tanveer Ahmad Nisha Chaudhary and Deepak Kumar Singh
Multidisciplinary Centre for Advanced Research & Studies, Jamia Millia Islamia, New Delhi, India

Rohit Kumar and Siddharth Raj Yadav
Department of Pulmonary Medicine and Sleep Disorders, Vardhman Mahavir Medical College, Safdarjung Hospital, New Delhi, India

Ruchika Butola
360 Diagnostic and Health Services, Noida, India

Aryan Ganotra
Department of Computer Science & Engineering, Delhi Technological University, Delhi, India

Gopal Datt Joshi
Noodle Analytics Pvt Ltd., Bangalore, India

Gagan Deep Jhingan
Valerian Chem Pvt. Ltd., New Delhi, India

Gabriel Augusto Pires de Souza, Ikram Omar Osman, Marion Le Bideau, Jean-Pierre Baudoin, Rita Jaafar and Bernard La Scola
Aix-Marseille Université, Institut de Recherche pour le Développement (IRD), Assistance Publique - Hôpitaux de Marseille (AP-HM), MEPHI, Marseille, France
Microbes, Evolution, Phylogénie et Infection (MEPHI), IHU - Méditerranée Infection, Marseille, France

Christian Devaux
Aix-Marseille Université, Institut de Recherche pour le Développement (IRD), Assistance Publique - Hôpitaux de Marseille (AP-HM), MEPHI, Marseille, France
Microbes, Evolution, Phylogénie et Infection (MEPHI), IHU - Méditerranée Infection, Marseille, France
Centre National de La Recherche Scientifique (CNRS), Marseille, France

Hayder M. Al-kuraishy and Ali I. Al-Gareeb
Department of Clinical Pharmacology and Medicine, College of Medicine, ALmustansiriyia University, Baghdad, Iraq

Hani Faidah
Faculty of Medicine, Umm Al Qura University, Mecca, Saudi Arabia

Athanasios Alexiou
Department of Science and Engineering, Novel Global Community Educational Foundation, Hebersham, NSW, Australia
AFNP Med Austria, Wien, Austria

Gaber El-Saber Batiha
Department of Pharmacology and Therapeutics, Faculty of Veterinary Medicine, Damanhour University, Damanhour, Egypt

Index

O

P

R

S

T

U

V